Complete Review of

Microbiology & Immunology

FOURTH EDITION

Sonu Panwar MBBS, MD
Professor and Head, Department of Microbiology
Krishna Mohan Medical College and Hospital, Mathura, U.P.

Sameer Singh Faujdar PhD (Med.)
Assistant Professor, Department of Microbiology
Maharishi Markandeshwar Medical College
and Hospital, Solan, H.P.

Peepee Publishers and Distributors (P) Ltd.®

Complete Review of Microbiology and Immunology

Published by
Pawaninder P. Vij and Anupam Vij

Peepee Publishers and Distributors (P) Ltd.
Head Office: 160, Shakti Vihar, Pitam Pura, Delhi-110 034 (India)

Correspondence Address:

7/31, First Floor, Ansari Road, Daryaganj
New Delhi-110 002 (India)

Ph: 011-41512412, 011-23246245, 9811156083

e-mail: peepee160@yahoo.co.in

e-mail: peepee160@gmail.com

www.peepeepub.com

join us on facebook.com/pp.publishers

First Edition: 2017

Fourth Edition: 2023

ISBN: 978-81-9523-444-8

DEDICATION

Dedicated to my family members: Dr. Kehar Singh and Mrs. Saroj Singh, Dr. Vandana Singh, Miss Jahnavi Panwar, Master Shobhit Panwar, my nephews Daksh and Kushu, Mrs. Seema and Mr. Sandeep Parmar.

Sonu Panwar

Dedicated to my family members: Er. Tejsingh Faujdar, Late Shrimati Sharda Faujdar, Er. Pawan Faujdar (IIS), Dr. Shalini Faujdar, Late Ritu Di, Er. Mausam Faujdar, Dr. Priya Mehrishi, Dr. Akansha Yadav, Aayaan Tej Faujdar, Chaitanya Faujdar, Sharth Faujdar and Risha.

Sameer Singh Faujdar

ACKNOWLEDGEMENTS

A special appreciation to Mr. Pawaninder Paul Vij, Director, Peepee Publishers and Distributors (P) Ltd., Dr. Deepanshu Goyal, Mr. Sahil Goyal, Mr. Vitul, Team Prepladder, Dr. Mukesh Bhatia, Director and Faculty Medicine at DBMCI and Dr. Nachiket Bhatia, DBMCI, who constantly motivated me to pen down my experience of teaching for so many years so that youngsters should get benefited by delivering our knowledge in the form of book.

How can I forget all of my teachers right from the beginning of my school who always believed in me and contributed in what I am today. Specially I want to thank my PG guide Dr. Ravindranath Gangane, my favourite Dr. Sunil Biradar and Dr. Sahil Jindal for constantly guiding me during my postgraduation in Microbiology.

I have special thanks to my friends, colleagues and fellow faculties:

Dr. Vishu Vijayant (DRM, DNB Nuclear Medicine), Dr. Amit Narayan (Spine Surgeon), Dr. Virendra Singh (DNB TB Chest), Dr. Apreesh Sharma (MD Anaesthesia), Dr. Deepak Guliani (Associate Professor, General Surgery), MAMC, Delhi, Dr. Ranjan Patel (MD Pharmacology), Dr. Vivek Jain (MD PSM), Dr. Rajat Jain (MD Radiology), Dr. Apurv Mehra (MS Orthopaedics), Dr. Praveen Jain (MD), Dr. Bhaskar Gupta, Dr. Devki Verma (MD Microbiology), Dr. Gobind Rai Garg, Mr. Dinesh Bhati, Mr. Pankaj Bhatia, Mr. Aayush, Mr. Abhinav Gupta and Dr. Gaurav Goel, Associate Consultant, Clinical Microbiology, Tata Medical Centre, Kolkata.

My students: Dr. Rachit Singhania, Dr. Javed Ali and Dr. Ranjusree Mandal.

Special thanks to: Dr. Hari Singh (MD Radiology), Head of Radiology Department, SNMC, Agra.

Dr. Sonu Panwar
drsonupanwar187@gmail.com

Co-Author Dr. Sameer Singh Faujdar

Sincere gratitude to Dr. Ravi Chand Sharma (Principal of MMMCH, Solan), Dr. J.S. Sandhu (Vice-Principal of MMMCH, Solan), Dr. Manpreet S. Nanda (MS of MMMCH, Solan), Dr. Paramjit Singh (Ex-HOD Micro, MMCH, Muzaffarnagar), Dr. Dakshina Bisht (IQAC Director, Santosh Medical College and Hospital, UP), Dr. Varsha A. Singh (HOD Microbiology, RVRS GMC, Bhilwara), Dr. Satish Kumar (HOD Microbiology, MMMCH, Solan), Dr. Narinder Kaur (HOD Microbiology, MMIMSR, Mullana), Dr. Chaitanya Tellapragada (PostDoc K. I., Sweden), Dr. Subhabrata Sarkar (Scientist C, PGIMER), Dr. Rishab Garg (M.Ch Neuro.), Dr. Sumit Chawla (MD PSM), Dr. Bharti Mehta (MD PSM), Dr. Prashant Bansal (M.Ch Urology), Dr. Tushar Shaw (Assist. Prof.), Dr. Lokendra Yadav (M.Ch Urology), Dr. Anil Yadav (MD Psychiatry AIIMS), Dr. Garima Yadav (MS ENT LHMC), Dr. Amandeep Singh (PhD PGIMER), Dr. Manpreet Shandu (MDS), Dr. Girraj Soni (MS OBG), Dr. Ankur Nama (MS OBG), Dr. Rajaram (MD Radio.), Dr. Banesh Jain (M.Ch Neuro.), Dr. K.C. Gupta (PostDoc), Dr. Sharad Lodhi (MD Medicine, LDMC, Delhi), Dr. Amandeep Badhan (MD Pediatrics), Dr. Shwaita Goyal (MD), Dr. Ranjit Bajwa (MD Medicine), Dr. Sahil Garg (MD Radio), Dr. Shabnum Thakur, Dr. Deepak, Dr. Ankit Jain, Dr. Anil, Dr. Rajdeep Bajwa, Dr. Shivendra Shukla, Mr. Sunil Kawat for encouraging us to write this book.

My students: Dr. Vijay Rana, Dr. Madhav Verma, Dr. Shivanshi Sharma, Dr. Sandeep, Dr. Gaurav Kherwal, Dr. Panya Kapoor, Dr. Shubhamshree P., Dr. Garima Verma, Dr. Akul and others.

Special thanks to: Dr. Avinash Laghawe, Dr. Amisha Sharma, Dr. Rakesh Agarwal, Dr. Hemant Saini, Dr. Dinesh Bhati, Dr. Seema Solanki, Dr. Rakesh Sadhu, Dr. Monika Jindal, Dr. Rajwinder Singh, Dr. Jaswinder Kaur, Dr. Priyam Chawla and Dr. Saurabh Jain.

August 2022

Dr. Sameer Singh Faujdar

PREFACE TO THE FOURTH EDITION

I am thankful to all my students for appreciation of the 3rd edition of **"Complete Review of Microbiology and Immunology"**. As per their suggestions, we have incorporated Covid19 and Mucormycosis chapters along with MCQs.

This 4th edition is thoroughly revised and updated completely. Latest questions of recent INI CET, NEET pattern and FMGE pattern with explanatory answers also incorporated in this edition.

New coloured recently asked images based questions are also included at the end of book.

Your suggestions, appreciation and criticism are most welcome.

Wishing you all the best for exams.

You can download my Microbiology App on Google Play Store and Apple Store for daily MCQs and Updates.

New Delhi
August 2022

Dr. Sonu Panwar
Dr. Sameer Singh Faujdar
drsonupanwar187@gmail.com

PREFACE TO THE FIRST EDITION

I am really thankful to all of my students who had been a real source of inspiration for me to write down the most demanded book of its kind in Microbiology by the subject experts with the name of **Complete Review of Microbiology and Immunology.** The book is a collection of my PG notes and vast experience of MCQ based teaching methods. Hence with my experience of teaching for the last 5 years I had tried my best to fulfil the demands and request of the students from all over India to write a conceptual based book to cover the pattern of each and every exam the student is going to give.

Microbiology always carries a major chunk of questions in every exam, so I hope this new edition of my book will serve you the best, most simplified and fruitful approach. A section of images based on recent trends incorporated, which will help you to tackle all sorts of recent Image-based Questions asked in recent past in most of the exams.

We must admit that despite our best efforts, some errors might have crept in inadvertently regarding factual information or typographical mistakes. You are all requested to send these errors and also send your valuable suggestions for improvement of the book, your suggestions, appreciation and criticism are most welcome. You can follow my Facebook **"PG Microbiology made easy by Dr. Panwar"** for recent updates and discussion.

New Delhi
July 2017

Dr. Sonu Panwar
Dr. Sameer Singh Faujdar

CONTENTS

Chapter 1

INI CET QUESTIONS

1. **In a completely and adequately immunized child against Diphtheria, the throat swab was collected. It showed the presence of following organism (shown in image) what is the Staining Protocol for the following image?**

   (a) Gram stain
   (b) Acid fast stain
   (c) Albert stain
   (d) None

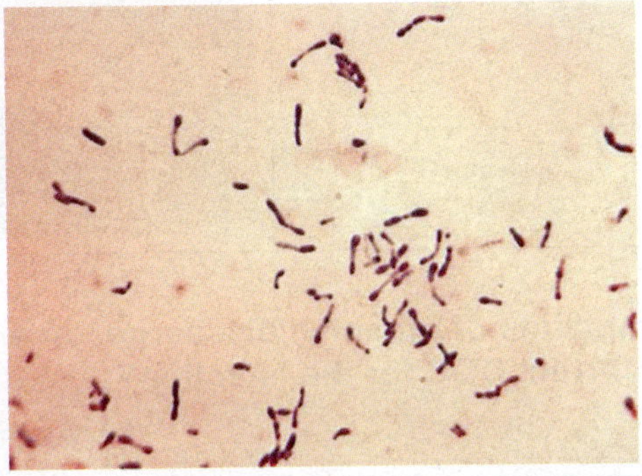

2. **What is the basis of Paul Bunnel Test for EBV?**

   (a) Heterophile antibody
   (b) Cell mediated hypersensitivity
   (c) Immune complex mediated
   (d) None

3. **Match the following eggs:**

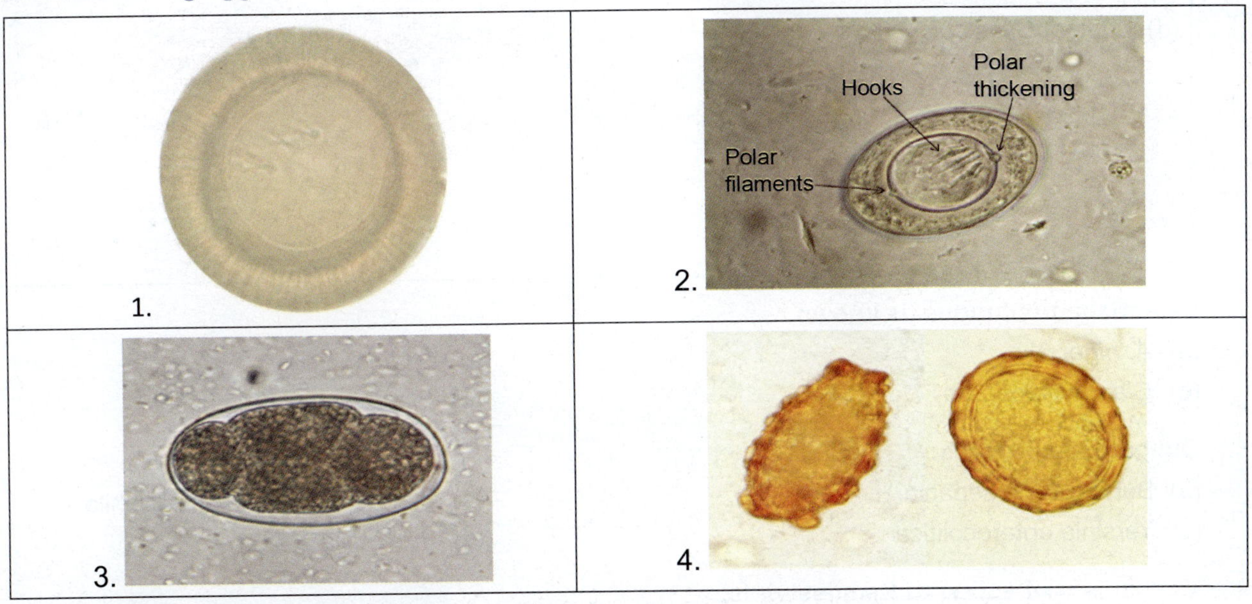

   (a) 1- H. nana; 2- Taenia; 3- Hookworm; 4- Ascaris
   (b) 1- Ascaris; 2- H. nana; 3- Hookworm; 4- Taenia
   (c) 1- Taenia; 2- H. nana; 3- Hookworm; 4- Ascaris
   (d) 1- Hookworm; 2- Ascaris; 3-Taenia; 4- H. nana

4. **A Forest worker/Rose Gardner got thorn prick which later developed with linear lesions and lymphatic spread. What will be the correct diagnosis?**

(a) Insect Bite
(b) Mycetoma
(c) Sporotrichosis
(d) Scabies

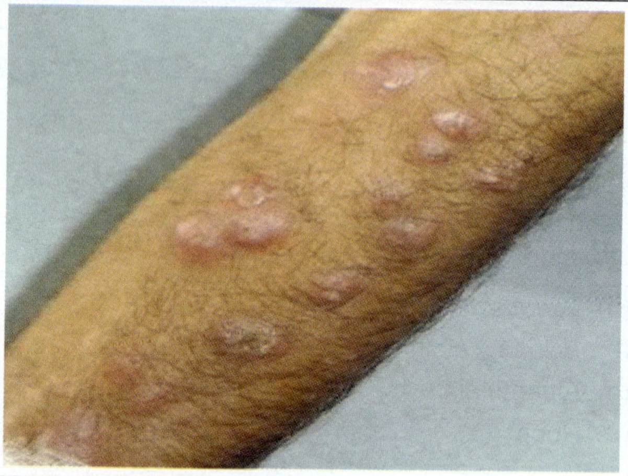

5. **A woman presented with complaints of greenish discharge, on examination she had strawberry cervix and vagina, what will be the correct DOC for the infection?**

(a) Ceftriaxone
(b) Azithromycin
(c) Chloramphenicol
(d) Metronidazole

6. **Identify the organism associated with given Image:**

(a) MTB
(b) *C. diphtheriae*
(c) *Gardnerella vaginalis*
(d) *Lactobacillus acidophilus*

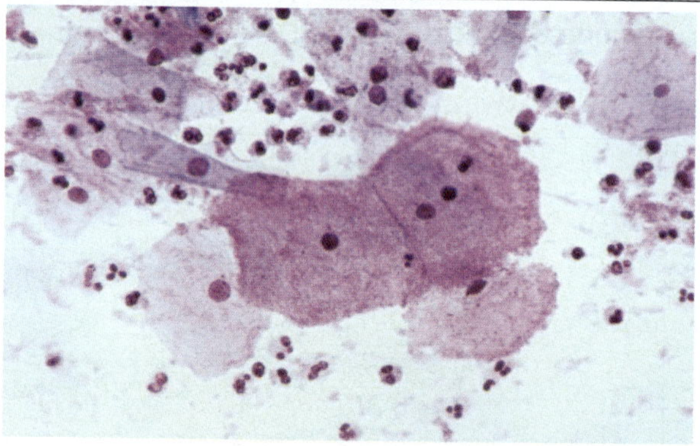

7. **Dematiaceous fungus is known as:**

(a) *A. niger*
(b) *Mucor*
(c) *Cladophialophora*
(d) *Blastomyces dermatitidis*

8. **Obligate anaerobe is:**

(a) Burkholderia cepacia
(b) Stenotrophomonas maltophila
(c) Yersinia enterocolitica
(d) Prevotella

9. **Mechanism of action of Remdesivir is:**

(a) Inhibits the fusion
(b) Inhibits the RNA-dependent RNA polymerase (RdRp)
(c) Inhibits the phagocytosis
(d) Inhibits the translation

10. Hepatitis B subunit vaccine is derived from which antigen?

(a) HBeAg
(b) HBsAg
(c) HBcAg
(d) HBV DNA

11. In this image given life cycle is of which virus?

(a) HSV
(b) HIV
(c) HBV
(d) All of the above

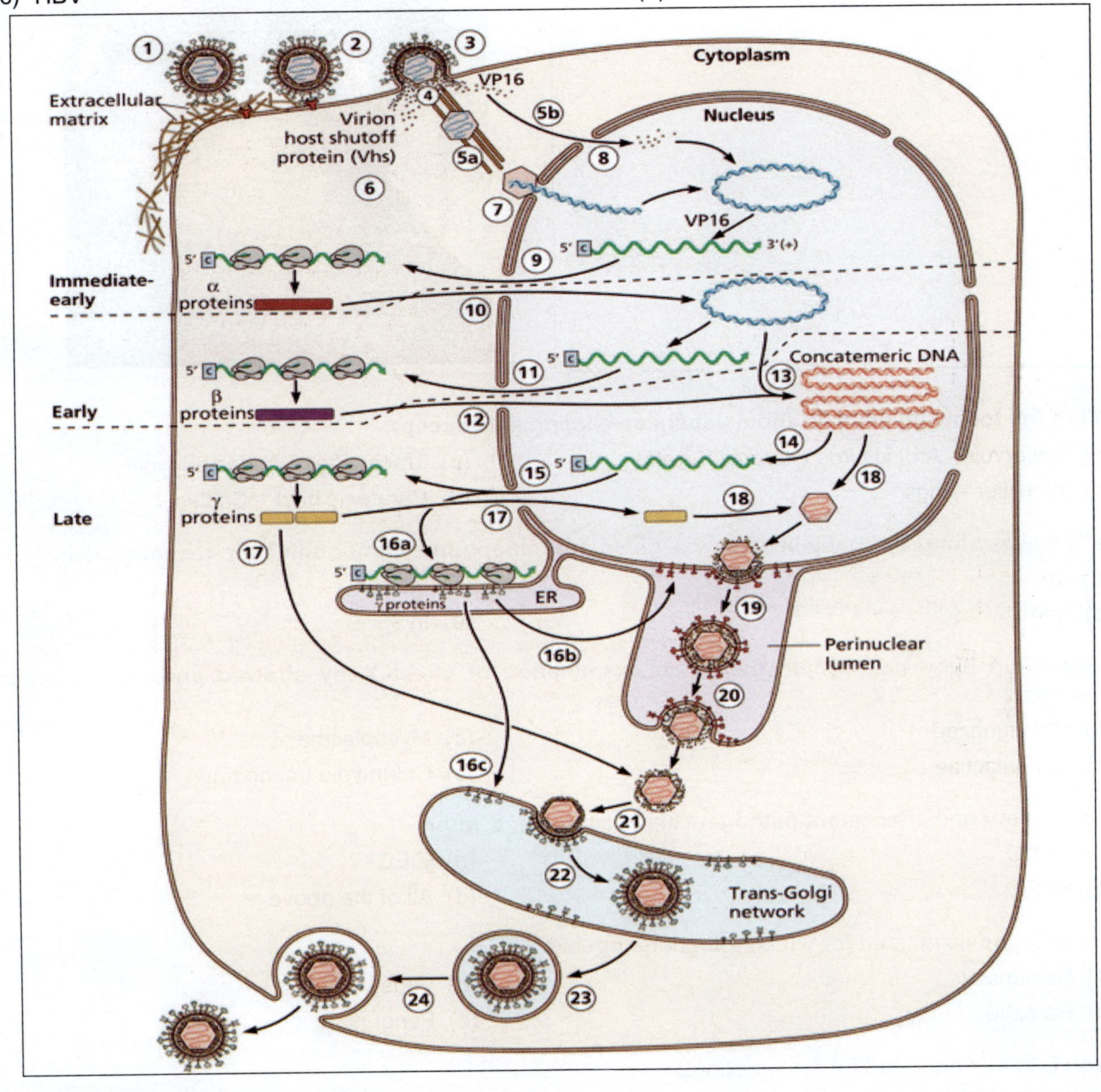

12. Most common ocular manifestation in COVID-19:

(a) Pseudomembrane conjunctivitis
(b) Follicular conjunctivitis
(c) Retinal vein occlusion
(d) Cellulitis

13. A patient from Bihar with hypopigmented and normoaesthetic patches on the back (image given). He gave history of long-term fever in his childhood. Which of the following is the likely diagnosis?

(a) Tuberculosis leprosy
(b) Indeterminate leprosy
(c) Lepromatous leprosy
(d) PKDL

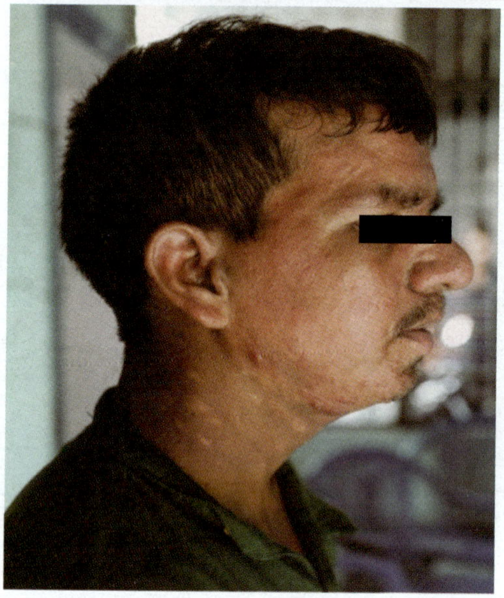

14. All of the following are true about Japanese encephalitis except:

(a) Reservoir – Ardeid birds (Herons, Egrets)
(b) Transmitter – Aedes aegyptii
(c) Amplifier – Pigs
(d) Paratenic host – Cattles

15. A man was stung by honey bee, he was given norepinephrine, immunoglobulin responsible is:

(a) IgA
(b) IgE
(c) IgM
(d) IgG

16. 2-week-old baby had conjunctivitis, on examination of chest X-ray showed pneumonia, probable diagnosis:

(a) H. influenzae
(b) Mycoplasma
(c) S. agalactiae
(d) Chlamydia trachomatis

17. Attachment and effacement pathogenesis is associated with:

(a) EPEC
(b) EIEC
(c) EAEC
(d) All of the above

18. Xenodiagnosis is used for which infectious agent?

(a) Bacteria
(b) Virus
(c) Parasite
(d) Fungi

19. Which test is not used for milk testing?

(a) Alkaline Phosphatase test
(b) Standard plate count
(c) Methylene Blue Reduction Test
(d) Most Probable Number (MPN) Test

ANSWERS AND EXPLANATIONS

1. Ans.: (a)

Gram staining of the smear showing Gram-positive bacilli with V and L formation or Chinese letter pattern formation or cuneiform arrangement. Albert, Neisser, or Ponder stain of direct smears shows metachromatic granules. However, diphtheria bacilli may not always be demonstrated in the smears, and also it may be difficult to differentiate the bacilli from those of commensal corynebacterial frequently found in the throat.

2. Ans.: (a)

Paul-Bunnell Test: Infectious mononucleosis is accompanied by production of heterophile agglutinins. These antibodies are IgM heterophile antibodies elicited by EBV infection and appear in 85-90% of patient's sera during the acute phase of illness. The Paul-Bunnel antibody develops early during the course of infectious mononucleosis, and disappears within about two months. These can be detected by the Paul-Bunnell test or a rapid slide agglutination test. Agglutination of horse or sheep red cells by serum absorbed to exclude a natural antibody is the basis of this test.

3. Ans.: (c)

Taenia species eggs are indistinguishable from each other.

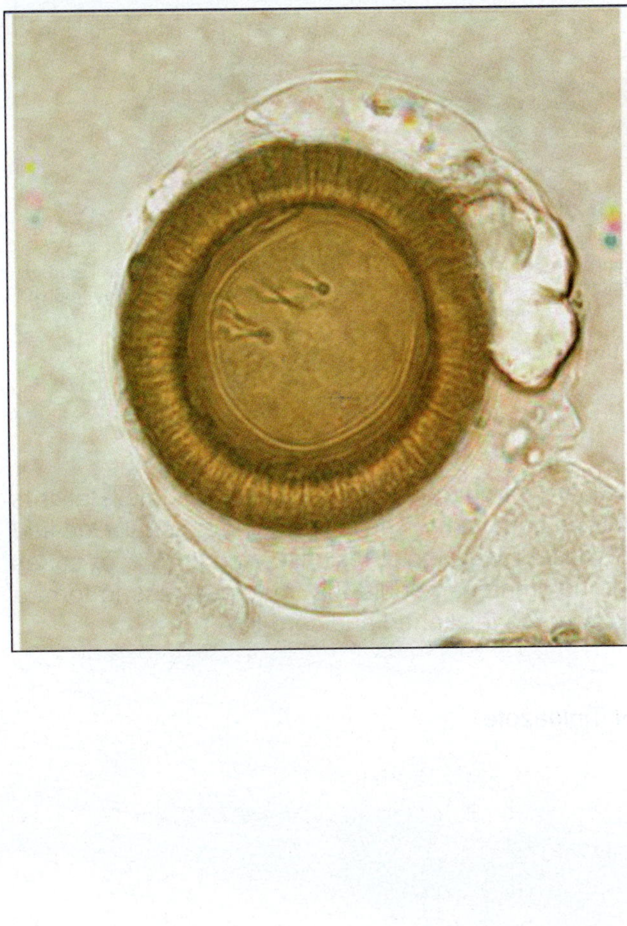

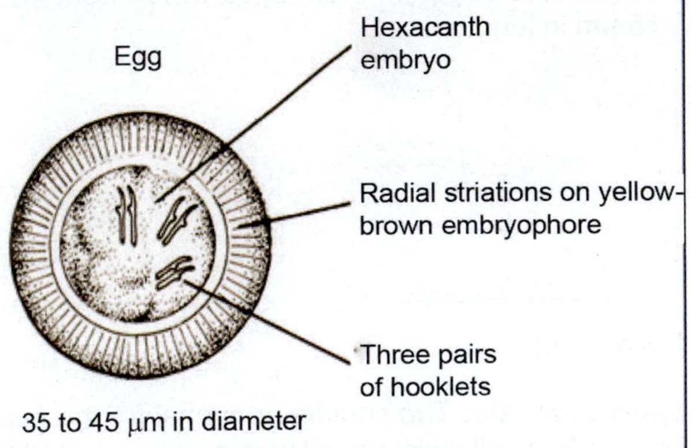

Hymenolepis nana eggs are oval and smaller than those of *H. diminuta*, with a size range of 30 to 50 µm. On the inner membrane are two poles, from which 4-8 polar filaments spread out between the two membranes.	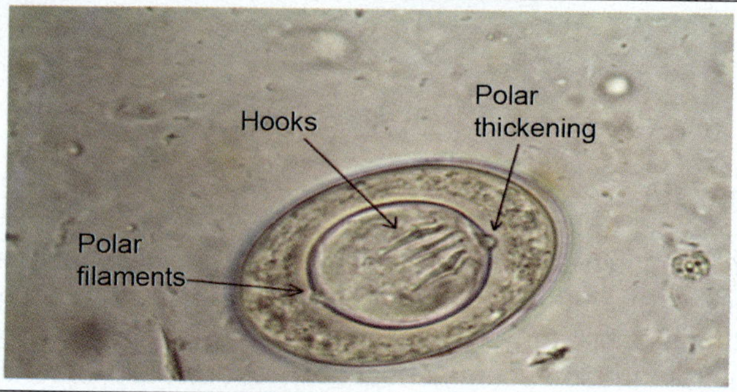
Hookworm eggs of *Ancylostoma* and *Necator* cannot be differentiated microscopically. The eggs are thin-shelled, colourless and measure 60-75 µm by 35-40 µm.	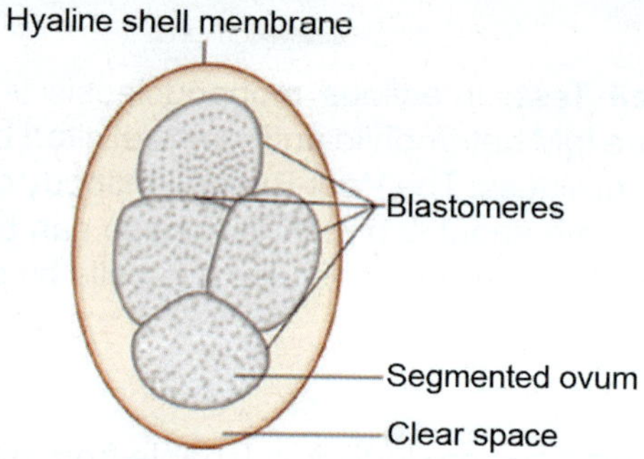
Ascaris lumbricoides: Fertilized eggs are rounded and have a thick shell with an external mammillated layer that is often stained brown by bile. In some cases, the outer layer is absent (known as decorticated eggs). Fertile eggs range from 45 to 75 µm in length.	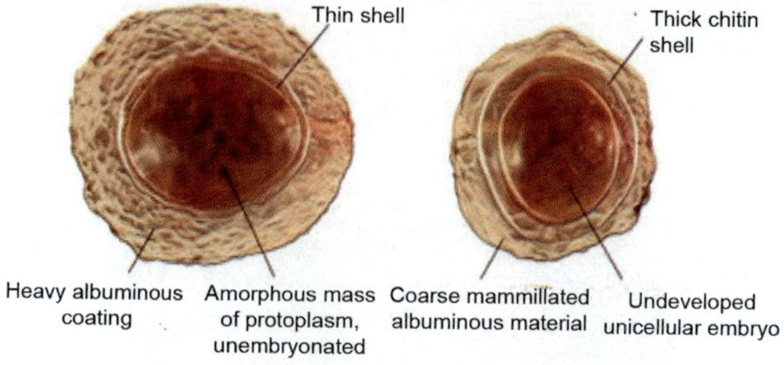 **Unfertilized egg** **Fertilized egg**

4. Ans.: (c)

Sporotrichosis: The conidia or hyphal fragments of *S. schenckii* are introduced into the skin by trauma. Patients frequently recall a history of trauma associated with outdoor activities and plants. The initial lesion is usually located on the extremities but can be found anywhere (children often present with facial lesions). About 75% of cases are lymphocutaneous; that is, the initial lesion develops as a granulomatous nodule that may progress to form a necrotic or ulcerative lesion. Meanwhile, the draining lymphatics become thickened and cord-like.

5. Ans.: (d)

This is the case of Trichomoniasis and DOC is Metronidazole or Tinidazole.

6. Ans.: (c)

Bacterial vaginosis is characterized by the presence of clue cells, which are epithelial cells of the cervix that are covered with rod-shaped bacteria (*Gardnerella vaginalis*). The normal vaginal squamous epithelial cells have distinct cell margins and lack granularity. Clue cells are seen as squamous epithelial cells with a large number of coccobacillus organisms densely attached in clusters to their surfaces, giving them a granular appearance. The edges of squamous epithelial cells, which normally have a sharply defined cell border, become indistinct or stippled.

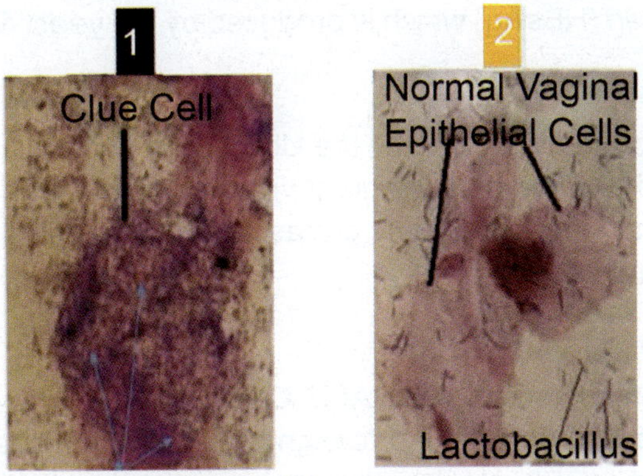

Gram-variable, coccobacilli
(Gardnerella vaginalis)

7. Ans.: (c)

The dematiaceous (brown-pigmented) fungi are a large and heterogenous group of moulds that cause a wide range of diseases including phaeohyphomycosis, chromoblastomycosis, and eumycotic mycetoma. Among the more important human pathogens are Alternaria species, Bipolaris species, Cladophialophora bantiana, Curvularia species, Exophiala species, Fonsecaea pedrosoi, Madurella species, Phialophora species, Scedosporium prolificans, Scytalidium dimidiatum and Wangiella dermatitidis. These organisms are widespread in the environment, being found in soil, wood, and decomposing plant debris.

8. Ans.: (d)

Prevotella species are gram-negative bacilli and may appear as slender rods or coccobacilli. Most commonly isolated are P melaninogenica, Prevotella bivia, and Prevotella disiens. P melaninogenica and similar species are found in infections associated with the upper respiratory tract. P bivia and P disiens occur in the female genital tract. Prevotella species are found in brain and lung abscesses, in empyema, and in pelvic inflammatory disease and tuboovarian abscesses.

Anaerobic Bacteria of Clinical Importance

Genera	Anatomic Site
Bacilli (rods)	
• Gram negative	
– *Bacteroides fragilis* group	Colon, mouth
– *Prevotella melaninogenica*	Mouth, colon, genitourinary tract
– *Fusobacterium*	Mouth
• Gram positive	
– *Actinomyces*	Mouth
– *Propionibacterium*	Skin
– *Clostridium*	Colon
Cocci (spheres)	
• Gram positive	
– *Peptoniphilus*	Colon, mouth, skin, genitourinary tract
– *Peptostreptococcus*	Colon, mouth, skin, genitourinary tract
– Peptococcus	

9. Ans.: (b)

Remdesivir is the first drug that has been approved by the US Food and Drug Administration (FDA) for clinical use in hospitalized patients with COVID-19 illness. Remdesivir is a phosphoramidite prodrug of a monophosphate nucleoside analog and acts as a viral RNA-dependent RNA polymerase (RdRp) inhibitor, targeting the viral genome replication process.

10. Ans.: (b)

Recombinant hepatitis B vaccine is a non-infectious subunit hepatitis B viral vaccine. It contains hepatitis B surface antigen (HBsAg) which is produced by the yeast *Saccharomyces cerevisiae* by use of recombinant DNA technology.

11. Ans.: (a)

The protein encoded by the UL48 gene of alphaherpesviruses is named VP16 or alpha-gene-transactivating factor (α-TIF). In the early stage of viral replication, VP16 is an important transactivator that can activate the transcription of viral immediate-early genes, and in the late stage of viral replication, VP16, as a tegument, is involved in viral assembly.

12. Ans.: (b)

Patients infected with SARS-CoV-2 can present with acute conjunctivitis symptoms, including eye redness, ocular irritation, eye soreness, foreign body sensation, tearing, mucoid discharge, eyelid swelling, congestion and chemosis. The most prevalent ocular disease is conjunctivitis (88.8%).

13. Ans.: (d)

Post-kala-azar dermal leishmaniasis (PKDL) is a complication of visceral leishmaniasis (VL). It is characterised by a macular, maculopapular, and nodular rash in a patient who has recovered from VL and who is otherwise well. The rash usually starts around the mouth from where it spreads to other parts of the body depending on severity.

14. Ans.: (b)

An intermediate host which is not needed for the development of the parasite, but nonetheless serves to maintain the life cycle of the parasite. The difference between a paratenic and reservoir host is that the reservoir host is a primary host, whereas paratenic host serves as "dumps" for non-mature stages of a parasite which they can accumulate in high numbers. Two transmission cycles are predominant:

- Pig – culex – Pig
- Ardeid birds – Culex - Ardeid birds

15. Ans.: (b)

Honeybee stings can induce a Th2 cell-mediated immune response associated with BV-specific IgE antibodies.

16. Ans.: (d)

Ophthalmia neonatorum and Pneumonia are caused by *Chlamydia trachomatis*.

17. Ans.: (a)

Enteropathogenic *E. coli* (EPEC) and enterohaemorrhagic *E. coli* (EHEC) are attaching and effacing (A/E) pathogens that efface the microvilli and subvert host cell actin to form pedestals beneath the attachment site.

18. Ans.: (c)

Xenodiagnosis (XD) is a sophisticated procedure – developed by Brumpt in 1914 – which utilize the vector, acting as a biological culture medium, for the detection of *Trypanosoma cruzi* infection in man and other mammals.

19. Ans.: (d)

MPN is most commonly applied for quality testing of water i.e. to ensure whether the water is safe or not in terms of bacteria present in it. A group of bacteria commonly referred to as fecal coliforms act as an indicator of fecal contamination of water. The presence of very few fecal coliform bacteria would indicate that water probably contains no disease-causing organisms, while the presence of large numbers of fecal coliform bacteria would indicate a very high probability that the water could contain disease-producing organisms making the water unsafe for consumption.

NEET MAY 2022 QUESTIONS

1. A female presented with curdy white vaginal discharge. Gram staining of discharge showed budding yeast cell. Which medium is used to differentiate the species of the causative organism?

(a) Bird seed agar
(b) Chrome agar
(c) SDA
(d) PDA

2. A farmer is presented with sinuses with a discharging granule on the leg. The granules were crushed and further examined macroscopically and microscopically, which of the following statement is correct regarding this scenario?

(a) Can be caused by Bacteria and Fungi
(b) Involves Skin only, no deeper tissue involvement
(c) Lymphocyte accumulation is present
(d) Spread by hematogenous route

3. A woodworker presented with chronic localized infection of the skin on lower legs and feet which were irregular, rough, cauliflower-like lesions, microscopy (10% KOH) of lesion scrapings shows copper penny/muriform cells/medlar bodies, probable diagnosis is:

(a) Chromoblastomycosis
(b) Phaeohyphomycosis
(c) Chromomycosis
(d) Rhinosporidiosis

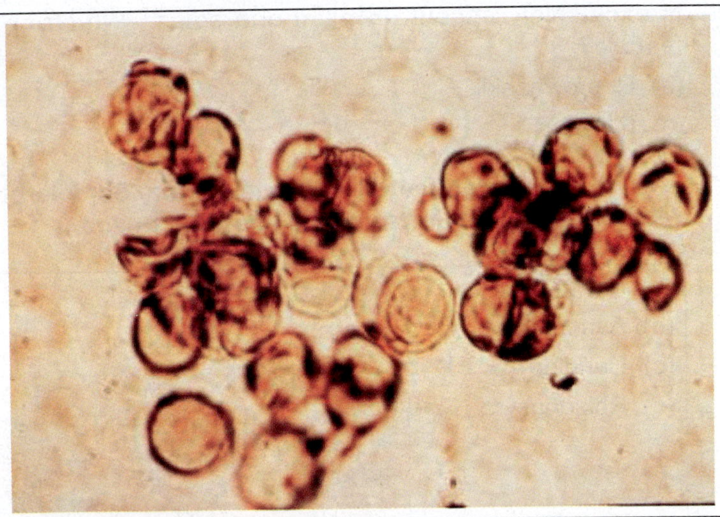

4. In a patient with rice water diarrhea, which will be involved?

(a) GM1 ganglioside
(b) GM2 ganglioside
(c) Both A and B
(d) None of the above

5. A young boy presented with fever, sore throat, malaise and abdominal pain, conjunctival suffusion and calf tenderness. No history of cough, vomiting, hemorrhage and travel. What is the diagnosis?

(a) Chikungunya
(b) Leptospirosis
(c) Dengue hemorrhagic fever
(d) Hepatic encephalopathy with hepatitis A

6. Which of the following is the best way to diagnose a Clostridium associated diarrhea?

(a) Stool culture
(b) Toxin demonstration
(c) Blood culture
(d) Stool anerobic culture and toxin demonstration

7. A 26 years old lady came to OPD with a case of anogenital warts. With the help of genetic study, it has come to their knowledge that she's having high risk of Cervical cancer. Which will be most responsible?

(a) HPV 5
(b) HPV 18
(c) HPV 11
(d) HPV 1

8. A patient died of Botulinum intoxication. What will be the most probable mechanism?

(a) Prevents the release of inhibitory neurotransmitters
(b) Blockage of ACh release
(c) Inhibition of glycine dependent postsynaptic nicotinic receptor
(d) None of the above

9. A 24-year-old male who recently returned from Africa reported with Jaundice and Hemorrhagic fever and having torres body, Symptomatic treatment was given but the patient died. Which vaccine must have prevented this occurrence?

(a) Edmonston jagreb vaccine
(b) RA27/3 Vaccine
(c) Jerryl Lynn vaccine
(d) 17 D Vaccine

10. A police officer admitted to hospital with fever and myalgia. Physical examination revealed rash which is exclusively absent on palm and soles. Which of the following lice infestation best explains this feature?

(a) R. prowazekii
(b) R. akari
(c) R. typhi
(d) R. conorii

11. A truck driver manifested with pneumonia. Sample histopathology (H&E) showed the septate hyphae with 45-degree angle branch as shown in image.

(a) Mucor
(b) Aspergillus
(c) Candida
(d) Rhizopus

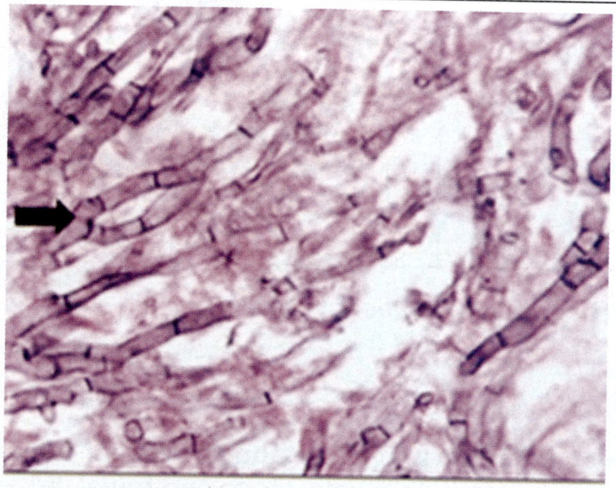

Narrow, septate hyphae
Acute angled branching

12. An HIV patient presented with fever, cough and breathlessness, red pigment with TLC -2500. The isolated organism was a fungus showing yeast from at 37°C and mold form at 25°C as shown in the image (LBCM mount). What is the causative agent?

(a) Pneumocystis jirovecii
(b) Talaromyces marneffei
(c) Blastomyces
(d) Aspergillus versicolor

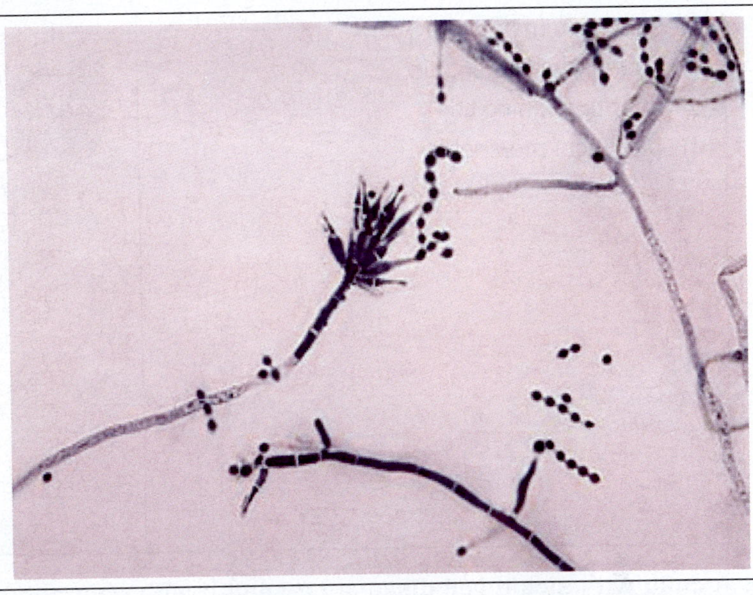

13. A newborn of an HIV infected mother has diarrhea. Which test is to be done to identify causative organism?

(a) HIV antibody in neonate
(b) GDH
(c) Stool microscopy
(d) HIV RNA RT-PCR to determine viral load

14. A red pigment producing pencil shaped macroconidia?

(a) Trichophyton rubrum
(b) Trichophyton violaceum
(c) Trichophyton tonsurans
(d) Trichophyton schoenleinii

15. A diabetic patient recovered from covid-19 presented with facial pain and teeth pain. What is the next best investigation?

(a) KOH mount of nasal swab
(b) MRI of head
(c) Serum ferritin
(d) HBA1c

16. Microfilaria with a sheath surrounding it and two big nuclei at its tail tip. Identify:

(a) Wuchereria bancrofti
(b) Brugyia malayi
(c) Loa Loa
(d) Onchocerca volvulus

17. A 28-year-old lady with HBsAg positive, IgM HBc positive, IgG HBs and IgG HBe negative, Anti HCV negative. What is the diagnosis?

(a) Acute HBV infection
(b) Chronic HBV infection
(c) Acute HCV Infection
(d) Chronic HCV infection

18. Broken vaccine vials to be segregated in which colour bag?

(a) Yellow
(b) Puncture proof blue
(c) White
(d) Red

19. A person manifested with fever, headache, vomiting and neck rigidity. CSF sample analysis showed slight decrease in glucose and highly elevated proteins with cob web coagulum as shown in the image. What is the condition?

(a) Pyogenic meningitis
(b) Tubercular meningitis
(c) Aseptic meningitis
(d) Chemical meningitis

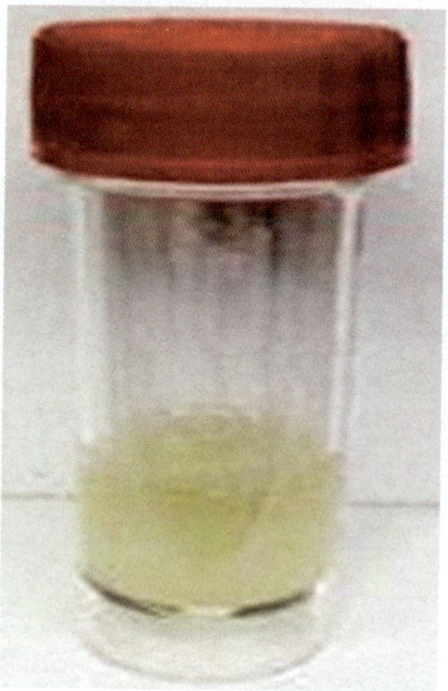

20. A child with sickle cell disease presented with pain and swelling of the knee joint. X-ray showed lytic lesions and sclerotic borders. Joint aspirate was collected which showed the following picture. What is the causative agent?

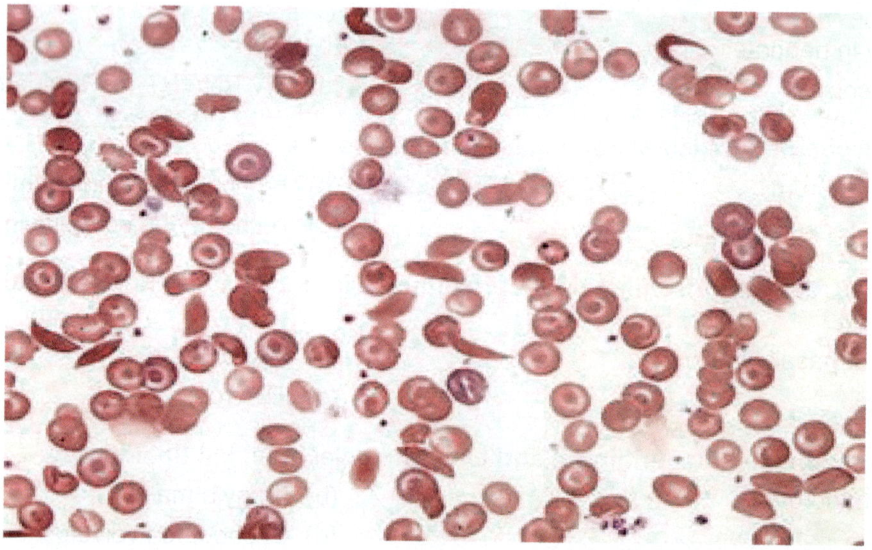

(a) Staphylococcus
(b) Streptococcus
(c) Salmonella
(d) E. coli

21. MDR Tb resistant to:

(a) Isoniazid and rifampicin
(b) Kanamycin
(c) Isoniazid and fluoroquinolones
(d) Isoniazid and kanamycin

ANSWERS AND EXPLANATIONS

1. Ans.: (b)

Probable diagnosis: Genital-vulvovaginal candidiasis (VVC).

Chromagar: It is a selective and differential medium, which facilitates rapid isolation of yeasts from mixed cultures and allows differentiation of Candida species on the basis of coloration and colony morphology.

Image: Gram-positive, darkly stained yeast cells, one of which was designated by an arrowhead	**Image:** Chromagar
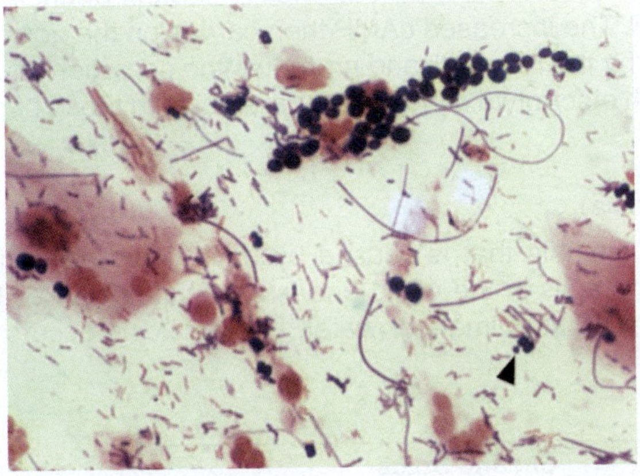	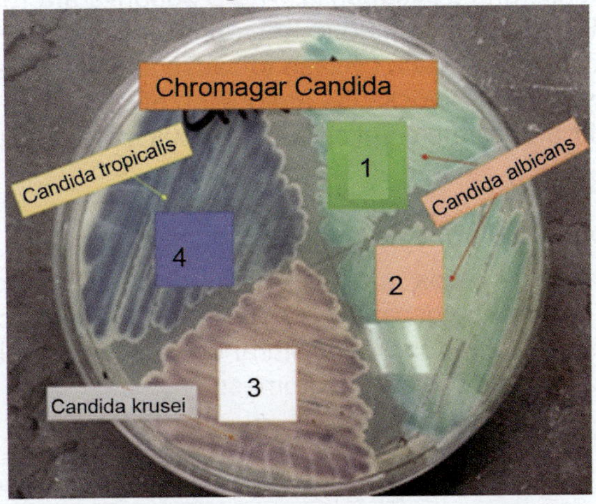

2. Ans.: (a)

Probable diagnosis: Mycetoma, it is a chronic, granulomatous disease of the skin and subcutaneous tissue, which sometimes involves muscle, bone and neighboring organs. It is characterized by tumefaction, abscess formation and fistulae. It typically affects the lower extremities, but it can occur in almost any region of the body. Infection is most probably acquired by traumatic inoculation of fungi (eumycetoma) or bacteria (actinomycetoma) into the subcutaneous tissue.

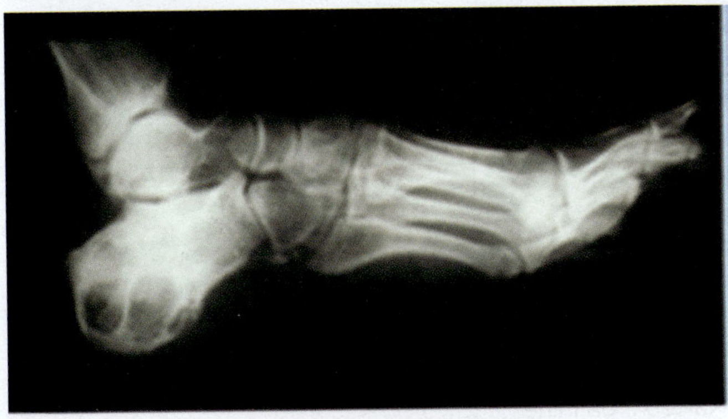

X-ray of a patient with eumycetoma of the foot, showing multiple big cavities

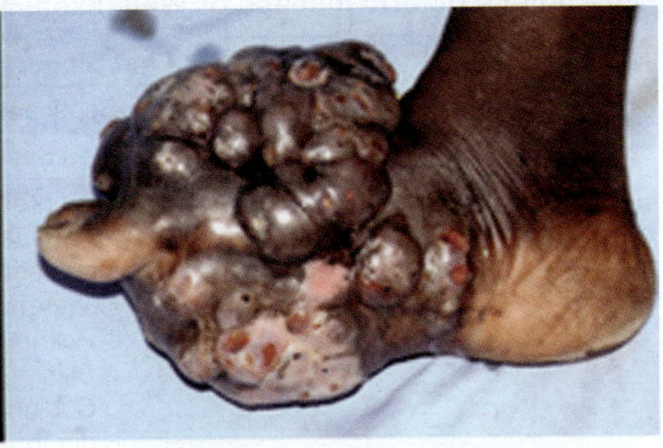

Late stage eumycetoma of the foot

3. Ans.: (a)

Probable diagnosis: Chromoblastomycosis, it is a chronic fungal infection of the skin and the subcutaneous tissue caused by traumatic inoculation of a specific group of dematiaceous (phaeoid) fungi (usually *Fonsecaea pedrosoi*, *Phialophora verrucosa*, *Cladosporium carrionii*, or *Fonsecaea compacta*) through the skin.

Direct examination of 10% potassium hydroxide cleared lesion scrapings is by far the most useful. Typical, thick-walled, cigar-colored, sclerotic cells, also known as Medlar bodies, are readily seen, sometimes more colorfully referred to as golden-brown septate "copper pennies." Although these cells are pathognomonic of chromoblastomycosis, they do not give specific information on the agent.

4. Ans.: (a)

Probable diagnosis: Cholera.

V. cholerae O1 and O139 cause clinical disease by producing an enterotoxin that promotes the secretion of fluid and electrolytes into the lumen of the small intestine. The enterotoxin is a protein molecule composed of 5 B subunits and 2 A subunits. The B subunits are responsible for binding to a ganglioside (monosialosyl ganglioside, GM1) receptor located on the surface of the cells that line the intestinal mucosa. The A1 subunit of cholera toxin activates adenylate cyclase to cause a net increase in cAMP. The increased cAMP then carries on the downstream effects. cAMP blocks the absorption of sodium and chloride by the microvilli and promotes the secretion of chloride and water by the crypt cells. The result is watery diarrhea with electrolyte concentrations isotonic to those of plasma.

5. Ans.: (b)

Probable diagnosis: Mild anicteric febrile illness (leptospirosis).

Leptospirosis is an infectious disease of humans and animals that is caused by pathogenic spirochetes of the genus Leptospira. It is considered the most common zoonosis in the world and is associated with settings of poor sanitation and agricultural occupations involving contact with animals or water. Leptospirosis occurs as two recognizable clinical syndromes:

1. **Mild illness (Anicteric disease):**

	First Stage	**Second Stage**
	– Septicaemic phase	– Immune phase
	– 3-10 days	–
Features	– Fever, Myalgia, Conjunctival suffusion, Abdominal pain, Vomiting	– Meningitis, Uveitis, Chorioretinitis, Rash, Fever, Peripheral neuropathy

2. **Severe illness (Icteric disease or Weil disease):**

	First Stage	**Second Stage**
	– Septicaemic phase	– Immune phase
	– 3-10 days	– 10-30 days
Features	– High grade fever – Liver→Jaundice and increased liver enzymes – Hemorrhages o Pulmonary o Skin o Conjunctival – Kidney→Raised creatinine level	– All features of septicaemic phase can be present

6. Ans.: (d)

Probable diagnosis: *Clostridium difficile* associated diarrhoea or *Cl. difficile* colitis.

Combination of tests are used in diagnosis of *Clostridium difficile* associated diarrhea as single test has got very less reliability.

7. Ans.: (b)

Diagnosis: Cervical carcinoma.

Low-risk HPVs mostly cause no disease. However, a few low-risk HPV types can cause warts on or around the genitals, anus, mouth or throat.

High-risk HPVs can cause several types of cancer. There are about 14 high-risk HPV types including HPV 16, 18, 31, 33, 35, 39, 45, 51, 52, 56, 58, 59, 66 and 68. Two of these, HPV16 and HPV18, are responsible for most HPV-related cancers.

8. Ans.: (b)

Diagnosis: Botulism.

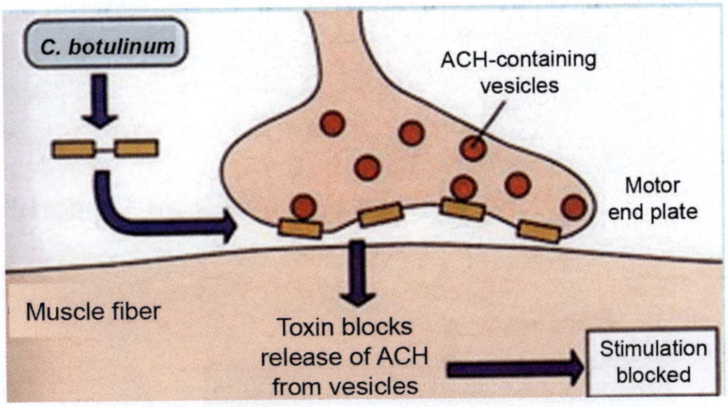

9. Ans.: (d)

Probable diagnosis: Yellow fever.

Yellow fever is an arthropod-borne viral hemorrhagic fever syndrome caused by the yellow fever virus. Yellow fever virus is unique among the viral hemorrhagic fevers in its capacity to cause hepatitis and jaundice.

Torres body: An intranuclear eosinophilic inclusion body of host protein seen in liver cells infected with yellow fever virus.

There are no specific antiviral therapies available for yellow fever. A 17D live-attenuated vaccine is available for travelers to endemic regions, but is contraindicated in pregnancy and immunosuppressed persons.

10. Ans.: (a)

Probable diagnosis: Epidemic typhus.

Louse-borne typhus (epidemic typhus or exanthematic typhus) is a vector-borne disease caused by *Rickettsia prowazekii* and transmitted through infected faeces of the body louse *Pediculus humanus humanus*.

11. Ans.: (b)

Probable diagnosis: Pulmonary Aspergillosis.

Aspergillus hyphae tend to have dichotomous branching that is progressive and primarily at acute angles of around 45°.

12. Ans.: (b)

Probable diagnosis: Talaromycosis (formerly Penicilliosis).

In general, talaromycosis occurs in person with immunocompromised status like AIDS and other conditions. *Talaromyces marneffei* is a dimorphic fungus which also produces red pigment.

13. Ans.: (d)

Probable diagnosis: Neonatal HIV.

Neonatal HIV diagnostics differs from that of adults and older children. It is not appropriate to test for HIV antibodies. The utilization of novel combination antigen/antibody immunoassays to confirm the diagnosis of HIV in neonates is not recommended as positive results confer passive transfer of maternal antibodies. Maternal HIV antibodies persist until 18 months. The use of viral load assays or nucleic acid tests (NATs), which include qualitative RNA assays, quantitative HIV RNA assay, or DNA polymerase chain reaction (PCR) assays, are more appropriate to confirm the diagnosis of HIV in neonates.

14. Ans.: (a)

Trichophyton rubrum: As a dermatophyte it causes athlete's foot, fungal infection of nails, jock itch and ringworm. The pigmentation of *T. rubrum* is variable and can range from white or yellow to wine-red.

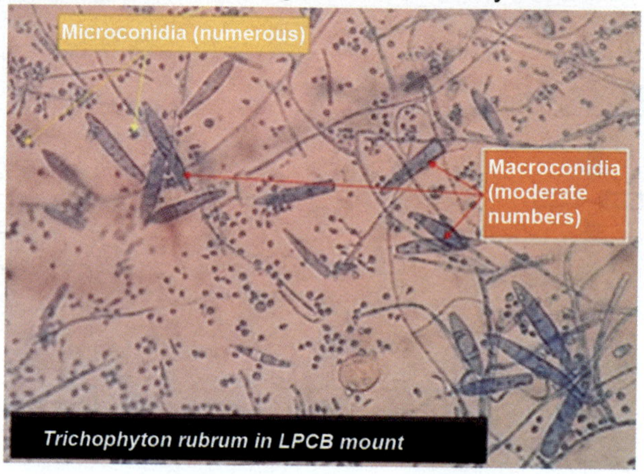

Trichophyton rubrum in LPCB mount

15. Ans.: (b)

Probable diagnosis: Post Covid Mucormycosis.

Diagnostic methods include biopsy, which remains the mainstay of laboratory diagnosis. Facilities where fungal culture and susceptibility testing are available can help to confirm the species of mucormycosis. Imaging tests (MRI) of infected area, may also be used to support the diagnosis.

16. Ans.: (b)

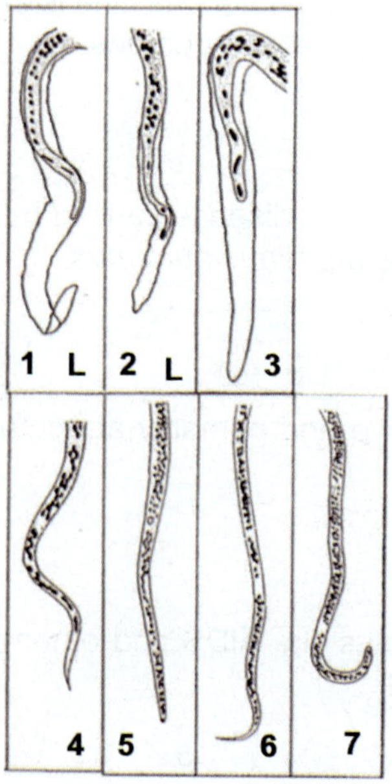

1. ***Wuchereria bancrofti*** **(lymphatic)**
   Sheath, no nuclei in the tip of the tail
2. ***Brugia malayi*** **(lymphatic)**
   Sheath, 2 distinct nuclei in the tip of the tail
3. ***Loa loa*** **(tissue and "eye worm")**
   Sheath, nuclei extending to the tip of the tail
4. ***Onchocerca volvulus*** **(skin)**
   No sheath, no nuclei in the tip of the tail
5. ***Mansonella perstans***
   No sheath, nuclei extending to the tip of the tail
6. ***Mansonella ozzardi***
   No sheath, no nuclei in the tip of the tail
7. ***Mansonella streptocerca*** **(skin)**
   No sheath, nuclei extending to the tip of the hooked tail

17. Ans.: (a)

Probable diagnosis: Acute HBV infection.

Interpretation of Serologic Markers of Hepatitis B Virus Infection

Serologic Reactivity	Disease State					Healthy State	
	Early (Pre-symptomatic)	Early Acute	Acute	Chronic	Late Acute	Resolved	Vaccinated
Anti-HBc	–	–	+*	+	+/-	+	–
Anti-HBe	–	–	–	–	+/-	+/–†	–
Anti-HBs	–	–	–	–	–	+	+
HBeAg	–	+	+	+	–	–	–
HBsAg	+	+	+	+	+	–	–
Infectious virus	+	+	+	+	+	–	–

HBC, Hepatitis B core; *HBeAG*, hepatitis Be antigen; *HBsAg*, hepatitis B surface antigen.
*Anti-HBc immunoglobulin M should be present.
†Anti-HBe may be negative after chronic disease.

18. Ans.: (b)

19. Ans.: (b)

Probable diagnosis: Tubercular meningitis (TBM).

CSF examination in case of TBM showed **cobweb coagulum** in majority cases. Inspect the CSF visually and note its gross appearance. It typically is clear or slightly turbid. If the CSF is left to stand, a fine clot resembling a pellicle or cobweb may form. This faintly visible "**cobweb coagulum/spider's web clot**" is due to the very high level of protein in the CSF (1–8 g/L, or 1000–8000 mg/dL) typical of this condition.

Character	Normal individual	Pyogenic meningitis	Tuberculous meningitis	Viral meningitis
CSF pressure (mm of water)	Normal (50-150)	Highly elevated (>180)	Moderately elevated	Slightly elevated/ normal
Total leukocyte count (per mm^3)	0-5	100-10,000	10-500	25-500
Predominant cell type	Lymphocytes	Neutrophils	Lymphocytes	Lymphocytes
Glucose (mg%)	40-70	(<40 mg/dL) (decreased to absent	20-40 mg/dL (slightly decreased)	Normal
Total protein (mg%)	15-45	>45 mg/dL (usually >250) (markedly increased)	100-500 mg/dL (moderate to markedly increased)	20-80 mg/dL (normal or slightly elevated)

20. Ans.: (c)

Probable diagnosis: *Salmonella* osteomyelitis.

Patients with sickle cell disease are prone to infection of the bone and bone marrow in areas of infarction and necrosis. Although *Staph aureus* is the most common cause of osteomyelitis in the general population but in patients (often children) with sickle cell disease, *Salmonella* osteomyelitis is quite common. There are several factors which make Salmonella susceptible to cause osteomyelitis in patients with Sickle Cell Disease:

- Poor sanitation.
- Bowel infarction.
- Bone marrow infarction.

- RES dysfunction.
- Hepatic dysfunction.

21. Ans.: (a)

Multidrug-resistant TB (MDR TB) is caused by TB bacteria that are resistant to at least isoniazid and rifampin the two most potent TB drugs. These drugs are used to treat all persons with TB disease.

Pre-Extensively Drug-resistant TB (pre-XDR TB) is a type of MDR TB caused by TB bacteria that are resistant to isoniazid, rifampin, and a fluoroquinolone OR by TB bacteria that are resistant to isoniazid rifampin and a second-line injectable (amikacin, capreomycin and kanamycin).

Extensively drug-resistant TB (XDR TB) is a rare type of multidrug-resistant tuberculosis (MDR TB) that is resistant to isoniazid and rifampin, plus any fluoroquinolone and at least one of three injectable second-line drugs (i.e., amikacin, kanamycin, or capreomycin). MDR TB is caused by an organism that is resistant to at least isoniazid and rifampin, the two most potent TB drugs.

RECENT NEET MCQs

1. **A child presented with abdominal pain and blood in stool. Which enrichment media should be used to culture following organism?**
   (a) Selenite F broth
   (b) Alkaline Peptone water
   (c) Robertson cooked media
   (d) BHI

2. **Pus sample was collected from burn patient and isolated organism was found to be obligate aerobe and oxidase positive. Probable causative agent is:**
   (a) Staphylococcus epidermidis
   (b) Corynebacterium species
   (c) Pseudomonas aeruginosa
   (d) Candida albicans

3. **An HIV positive patient presented with fever, chills, his CD4 count is less than 55. Examination findings of consolidation in right intrascapular area with X-ray showing right lower consolidation. Most probable diagnosis of the infection is:**
   (a) S. aureus
   (b) S. pneumoniae
   (c) Pseudomonas aeruginosa
   (d) P. jiroveci

4. **A child presented to emergency department with history of 4-day fever, on examination white lesions seen on buccal mucosa. Probable causative agent is:**
   (a) SS RNA enveloped
   (b) DS RNA enveloped
   (c) SS DNA enveloped
   (d) DS DNA non-enveloped

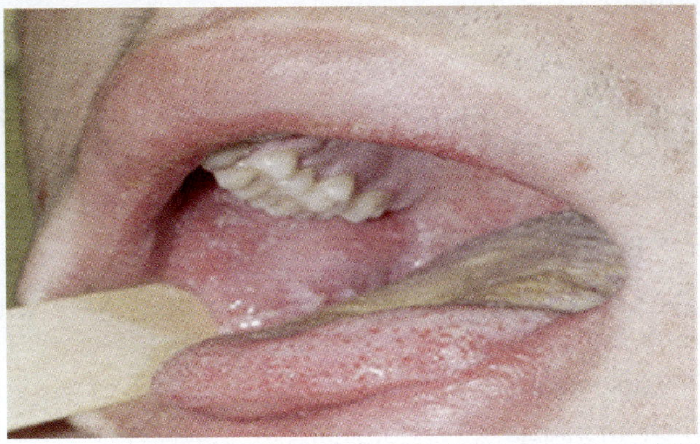

5. **A young girl who has pet dog presented with Deep boggy red areas characterized by a severe acute inflammatory infiltrate with pustule. Probable diagnosis is:**
   (a) Folliculitis
   (b) Abscess
   (c) Kerion
   (d) Epidermal cyst

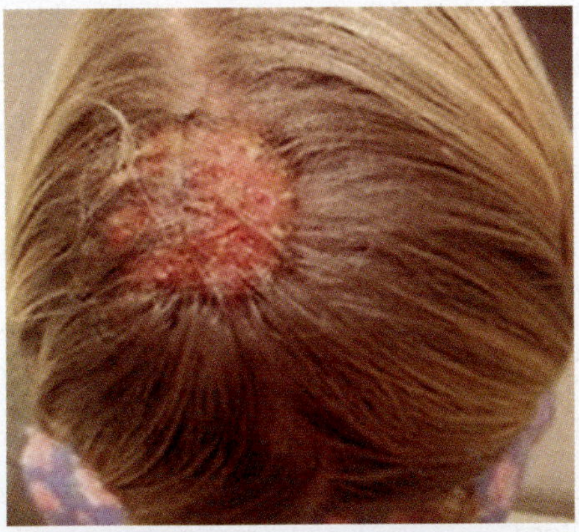

6. One group of friends had late night dinner. Next day early morning one of them started vomiting followed by another friend. On history taking, both of them revealed that they had pastry in restaurant. Most probable organism associated with this clinical condition is:

(a) Vero toxin producing Strain
(b) Bacillus cereus
(c) Staph aureus
(d) Salmonella

7. A child is presented with history of Pharyngitis. Throat swab was taken and sent for microscopy and culture. After the sample processing, where should be swab sample discarded?

(a) Yellow bag
(b) Red bag
(c) White box
(d) None of these

8. Tube agglutination test for Brucellosis was done, initially tested negative but after dilution test came positive, what could be the reason for that:

(a) Post zone phenomenon
(b) Pro zone phenomenon
(c) Complement inactivation
(d) None of these

9. Blood spillage management is done by:

(a) Ethyl alcohol
(b) Chlorhexidine
(c) Formaldehyde
(d) Sodium hypochlorite

10. Wedge shaped perforations in the hair shaft is seen in infection with:

(a) T. rubrum
(b) T. mentagrophytes
(c) M. audouinii
(d) M. canis

11. There is Endemic encephalitis in a community, according to universal immunization schedule, which type of vaccine is used?

(a) Killed SC
(b) Oral live
(c) Live subcutaneous
(d) Killed IM

12. Female presenting with profuse white discharge without itching, on 13th day of menstruation, what could be the probable reason for it?

(a) Physiological
(b) Candidiasis
(c) Trichomoniasis
(d) Bacterial vaginosis

13. Child with hydrocephalus underwent operative correction 4 months ago, later presents with frequent episodes of headache, irritability, loss of appetite.

(a) Culture from lumbar puncture and isolate the organism
(b) Culture from CSF shunt and isolate the causative organism
(c) Culture is not needed for the same, remove the shunt as soon as possible
(d) Observe the child

14. A pregnant woman, whose niece contracted varicella, pregnant woman serum negative for antibodies:

(a) She is susceptible to zoster
(b) She is susceptible to chickenpox
(c) She is immune to chickenpox
(d) She is immune to zoster

15. Name the parasite whose microfilariae have a sheath with no nucleus seen at the end/tail:

(a) Brugia malayi
(b) W. bancrofti
(c) Loa loa
(d) O. volvulus

16. A woman aged 47 years with a 3-year history of nasal obstruction, fetid odour and anosmia was admitted. The fetid odour was detectable as soon as she entered the room. Diagnostic nasal endoscopy revealed green-yellow crusts in the nasal cavity and atrophy of the turbinates (Roomy nose), what is the probable diagnosis?

(a) Atropic rhinitis
(b) Nasal mass
(c) Nasal polyp
(d) GDM

17. A patient was on steroids for chronic urticaria for 2 years, was having nocturnal cough and chronic urticaria, BAL done showed small larvae, recurrent eczema is due to:

(a) Ancyclostoma caninum
(b) S. stercoralis
(c) Enterobius vermicularis
(d) Capillaria philipinensis

18. A man presented with painless, demarcated ulcer on penis with inguinal lymphadenopathy. Which type of best method is used to see motility of organism?

(a) Fluorescent microscope
(b) Dark Field microscopy
(c) Electron microscope
(d) Light microscope

19. What is the vector for a parasite which has kinetoplast in infective and other forms?

(a) Tsetse fly
(b) Sand fly
(c) Anopheles mosquito
(d) Triatomine bug

20. A child had myoclonic seizures, recent decline in school activities, no past history except for fever with rash on first year of life, EEG shows burst wave? How to go for diagnosis of the same?

(a) Anti AQ4
(b) Measle IgG
(c) CSF globulin is not elevated
(d) CSF examination usually reveals increased pressure, cell count and total protein content

21. A man presented with profuse urethral discharge as seen in image given, which is the causative agent?

(a) Gonococcus
(b) Herpes
(c) Chlamydia
(d) None

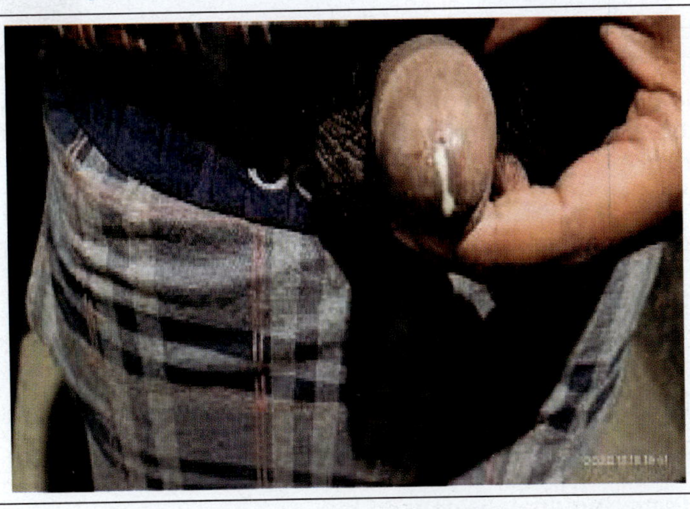

22. What is the most probable diagnosis?

(a) Exanthem subitum
(b) Erythema infectiosum
(c) Hand-foot-and-mouth disease
(d) Mumps

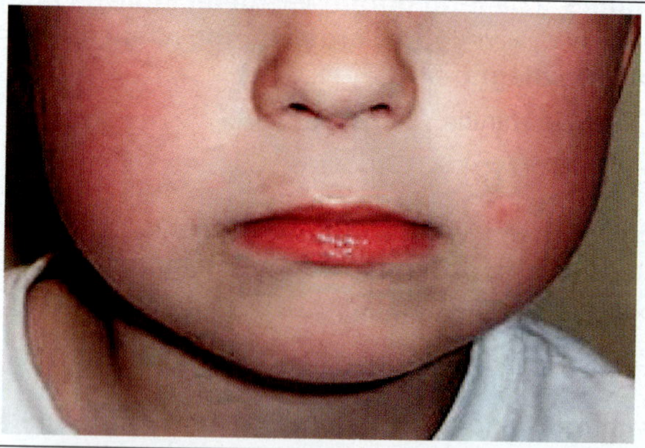

23. An 8-year-old child is presented with swelling on face and swelling on scrotum after few weeks. Which of the following is causative agent?

(a) Measles virus
(b) Polio virus
(c) Mumps virus
(d) Cox virus

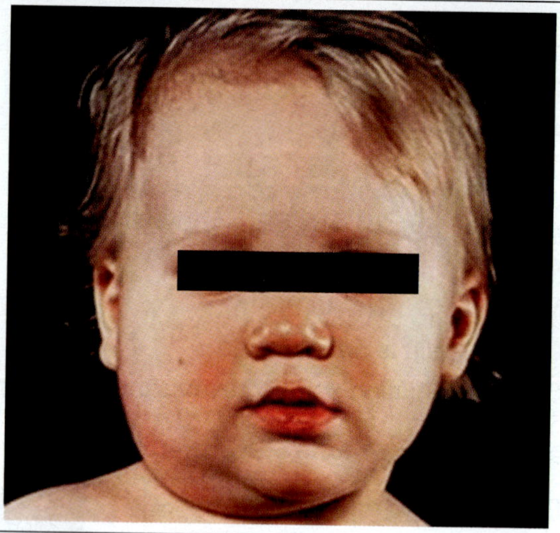

24. A patient presented with multiple episodes of bloody diarrhea. On investigations of blood sample Enterohemorrhagic strain of *E. coli* was isolated. On which of the following media this organism can be cultured?

(a) TCBS
(b) Selenite F broth
(c) Robertson cooked meat media
(d) Sorbitol MacConkey agar

25. A patient presented with multiple asymptomatic scaly patches varying in color from white to tan to brown to pink. On potassium hydroxide wet mount spaghetti and meat ball appearance is seen. Which of the following is causative organism for this disease?

(a) Tinea corporis
(b) Malassezia furfur
(c) Sporotrichosis
(d) Blastomycosis

26. Granuloma inguinale is caused by:

(a) T. pallidum
(b) Chlamydia
(c) HSV
(d) Klebsiella granulomatis

27. Tumbling motility is seen in:

(a) Vibrio
(b) Listeria
(c) Proteus
(d) Treponema pallidum

28. A worker got flea bite in wheat godown. Patient developed axillary lymphadenopathy. What is best method to examine the smear from lymph node?

(a) Gram stain
(b) Giemsa
(c) Acid fast
(d) None

29. Identify the organism:

(a) P. falciparum
(b) P. vivax
(c) P. knowlesi
(d) P. malariae

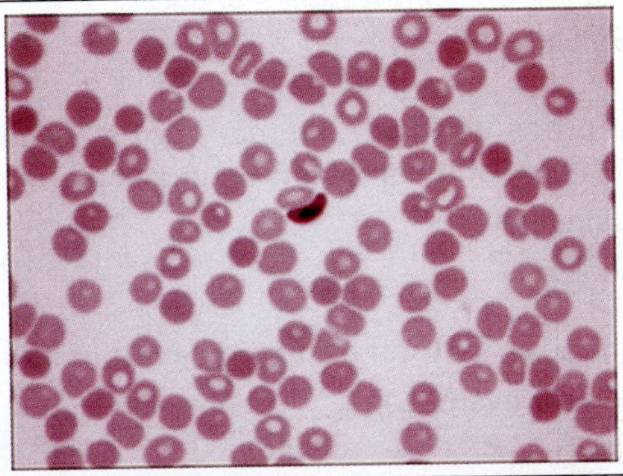

30. Which of the following is strongly associated with Mucormycosis?

(a) Diabetic ketoacidosis
(b) Pregnancy
(c) Pneumocystis
(d) Histoplasmosis

31. A patient is taking Clindamycin for a long period of time presented with diarrhea. Which of the following is causative organism for this?

(a) Cl. botulinum
(b) Cl. tetani
(c) Cl. difficile
(d) Cl. perfringens

32. A lady presented with foul smelling greyish white discharge and whiff test was positive. On examination following cells were seen as shown in image given below. Identify the causative organism and drug of choice:

(a) Candida, Fluconazole
(b) Trichomonas, metronidazole
(c) Gardnerella vaginalis, metronidazole
(d) Gonococci, Doxycycline

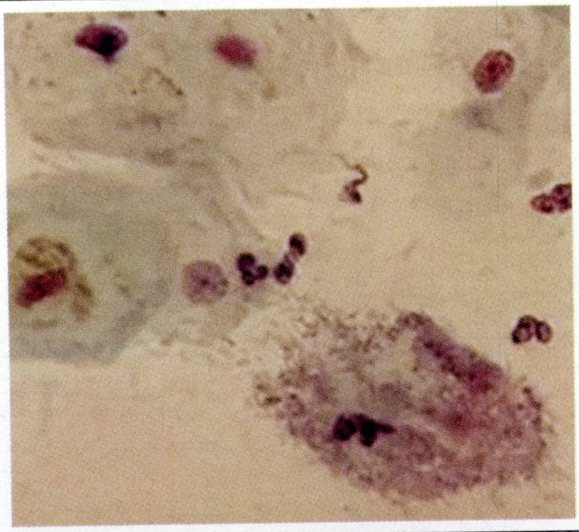

33. Reinfection with which of the following virus can lead to more severe disease with complications (Antibody dependent enhancement)?

(a) Dengue
(b) Rabies
(c) Measles
(d) Mumps

34. Gram positive alpha hemolytic cocci with catalase negative and optochin resistant causing endocarditis:

(a) Streptococcus pneumoniae
(b) Streptococcus agalactiae
(c) Staphylococcus epidermidis
(d) Streptococcus sanguis

35. Which can cause condyloma acuminata?

(a) HPV 1, 6
(b) HPV 16, 18
(c) HPV 31, 33
(d) HPV 6, 11

36. A child presented with complaint of dysphagia, cough and greyish white membrane over the tonsils. Which of the following is causative organism?

(a) Clostridium
(b) Corynebacterium diphtheriae
(c) Candida
(d) Pneumococcus

37. Cost effective method to test for syphilis (spirochetes) in village with poor resources?

(a) Darkfield microscopy
(b) Immunofluorescence
(c) Culture
(d) Simple microscopy

38. Rh+ve father and Rh -ve mother had Rh +ve child. This Rh incompatibility is which type of hypersensitivity reaction?

(a) Type 1
(b) Type 2
(c) Type 3
(d) Type 4

ANSWERS AND EXPLANATIONS

1. Ans.: (a)

Selenite F broth (enrichment broth): It inhibits coliform bacilli while permitting salmonellae and many shigellae to grow.

2. Ans.: (c)

P. aeruginosa is one of the common bacteria that causes skin and soft tissue infection in burn patients. Mnemonics for Oxidase Positive Organisms–**PVNCH** (It's just an acronym inspired by the famous mnemonic for Urease Positive organisms–**PUNCH**).

1. **P**: *Pseudomonas* spp.
2. **V**: *Vibrio cholerae.*
3. **N**: *Neisseria* spp.
4. **C**: *Campylobacter* spp.
5. **H**: *Helicobacter* spp/*Haemophilus* spp.
6. ***A****eromonas* spp.
7. ***A****lcaligens.*

3. Ans.: (b)

4. Ans.: (a)

Measles virus (MV) is an enveloped, non-segmented, negative-strand RNA virus belonging to the Morbillivirus genus in the Paramyxoviridae family. Koplik spots—pathognomonic for measles—are small, bluish white ulcerations on the buccal mucosa opposite the lower molars. These spots contain giant cells and viral antigens and appear slightly before the rash.

5. Ans.: (c)

Hair follicle inflammation can be superficial, involving just the ostium of the follicle (folliculitis), or deep (furuncles and carbuncles). *S. aureus* infections cause ecthyma, folliculitis, furuncles, carbuncles, bullous impetigo and the scalded skin syndrome.

6. Ans.: (c)

The foods that have been most frequently implicated in cases of staphylococcal food poisoning are poultry and cooked meat products such as ham or corned beef. Other foods implicated were milk and milk products, canned food and bakery products. Food poisoning caused by staphylococcal enterotoxin is characterized by a short incubation period (1–8 hours); violent nausea, vomiting and diarrhea; and rapid convalescence. There is no fever.

7. Ans.: (a)

Yellow bag–for infectious non plastic waste.

Red bag–for infectious plastic waste.

White bag–for metal sharps and its puncture proof box.

Bule bad–for broken glass items and metal implants, its puncture proof box.

8. Ans.: (b)

Since prozone is a well-known phenomenon in the serologic diagnosis of Brucella infections, it is necessary to prepare higher serum dilutions in the standard tube agglutination (STA) test for the brucellosis suspected patients to avoid false negativity.

9. Ans.: (d)

Different concentration (0.5-1%) of Sodium hypochlorite is used for blood spillage management in hospitals.

10. Ans.: (b)

Hair perforation test: In this test *T. mentagrophyte* and *M. canis* pierce the hair producing wedge shaped perforation.

11. Ans.: (c)

Live attenuated SA-14-14-2 vaccine is used to give children (1-15 years) in endemic areas of India such as UP, Bihar, Assam, West Bengal and Karnataka. It is given subcutaneously at left upper arm.

12. Ans.: (a)

A bit of white discharge, especially at the beginning or end of your menstrual cycle, is normal. However, if the discharge is accompanied by itching and has a thick, cottage cheese-like consistency or appearance, it's not normal and needs treatment. This type of discharge may be a sign of a Candida yeast infection.

13. Ans.: (b)

It's a case of CSF shunt associated infection. The most common organisms infecting CSF shunts are staphylococci. Approximately 40% of shunt infections are caused by *Staphylococcus epidermidis* infections and 20% by *S. aureus*.

14. Ans.: (b)

15. Ans.: (b)

Microfilaria	Head end	Tail end
Wuchereria bancrofti	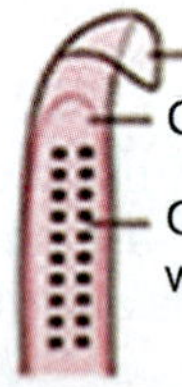	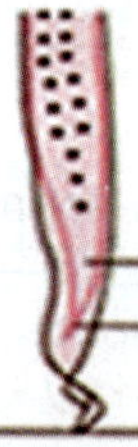
Brugia malayi	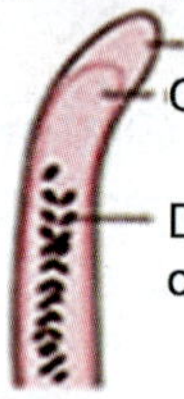	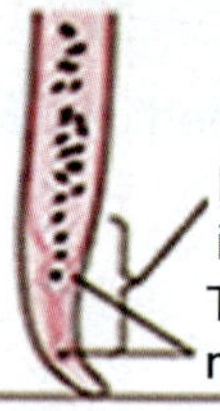
Loa loa	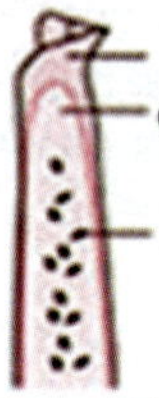	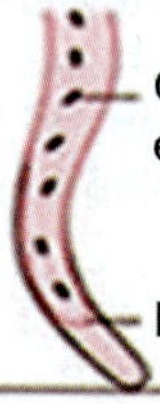
Onchocerca volvulus	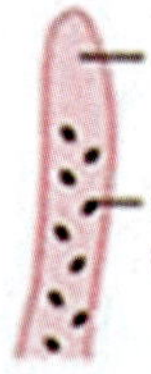	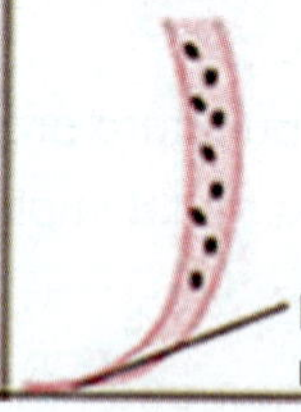

16. Ans.: (a)

Atrophic rhinitis is a chronic disease of the nasal mucosa. The disease is characterized by abnormally wide nasal cavities, and its main symptoms are dryness, crusting, atrophy, fetor, and a paradoxical sensation of nasal congestion.

17. Ans.: (b)

S. stercoralis pulmonary disease secondary to larval migration through the lung rarely occurs and may resemble Loeffler syndrome (cough, wheezing, shortness of breath, transient pulmonary infiltrates accompanied by eosinophilia).

18. Ans.: (b)

It's a case of primary syphilis. Darkfield microscopy is used for the demonstration of live *T. pallidum* in specimen.

19. Ans.: (b)

The causative agent of leishmaniasis is transmitted from man to man by a tiny insect called sandfly.

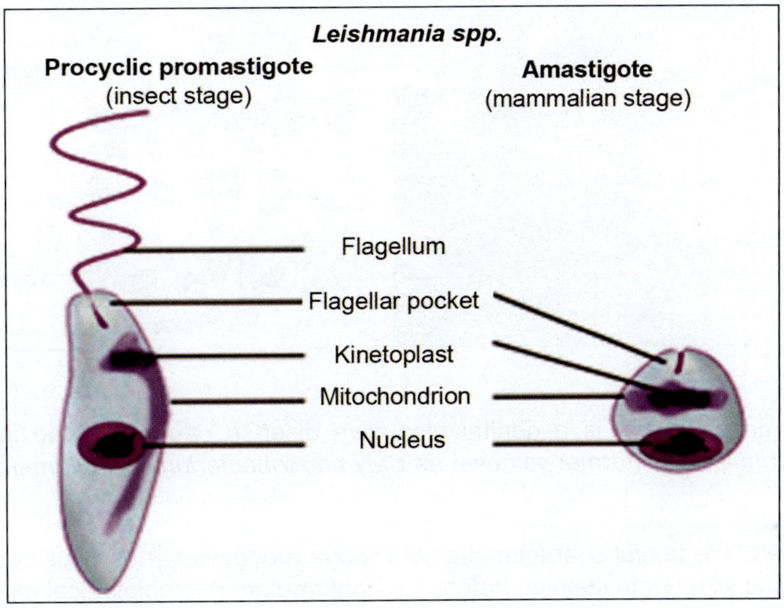

20. Ans.: (b)

SSPE is a rare late complication of measles, caused by persistent nonproductive measles virus infection of neurons and glia in immunocompetent patients. At the time neurological symptoms occur, neurons and glia contain nuclear and cytoplasmic viral inclusion bodies, and high titers of antimeasles antibody is found in both serum and CSF. The CSF/serum antibody ratio is consistent with high levels of intrathecal synthesis of measles antibody. CSF pleocytosis is absent, glucose is normal, and total protein is normal or elevated.

21. Ans.: (a)

In gonococcal urethritis, *Neisseria gonorrhoeae* (Gonococcus) produces an acute inflammation of the urethra. Following a short incubation period of 2 to 5 days after intercourse, a purulent urethral discharge develops, with pain on passing urine.

22. Ans.: (b)

Erythema infectiosum (fifth disease) is usually a benign childhood condition characterized by a classic slapped-cheek appearance (see the image below) and lacy exanthem. It caused by parvovirus B19.

23. Ans.: (c)

Mumps is characterized by swollen, painful salivary glands in the face, causing the cheeks to puff out. Pain and swelling of the testicle (orchitis) affect up to 1 in 3 males who get mumps after puberty. The swelling is usually sudden and affects only one testicle. The testicle may also feel warm and tender.

24. Ans.: (d)

Sorbitol MacConkey agar is recommended for isolation of Enterohemorrhagic *E. coli* O157:H7, which ferments lactose but does not ferment sorbitol, hence produces colourless colonies. Rainbow agar is also used for isolation of EHEC.

25. Ans.: (b)

Tinea versicolor (Pityriasis versicolor) is a chronic, usually asymptomatic, involvement of the stratum corneum, characterized by discrete or confluent macular areas of discoloration or depigmentation of the skin, caused by *M. furfur* (lipophilic fungi). 10% KOH mount of scrapings from the lesion shows yeast cells along with short curved hyphae (banana and grapes; spaghetti and meat ball appearance).

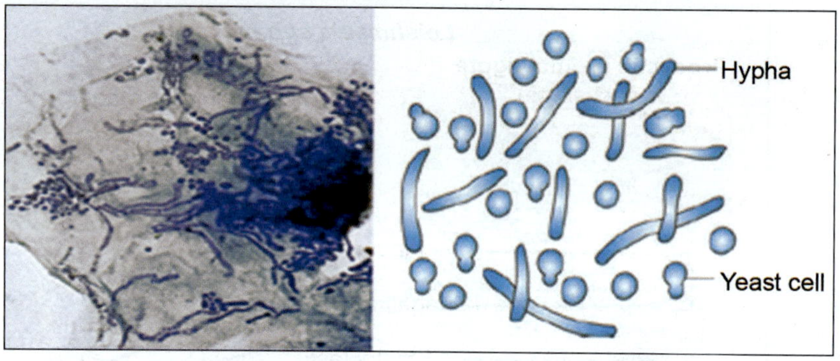

26. Ans.: (b)

Granuloma inguinale (donovanosis) is a genital ulcerative disease caused by the intracellular gram-negative bacterium *Klebsiella granulomatis* (formerly known as *Calymmatobacterium granulomatis*).

27. Ans.: (b)

Tumbling motility is one of the useful characteristics of Listeria monocytogenes. This can be helpful to identify the causative pathogen along with Gram staining before the confirmatory microbiological examination.

28. Ans.: (b)

Endemic typhus or murine typhus (*Rickettsia typhi*)—Infected flea feces rubbed into the bite wound is the method of transmission. Skin biopsies taken from patients may reveal *R. typhi* by histology and Immunohistochemical Analyses.

29. Ans.: (a)

P. falciparum gametocytes are crescent or sausage or banana shaped.

30. Ans.: (a)

The major risk factors for mucormycosis include uncontrolled diabetes mellitus in ketoacidosis, other forms of metabolic acidosis, treatment with corticosteroids, organ or bone marrow transplantation, neutropenia, trauma and burns, malignant hematologic disorders, and deferoxamine therapy in patients receiving hemodialysis.

31. Ans.: (c)

Antibiotic associated diarrhoea is cause by *Cl. difficile.*

32. Ans.: (c)

A whiff test is performed by adding several drops of 10% potassium hydroxide to a sample of vaginal discharge. A strong fishy odor is indicative of a positive test result. Such a result may suggest either trichomoniasis or bacterial vaginosis. **Clue cells** are epithelial cells of the vagina which obtain their distinctive speckled appearance by being coated with bacteria (The etymology behind the term "clue cells" comes from the original research article by Gardner and Dukes). They are a medical sign of bacterial vaginosis, especially that caused by Gardnerella vaginalis, a group of Gram variable bacteria.

33. Ans.: (a)

Patients experiencing a second infection with a heterologous dengue virus serotype have a significantly higher risk for developing dengue haemorrhagic fever (DHF). DHF is currently defined by the following four World Health Organization (WHO) criteria:

- Fever or recent history of fever lasting 2–7 days.
- Any haemorrhagic manifestation.
- Thrombocytopenia (platelet count of $<100{,}000/mm^3$).
- Evidence of increased vascular permeability.

34. Ans.: (d)

The viridans streptococci cause a significant percentage of all cases of infective endocarditis (IE). There are at least 30 recognized species of VGS, which are classified into six major groups: S. mutans group, Streptococcus salivarius group, Streptococcus mitis group, Streptococcus sanguinis group, Streptococcus anginosus group and Streptococcus bovis group.

35. Ans.: (d)

HPV strains 6 and 11 are the most prevalent strains that cause condyloma acuminata.

36. Ans.: (b)

It's a case of diphtheria as description of pseudo-membrane is there.

37. Ans.: (a)

Darkfield microscopy is used for the demonstration of live *T. pallidum* in specimen and it's a cost-effective method than given other methods.

38. Ans.: (b)

In complement-mediated Type II hypersensitivity, IgG isotype antibody recognition of cell surface epitopes leads to the assembly of the complement C5–C9 membrane attack complex (MAC) and subsequent lysis of the cell. This reaction is the underlying mechanism in multiple disease states, including those seen in autoimmune hemolytic anemia and Rh incompatibility leading to erythroblastosis fetalis.

LATEST FMGE MCQs

1. **Diagnosis of typhoid fever in 3rd days is best done by:**
   (a) Blood culture
   (b) Urine culture
   (c) Stool culture
   (d) Widal test
2. **Which organism cannot be cultured on artificial media?**
   (a) S. aureus
   (b) M. tuberculosis
   (c) M. leprae
   (d) Listeria
3. **An IV drug abuser presented with splinter haemorrhage on nails and tricuspid valve vegetation, murmur was described in the question, most common cause is:**
   (a) Staph aureus
   (b) Pseudomonas
   (c) Candida albicans
   (d) Strep. viridans
4. **There was a pneumonia outbreak in a nursery, negative sense single stranded RNA was found for outbreak, which is neuraminidase and haemagglutinin negative. Which of the following is causative agent?**
   (a) Influenza A
   (b) Adenovirus
   (c) Paramyxovirus
   (d) RSV
5. **A child presented with fever, headache, neck rigidity, gram stain found to be negative for any organism, in CSF examination neutrophils are predominant, CSF sugar is markedly decreased and protein levels increased. All these features suggestive of which meningitis?**
   (a) TBM
   (b) Viral meningitis
   (c) Pyogenic meningitis
   (d) Fungal meningitis
6. **DOC for legionella infection:**
   (a) Azithromycin
   (b) Clindamycin
   (c) Ampicillin + Gentamycin
   (d) None of these
7. **Causative agent for acne:**
   (a) Propionibacterium Acne
   (b) Mobiluncus
   (c) Prevotella
   (d) Actinomyces
8. **Blood bags are disposed in:**
   (a) Yellow
   (b) Red
   (c) Blue
   (d) Green
9. **Causative agent for cat scratch disease:**
   (a) B. quintana
   (b) B. henselae
   (c) B. baciliformis
   (d) None of these
10. **Which of the following do not have cystic stage?**
   (a) Trichomonas
   (b) Giardia
   (c) Trypanosoma
   (d) Leishmania
11. **Sclerotic bodies are found in:**
   (a) Chromoblastomycosis
   (b) Sporotrichosis
   (c) Coccidiomycosis
   (d) Talaromycosis

12. In emergency patient relative donated blood, it was further tested in lab before blood transfusion, which of the following disease will be tested except:

(a) Hep B
(b) Hep A
(c) HIV 1 and HIV 2
(d) Hep C

13. E coli O antigen present in:

(a) Lipopolysaccharide
(b) Peptidoglycan
(c) Flagella
(d) Pili

14. Which of the following shows food poisoning associated with Chinese fried rice?

(a) Bacillus cereus
(b) S. aureus
(c) Clostridium
(d) Salmonella

15. An HIV positive patient developed lung infection, cultured on LJ media and found to be acid fast in ZN staining of sputum?

(a) Bacillus cereus
(b) MTB
(c) Candida
(d) None of the above

16. A farmer presents with multiple discharging sinuses in the leg not responding to antibiotics. Most likely causative agent is:

(a) Sporothrix
(b) Actinomycetes
(c) Nocardia
(d) Madurella

17. Which of the following method is used for sterilization of disposable plastic petri dish?

(a) Glutaraldehyde
(b) Ethylene oxide
(c) Autoclave
(d) Hot air oven

18. Bee sting is which type of hypersensitivity?

(a) Type 1 HS
(b) Type 2 HS
(c) Type 3 HS
(d) Type 4 HS

19. Myasthenia gravis is which hypersensitivity?

(a) Type 1 HS
(b) Type 2 HS
(c) Type 3 HS
(d) Type 4 HS

20. Multiple myeloma light chains type:

(a) Kappa IgG
(b) Kappa IgM
(c) Beta IgG
(d) Alpha IgM

21. Antigenic shift in influenza virus is by:

(a) Point mutation
(b) Frame shift mutation
(c) Minor antigenic changes
(d) Reassortment

22. Drug of choice for Mucormycosis?

(a) LAMB
(b) Terbinafine
(c) Ketoconazole
(d) None of them

23. Difference between Gram-positive and Gram-negative bacteria is mainly based on:

(a) LPS
(b) Protein A
(c) Peptidoglycan
(d) Beta 1,3 glucan

ANSWERS AND EXPLANATIONS

1. Ans.: (a)

Widal test: Blood culture: 1st week of illness.

BASU [1st week: Blood culture (Best method: Bone marrow culture); **2nd week: A**gglutination (Widal test)/ Serology; **3rd week: S**tool culture; **4th week: U**rine culture**].**

2. Ans.: (c)

Mouse (foot-pad) and Nine-banded armadillos are commonly used for the isolation.

3. Ans.: (a)

Staphylococcus aureus is most common cause of Endocarditis in IV drug abusers.

4. Ans.: (d)

DNA virus: Adenovirus

RNA (-ve sense, ss): Influenza virus, Parainfluenza virus, Respiratory syncytial virus (RSV).

RSV possesses three integral membrane proteins: the receptor attachment glycoprotein (G), the fusion protein (F), and a short hydrophobic (SH) protein. The G protein is involved in viral attachment to the host cell, while the F protein is responsible for fusion.

5. Ans.: (c)

Character	Normal individual	Pyogenic meningitis	Tuberculous meningitis	Viral meningitis
CSF pressure (mm of water)	Normal (50-150)	Highly elevated (> 180)	Moderately elevated	Slightly elevated/normal
Total leukocyte count (per mm^3)	0-5	100-10000	10-500	25-500
Predominant cell type	Lymphocytes	Neutrophils	Lymphocytes	Lymphocytes
Glucose (mg%)	40-70	(< 40 mg/dl) (decreased to absent)	20-40 mg/dl (slightly decreased)	Normal
Total proteins (mg%)	15-45	>45 mg/dl (usually >250) (markedly increased)	100-500 mg/dl (moderate to markedly increased)	20-80 mg/dl (normal or slightly elevated)

6. Ans.: (a)

DOC for legionella infection:

- Macrolides like azithromycin, clarithromycin.
- Fluoroquinolones such as levofloxacin and moxifloxacin.

7. Ans.: (a)

Acne is a chronic, inflammatory skin condition that causes spots and pimples, especially on the face, shoulders, back, neck, chest and upper arms. ***Propionibacterium acnes*** is a gram-positive human skin commensal that prefers anaerobic growth conditions and is involved in the pathogenesis of acne.

8. Ans.: (a)

9. Ans.: (b)

Cat scratch disease (CSD), also known as cat scratch fever or subacute regional lymphadenitis, is a bacterial infection affecting lymph nodes that drain the sites of inoculation. ***Bartonella henselae***, a gram-negative rod, is considered the principal etiologic agent. CSD is one of the most common causes of chronic lymphadenopathy in children and adolescents.

10. Ans.: (a)

Trichomonas vaginalis resides in the female lower genital tract and the male urethra and prostate, where it replicates by binary fission. The parasite does not appear to have a cyst form, and does not survive well in the external environment.

11. Ans.: (a)

Chromoblastomycosis is a chronic fungal infection of the skin and the subcutaneous tissue caused by traumatic inoculation of a specific group of dematiaceous fungi (usually Fonsecaea pedrosoi, Phialophora verrucosa, Cladosporium carrionii, or Fonsecaea compacta) through the skin.

Sclerotic bodies are found in the stratum corneum and the following layers of the epidermis and the skin. Sclerotic cells, also known as Medlar bodies, are globe-shaped, cigar-colored, thick-walled structures of fungi.

12. Ans.: (b)

The hepatitis A virus (HAV) is transmitted through ingestion of contaminated food and water or through direct contact with an infectious person.

13. Ans.: (a)

Lipopolysaccharide on the surface of Escherichia coli constitutes the O antigens which are important virulence factors that are targets of both the innate and adaptive immune systems and play a major role in host-pathogen interactions.

14. Ans.: (a)

Bacillus cereus is a toxin-producing bacteria that is one of the most common causes of food poisoning, also called **fried rice syndrome**.

15. Ans.: (b)

HIV weakens the immune system, increasing the risk of TB in people with HIV. Infection with both HIV and TB is called HIV/TB coinfection. Untreated latent TB infection is more likely to advance to TB disease in people with HIV than in people without HIV. Lowenstein-Jensen (LJ) Medium is a selective media for isolation of *M. tuberculosis*. Ziehl-Neelsen (ZN) staining is used for the demonstration of acid-fast nature of *M. tuberculosis*.

16. Ans.: (d)

Madurella mycetomatis (Fungi) is the most common cause of eumycotic mycetoma worldwide therefore it would not respond to any antibiotics.

17. Ans.: (b)

ETO is used for the items which are moisture and heat sensitive.

18. Ans.: (a)

19. Ans.: (d)

20. Ans.: (a)

The most common type of myeloma is IgG kappa. This means the myeloma cells produce immunoglobulins made of two IgG heavy chains and two kappa light chains.

21. Ans.: (d)

Human influenza A viruses evolve rapidly by antigenic shift and antigenic drift. Antigenic shift occurs by genetic reassortment between currently circulating human viruses and influenza viruses of other origin and by re-emergence of a previously circulating virus.

22. Ans.: (d)

Mucormycosis is a serious infection and needs to be treated with antifungal medicine, usually amphotericin B, posaconazole, or isavuconazole.

23. Ans.: (c)

Gram staining technique was proposed by Christian Gram to distinguish the two types of bacteria (gram +ve and -ve) based on the difference in their cell wall structures.

CORONA VIRUS DISEASE 19 (COVID-19)

COVID-19 is an acute respiratory disease caused by severe acute respiratory syndrome coronavirus–2 (SARS-CoV2). Coronaviruses are members of the sub-family Coronavirinae from the family Coronaviridae and the order Nidovirales. Based on phylogenetic relationships and genomic structures, the sub-family Coronavirinae is divided into four genera namely, Alpha-coronavirus, Beta-coronavirus, Gamma-coronavirus and Delta-coronavirus. Beta-coronavirus includes the SARS-CoV2.

A. MORPHOLOGY OF SARS-COV2

The SARS-CoV2 made up of a nucleocapsid, surrounded by an envelope. It measures 100-120 nm in size and has a helical symmetry. It possesses 4 structural proteins (N, S, M, E), 16 non-structural proteins and several other accessory proteins. Most often, the virion of SARS-CoV2 has a spherical form, but also pleomorphic and oval shapes occur. The viral envelope is built of three proteins: the S-spike protein is a club-shaped surface projection that forms the peplomers and gives the virus a characteristic **crown shape**, M-membrane protein, and E-envelope protein, which provide the ring structure. There is also a fourth protein, N-nucleocapsid protein, a phosphoprotein, which is a structural component of the nucleocapsid. Nucleocapsid consists of +ve sense ssRNA.

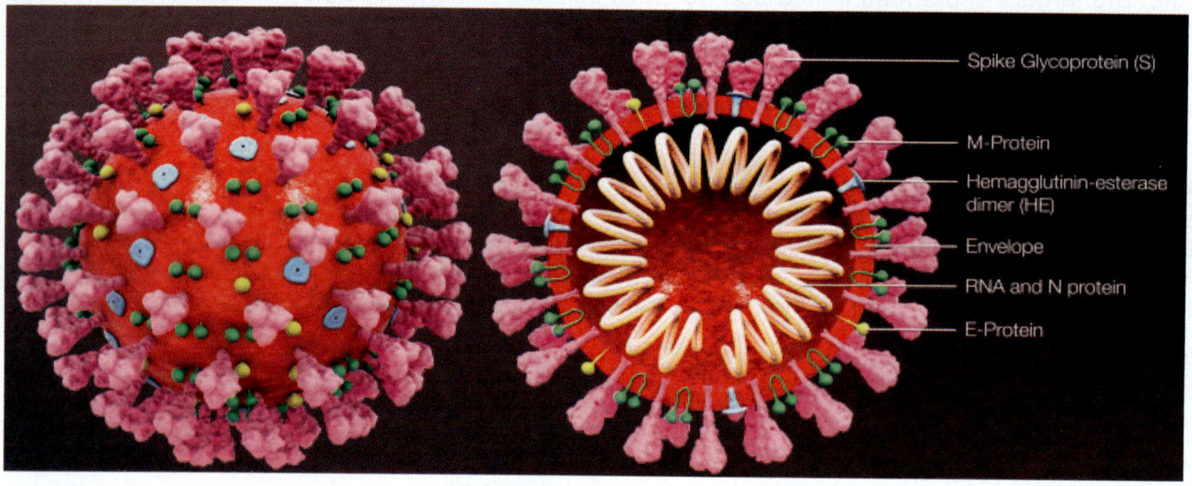

Fig: Structure of SARS-CoV2

- **N-nucleocapsid protein** aids in the regulation of viral RNA synthesis.
- **S-spike protein** helps in attachment to the host cells. Neutralizing antibodies are produced against S-spike protein are protective in nature.
- **M-membrane protein** is most abundant structural protein. M protein projects on the external surface of the envelope, spans the envelope 3 times, and is important in viral assembly.
- **E-envelope protein** is a transmembrane protein and participates in the formation of new virions that are mostly built from the host cell material.
- **Non-structural proteins** include several enzymes which help in replication of virus like RdRp, helicase etc.

B. PATHOGENESIS

Transmission

SARS-CoV2 spreads from an infected person to others through respiratory droplets and aerosols when an infected person breathes, coughs, sneezes, sings, shouts, or talks. The droplets vary in size, from large droplets that fall to the ground rapidly (within seconds or minutes) near the infected person, to smaller droplets, sometimes called aerosols, which linger in the air, especially in indoor spaces.

Infectious droplets or aerosols may come into direct contact with the mucous membranes of another person's nose, mouth or eyes, or they may be inhaled into their nose, mouth, airways and lungs. The virus may also spread when a person touches another person (i.e., a handshake) or a surface or an object (also referred to as a fomite) that has the virus on it, and then touches their mouth, nose or eyes with unwashed hands.

Incubation period: Average of 5 to 14 days.

Entry and replication of SARS-CoV2: Entry of SARS-CoV-2 into host target cells depends on the binding of spike glycoprotein to the cellular receptor angiotensin-converting enzyme 2 (ACE2) for internalization. ACE2 is expressed by epithelial cells of the intestine, kidney, blood vessels, and, most abundantly, in type II alveolar cells of the lungs. The human enzyme transmembrane protease, serine 2 (TMPRSS2), is also used by the virus for S protein priming and to aid in membrane fusion. The virus then enters the host cell via endocytosis. Internalization results in uncoating of viral RNA into cytoplasm that undergoes translation and generates replicase polyproteins pp1a and pp1b, which is further cleaved by virus-encoded proteinases into small proteins. The replication of SARS-CoV-2 involves ribosomal frame shifting during the translation process and generates both genomic and multiple copies of subgenomic RNA species by discontinuous transcription required for relevant viral proteins. Assembly of virion takes place via interaction of viral RNA and protein at endoplasmic reticulum (ER) and Golgi complex. These virions are subsequently released out of the cells via vesicles via exocytosis.

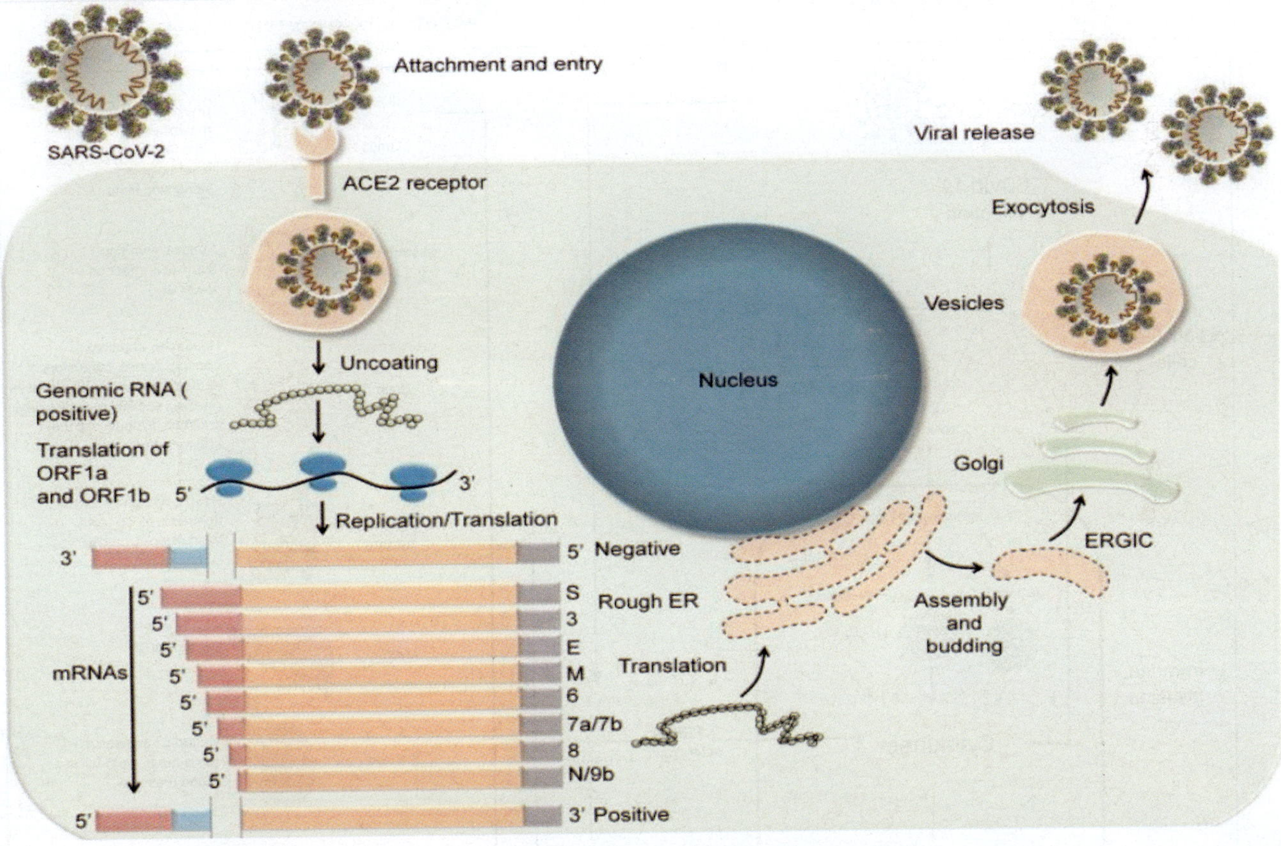

Fig: Entry and replication of SARS-CoV2 in host cells

Cytokines Storm: An over-reaction of immune system to COVID-19

COVID-19 infection is accompanied by an aggressive inflammatory response with the release of a large amount of pro-inflammatory cytokines in an event known as "cytokine storm". The host immune response to the SARS-CoV-2 virus is hyperactive resulting in an excessive inflammatory reaction. Several immune cells like neutrophils, T-lymphocytes, macrophages are recruited to the lung.

Acute influx of cytokines: Tissue macrophages, mast cells, endothelial, and epithelial cells are the major source of cytokines during innate immune response. Three of the most important pro-inflammatory cytokines of the innate immune response are IL-2, IL-2R, IL-6, IL-7, IL-8, IL-10 and TNF-α (Others being IFNα, IFNγ, IL-1β,

IL-12, IL-18, IL-33). The "cytokine storm" results in influx of more immune cells from the circulation into the site of infection leading to destabilization of endothelial cell to cell interactions, damage of vascular barrier, capillary damage, diffuse alveolar damage, multiorgan failure and ultimately death. Lung injury is one consequence of the cytokine storm that can progress into acute lung injury or its more severe form acute respiratory distress syndrome (ARDS).

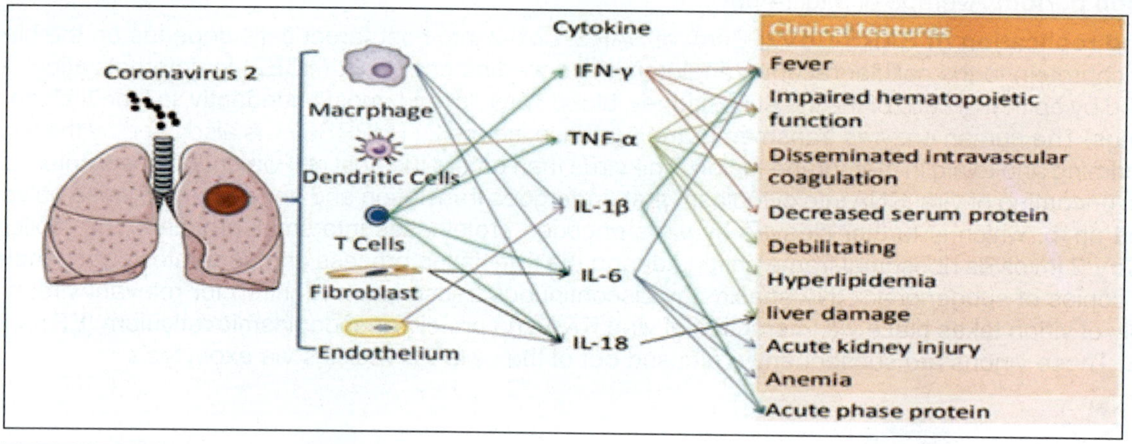

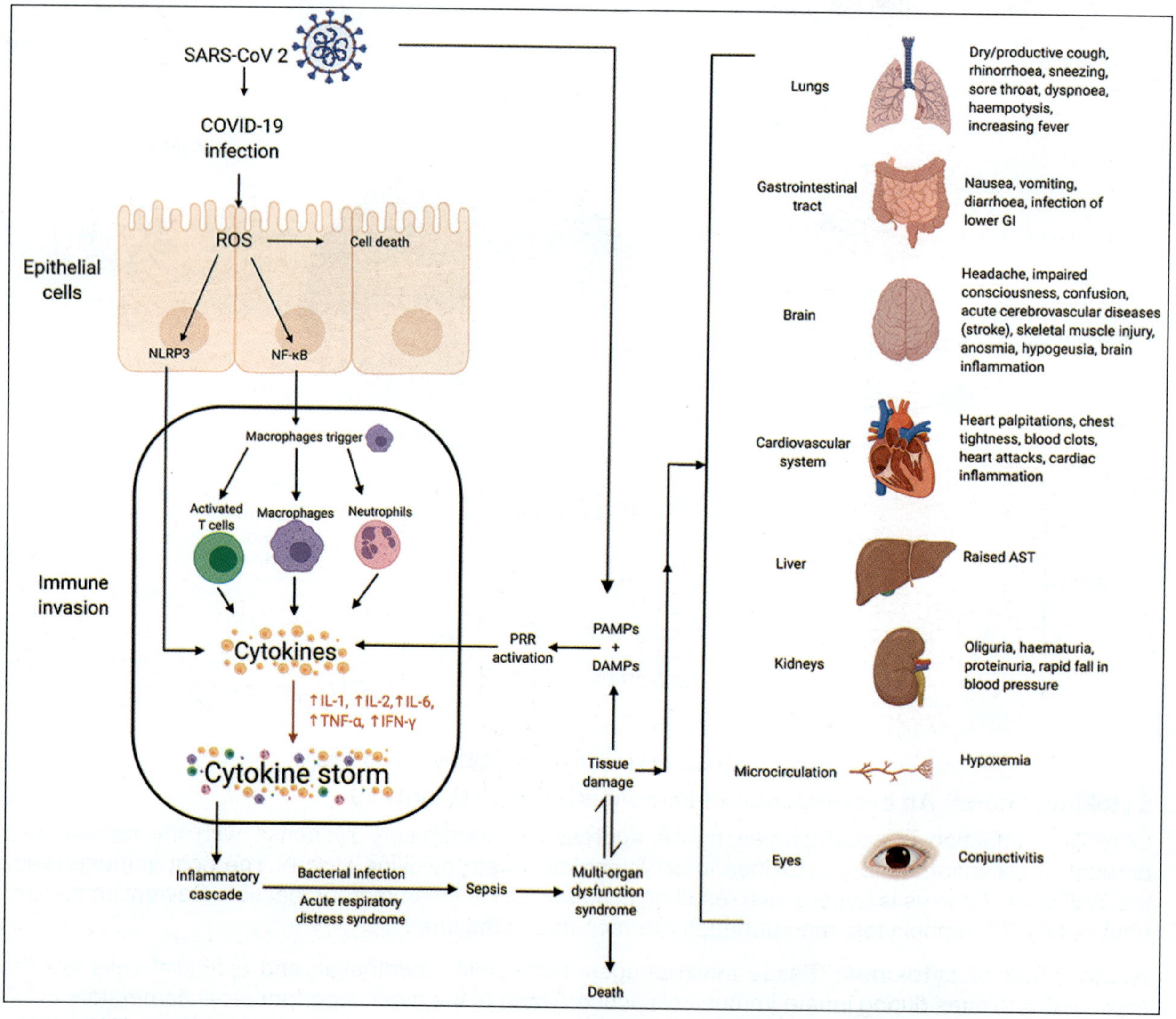

C. CLINICAL MANIFESTATION

1. **Mild Disease**

Influenza like illness (ILI):

It is occurred at the beginning of the stage of most of the symptomatic cases.

- **Cardinal symptoms of Influenza like illness–**ILI – an acute respiratory infection (sudden cough and sore throat) with measured fever of ≥ 100.4 F; with onset within the last 10 days.
- **Other associated symptoms–**Muscle or body aches, Headaches, Fatigue, Vomiting and diarrhea (more common in children than adults) and Running or stuffy nose.

Loss of taste and/or smell may occasionally occur preceding the onset of respiratory symptoms.

2. **Moderate Disease**

Pneumonia with no sign of severe disease:

Dyspnoea, fever cough, hypoxia, SpO_2 <94%, respiratory rate (RR) >24/min.

3. **Severe disease (Severe Acute Respiratory Illness–SARI)**

Severe pneumonia:

Pneumonia plus one of the following sign: (1) RR >30/min (2) SpO_2 <90%.

Acute respiratory distress syndrome (ARDS): One of the most common causes of mortality in COVID-19 patients is hypoxenic respiratory failure which can result in ARDS.

Sepsis: Acute life threatening multi organ dysfunction.

Septic shock: Persisting hypotension despite volume resuscitation.

D. LABORATORY DIAGNOSIS

1. **Specimens:** Throat and nasal swab.
2. **Nucleic acid amplification test (NAAT):** RT-PCR and CBNAAT.

a. Gene targets for RT-PCR:

- Gene targets for Screening are genus specific (Beta-coronavirus).
- Spike protein (S).
- Envelope protein (E).
- Nucleocapsid protein (N).
- Membrane protein (M).
- Gene targets for confirmation are species specific (SARS-CoV2).
- RNA-dependent RNA polymerase (RdRp).
- Open Reading Frames (ORF1a/b).
- N2 nucleocapsid.

b. Gene targets for CBNAAT:

- Gene target for screening are genus specific (Beta-coronavirus)–E gene.
- Gene target for confirmation are species specific (SARS-CoV2)–N2 gene.

c. Gene targets for Truenat:

- Gene target for screening are genus specific (Beta-coronavirus)–E gene.
- Gene target for confirmation are species specific (SARS-CoV2)–RdRp gene.

3. **Antigen detection test:** Point of care (Rapid ICT) test and it detects Nucleocapsid protein antigen in nasopharyngeal swab.
4. **IgG antibody detection assay:** It is used for serosurveillance and survey but not used for clinical diagnosis.
5. **Sequencing:** To detect different variant of SARS-CoV2.

6. **Viral culture:** It is used for research purpose.
7. **Nonspecific tests:**
   - **Chest CT scan**–Ground-glass appearance.
   - **Biomarkers**–IL-6, D-dimer.

E. SARS-CoV-2 VARIANT CLASSIFICATIONS

Viruses like SARS-CoV-2 continuously evolve as changes in the genetic code (genetic mutations) occur during replication of the genome. A lineage is a genetically closely related group of virus variants derived from a common ancestor. A variant has one or more mutations that differentiate it from other variants of the SARS-CoV-2 viruses.

SARS-CoV-2 Interagency Group (SIG): The U.S. Department of Health and Human Services (HHS) established a SARS-CoV-2 Interagency Group (SIG) to classify the different SARS-CoV-2 variants. This interagency group is focussed on the rapid characterization of emerging variants and actively monitors their potential impact on critical SARS-CoV-2 countermeasures, including vaccines, therapeutics and diagnostics. SARS-CoV-2 variants may be classified and reclassified based on their attributes and prevalence across the globe as:

- **Variants being monitored (VBM).**
- **Variant of interest (VOI).**
- **Variant of Concern (VOC).**
- **Variant of high consequence (VOHC).**

(a) **Variants Being Monitored (VBM):** These variants do not pose a significant and imminent risk to public health. Examples are Alpha, Beta, Gamma, Epsilon, Eta, Iota, Kappa, Mu, Zeta.

(b) **Variant of Interest (VOI):** A variant with specific genetic markers that have been associated with changes to receptor binding, reduced neutralization by antibodies generated against previous infection or vaccination, reduced efficacy of treatments, potential diagnostic impact, or predicted increase in transmissibility or disease severity. Currently, no SARS-CoV-2 variants are designated as VOI.

(c) **Variant of Concern (VOC):** A variant for which there is evidence of an increase in transmissibility, more severe disease (for example, increased hospitalizations or deaths), significant reduction in neutralization by antibodies generated during previous infection or vaccination, reduced effectiveness of treatments or vaccines, or diagnostic detection failures. Examples are:

1. **Delta**

   WHO Label: Delta.

   Pango Lineage: B.1.617.2 and AY lineages.

   First Identified: India.

   Attributes:

   - Increased transmissibility.
   - Nearly all lineages designated as Delta are susceptible to Emergency Use Authorization (EUA) monoclonal antibody treatments. AY.1 and AY.2 lineages are not susceptible to some monoclonal antibody treatments.
   - Reduction in neutralization by post-vaccination sera.

2. **Omicron**

   WHO Label: Omicron.

   Pango Lineage: B.1.1.529 and BA lineages.

   First Identified: South Africa.

Attributes:

- Potential increased transmissibility.
- Potential reduction in neutralization by some EUA monoclonal antibody treatments.
- Potential reduction in neutralization by post-vaccination sera.

(d) Variant of High Consequence (VOHC): A VOHC has clear evidence that prevention measures or medical countermeasures (MCMs) have significantly reduced effectiveness relative to previously circulating variants. Currently, no SARS-CoV-2 variants are designated as VOHC.

F. VACCINES

There are several COVID-19 vaccines validated for use by WHO (given EUL: Emergency Use Listing).

1. **The Pfizer/BioNTech Comirnaty vaccine**
   - **Type of vaccine:** mRNA Vaccine.
2. **The SII/COVISHIELD and AstraZeneca/AZD1222 vaccines**
   - **Type of vaccine:** Recombinant vaccine (replication-deficient chimpanzee adenovirus vector encoding the SARS-CoV-2 Spike (S) glycoprotein).
3. **The Janssen/Ad26.COV 2.S vaccine developed by Johnson and Johnson**
   - **Type of vaccine:** Non-Replicating Viral Vector.
4. **The Moderna COVID-19 vaccine**
   - **Type of vaccine:** mRNA 1273 Vaccine.
5. **The Sinopharm COVID-19 vaccine**
   - **Type of vaccine:** An inactivated vaccine with an adjuvant.
6. **The Sinovac-CoronaVac vaccine**
   - **Type of vaccine:** An inactivated whole virus vaccine.
7. **The Bharat Biotech BBV152 COVAXIN vaccine**
   - **Type of vaccine:** An inactivated whole virus vaccine.
8. **The Covovax/Nuvaxovid (NVX-CoV2373) vaccine**
   - **Type of vaccine:** Recombinant Protein vaccine: SARS-CoV-2 rS (Recombinant, adjuvanted) is a protein-based vaccine candidate engineered from the genetic sequence of the first strain of the SARS-CoV-2 beta coronavirus.

MUCORMYCOSIS IN COVID-19

COVID-19 is caused by SARS-CoV-2 has been associated with a wide range of opportunistic fungal infections and Mucormycosis is one of them. Fungal infections, including mucormycosis, aspergillosis and invasive candidiasis, have been reported in patients with severe COVID-19 or those recovering from the disease and have been associated with severe illness and death.

Immunocompromised Hosts are Predisposed to Mucormycosis

The primary reason that appears to be facilitating Mucorales spores to germinate in people with COVID-19 is an ideal environment of low oxygen (hypoxia), high glucose (diabetes, new-onset hyperglycemia, steroid-induced hyperglycemia), acidic medium (metabolic acidosis, diabetic ketoacidosis), high iron levels (increased ferritins) and decreased phagocytic activity of WBC due to immunosuppression (SARS-CoV-2 mediated, steroid-mediated or background comorbidities) coupled with several other shared risk factors including prolonged hospitalization with or without mechanical ventilators.

Transmission of Mucormycosis

1. It is not contagious and does not spread by contact of person to person.
2. This fungus is found in the environment. Transmission occurs through inhalation, inoculation, or ingestion of spores from the environment.
3. Although most cases are sporadic, health care-associated outbreaks have been linked to adhesive bandages, wooden tongue depressors, hospital linens, negative pressure rooms, water leaks, poor air filtration, non-sterile medical devices and building construction.
4. It most commonly affects the sinuses or the lungs after inhaling fungal spores from the air. In such cases, it may spread to brain and eyes.
5. It may also occur on the skin after a cut, burn, or other type of skin injury gets infected.

When to Suspect Mucormycosis (in COVID-19 patients, diabetics or immunosuppressed individuals)

- Sinusitis – nasal blockade or congestion, nasal discharge (blackish/bloody), local pain on the cheek bone.
- One sided facial pain, numbness or swelling.
- Blackish discoloration over bridge of nose/palate.
- Toothache, loosening of teeth, jaw involvement.
- Blurred or double vision with pain; fever, skin lesion; thrombosis and necrosis (eschar).
- Chest pain, pleural effusion, haemoptysis, worsening of respiratory symptoms.

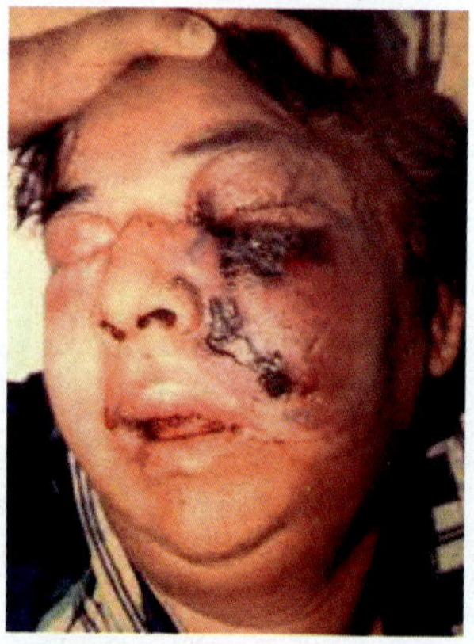

Fig.: Rhinocerebral mucormycosis

Common Misconceptions

The term **"black fungus"** has been used by the public to describe mucormycosis; however black fungus is actually a different category of fungus (fungi causing Chromoblastomycosis and Phaeohyphomycosis) that is not associated with COVID-19 associated pulmonary aspergillosis (CAPA) or COVID-19 associated mucormycosis (CAM). From a mycological point of view, the term 'black fungus' (or 'black yeasts') is restricted to fungi called dematiaceous, which have melanin in their cell walls. Instead of black fungus, the medical community prefers to use **"mucor fungi"**.

Diagnosis

Diagnostic methods include biopsy and fungal staining (KOH mount), which remains the mainstay of laboratory diagnosis. Facilities where fungal culture and susceptibility testing are available can help to confirm the species of mucormycosis. Treatment initiation, however, should not wait for fungal culture results.

A. **Specimen collection:** Depends on site of infection like infected tissue, nasal discharge or nasal swab.

B. **Direct Microscopy**

10% KOH mount may reveal hyaline, broad shaped, ribbon-like with uneven thickness, aseptate, obtuse angle branched hyphae with irregular branching.

Histopathological staining (H and E, methenamine silver) of biopsies shows characteristic broad with uneven thickness, aseptate, obtuse angle branched hyphae with irregular branching.

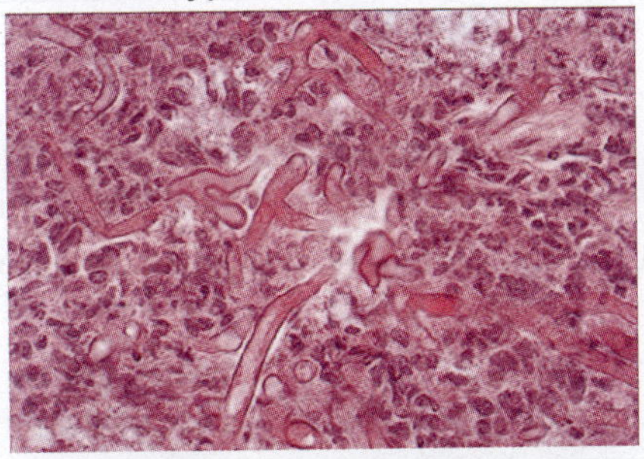

Fig.: Histopathology smear of Rhino-oculo-cerebral patient showing broad nonseptate hyphae of Mucor

C. **Culture and Identification**

The fungi are readily isolated on SDA without cycloheximide at 25°C, producing abundant cottony colonies hence known as **lid lifter fungi**. In SDA slant they show **tube filling** cottony growth.

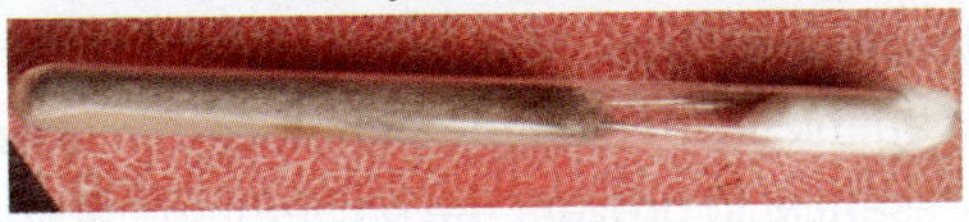

Fig.: Tube filling cottony growth of *Rhizopus*

Microscopic appearance (LBCB mount): Identification is based on the sporangial structures and rhizoids.

- **Mucor:** Shows nonseptate mycelium without rhizoids (root like structures). Sporangiophores, which may be branched, terminate in large globose sporangia containing numerous spores.
- **Rhizopus:** Shows nonseptate mycelium with rhizoids. Unbranched sporangiophores arise in groups directly above the rhizoids.
- **Absidia:** Has also rhizoids but sporangiophores arise from the aerial mycelium in between the rhizoids.

D. Blood cultures are of no value.

E. No serological tests are available.

F. **Imaging tests** such as a CT scan of lungs, sinuses, or other parts of body, depending on the location of the suspected infection, may also be used to support the diagnosis.

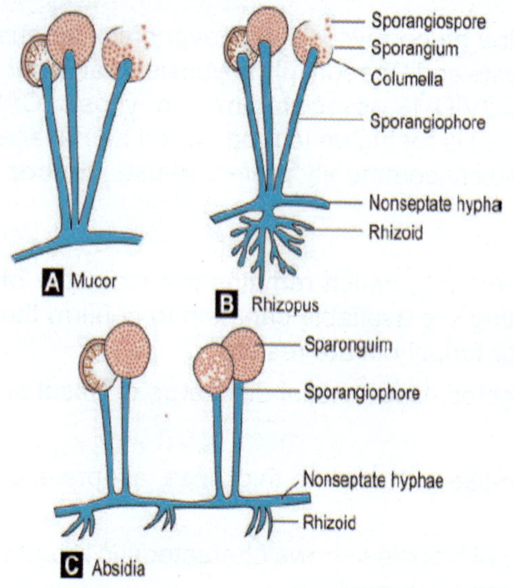

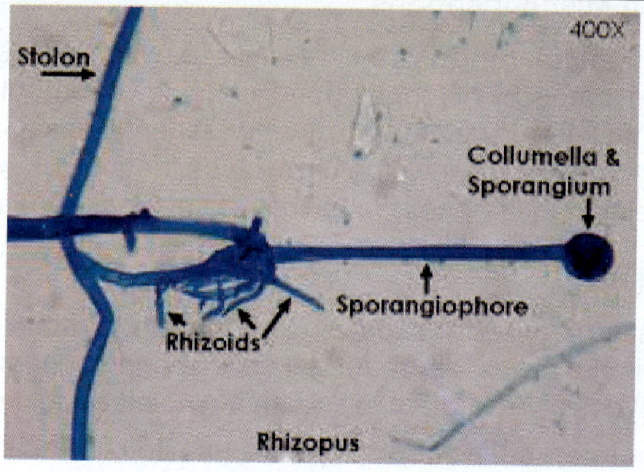

Fig.: LBCB mount of Rhizopus

Treatment

- Early recognition, diagnosis and prompt administration of appropriate antifungal treatment and surgical debridement (as needed) are important for improving outcomes for patients with mucormycosis.
- Mucormycosis is difficult to treat. It may sometimes require both intravenous antifungal therapy and surgical excision.
- Liposomal amphotericin B is the drug of choice and needs to be initiated early. Other antifungals like posaconazole, or isavuconazole have also been described for treatment.

Disease Prevention

Prevention of COVID-associated mucormycosis needs to focus on addressing the underlying risk factors:

- Aiming for better glycemic control in those with diabetes.
- Appropriate use of systemic corticosteroids; and
- Prevention of unnecessary use of antibiotic, antifungal and other immunomodulators.

IPC measures at the facility level are essential to prevent the environmental spread of this pathogen. These include:

- Sterilization and disinfection of the equipment used by multiple patients (tracheal tubes, ventilators), ventilation systems (if there is poor ventilation in the hospital that can contribute to dampness and dust).
- Proper wound management (bandage, tape, adhesives, including tapes to secure medical devices such as endotracheal tubes, ostomy devices must be sterilized and changed regularly).
- Proper line management in health facilities.

QUESTIONS AND ANSWERS

1. **Which one is not the causative agent of mucormycosis?**
   (a) Rhizopus
   (b) Mucor
   (c) Aspergillus
   (d) Absidia

2. **Which one is the predisposing factor of mucormycosis in COVID-19 patients?**
   (a) Diabetic ketoacidosis
   (b) Neutropenia
   (c) Long-term systemic corticosteroid use
   (d) Hemochromatosis
   (e) All of the above

3. **Most common form of mucormycosis in COVID-19 patients?**
   (a) Pulmonary mucormycosis
   (b) Cutaneous mucormycosis
   (c) Rhino-orbito-cerebral mucormycosis
   (d) Gastrointestinal mucormycosis

4. **Which fungi is not the black fungi?**
   (a) Alternaria
   (b) Bipolaris
   (c) Curvularia
   (d) Mucor

5. **Which fungi is commonly associated with mucormycosis in COVID-19 patients?**
   (a) Rhizopus
   (b) Mucor
   (c) Apophysomyces
   (d) a and b

Answers:

1. (c)	2. (e)	3. (c)	4. (d)	5. (d)

AIIMS MAY 2019

1. **Medlar bodies is associated with:**
   (a) Chromoblastomycosis
   (b) Rhinoproridiosis
   (c) Sporothrix
   (d) Mycetoma

2. **In chronic allergy which Ig are more persistent in the body?**
   (a) IgG
   (b) IgE
   (c) IgA
   (d) IgM

3. **Steps of Gram stain sequence arrangement:**
   (1) Mordant-iodine treatment
   (2) Safranin
   (3) Crystal violet
   (4) Alcohol wash
   (a) 3 – 4 – 1 – 2
   (b) 3 – 1 – 4 – 2
   (c) 2 – 1 – 4 – 3
   (d) 2 – 4 – 1 – 3

4. **Which of the following exists as yeast at 37° and hyphae at 25°?**
   (a) Histoplasma capsulatum
   (b) Penicillum species
   (c) Candida
   (d) Cryptococcus

5. **A person working in which of the following profession can have the problem shown in the image?**

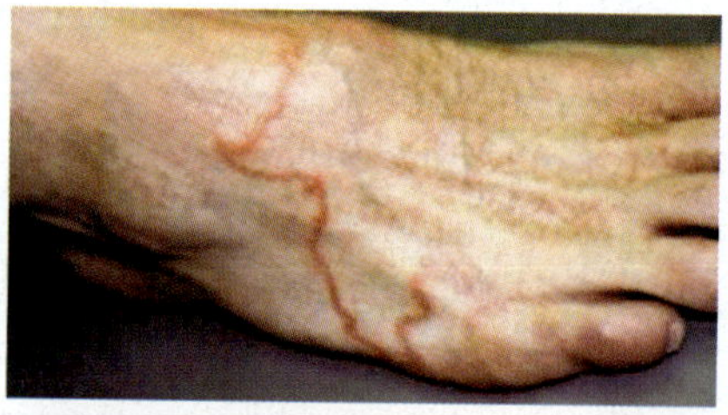

   (a) Person is working in the butcher house
   (b) Lifeguard in swimming pool
   (c) Kennel worker
   (d) Poultry farm worker

6. **A 22-year-old college boy with history of sex with commercial workers came to Derma OPD with lesions in genital region, tissue from this lesion was examined, which is the most likely finding?**

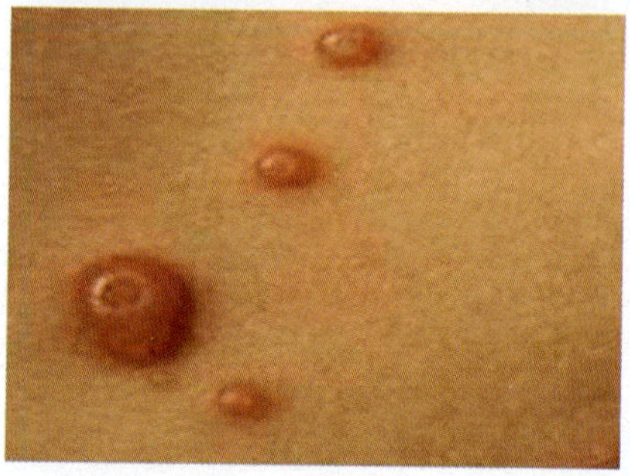

   (a) Intracytoplasmic vacuolations
   (b) Multinucleated gianty cells
   (c) Intranuclear inclusion bodies
   (d) Lipschultz body

7. **Which of the following marker persists in chronic hepatitis and recurrent hepatitis?**
   (a) IgG Anti HbcAg
   (b) HBsAg
   (c) IgG Anti HBsAg
   (d) HBeAg

8. **Patient had rashes on body, sores in mouth. Which of the following is the true statement in view of this image?**

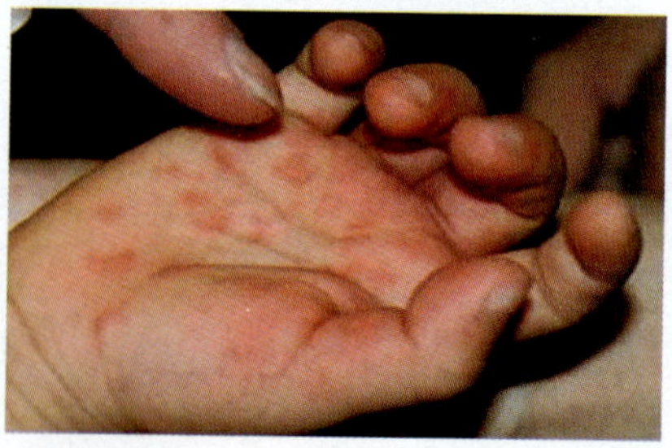

   (a) It belongs to family of picornaviridae
   (b) Herpes simplex virus 1
   (c) Herpes simplex virus 2
   (d) It belong to family of parvoviruses

9. A forest guard of Uttrakhand region had myalgia (c/c of fever, body pains) for few days. He came to OPD and was given ceftriaxone. He later deteriorates and comes back with a lesion in the armpit as shown in the image. What is the diagnosis?

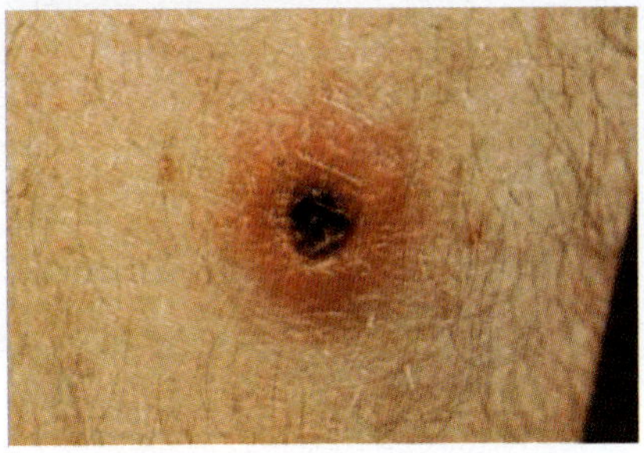

(a) Kyasanur forest disease
(b) Scrub typhus
(c) Cutaneous anthrax
(d) Cutaneous Diphtheria

10. Mw vaccine is prepared from:

(a) Mycobacterium bovis
(b) Mycobacterium indicus pranii
(c) Mycobacterium welchii

11. Which of the following statement regarding Regulatory T cells is correct?

(a) Regulation by CD8 cells
(b) Regulation by CD25
(c) FOXP3 receptors are involved in autoimmune diseases
(d) Regulation by CD4 cells

12. True and False question regarding community acquired UTI:

(a) Most common cause in the world is enterococci
(b) Urine is refrigerated before testing
(c) Most common cause of UTI is E. coli
(d) Most common Gram-positive cocci cause of UTI in young females is Staphylococcus saprophytic

13. Patient post-transplant developed diarrhea and stool examination was done. There were 3 histo-pathological images were given and the steps were given in the options.

(a) Safranin – Acetone – Crystal violet
(b) Neutral red – Acetone – Methylene blue
(c) *Cold method:* Carbol Fuchsin – Sulphuric acid – Methylene blue
(d) Methylene Blue with phenol – Sulphuric acid – Dilute Carbol Fuchsin

Answers:

1. (a)	2. (b)	3. (b)	4. (a)	5. (c)	6. (a)	7. (a)
8. (a)	9. (b)	10. (b)	11. (c)	12. (a) False (b) False (c) True (d) True		13. (c)

AIIMS NOVEMBER 2018

1. **Which virus does the following cycle depict?**

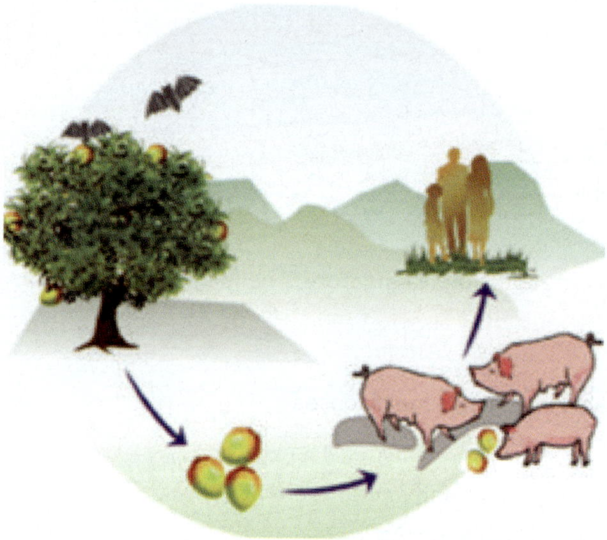

   (a) Swine flu virus
   (b) Nipah virus
   (c) Polio virus
   (d) West nile encephalitis

2. **What is the isolation period of measles?**
   (a) From the day of appearance of rash to the resolution of the rash
   (b) From the day of the appearance of kopliks spots to their disappearance
   (c) From the appearance of rash to appearance of Koplik's spots
   (d) Isolation from the onset of the prodromal stage to the 3rd day of rash

3. **A patient comes to casualty with signs and symptoms of food poisoning. He gives a history of consuming oysters more than 16 hours before the start of symptoms. Which of the following is the most likely pathogen?**
   (a) Staphylococcus
   (b) Vibrio paraaureus haemolyticus
   (c) Bacillus cereus
   (d) Clostridium welchii

4. **Presence of fecal leucocytes along with mucus is typically seen associated with:**
   (a) Entamoeba histolytica
   (b) Hookworm infection
   (c) Tenia infection
   (d) Trichomonas infection

5. **Lieshman's stain of the blood of a patient shows the following picture. Rk39 was positive. What is the organism responsible?**

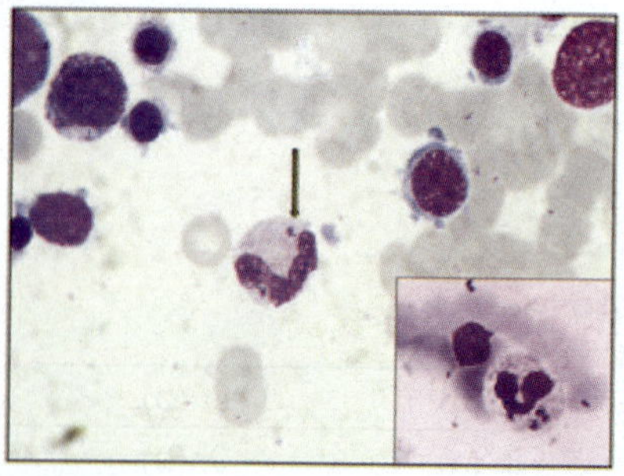

   (a) Babesia
   (b) Toxoplasma
   (c) Leishmania
   (d) Plasmodium

6. **Zn staining of the stool sample shows the following. What is the causative agent?**

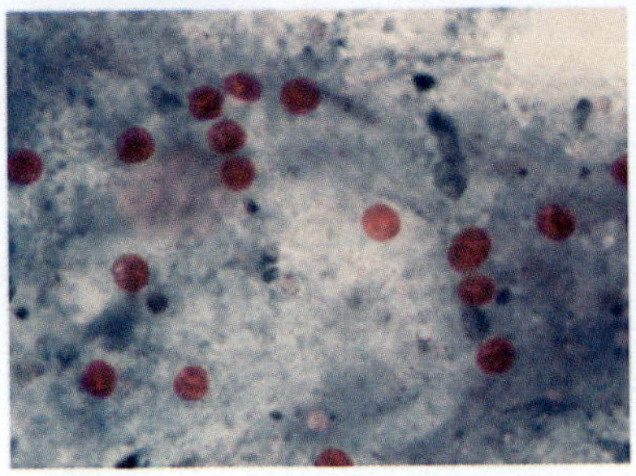

(a) Isospora belli
(b) Sarcocystis
(c) Cyclospora
(d) Cryptosporidium

7. **Which is the correct protocol to manage a blood spill?**
   (a) Put appropriate signage in the area and cordon of the area→Saturate the area again with sodium hypochlorite (bleach) 1% for about 20 minutes→Wear a pair of non-sterile gloves→Use disposable paper towels to absorb as much of the body fluids as possible
   (b) Use disposable paper towels to absorb as much of the body fluids as possible→Saturate the area again with sodium hypochlorite (bleach) 1% for about 20 minutes→Wear a pair of non-sterile gloves→Put appropriate signage in the area and cordon of the area
   (c) Wear a pair of non-sterile gloves→Use disposable paper towels to absorb as much of the body fluids as possible→Saturate the area again with sodium hypochlorite (bleach) 1% for about 20 minutes→Put appropriate signage in the area and cordon of the area
   (d) Put appropriate signage in the area and cordon of the area→Wear a pair of non-sterile gloves→Use disposable paper towels to absorb as much of the body fluids as possible→Saturate the area again with sodium hypochlorite (bleach) 1% for about 20 minutes

8. **Which of the following is not a part of Albert's stain?**
   (a) Toludiene blue
   (b) Malachite green
   (c) Crystal violet
   (d) Iodine

9. **Which is the most likely cause of bloody diarrhea in an immunocompromised patient?**
   (a) Cytomegalovirus
   (b) Hepatitis A virus
   (c) RSV
   (d) Hepatitis E virus

10. **Which of the following is not a mode of transmission of zika virus?**
   (a) Aedes mosquito
   (b) Feco oral route
   (c) Sexually
   (d) From mother to child

Answers:

1. (b)	2. (d)	3. (b)	4. (a)	5. (c)	6. (d)	7. (d)
8. (c)	9. (a)	10. (b)				

ALL INDIA JANUARY 2019 QUESTIONS

1. **Flask shaped ulcers in intestine caused by:**
   (a) Giardia lamblia
   (b) Entamoeba histolytica
   (c) Helicobacter pylori (H. pylori)
   (d) E. vermicularis
2. **What type of culture media is used for Legionella?**
   (a) (BCYE) agar media
   (b) MacConkey agar
   (c) Baird–Parker agar
   (d) Sabouraud's agar
3. **Special Stain for cryptococcus:**
   (a) ZN stain
   (b) Gram stain
   (c) Mucicarmine stain
   (d) Malachite green
4. **A 36 years old male patient c/o cough, cold, fever/rusty sputum/sputum neg for TB, history of travel in China and eaten crab. Name the infection:**
   (a) Paragonimus westermani
   (b) Faciola hepatica
   (c) Fasciolopsis buski
   (d) Entamoeba histolytica
5. **Microbiological test for diagnosing leptospira infection:**
   (a) Cold agglutination
   (b) Standard agglutination
   (c) Microscopic agglutination test (MAT)
   (d) None of these
6. **Identify the picture:**

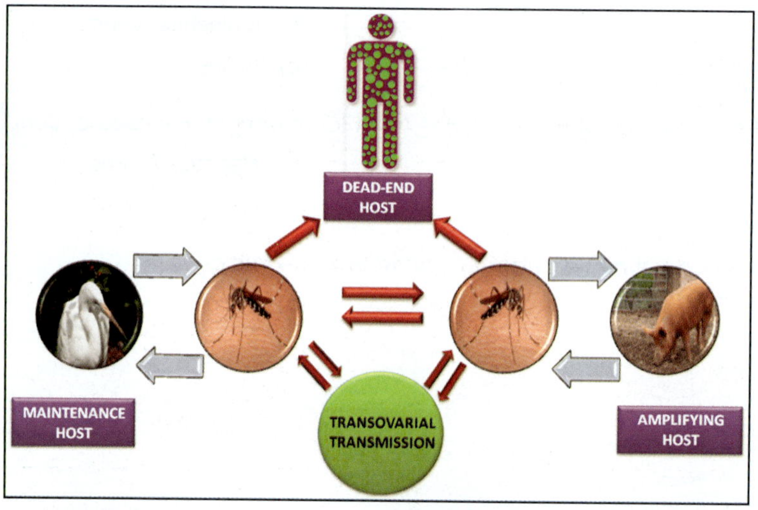

   (a) Malaria
   (b) Plague
   (c) Japanese encephalitis
   (d) Paragonimus
7. **Disc diffusion method is also known as:**
   (a) Kirby Bauer
   (b) VDRL
   (c) Darkfield microscopy
   (d) None of these
8. **Rubella virus belongs to which family?**
   (a) Rheovirus
   (b) Togavirus
   (c) Picornavirus
   (d) Orthomyxo
9. **Which of the following infection resembles erythroblastosis?**
   (a) EBV
   (b) CMV
   (c) HSV
   (d) Staphylococcus

10. Diagnostic test for neurosyphilis:

(a) VDRL (b) RPR

(c) TPI (d) FTA-ABS

11. A 6-year-old boy is having symptoms such as fever and chills, cough, rapid breathing, difficulty in breathing and chest pain, culture from a sample shows gram-positive culture. Identify the image:

(a) Streptococcus pneumoniae

(b) Staphylococcus

(c) Propionibacterium

(d) Mycobacterium

Q. 11.

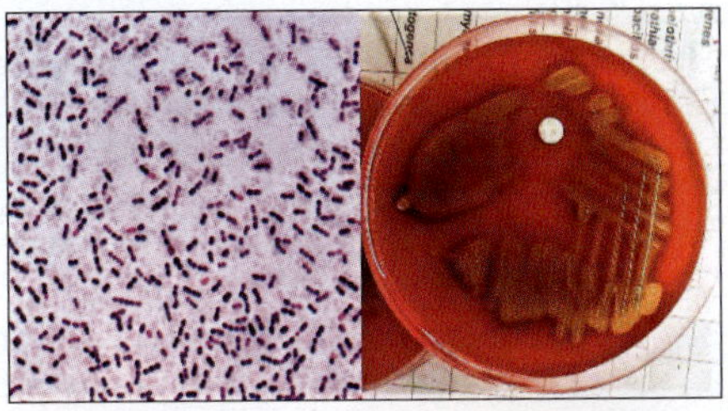

12. Identify the picture:

(a) Herpes zoster

(b) Smallpox

(c) Chickenpox

(d) Atopic dermatitis

Q. 12.

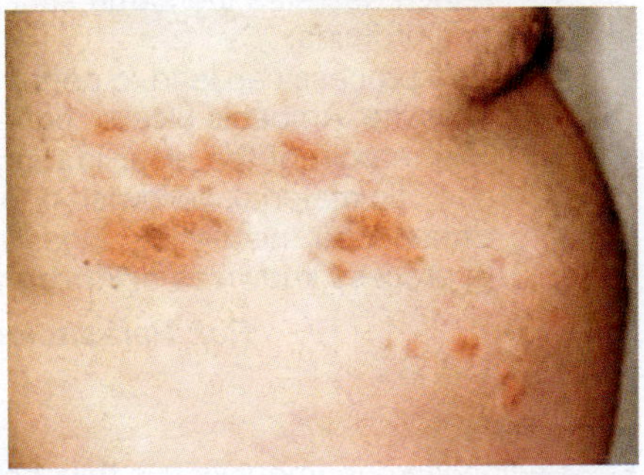

13. A patient is having gastrointestinal problems including abdominal pain and distension, bloody or mucus-filled diarrhea and tenesmus, with rectal prolapse, a stool, ova and parasites exam reveals the presence of typical Barrel shaped eggs, possible causative agent is:

(a) Campylobacter (b) Clostridium difficile

(c) Giardia lamblia (d) Trichuris

14. Contact isolation is done for:

(a) MRSA (b) Mumps

(c) Diphtheria (d) Asthma

15. A child is suffering from recurrent chronic infections with encapsulated bacteria is due to deficiency of subclass:

(a) IgG1 (b) IgG2

(c) IgG3 (d) IgG4

16. D.O.C. for isospora:

(a) Penicillin G (b) Benzathine penicillin

(c) Cotrimoxazole (d) Albendazole

17. Coxsackievirus A16 causes:

(a) Yellow fever (b) Hand-foot-mouth disease

(c) Rocky mountain spotted fever (d) Encephalomyocarditis

18. Pneumocystis jiroveci is:

(a) Associated with CMV (b) Diagnosis is by sputum microscopy

(c) Seen only in immunocompromised patients (d) Always associated with pneumatocele

19. All are true about congenital Toxoplasmosis:

(a) Chorioretinitis (b) Conjunctivitis

(c) Hydrocephalus (d) Cerebral calcification

20. True about TRIAD congenital rubella syndrome:

(a) PDA, cataract and deafness is seen (b) Hepatosplenomegaly, mental retardation, deafness

(c) Chorioretinitis, multiorgan failure, pneumonitis (d) None of these

ANSWERS AND EXPLANATIONS

Ans. 1 (b)

The only member of **the subphylum Sarcodina** that is pathogenic to humans and causes intestinal amoebiasis E. histolytica. It is found worldwide.

It has 3 morphological stages:

1. **Trophozoite**–Growing or feeding stage – has a clear translucent ectoplasm and a granular endoplasm. RBCs, leucocytes and tissue debris are found in the endoplasm. It contains a single large nucleus.
2. **Precystic Stage**–10 to 20 mcg.
3. **Cystic Stage**–Surrounded by a cyst wall, quadrinucleate.
   - Disease occurs when amoeba comes in contact with the cells lining the intestine.
   - It then secretes the same substances it uses to digest bacteria, which include enzymes that destroy cell membranes and proteins.
   - This process can lead to penetration and digestion of human tissues, resulting first **in flask-shaped ulcerations** in the intestine. Amoebic ulcers confined to the large intestines and mostly found in the ileocaecal region.
   - The margin of the ulcer is ragged and undermined and the base is formed by the muscular coat and is filled up by necrotic material, yellowish or blackish slough.
   - Entamoeba histolytica ingests the destroyed cells by phagocytosis and is often seen with red blood cells (a process known as **erythrophagocytosis**) inside when viewed in stool samples, this feature is confirmatory.

Ref: Parasitology–Protozoology and Helminthology by K.D. Chatterjee, 13th edition, page 18-26

Ans. 2 (a)

Legionella

- Legionella pneumophila is a thin, aerobic, pleomorphic, flagellated, non-spore forming, Gram-negative bacterium.
- Primary human pathogenic bacterium and is the causative agent of legionellosis or Legionnaires' disease.
- **Transmission:** Legionella come from natural fresh water reservoirs, such as lakes, ponds and puddles, where they parasitize on a broad range of protozoan species as hosts. The availability of the hosts plays a major role in the reproduction and mass release of highly infectious Legionella forms into environments where they can be spread by airborne water caplets and inhaled by people
- **Risk population:** Most healthy individuals do not become infected with Legionella bacteria after exposure. People at higher risk of getting sick are: Older people (usually 50 years of age or older) Current or former smokers, those with a chronic lung disease (like COPD or emphysema) and immunocompromised.
- Legionella bacteria are not transmitted from person to person.
- Most people with Legionnaires' disease will have pneumonia (lung infection) since the Legionella bacteria grow and thrive in the lungs. Pneumonia is confirmed either by chest X-ray or on physical exam.
- People get **Legionnaires' disease or Pontiac fever** (non-pneumonic form) when they breathe in a mist or vapor (small droplets of water in the air) that has been contaminated with Legionella bacteria.
- **Pathogenesis:** Bacteria enter through alveoli and multiply inside the Monocytes and Macrophages. CMI effective.
- **Reservoirs of Infection:** L. pneumophila is a **facultative intracellular bacterium** that can invade and replicate inside amoebae in the environment, which can thus serve as a reservoir for L. pneumophila, as well as provide protection from environmental stresses, such as chlorination.
- **Diagnosis:**
  – Culturing Grown on **Buffered charcoal yeast extract agar with L cysteine, iron and with antibiotics.**
  – **Urine Antigen Test**–detects a part of the Legionella bacteria in urine. If the patient has pneumonia and the test is positive, then the patient is considered to have Legionnaires' disease.
  – Testing the Serum Paired sera (blood specimens) that show a four-fold increase in antibody.

Ref: Ananthanarayan and Paniker's Textbook of Microbiology, 7th edition, page 403-412

Ans. 3 (c)

Staining for Cryptococcus

1. With **India ink or 10% Nigrosin with formalin** as wet mount→shows round budding yeast cells ranging from 5-20 mcm with DISTINCT HALO capsule is twice as thick as diameter of the yeast.
   India ink staining is positive in 75% cases.
   Modified India ink – adding 2% chromium mercury→ clear identification of internal and external structures.
2. Gram staining → gram positive budding yeast cells.
3. Histopathological examination with → periodic acid-Schiff, H and E and GMS stain show budding yeast cell.
4. Alcian blue → capsule.
5. Mayer's muciramine→rose colored capsule, mucicarmine stain provides specific staining of polysaccharide cell wall in C. neoformans.
6. Cryptococcus is **Carminophilic** (like rhinosporidium).

7. Masson Fontana→production of melanin (highly significant for detecting capsule–deficient cryptococcus.

Ref: Bailey and Scott's Textbook of Diagnostic Microbiology, 12th edition, page 629-689

Ans. 4 (a)

Paragonimus Westermani

- **Geographic distribution:** Infections occur in limited areas where local people eat improperly cooked crustaceans occurs in the Far East specifically in the countries of Korea, Japan, China, Taiwan, Far East Russia, Malaysia, India, the Philippines and Indonesia.
- Also known as the **oriental lung fluke**.
- **Transmission:** Eating raw, undercooked or pickled crustaceans such as crab or crayfish.
- **Life cycle**.
- **Infective stage:** Metacercariae.
- **Infective mode:** Eating raw fresh water crabs and crayfish with metacercariae.
- **Infective route:** By mouth.
- **Site of inhabitation:** Lungs.
- **Intermediate hosts: 1st int. host**–Melania snail, **2nd int. hosts** – Crab and crayfish.
- **Reservoir hosts:** Carnivores such as tiger, lion, wolf, fox, dog, leopard, cat and etc.
- **Eggs:** Operculated and golden yellow in color. The shell is uneven in thickness.
- **Pathophysiology:** When humans ingest raw infected crustaceans, larval flukes develop in the small intestine, penetrate the intestinal wall into the peritoneal cavity 30 minutes to 48 hours after excysting → They then migrate into the abdominal wall or liver, where they undergo further development.

  Approximately 1 week later, adult flukes reenter from the abdominal cavity and penetrate the diaphragm to reach the pleural space and lungs.

  Flukes mature, a fibrous cyst wall develops around them, and then egg deposition starts 5-6 weeks after infection.
- **Clinical features:** During invasion and migration of the flukes, diarrhea, abdominal pain, fever, cough, urticaria, hepatosplenomegaly, pulmonary abnormalities, and eosinophilia may develop. During the chronic phase, the lungs are damaged most, but other organs may be involved. The clinical picture resembles and is often confused with TB.
- Praziquantel is the treatment of choice.

Ref: Parasitology–Protozoology and Helminthology by K.D. Chatterjee, 13th edition, page 196-198

Ans. 5 (c)

Leptospirosis

- **Zoonotic disease** caused by **spirochetes of the genus Leptospira.**
- **Weils disease:** A severe leptospirosis characterized by: fever, jaundice, acute renal injury, refractory shock and hemorrhage (especially pulmonary hemorrhage).
- Human-to-human transmission does not occur.
- Sources of transmission to humans: rats, dogs, cattle and pigs.
- **Transmission:**
  1. Indirect contact with contaminated animal urine through surface waters, moist soil, or other wet environments.
  2. Direct contact with urine and other excreta (e.g., products of parturition, placenta) of infected animals.
- Leptospires are difficult to culture from blood, urine and (CSF), although certain species and serovars (e.g., L. interrogans serovar Copenhageni) are grown more easily than others.
- Classic Weils disease: Suggested by elevated BUN and serum creatinine with mixed conjugated and unconjugated hyperbilirubinemia with SGPT elevation to less than five times the upper limit of normal.
- **Definitive DX:** Presence of the organism by culture isolation, detection of nucleic acids or antigen in body fluids, or immunohistochemical visualization in tissue. Leptospiral cultures do not become positive for weeks and therefore cannot guide clinical care.

  PCR–based assays have been used in research laboratories to detect leptospiral DNA.
- **Gold standard: Microscopic agglutination test (MAT)**–Darkfield microscopy or by immunofluorescence or light microscopy after appropriate staining used.

Ref: Ananthanarayan and Paniker's Textbook of Microbiology, 7th edition, page 377-395

Ans. 6 (c)

Japanese Encephalitis

- **Infectious Agent:** Japanese encephalitis (JE) virus is a **single-stranded RNA virus** that belongs to the genus ***Flavivirus*** and is closely related to West Nile and Saint Louis encephalitis viruses.
- **Transmission:** Transmitted to humans through the bite of an infected mosquito, primarily ***Culex*** species.
- The virus is maintained in an enzootic cycle between mosquitoes and **amplifying vertebrate hosts, primarily pigs and wading birds. Humans are incidental or dead-end hosts**, because they usually do not develop a level or duration of viremia sufficient to infect mosquitoes.
- **Epidemiology:** JE virus is the **most common vaccine-preventable cause of encephalitis in Asia**, occurring throughout most of Asia and parts of the western Pacific.
- Transmission principally occurs in rural agricultural areas, often associated with rice cultivation and flood irrigation.

- **Clinical Presentation:** Most human infections with JE virus are asymptomatic; <1% of people infected with JE virus develop clinical disease. Acute encephalitis is the most commonly recognized clinical manifestation of JE virus infection. The classical description of JE includes a parkinsonian syndrome with mask-like facies, tremor, cogwheel rigidity, and choreoathetoid movements.
- **Diagnosis:** JE should be suspected in a patient with evidence of a neurologic infection (such as encephalitis, meningitis, or acute flaccid paralysis) who has recently traveled to or resided in an endemic country in Asia or the western Pacific.
- **Laboratory diagnosis** – Using a JE virus–specific IgM-capture ELISA on CSF or serum.
- **Plaque reduction neutralization tests** can be performed to confirm the presence of JE virus–specific neutralizing antibodies and discriminate between cross-reacting antibodies from closely related flaviviruses (such as dengue and West Nile viruses). A **≥4-fold ris**e in JE virus–specific neutralizing antibodies between acute- and convalescent-phase serum specimens may be used to confirm recent infection.
- **Vaccine** – JE vaccine an inactivated Vero cell culture– derived vaccine.

Ref: Fields Virology, 5th edition, chapter 33

Ans. 7 (a)

Methods of Testing Antibiotic Sensitivity Testing

Kirby-Bauer Antibiotic Testing

- Uses antibiotic-impregnated paper disks to test whether particular bacteria are susceptible to specific antibiotics.
- A known quantity of bacteria are grown on agar plates in the presence of thin filter paper discs containing relevant antibiotics.
- If the bacteria are susceptible to a particular antibiotic, an area of clearing surrounds the wafer where bacteria are not capable of growing (called a zone of inhibition).

Macrobroth Dilution Tests

A serial two-fold dilution of antibiotic are made in test tubes from 0 to maximum concentration that is achieved. The inoculum density of bacterial isolate to be tested is standardized with 0.5 McFarland turbidity standard. The suspension should have a final inoculum of 5 × 105 cfu/ml. 1 ml of bacterial suspension is added to rows of antibiotic solution and incubated at 37°C overnight. The lowest concentration of antibiotic that completely inhibits visual growth of bacteria (no turbidity) is recorded as MIC.

Microbroth dilution tests: A polystyrene tray containing 80 wells is filled with small volumes of serial two-fold dilutions of different antibiotics. The inoculum suspension and standardization is done according to McFarland standard. The bacterial inoculum is then inoculated into the wells and incubated at 37°C overnight. MIC is determined as in macrobroth dilution test.

Agar dilution method: A serial two-fold dilution of the antibiotic is prepared in Mueller-Hinton agar.The bacterial inoculum is standardized according to McFarland standard. Using calibrated loops a volume of 0.001-0.002 ml is inoculated on the surface of agar and incubated at 37°C overnight. The lowest concentration of antibiotic that inhibits visible growth on surface of agar is taken as MIC.

Automated Susceptibility Methods: VITEK (report ready in 4-15 hours), Flourimetric detection: AutoSCAN Walkaway (report ready in 3.5-7 hours), Video Image processing: ALADIN (report ready in 18-24 hours).

Newer Non-Automated Susceptibility Tests: E-test and Spiral gradient endpoint system.

Molecular Techniques: Detection of gene coding for resistance to one or several drugs by techniques such as PCR and DNA hybridization.

Ref: Bailey and Scott's Textbook of Diagnostic Microbiology, 12th edition, page 93-111

Ans. 8 (b)

- **Rubella (German measles**) is a disease caused by the rubella virus.
- Because of routine vaccination against rubella since 1970, rubella is now rarely reported.
- Family – **Togaviridae,** Genus-Rubivirus.
- **ss–RNA virus**, **Enveloped Spherical,** Virus carry hemagglutinin, Virus multiply in the cytoplasm of infected cell.
- Virus can be cultured and adopted to continuous cell lines, Rabbit kidney cells (RK 13) and Vero cells.
- The clinical events occurring in the neonatal age is more important and divided into two major groups:
  1. Post Natal Rubella.
  2. Congenital Rubella.
- Adults acquire Infection–Acquired (i.e. not congenital), rubella is transmitted via airborne droplet emission from the upper respiratory tract of active cases.
- **Congenital Rubella Syndrome:** Maternal viremia with Rubella infection during pregnancy may result in infection of placenta and fetus. The growth rate of fetal cells are reduced→Lead to deranged and hypoplastic organ development.
- **Classical Triad of Rubella:** Cataract, Cardiac abnormalities and Deafness.
- **Diagnosis of Congenital Rubella Syndrome:** Demonstration of Rubella antibodies of IgM in a newborn is diagnostic value. As IgM group donot cross the placenta and they are produced in the infected fetus.
- **MMR Vaccine** is a mixture of three live attenuated viruses, administered via injection for immunization against measles, mumps and rubella. It is generally administered to children around the age of one year, with a second dose before starting school (i.e. age 4/5). The second dose is not a booster; it is a dose to produce immunity in the small number of persons (2-5%) who fail to develop measles immunity after the first dose.

Ref: Fields Virology, 5th edition, chapter 32

Ans. 9 (b)

Cytomegalovirus is a herpesvirus V.

Clinical Features: Most people with CMV infection have no symptoms and aren't aware that they have been infected. In some cases, infection in healthy people can cause mild illness that may include:

- Fever.
- Sore throat.
- Fatigue.
- Swollen glands.

Occasionally, CMV can cause mononucleosis or hepatitis. Babies born with CMV can have brain, liver, spleen, lung and growth problems. Important feature is hepatosplenomegaly. The most common problem in babies born with congenital CMV infection is hearing loss, which may be detected soon after birth or may develop later in childhood.

Transmission and Prevention: People with CMV may pass the virus in body fluids, such as saliva, urine, blood, tears, semen and breast milk. CMV is spread from an infected person in the following ways:

- From direct contact with saliva or urine, especially from babies and young children.
- Through sexual contact.
- From breast milk to nursing infants.
- Through transplanted organs and blood transfusions.

A woman who is infected with CMV can pass the virus to her developing baby during pregnancy. Women may be able to lessen their risk of getting CMV by reducing contact with saliva and urine from babies and young children. The saliva and urine of children with CMV have high amounts of the virus.

Ref: Fields Virology, 5th edition, chapter 69

Ans. 10 (a)

Venereal Disease Research Laboratory (VDRL) Test is a **slide flocculation test** employed in the diagnosis of syphilis. Since the **antigen used** in this test is **cardiolipin**, which is a lipoidal extracted from beef heart, it is not a specific test. This test is also classified as **non-specific or non-treponemal or standard test**. The antibodies reacting with cardiolipin antibodies have been traditionally termed "regain".

Principle: Patients suffering from syphilis produce antibodies that react with cardiolipin antigen in a slide flocculation test, which are read using a microscope.

VDRL antigen: The cardiolipin antigen is an alcoholic solution composed of 0.03% cardiolipin, 0.21% lecithin and 0.9% cholesterol. The cardiolipin antigen must be freshly constituted each day of test. The working antigen is a buffered saline suspension of cardiolipin.

Procedure: Patients' **serum is inactivated** by heating at 56°C for 30 minutes in a water bath to remove non-specific inhibitors (such as complement). The test can be performed both **qualitatively and quantitatively**. Those tests that are reactive by qualitative test are subjected to quantitative test to determine the antibody titres.

CSF VDRL: VDRL test may also be performed on CSF samples in the **diagnosis of neurosyphilis. Quantitative VDRL is the test of choice on CSF specimens.** A positive test confirms neurosyphilis but a negative result does not rule out neurosyphilis.

Significance of VDRL test: VDRL test becomes positive 1-2 weeks after appearance of (primary lesion) chancre. The test becomes reactive (50-75%) in the late phase of primary syphilis, becomes highly reactive (100%) in the secondary syphilis and reactivity decreases (75%) thereafter.

Treatment in the early stages of infection may completely suppress production of antibodies and result in non-reactive tests. Effective treatment in the primary or secondary stages results in rapid fall in titre and the test may turn non-reactive in few months. Treatment in latent or late syphilis has very little effect on the titre and the titres may persist at low levels for long periods. Since the titre falls with effective treatment, it can be used for assessment of prognosis.

VDRL test is more suitable as a screening agent than a diagnostic tool. VDRL test is also helpful in the diagnosis of congenital syphilis. Since passively transferred antibodies through placenta may give false reactive test in serum of the infant, a repeat test after a month showing no increase in titre may help rule out congenital syphilis. If both test, i.e., VDRL and FTA-ABS IgM (specific) test are positive in the infant then congenital syphilis should be strongly suspected and the child should be treated.

Since the test employs a non-treponemal antigen, there are many chances of false positive results. False positivity may be due to physiological of pathological conditions. These are called biological false positives (BFP). If the remain positive for less than 6 months it is considered acute and they remain positive for longer than 6 months it is called chronic BFP. **The physiological reasons for BFP include pregnancy, menstruation, repeated blood loss, vaccination, severe trauma etc while the reasons for pathological BFP include malaria, infectious mononucleosis, hepatitis, relapsing fever, tropical eosinophilia, lepromatous leprosy, SLE, rheumatoid arthritis** etc. A reactive VDRL test does not necessarily imply that the person is syphilitic. The diagnosis must be made in conjunction with clinical findings. **Any reactive VDRL test must be confirmed with a specific or treponemal test such as TPHA, FTA-ABS test.**

Ref: Bailey and Scott's Textbook of Diagnostic Microbiology, 12th edition, page 533-542

Ans. 11 (a)

- **Bacterial etiological agents of pneumonia are:**
  - Streptococcus pneumoniae.
  - Hemophilus influenzae.

- Klebsiella pneumoniae.
- Staphylococcus aureus.
- Rarer pathogenic bacteria–Legionella pneumophila and Pseudomonas aeruginosa.
- People with poor oral hygiene, altered swallowing reflexes, or impaired consciousness are predisposed to infection by anaerobes due to aspiration of oral fluids. Mycoplasma pneumoniae is known to cause primary atypical pneumonia.

- **Specimens collected:** Expectorated **sputum**, bronchial washing specimen or transtracheal aspirate. Urine may also be collected for demonstration of pneumococcal antigens.
- Sputum specimen is processed and a gram stained smear should be made from the thick part of the sputum and observed for pus cells and bacteria. The sputum should also be inoculated on to **Blood agar** or **chocolate agar** and incubated at 37°C in 5-10% CO_2, preferably in a **candle jar**.
- **Gram smear of sputum** showed plenty of pus cells along with gram positive lanceolate shaped cocci in pairs. Small, circular, smooth, **draughtsman-type** colonies with **alpha hemolysis** were seen on blood/chocolate agar.
- **Gram stained smear of the colonies** revealed gram positive lanceolate shaped cocci in pairs suggestive of pneumococci. These colonies were **catalase negative**. Bile solubility, inulin fermentation, optochin susceptibility, quellung reaction and mouse intraperitoneal inoculation may be done to differentiate pneumococci from viridans streptococci. Pneumococci are positive for **bile solubility**, **inulin fermentation**, quellung reaction, are **susceptible to optochin** and are pathogenic to mouse. The capsular antgien may be detected by **latex agglutination** or coagglutination.
- The Neufeld's **quellung reaction** is also known as "capsule swelling" reaction. When a suspension of pneumococcal colonies are treated with a loop of serum containing anitbodies to capsular polysaccharide and observed under microscope, the capsule appears swollen. The binding of antibodies to capsular antigen brings about a change in its refractive index, making it appear swollen. A drop of methylene blue may also be added to the suspension to provide contrast. The serum used may be monovalent or polyvalent (omniserum).
- **Optochin** is ethyl hydrocuprein hydrochloride, a disc 5 µg of strength is placed on the lawn culture of pneumococci and incubated. A wide zone of inhibition around the disc indicates susceptibility.
- **Bile solubility test:** Pneumococci have amidase enzymes that result in autolysis. These enzymes can be activated by surface active agents such as bile salts. Bile solubility test can be done in **test tube** or in **culture plates**. The disappearance of colonies leaving behind an area of alpha hemolysis indicates positive test.
- **Pathogenesis:** Streptococcus pneumoniae reach the lungs after first colonizing the oropharynx. S pneumoniae generally resides in the nasopharynx and is carried asymptomatically in approximately 50% of healthy individuals. Viral infections increase pneumococcal attachment to the receptors on activated respiratory epithelium. Presence of capsule is a major virulence factor as it helps the bacterium to evade phagocytosis. The pneumonic lesion progresses as pneumococci multiply in the alveolus and invade alveolar epithelium. Pneumococci spread from alveolus to alveolus, thereby producing inflammation and consolidation along lobar compartments. A patchy bronchopneumonic pattern involving the lower lobes is seen in the elderly. Since S. pneumoniae infection has a tendency to involve the pleura, pleural effusion is often seen.
- **Other infections produced by pneumococci:** Pneumococci is known to cause sinusitis, otitis media, bronchitis, lung abscess, septic arthritis, septicemia, meningitis, peritonitis and endocarditis.
- **Treatment: Penicillin** used to be the drug of choice but large number of strains are now developing resistance due to alteration in the penicillin binding proteins. Alternate choices include **macrolides (erythromycin, roxithromycin, clindamycin), quinolones (ciprofloxacin, levofloxacin), cephalosporins (cefuroxime, cefpodoxime, cefotaxime**). Many of the penicillin-resistant strains are also resistant to erythromycin, cotrimoxazole, tetracycline and chloramphenicol.
- **Conditions predisposing to pneumococcal infections:** Chronic alcoholism, splenectomy, previous viral respiratory illness, malnutrition, chronic smoking, cirrhosis of liver, coronary artery disease etc.
- **Vaccines:** A **23-valent polysaccharide vaccine** against 23 common serotypes has been in use in some countries. 23-valent pneumococcal polysaccharide vaccines has been recommended for use among children aged **≥2 years** who have high rates of disease, including those with sickle cell disease (SCD), chronic underlying diseases, human immunodeficiency virus (HIV) infection, or others who are immunocompromised. 23-valent pneumococcal polysaccharide vaccines are effective in preventing invasive pneumococcal disease among older children and adults, these vaccines do not protect children aged <2 years. A **7-valent pneumococcal polysaccharide-protein conjugate** vaccine was licensed for use among infants and young children as it decreases colonization and prevents pneumococcal disease among children aged **≤2 years.**

Ref: Bailey and Scott's Textbook of Diagnostic Microbiology 12th edition, page 798-813

Ans. 12 (a)

Herpes Zoster–Also known as Shingles.

- An acute viral infection of the nerve cells and surrounding skin.
- Characterized by a rash of blisters, can be very painful but is not life-threatening.
- **Caused by the varicella zoster virus that also causes chickenpox.**
- Shingles usually appears, band of blisters on one side of the chest or back, but it can occur anywhere on the body, including on the face and near the eyes.
- Herpes virus **(DNA)** → Primary infection results in varicella (chickenpox) and Recurrent infection results in herpes zoster (shingles).
- **Transmission** → Direct contact with open sores of shingles rash. Can pass to someone who has never had the chickenpox. High incidence groups.
- **Pathophysiology–Reactivation of virus in dorsal root ganglia.**

- **Clinical Symptoms:** The first signs of shingles may include–Headache, Feeling generally unwell, Myalgia, Fever and in the Acute stage–A rash will begin to develop, often causing a pain, itching or tingling sensation in the area of the affected nerve. A fluid-filled painful rash then develops a few days after and commonly occurs either on one side of the face or body. Fluid-filled blisters that break open and crust over in 7-10 days and this clears within 2-4 weeks.
- **Complications:** 1. Post herpetic neuralgia (PHN). 2. Ophthalmic. 3. Ramsay Hunt syndrome (known as herpes zoster oticus), inflammation of several of the nerves that come out of the brain.
- **Prevention of Shingles – vaccine (Zostavax):** It is given to people 60 years of age and older who have already had the chickenpox. The **shingles vaccine is a live vaccine** given as a single injection, usually in the upper arm. The most common side effects of the shingles vaccine are redness, pain, tenderness and swelling at the injection site and headaches.

Ref: Fields Virology, 5th edition, chapter 67

Ans. 13 (d)

Trichuris Trichiura (Whipworm)–Very common intestinal helminthic (nematode) infection.
- About one quarter of the world's population is thought to carry the parasite.
- Tropical Asia and to a lesser degree, in Africa and South America.
- Only patients with heavy parasite burden become symptomatic.
- Poor hygiene is associated with trichuriasis transmission and children are especially vulnerable because of their high exposure risk.
- Adults reside in the large intestine, **cecum and appendix of the host**→buries its thin, threadlike anterior half into the intestinal mucosa and feeds on tissue secretions, not blood.
- **Transmission: Fecal-oral via embryonated ova.**
- **Reservoir:** Mainly human.
- **Pathology:** Resembles that of inflammatory bowel disease due to mechanical disruption and toxicity of whipworms.The pathological changes include: hyperemia, edema, hemorrhage/bleeding.
- **Clinical manifestations:** Light infestations (<100 worms) are frequently asymptomatic. Heavy infestations may have **bloody diarrhea**. Long-standing blood loss may lead to **iron-deficiency anemia**. **Rectal prolapse** is possible in severe cases. **Vitamin A deficiency** may also result due to infection. Mechanical damage to the mucosa may occur as well as toxic or inflammatory damage to the intestines of the host.
- **Diagnosis:** T. trichiura eggs are detected in stool examination. Eggs will appear **barrel-shaped** and **unembryonated, having bipolar plugs and a smooth shell.**

Ref: Parasitology–Protozoology and Helminthology by K.D. Chatterjee, 13th edition, page 205-206

Ans. 14 (d)
- Corynebacterium diphtheriae causes diphtheria.
- The condition is typically spread through person-to-person contact or through contact with objects that have the bacteria on them, such as a cup or used tissue.
- Even if an infected person doesn't show any signs or symptoms of diphtheria, they're still able to transmit the bacterial infection for up to six weeks after the initial infection.
- The bacteria most commonly infect your nose and throat. Once you're infected, the bacteria release toxins. The toxins spread through your bloodstream and often cause a thick, gray coating in nose, throat, lungs.
- **Diphtheria prophylaxis** can be active, passive or combined. **Active immunization** using diphtheria toxoid is given to the unvaccinated (as DTP or DTaP in children) or as DT or Td (tetanus toxoid and a low dose of diphtheria) to the traveler. It is a **part of the national immunization schedule** in India to immunize infants, where it is given in three doses of DPT are given at intervals of 4-6 weeks and followed by a fourth dose a year later. A booster dose may be given every five years.
- **Schick test** was used in the past to determine if a subject needed to be immunized.
- **Passive immunization** involves subcutaneous administration of 500-1000 units of anti-diphtheritic serum as an emergency measure to the exposed unvaccinated susceptible individuals. Such people should be followed up with active immunization. Combined immunization consists of administration of the first dose of diphtheria toxoid on one arm and anti-diphtheritic serum on the other arm, which is followed up by full course of active immunization

Ref: Bailey and Scott's Textbook of Diagnostic Microbiology, 12th edition, page 228-300

Ans. 15 (b)
- Most of the antibodies in the blood and the fluid that surround the tissues and cells of the body are of the IgG class. The IgG class of antibodies is composed of four different subtypes-IgG1, IgG2, IgG3 and IgG4.
- IgG1 and IgG3 subclasses are rich in antibodies against proteins such as the toxins produced by the diphtheria and tetanus bacteria, as well as antibodies against viral proteins.
- IgG2 antibodies are predominantly against the polysaccharide (complex sugar) coating (capsule) of certain disease-producing bacteria (such as, *Streptococcus pneumoniae* and *Haemophilus influenzae*).

Ref: Bailey and Scott's Textbook of Diagnostic Microbiology, 12th edition, page 147-158

Ans. 16 (c)
- Isosporiasis does not respond well to most antibiotics used to treat diarrhea.
- Cotrimoxazole is the drug of choice because it is the best-studied and most readily available agent.
- Oral TMP-SMZ is well absorbed, even in patients with enteritis.

- A combination of 160 mg of TMP with 800 mg of SMZ (1 double-strength tablet PO q6h for 2-4 weeks) is the preferred regimen.
- In patients who are intolerant to sulfonamides, pyrimethamine (50-75 mg PO q24h) with folinic acid (5-10 mg PO q24h) may be given for 2-4 weeks.

Ref: Parasitology–Protozoology and Helminthology by K.D. Chatterjee, 13th edition, page 128-129

Ans. 17 (b)

- Coxsackieviruses – part of the **enterovirus** family of viruses (which also includes polioviruses and hepatitis A virus).
- Spread from person to person, usually on unwashed hands and surfaces contaminated by feces, where they can live for several days.
- Coxsackievirus are divided into group A and group B viruses.
- Coxsackie's virus infects suckling mice but not adult mice.
- Several Serotypes–At least 23 serotypes (1-22, 24) of group A and 6 serotypes (1-6) of group B are recognized.
- **Diseases Caused by Coxsackievirus**
  - Herpangina–coxsackie A virus.
  - Hand-foot-and-mouth disease–Coxsackievirus A16 and enterovirus 71.
  - Pleurodynia–Coxsackie B virus.
  - Myocardial and pericardial infections–Coxsackie B virus (B3).
  - Viral meningitis–Coxsackievirus or echovirus.
- Hand-foot-and-mouth disease–It typically begins with a fever and feeling generally unwell. This is followed a day or two later by flat discolored spots or bumps that may blister, on the hands, feet and mouth and occasionally buttocks and groin.

Ref: Fields Virology, 5th edition, chapter 25

Ans. 18 (b)

- Human isolate of Pneumocystis which is associated with severe pneumonia in immunocompromised state particularly AIDS.
- P. jerovici is an extracellular pathogen. Growth in the lung is limited to surfactant layer above alveolar epithelium.
- Serologic evidence suggest that most individuals are infected in early childhood (thus option "C" is wrong) but the pneumonia is seen only in immunocompromised state.
- Diagnosis is made by detection of organism in proper specimen.
- Sputum: Quick and non-invasive.
- Bronchoalveolar lavage (BAL) fluid: Mainstay of pneumocystis diagnosis.
- Transbronchial biopsy: If diagnosis cannot be made by BAL.

Ref: Parasitology–Protozoology and helminthology by K.D.Chatterjee, 13th edition, page 135-136

Ans. 19 (b)

- Toxoplasmosis is caused by infection with the protozoan parasite **Toxoplasma gondii**.
- Cogenital toxoplasmosis is an infection resulting from the **transplacental passage** of the parasites from an infected mother to the foetus.
- An acute infection in pregnant women is associated with a range of outcomes from subclinical infection to intrauterine death.
- Damage to the central nervous system (**cerebral calcification, hydrocephalus, microcephaly**) and **chorioretinitis** accounts for most of the non-fatal morbidity. The newborn often has a low birth weight, enlarged liver and spleen, jaundice, anemia, petechiae, and eye damage evidenced by inflammation of the retina.
- Children who are apparently normal at birth may subsequently develop toxoplasmosis-associated injuries.
- The diagnosis of congenital toxoplasmosis frequently relies on **PCR tests of amniotic fluid**.
- The rate of transplacental transmission of the toxoplasma varies from 6% at 13 weeks gestation to 72% at 36 weeks. As **gestational age is increased, risk of transmission to fetus increased, i.e., max. in 3rd trimester while severity of fetal damage is decreased, i.e., infant is usually asymptomatic if infection transmit in 3rd trimester**.
- Although the efficacy of therapy is debated, early treatment may prevent the further progress of the infectious process and the development of handicaps in children.

Ref: Parasitology–Protozoology and Helminthology by K.D.Chatterjee, 13th edition, page 129-130

Ans. 20 (a)

- Congenital rubella syndrome (CRS) can occur in a developing fetus of a pregnant woman who has contracted rubella (GERMAN MEASLES), usually in the first trimester.
- After the fourth month, the mother's rubella infection is less likely to harm the developing baby.
- The classic triad for congenital rubella syndrome is: **Sensorineural deafness** (58% of patients) **Eye abnormalities especially pigmentary retinopathy, cataract and microphthalmia** (43% of patients). Congenital **heart disease—especially pulmonary artery stenosis and patent ductus arteriosus** (50% of patients).
- Rubella vaccine is given to children at 15 months of age as a part of the MMR (measles-mumps-rubella) immunization. The vaccine is **live and attenuated and confers lifelong immunity**. Given to children 09 and 15 months and again between 3 and 6 years of age.

Ref: Fields Virology, 5th edition, chapter 32

Chapter 2

MUST KNOW

BACTERIOLOGY

1. ALTERNATE NAMES OF IMPORTANT BACTERIA

Bacteria	Alternate Name
• Bordetella	Bordet Gengou bacillus
• Clostridium tetani	Nicolaire's bacillus
• Corynebacterium diphtheria	Klebs-Loeffler's bacillusQ
• Corynebacterium pseudotuberculosis	Preisz-Nocard bacillusQ
• Haemophilus aegypticus	Koch-Weeks bacillus
• Haemophilus influenza	Pfeiffer's bacillusQ
• Klebsiella pneumoniae	Friedlander's bacillusQ
• Klebsiella ozaenae	Abel's bacillus
• Klebsiella rhinoscleromatis	Frisch's bacillusQ
• Mycobacterium tuberculosis	Koch's bacillus
• Mycobacterium intracellulare	Battey's bacillusQ
• Mycobacterium paratuberculosis	Johne's bacillusQ

2. TYPES OF CULTURE MEDIUM

Type of medium	Name of medium	Laboratory use
Liquid Media		
A. Basal (simple)	1. Peptone water	Routine culture, basal medium for sugar fermentation test
	2. Nutrient broth	Routine culture
B. Special (complex)		
(a) Enriched	1. Glucose broth	Blood culture
(b) Enrichment	1. Robertson's cooked meat medium	Culture of anaerobic bacteria
	2. Tetrathionate broth	Enrichment culture for salmonella
	3. Selenite F broth	Enrichment culture for salmonella and shigella
	4. Thioglycollate broth	Culture of anaerobic bacteria
	5. Alkaline peptone water	Enrichment culture for vibrio
Solid media A. Simple, B. Special	Nutrient agar (2-3%)	Routine culture
(a) Enriched	1. Blood agar	General culture, Streptococcus; Most widely use medium, demonstration of Hemol[illegible] used in: • CAMP • Reverse CAMP

Contd.

	2. Chocolate agar	Culture of H. influenzae, N. gonorrheae
	3. Loeffler's serum slope	Culture of C. diphtheriae
	4. Dorset egg medium	Culture of Mycobacteria tuberculosis
(b) Selective (contains inhibitory substance)	1. MacConkey agar (also indicator and differential medium)	Enterobacteriacea (Lactose fermenters produce pink colonies)
	2. Deoxycholate citrate agar (DCA)	Selective medium for Salmonella and Shigella
	3. Lowenstein Jensen (L J)	Culture of M. tuberculosis

3. IMPORTANT MEDIAS IN MICROBIOLOGY

S. aureus	Mannitol salt agar Q, Milk salt agar, Ludlam's medium
Enterococcus	Bile esculin agarQ
Neisseria (gonococcus/ meningococus)	Thayer Martin medium, chocolate agar, modified New York agar
Corynebacterium Diphtheriae	Loeffler's serum slope, Potassium tellurite agar
Bacillus Anthracis	PLET (Polymyxin Lithium EDTA thallous acetate)
Bacillus Cereus	MYPA (Mannitol egg Yolk Phenol red polymxin agar)
M. Tuberculosis	LJ medium, Middle Brook's medium, Dorset egg medium
Listeria	PALCAM agarQ, Chocolate agar
Actinomyces	Thioglycollate medium, Brain heart infusion agar
M. Tuberculosis	LJ medium, Middle Brook's 7H9 medium, Dorset egg medium
Lactose fermenting Enteric pathogens (E. coli and others)	MacConkey agar, Eosin-methylene blue (EMB), Deoxycholate agar, CLED in urine culture
Salmonella	Tetrathionate broth, Selenite F. broth
Salmonella, Shigella	Deoxycholate medium, Hektoen enteric agar (Salmonella-Shigella agar)
Pseudomonas	Cetrimide AgarQ, (Kings media for pigment production)
Plating media for V cholera	TCBS (Thiosulfate Citrate Bile Salt sucrose), BSA (alkaline bile salt agar), GTTA (Gelatin Taurocholate Tellurite Agar)
Enrichment media for V cholera	Alkaline peptone water, Monsur's taurocholate peptone water
Hemophilus	Satellitism (Blood agar with staph streak), Levinthal's medium, Fildes agar, chocolate agar
Yersinia	CIN (Cefsulodin-Irgasan-Novobiocin) medium, Ghee broth for Y. pestis.Q
Bordetella	Regan Lowe medium, Bordet-Gengou medium, Lacey's DFP medium
Legionella	BCYE (Buffered Charcoal Yeast Extract)Q
Mycoplasma pneumoniae	PPLO agar (Fried egg appearance)Q

Organism	Transport media
Streptococcus pyogenes	Pike's medium
For stool specimen	Buffered glycerol saline, Cary-Blair, Stuart medium
Salmonella, Shigella	Sach's buffered glycerol saline
V cholerae	Venkat Raman Ramakrishna medium, Cary-Blair medium, Autoclaved sea water
Bordetella	Modified Stuart's, Mischulow's charcoal agar
Neisseria	Stuart's medium, Amies medium

4. IMPORTANT STAINS IN MICROBIOLOGY

Name of the stain	Importance
Gram stain	• Stains bacterial cell wall (peptidoglycan) • Distinguishes bacteria into Gram positive and Gram negative
(Ziehl-Neelsen) acid-fast stain	• Stains bacterial cell wall (mycolic acid) • Distinguishes bacteria into acid-fast and nonacid-fast
Kinyoun stain	Modification of acid-fast stain (no use of heat)
Auramine O stain	Fluorescent stain for Mycobacterium tuberculosis
Schaeffer-Fulton stain	Stains bacterial endospores
Albert stain Ponder stain Neisser stain	Stains metachromatic granules of Corynebacterium diphtheriae
India ink stain, Nigrosin stain	Stains bacterial capsules, Cryptococcus
Methylene blue with anticapsular sera	Stains capsules of Streptococcus penumoniae (Quellung Reaction)
Silver impregnation method Leifson stain	Stains bacterial flagella
Giemsa stain	Stains intracellular pathogens (e.g., elementary bodies of Chlamydia, Rickettsiae)
Fontana stain	Stains treponemes in smear
Levaditi stain	Stains treponemes in tissue sections
Diene's stain	Stains MycoplasmaQ
Macchiavello stain	Stains Rickettsia
Warthin-Starry stain	Stains H. pylori

5.

Motile by polar flagella	Motile by peritrichous flagella
• Vibrio • Pseudomonas • H. pylori • Campylobacter • Spirochaetes • Legionella	• E. coli • Proteus • Listeria monocytogenes • All clostridia except Cl. perfringens and Cl. Tetani VI • Bacillus except B. anthrax • Salmonella except S. gallinarum pullorum (Non motile)

6. IMPORTANT BACTERIAL TOXINS AND GENETIC CODING

Toxins	Mechanism of action
Botulinum toxin	Acts on the peripheral nervous system (i.e., neuromuscular junctions by inhibiting myoneural junction acetylcholine released and cause flaccid paralysis (many strains of Clostridium botulinum synthesized C2 toxin, that ADP-ribosylates actin, thereby inhibiting its polymerization, affecting the shape of target cells, and resulting in enterotoxin activity in vivo).
Diphtheria toxin	Inhibits protein synthesis in target cells by catalyzing the ADP ribosylation of elongation factor 2, a host protein required for translocation of ribosomal messenger RNA.
Pertussis toxin	Acts by ADP ribosylation of several members of the family of guanine nucleotide-binding (G) proteins involved in signal transduction, inhibiting their function and affecting a variety of effector systems, such as adenylate cyclase, phospholipases, and several types of icon channels.
ST of E. coli	Activates **G**uanyl cyclase to increase c**G**MP.
V. cholerae toxin LT of E. coli	Activates adenylate cyclase of the intestinal epithelial cell by **ADP ribosylation of the stimulatory G. protein**→ ↑cAMP.
Shiga toxin	Inhibits protein synthesis by enzymatic inactivation of the 28S RNA within the 60S ribosomal subnit.
Verocytotoxin of E. coli	Inhibit protein synthesis by inhibiting ribosomal function (same as shiga toxin).

Genetic material coding for different toxins
Plasmid borne • Tetanospasmin of C. tetani **(T P H A)** • Pertussis toxin of B. pertussis • Heat-labile toxin (LT) of ETEC • Anthrax toxin of B. anthracis
Chromosomal • Cholera toxin (CT) of V. cholera • Shiga toxin of S. dysenteriae • Pyrogenic toxin B of S. pyogenes • Pertussis toxin of B. pertussis • Exotoxin A of P. aeruginosa
Phage encoded • Botulinum toxin of C. botulinum **(Bottle vich drinks paa)** • Verotoxin (Shiga-like toxin) of EHEC • Diphtheria toxin of C. diphtheriae • Pyrogenic toxin (A, C) of S. pyogenes

7.

BIPOLAR STAINING – SAFETY PIN APPEARANCE
Yersinia pestis
Hemophilus ducreyi
Calymatobacter Granulomatis
Pseudomonas mallei
Pseudomonas pseudomallei
Vibrio parahemolyticus

PLEOMORPHIC ORGANISM
Mycoplasma
Clostridium
H.influenzae
V.cholerae
V.parahemolyticus
Proteus

Memory aid – (MCH Very Very Progressive)

8.

INTRACELLULAR BACTERIA	OBLIGATE INTRACELLULAR BACTERIA
Yersinia	1. M leprae
Rickettsiae	2. Rickettsiae
Mycobacterium sps	3. Chlamydia
Brucella, Bordetella	4. Coxiella burnetti
Chlamydia	5. T. pallidum
Salmonella	
Meningococcus	
Legionella	
Donovani granulomatis	

Memory aid – **Y**aar **R**itesh **me**rekoe **Br**u **C**offee **s**ale **m**ain **L**a **d**e

9. Spore producing Bacteria

A. Anthrax (Bacillus)
B. Burnetti (Coxiella)
C. Clostridia

Memory aid – A B C

10. Anaerobes

Obligate Anaerobe lack following enzyne:
- Superoxide dismutase.
- Catalase.
- Cytochrome–C oxidase → enzyme that destroy toxic products of O_2 metabolism.

Cocci

Gram positive – Peptostreptoccus

Gram negative – Veilonella

Bacilli

Endospore forming – Clostridia

Non sporing

Gram positive:

Eubacterium **(Engineers loe MBA Program)**

Lactobacillus

Mobiluncus

Bifidobacterium

Actinomyces

Propionibacterium

Gram negative nonsporing anaerobe:

BPL fuse (memory aid)

B- **B**acteroides

P- **P**revotella, prophyromonas

L- **l**eptotrichia

F- **F**usobacterium

11.

OXIDASE POSITIVE ORGANISMS Memory aid – (AL VC have PNH)
• Aeromonas
• Legionella micadedi
• Vibrio cholerae
• Campylobacter jejuni
• Pseudomonas
• Neisseria meningitides and gonorrhea
• Haemophilus influenzae

Oxidase reagent is (Tetra methyl para phenylene diamine dihydrochloride).Q

12. HACEK Group

Haemophilus species (mostly H. aphrophilus and H. para-influenzae)Q
• Actinobacillus actinomycetocomitansQ, Aggregatibacter
• Cardiobacterium hominisQ
• Eikenella corrodensQ
• Kingella kingae

HACEK bacteria normally inside in the oral cavity and have been associated with local infections in the Mouth and Culture negative endocarditis.

13. Catalase Positive Bacteria

- StaphylococciQ
- H. Pylori
- Yersinia and Pasteurella
- Shigella (except dysentriae-1)Q
- N. meningitidis

- H. influenzae
- L. monocytogenes
- Pseudomonas
- Atypical Mycobacteria
- Legionella
- Coliforms
- Nocardia
- Brucella

14. Urease Positive Bacteria

Staph – Staphylococcus
- Klub – Klebsiella
- Main – Morganella
- Urease–Ureaplasma urealyticum
- Program – Proteus
- Nahi – Nocardia
- Hai – H. pylori
- Mamta – Mycobacteria except MAC
- Cryptococcus neoformans
- Didi – Diphtheroides
- **Most powerful urease producer is by H. Pylori.**

15. Capsulated Bacteria (PAKIYB MCV)

- Pneumococcus
- Anthracis Bacillus
- Klebsiella
- Influenzae haemophilus
- Yersinia
- Bordetella
- Meningococci
- Cl. Perfringens and Cl. Butyricum
- V. parahemolyticus
- Fresh isolates of staphylococci, streptococci and E. coli also have capsule or slim layer.

16. Infective dose of bacteriaQ

Organism	Infective dose
• ETEC	10^6-10^{10}
• EIEC	10^8-10^{10}
• EHEC	10-100 (<10^3)
• Shigella	10-100
• Salmonella	10^3-10^6 Q
• Campylobacter jejuni	10^4
• Yersinia enterocolitica	10^8-10^9
• Vibrio	10^{10} (if source of infection is water) 10^2-10^4 (if source of infection is food)

17. Growth Requirement

1. Cholesterol, purines and pyrimidines–Mycoplasma.
2. Cysteine–Francisella, Burcella, Legionella, Pasteurella.
3. X (haemin/protoporphyrin) and V. (NAD)–H. influenzae.
   –H. aegypticus.

VIROLOGY

Virion – Extracellular infectious viral particle	**DNA-HHAPPPY**
Capsid – P for protein coat–protects nucleic acid	**H**erpes
Envelope – L for lipoprotein coat in some virus	**H**epadena (Hepatitis B)
Virioids – Protein free viral infectious agent	**A**–adeno
Prions are proteinaceous particle	**P**–pox
	P–parvo
	P–papilloma
	Y–polyoma
Parvo – smallest virus, Pox – largest virus	
Parvo – single strand DNA	
BORA – Bunyavirus, orthomyxovirus, Reovirus, Arenavirus	

DNA non-enveloped viruses (P A P) – Parvo, Adeno, Papova.Q

RNA non-enveloped viruses (P A R C) – (Picorna, Astro, Reo, Calci).Q

RNA Viruses: Negative Stranded

(FOR ABP News)

Filo

Orthomyxo

Rhabdo

Arena

Bunya

Paramyxo

News

Inclusion bodies – are nuclear or cytoplasmic aggregates of stainable substances, usually proteins. They typically represent sites of viral multiplication.

Intracytoplasmic

- **Negri body** – Rabies.
- **Guarnieri body** – Vaccinia.
- **Paschen body** – Variola.
- **Bollinger body** – Fowl pox.
- **Molluscum body** – Molluscum contagiosum virus.

Intranuclear

- Cowdry A **(HAY)** – herpes (Lipschultz body), yellow fever (Torres body).
- Cowdry B **(BAP)** – adeno, polio.

Both Intranuclear and Intracytoplasmic – Measles (Warthin finkeldy giant cell), CMV.

A large number of viruses agglutinate erythrocytes from different species by the process known as Hemagglutination.

Hemagglutination of influenza virus is due to presence of hemagglutinin spikes on the surface of virus.

Viruses causing Hemagglutination are:

RIPE MANGO cut

• **R**ubella (1)	• Rhino Virus
• **R**abies	• Reo Virus
• **I**nfluenza virus (2)	• **P**arainfluenza Virus (3)
• **E**ntero Virus (4)	• Echo Virus
• **M**easles (5)	• **C**oxsackie Virus (6)
• **T**oga virus (7)	

Elution (due to neuraminidase)–only in myxo (except RSV and Measles), also in Vibrio.

- **Hemadsorption**–RBC adsorbed onto virus infected cell surface.
- Mumps, Influenza, Parainfluenza.

Viral Interference

- When two viruses infect a cell, one inhibits the multiplication of the other virus.
- Seen in Rubella, Polio.Q

EBV Red Alerts

IM (Infectious mononucleosis)
Nasopharyngeal carcinoma
Burkitt lymphoma
Hodgkin's lymphoma
B cell lymphoma
CNS lymphoma
Oral hairy leukoplakia
Thymoma
Lymphoproliferative syndrome
Chronic fatigue syndrome

B cell R-CD21 Q
Kissing disease
Glandular fever
4-8 weeks (IP)
Sore throat
Post cervical LAP (lymphadenopathy)
Atypical lymphocytes are increased
Heterophile test-Paul-Bunnel test
IgM-VCA (specific)
MONO SPOT test (Confirmatory)

CYTOMEGALOVIRUS Red Alert Points

Salivary gland
Largest herpes virus

Cottage and cheese appearance app/pizza pie retinopathy
Count CD4<50-100

Most sensitive PCR for diagnosis
Maximum risk (1-4 months)

ROTA VIRUS

Most common cause of Diarrhoea–infant and children
Adult and older children–Most common-**Norwalk virusQ**
Genetic reassortment is seen
Group A>B (B-adult)

Destroys mature enterocyte (proximal intestine)
Peak age – 4-23 months
Viral antigen in feces
No growth in cell culture, ELISA and RT-PCR are more sensitive and specific

PARASITOLOGY

- **Prokaryotes – Monera (e.g., Bacteria, Blue green algae, archaebacteria.**
- **Eukaryotes – Protista (Protozoal parasite), Fungi (e.g., fungus), Plantae (e.g., plants), Animalia (e.g., Helminths, Arthropods and higher animals).**
- **KINGDOM – PHYLUM – CLASS – ORDER – FAMILY – GENUS – SPECIES.**

PROTOZOA

AMOEBAE – (a) Intestinal species – Entamoeba histolytica, E.coli.

(b) Free living – Acanthamoeba, Naegleria.

CILIATES – Balantidium coli.

FLAGELLATES – (a) Intestinal – Giardia lamblia, Trichomonas hominis.

(b) Oral and vaginal – Trichomonas vaginalis.

(c) Blood and tissue (Haemoflagellates).

SPOROZOA – (a) Blood species – Plasmodium sps, Babesia.

(b) Tissue sps. – Toxoplasma.

(c) Intestinal – Isospora, Cryptosporidium.

Helminths	Cestodes	Trematodes	Nematodes
Shape	Tape like	Leaf like (Flukes)	Cylindrical
Sex	Monoecious	Mainly monoecious but Schistosomes are dioecious	Dioecious
Head end	Suckers with hooks	Sucker without hooks	Buccal capsule
Alimentary canal	Present	Incomplete, anus absent	Complete
Body cavity	Absent	Absent	Present

Important Facts

- Largest protozoan – Balantidium coli.
- Smallest intestinal amoeba – Dientamoeba fragilis.
- Smallest tapeworm found in human intestine – H. nana.
- Largest helminth (largest worm) – T saginata (beef tapeworm).
- Largest liver fluke – F. hepatica.
- Largest trematode infecting man – Fasciolopsis buski.
- Largest Nematode – Ascaris.
- Smallest Nematode – Trichinella spiralis.
- Only protozoan parasite found in small intestine of man – Giardia lamblia.
- Only ciliate protozoan parasite of man – Balantidium coli.
- Parthenogenic worm (female is able to produce new individual without being fertilized by male gamete).
- Eggs or larvae without fertilization – Strongyloides stercoralis.

Non-Bile Stained Eggs (NEHA)

- Necator americanus.
- Enterobius vermicularis.
- Hymenolepis nana.
- Ancylostoma.

Auto Infection is Seen in (CHEST)

- Cryptosporidium parvum, capillaria philippinensis.
- H nana.
- Enterobius vermicularis.
- *S.stercoralis.*
- Taenia solium.

Name	Birth to	Example
Viviparous	Larva	Filarial worm Trichinella
Oviparous	Laying eggs	Hook worm Enterobius Ascaris Trichuris
Ovo-viviparous	Egg containing larva which immediately hatchout	Strongyloides

Feature	Ascaris (Roundworm)	Hookworm	Strongyloides stercoralis	Trichuris trichiura (Whipworm)	Enterobius vermicularis (Pinworm)	Trichinella
Infective stage	Egg	Filariform larva	Filariform larva	Egg	Egg	Larva L3
Route of infection	Oral	Percutaneous	Percutaneous or autoinfection.	Oral	Oral	Oral (uncooked pork)
Gastrointestinal location of worms	Jejunal lumen	Jejunal mucosa	Small-bowel mucosa	Cecum, colonic mucosa	Cecum, appendix	Jejunal muscle
Pulmonary passage of larvae	Yes	Yes	Yes	No	No	No
Diagnostic stage	Eggs in stool	Eggs in fresh stool, larvae in old stool	Larvae in stool or duodenal aspirate; sputum in hyperinfection	Eggs in stool	Eggs from perianal skin on cellulose acetate tape	Larva in muscle biopsy

MYCOLOGY

Yeast – Cryptococcus.

Yeast like – Candida.

Mould – Dermatophyte, Aspergillus, Zygomycetes.

Dimorphic – Mould at 25°C, Yeast at 37°C.

1. Histoplasma.Q
2. Blastomyces.Q
3. Coccidiodes.Q
4. Paracoccidiodes.
5. Sporothrix.
6. Penicillium marneffi.

Based on Sexual Spore Sexual Spore (ZAB)

- Zygospore.
- Ascospore.
- Basidiospore.
  1. Phycomycetes/zygomycetes – Zygospore, broad aseptate hyphae, e.g., Rhizopus, Mucor.
  2. Ascomycetes – Ascospores, Narrow septate hyphae, e.g., Aspergillus.
  3. Basidiomycetes – Basidiospore, e.g., Cryptococcus.
  4. Fungi imperfectii – Deuteromycetes/hypomycetes.Q
     – Sexual phase not found yet.
     – Candida, Dermatophyte, Dimorphic group.

Systemic Classification

I. **Superficial:** Tinea versicolor, Tinea nigra, Dermatophytes.

II. **Subcutaneous:** Mycetoma, Rhinosporidium, Chromoblastomycosis, Sporothrix.

III. **Systemic:**

1. Histoplasma.
2. Blastomyces.
3. Coccidioides.
4. Paracoccidioides.
5. Candida.
6. Cryptococcus.

IV. **Opportunistic fungi:**

- Aspergillus.
- Zygomycetes.
- Penicillium spp.
- Penicillium marneffi.
- Pneumocysts jirovecii.
- Fusarium.
- Candida.
- Cryptococcus.

Fungal Media

Sabouraud's Dextrose agar:

- Antibiotic – Cycloheximide, Chloramphenicol and Gentamicin pH – 5.6.
- Niger seed Agar – For Cryptococcus.
- BHI broth – Histoplasma and Cryptococcus.

Fungal Stains

- LPCB – Demonstrate the hyphae grown on SDA (Not from clinical samples).
- PAS – Periodic acid schiff.
- Mucicarmine – Cryptococcus and Rhinosporidium.
- India Ink and Nigrosin – Cryptococcus capsule.
- Gomori Methenamine Silver – Pneumocystis carnii.
- Calcofluor white – Fluorescent stain.

Not Cultivable Fungi

(a) Rhinosproridium.
(b) Pneumocystis jirovecii.
(c) Locazia.

Dermatophytes	**Macroconidia**	**Microconidia**
Trichophyton	Rare, thin walled, smooth, **pencil shaped**	**Abundant**
Microsporum	Numerous, thick walled, rough, **spindle shaped**	Rare
Epidermophyton	Numerous, smooth walled, **club shaped**	Absent

MORE HIGH YIELD IMPORTANT TABLES

IMPORTANT CONTRIBUTIONS IN MICROBIOLOGY

Scientists	Contribution
• Emil von Behring	• Developed diphtheria toxin
• Sir Ronald Ross	• Life cycle of malarial parasitesQ
• Robert Koch	• Tuberculosis – discovery of causative agentQ
• Laveran	• Discovery of malarial parasitesQ
• Har Gobind Khorana	• Interpretation of genetic code
• Karl Landsteiner	• Described ABO blood groups
• Marshall and Warren	• H. Pylori, its role in Peptic ulcer
• Watson and Crick	• Double helix structure of DNA Q
• Barbara Mcclintok	• Mobile genetic elementsQ
• Robert Koch	• Discovery of the causative agent of tuberculosis
• Paul Ehrlich and Elie Metchnikoff	• Selective theory of antibody formation and phagocytosis
• Charles Richet	• Discovered anaphylaxis
• Jules Bordet	• Discovered complement and developed complement fixation test
• Karl Landsteiner	• Described ABO blood group

Contd.

Contd.

• Sir Alexander Fleming	• Discovery of penicillin
• Enders, Robbins and Weller	• Cultivation of polio viruses
• Lederberg and Tatum	• First described conjugation in E.coli
• Blumberg	• Australian antigen (HBSAg)
• Rosalyn Yallow	• Developed radioimmunoassayQ
• Georges Kohler	• Developed hybridoma technology for monoclonal antibodies
• Kary B Mullis	• Polymerase Chain ReactionQ
• Stanley B. Prusiner	• Described Prion and PK ReactionQ

INCUBATION PERIOD OF IMPORTANT COMMUNICABLE DISEASES

Respiratory Tract Infections

Disease	Causative organism	Incubation period
Smallpox	Variola virus	7-14 days
Chickenpox	Human (alpha) herpes virus 3Q	14-16 days
Measles (Rubeolla)	RNA paramyxovirusQ	10-14 daysQ
Rubella (German Measles)	RNA TogavirusQ	14-24 days
Mumps	RNA Myxovirus	14-18 days
Influenza	Orthomyxovirus	18-72 hoursQ
Diphtheria	Corynebacterium diphtheriae	2-6 daysQ
Pertussis (Whooping cough)	Bordetella pertussis	7-14 days
Meningococcal meningitis	Neisseria meningitis	3-4 days
SARS	Corona virusQ	3-5 days
Tuberculosis	Mycobacterium tuberculosis	Weeks-years

GIT Infections

Disease	Causative organism	Incubation period
Poliomyelitis	Poliovirus	7-14 days
Hepatitis A	Enterovirus 72 (Picornavirus)	15-50 days
Hepatitis B	Hepadnavirus	50-150 days
Hepatitis C	Hepacivirus	15-150 days
Hepatitis D	Deltavirus	50-150 days
Hepatitis E	Calcivirus	21-45 days
Cholera	Vibrio cholerae	1-2 days
Typhoid fever	Salmonella typhi	10-14 days
Staphylococcal food poisoning	Staphylococcus aureus	1-6 hours
Ascariasis	Ascaris lumbricoides	2 months
Ancylostomiasis (Hookworm)	A.duodenale	5 weeks-9 months
Guinea worm disease (Dracunculiasis)	Dracunculus medinensis	1 year

Vector Borne Diseases

Disease	Causative organism	Incubation period
Dengue	Arbovirus	3-10 days
Malaria	Plasmodium vivax Plasmodium falciparum Plasmodium malariae Plasmodium ovale	8-17 days 9-14 days 18-40 days 16-18 days
Lymphatic filariasis	Wucheria bancrofti	8-16 months
Rabies	Lyssavirus type 1 (Rhabdovirus)	3-8 weeks
Yellow fever	Flavivirus fibricus	2-6 days
Japanese encephalitis	Group B arbovirus (Flavivirus)	5-15 days
KFD	Arbovirus (Flavivirus)	3-8 days
Chikungunya fever	Chikungunyavirus (Arbovirus A)	4-7 days
Bubonic plague	Yersinia pestis	2-7 days
Pneumonic plague	Yersinia pestis	1-3 days
Septicemic plague	Yersinia pestis	2-7 days
Scrub typhus	Rickettsia tsutsugamushi	10-12 days
Q. fever	Coxiella burnetii	2-3 days

Other Communicable Diseases

Leishmaniasis (Kala azar)	L. donovani	1-4 months
Trachoma	Chlamydia trachomatis	5-12 days
Tetanus	Clostridium tetani	6-10 days
Yaws	Treponema pertenue	3-5 weeks
HIV/AIDS	HIV/HTLV – III/LAV	Months-10 years
Leptospirosis	Leptospira interrogans	4-20 days
Swine flu	H1N1 Type A influenza	1-4 days
Crimean Congo Fever	Nairovirus	1-9 days

MODES OF TRANSMISSION OF COMMUNICABLE DISEASES

Disease	Modes of transmission	Communicable period
Chicken pox	Droplet infection, droplet nuclei	1-2 days before to 4-5 days after appearance of rash
Measles	Droplet infection, droplet nuclei, through conjunctiva	**4 days before rash to 5 days later**
Rubella	Droplet infection, droplet nuclei, vertical	1 week before rash to 1 week later
Mumps	Droplet infection, direct contact	4-6 days before symptoms to 7 days thereafter
Influenza	Droplet infection, droplet nuclei	1-2 days before to 1-2 days after onset of symptoms
Diphtheria	Droplet infection, direct contact, fomite borne	14-28 days from disease onset
Whooping cough	Droplet infection, direct contact, fomite	7 days after exposure to 3 weeks after paroxysmal stage

VECTOR BORNE DISEASES

Arthopods	Arthopod borne diseases	
1. Mosquito	1. Anopheles	Malaria Filaria[AI 12] (Not in India)
	2. Culex	Japanese encephalitis (BEWA) West nile fever Bancroftian filariasis[Q] Viral arthritis
	3. Aedes	Yellow feverQ (YDRC) Dengue[Q] Dengue hemorrhagic fever Chikungunya fever[Q] Rift valley fever[Q] Filaria[Q] (Not in India)
	4. Mansonoides	Brugian filariasis
2. Sandfly	Kala azar[Q] (Sandfly koe **KOSO)** Oriental sore[Q] Oraya fever[Q] Sandfly fever	
3. Tse-tse fly	Sleeping sickness	
4. Louse	Epidemic typhus[Q], relapsing fever[Q], trench fever[Q], pediculosis, vogabond disease[Q] **(T R E P)** the Louse	
5. Rat flea	Bubonic plague[Q], endemic typhus[Q], chiggerosis, hymenolepis diminuta[AI 95]	
6. Black fly	Onchocerciasis	
7. Reduvid bug	Chaga's disease[Q]	
8. Hard tick	Tick typhus[Q], viral encephalitis[Q], viral hemorrhagic fever, KFD[Q], Tularemia, tick paralysis, human babesiosis, Lyme's disease[Q]	
9. Soft tick	Q fever, relapsing fever[Q], KFD (QRS)	
10. Trombiculid mite	Scrub typhus[Q], Ricketssial pox[Q]	
11. Itch mite	Scabies[Q]	
12. Cyclops	Guinea worm disease, Fish tape worm (D. latum)	
13. Cockroaches	Enteric pathogens	
14. Housefly	Typhoid and paratyphoid fever, diarrhoea, dysentery, cholera, gastroenteritis, amoebiasis, helminthic infestations, poliomyelitis, conjunctivitis, trachoma, anthrax, yaws, etc.	

Note: KFD is mainly transmitted from hard tick, but soft tick can also transmit it[AI 95].

DRUGS OF CHOICE FOR TREATMENT

Infection	Drug of choice
• Anaerobes	Metronidazole
• Atypical pneumonia (mycoplasma)	Erythromycin
• Brucella	Doxycycline (DOC) + Rifampin
• Cholera	Doxycycline
• Gonorrhea	Ceftriaxone
• Staphylococci	Penicillin

Contd.

Contd.

• MRSA	Vancomycin
• VRSA	Linezolid
• P. Carinii (jiroveci)	Cotrimoxazole
• Pseudomonas	Antipseudomonal β-lactam + amino-glycoside
• Streptococcus	Penicillin
• Toxoplasma	Cotrimoxazole
• Toxoplasma in pregnancy	Spiramycin
• Rheumatic fever	Benzathine penicillin
• TB	INH with or without rifampicin
• Rickettsia	Tetracyclines
• Influenza A and B	Oseltamivir
• Diphtheria	Penicillin/Erythromycin
• Anthrax	Ciprofloxacin/Doxycycline
• Pertussis	Erythromycin
• HSV	Acyclovir
• Leptospirosis – Milder – Severe	 Oral amoxicillin IV penicillin G
• Lyme's disease	Doxycycline
• Syphillis	Penicillin G
• Pertussis	Erythromycin
• Actinomycosis	Penicillin G
• Lymphogranuloma venerum	Azithromycin or Doxycycline
• Legionella	Azithromycin or levofloxacin
• Plague	Streptomycin
• Typhoid fever	Ceftriaxone
• Listeria	Ampicillin + Gentamycin
• MAC	Azithromycin/clarithromycin
• Group B–streptococcus	Ampicillin
• Meningococcal meningitis	**Ciprofloxacin**/Rifampicin
• UTI	Cotrimoxazole
• Endocarditis	Amoxycillin/Clindamycin

DRUGS OF CHOICE FOR CHEMOPROPHYLAXIS

Infection	Drug of choice for chemoprophylaxis
• Cholera	Tetracycline
• Plague	Tetracycline
• P.carinii	Cotrimoxazole
• Whooping cough	Erythromycin
• Toxoplasmosis	Cotrimoxazole
• Rickettsia	Tetracyclines

Contd.

Contd.

• Bird flu	Oseltamivir
• Gonorrhoea/syphilis	Procaine penicillin
• Meningococci	Rifampicin (sulfadiazine if strain is sensitive)
• Diphtheria	Erythromycin
• Bacterial conjunctivitis	Erythromycin ointment
• TB	INH
• MAC	Clarithromycin/Azithromycin
• Malaria	Chloroquine

IMPORTANT BODIES IN MICROBIOLOGY

Name of the body	Disease/Infection
• Bollinger bodies	Fowlpox
• Chromatid bodies	Entamoeba histolytica precyst
• Citron bodies	Cl. SepticumQ
• Cigar bodies	Sporotrichosis
• Councilman bodies	Yellow fever/viral hepatitis
• Donovan bodies	Granuloma inguinale (LGV)
• Guarneri bodies	Inclusion bodies of vaccinia
• Henderson Paterson bodies	Molluscum contagiosumQ
• Levinthal coles lillie bodies	PsittacosisQ
• Mooser bodies	Endemic typhus
• Negri bodies	RabiesQ
• Paschen bodies	Vaccinia/variola
• Sclerotic bodies	ChromoblastomycosisQ
• Asteroid bodies	SporotrichosisQ
• Halbert Staedter Prowazek body	Chlamydia trachomatis
• Cowdry type A	Herpes, chicken pox, CMV, yellow fever (H **A** Y)
• Cowdry type B	Poliovirus, Adenovirus (**B**AP)
• Torres bodies	Yellow fever

IMPORTANT SEROLOGICAL TESTS

Serological Tests	Type	Use to diagnose
Paul Bunnell testQ	Tube agglutination	Infectious mononucleosis
Wasserman reactionQ	Complement fixation test	Syphilis
Rose Waaler testQ	Passive hemagglutination	Rheumatoid arthritis
Widal test	Slide/Tube agglutination	Typhoid
VDRL	Slide precipitation	Syphilis
Kahn's flocculation test	Tube precipitation	Syphilis
Weil Felix test	Heterophile tube agglutination	Rickettsiae
Lancefield test	Ring precipitation	Group of streptococci
Ascoli's testQ	Ring precipitation	Anthrax

Inhibit Na+ K+ ATPase	Increased cAMP	Increased GMP
Rota virus (secretory diarrhoea)	Cholera ETEC labile toxin Staph aureus Salmonella Bacillus cereus (diarrhoeal) Carcinoid Medullary carcinoma thyroid	E. histolytica ETEC – stable toxin Clostridium difficile

	Lecithinase	Lipase	Sacchrolytic	Proteolytic
Cl. perfringens	+	–	+	–
Cl. botulinum	–	+	–	+
Cl. tetani	–	–	–	±
Cl. septicum	–	–	+	–
Cl. difficile	–	–	–	–

CLINICAL MICROBIOLOGY

Meningitis

Etiology	
Age	Organisms
<1 month	• E.coli, Group B streptococci, Listeria.
1 month-18 years	• Neisseria meningitidis, Haemophilus influenzae, Streptococcus pneumoniae.
>20 years	• Streptococcus pneumoniae.

UTI

Non catheter associated (community acquired) – E.coli. proteus and Klebsiella

Obstruction or calculi associated – E.coli, proteus, Klebsiella, Serratia and Pseudomonas.

Catheter associated (nosocomial) – E.coli, proteus, pseudomonas, serratia, Staphylococcus saprophyticus

Food Poisoning

Onset: 1-6 hours – Bacillus cereus, Staphylococcus aureus.

Onset 8-16 hours – Clostridium perfringens, bacillus cereus (Diarrhoea).

Onset >16 hours – Vibrio parahemolyticus, Campylobacter jejuni, clostridium botulinum, E.coli, Salmonella sps, Shigella sps.

Chapter 3

HEALTH CARE-ASSOCIATED INFECTIONS

Health care-associated infection (HCAI), also referred to as "nosocomial" or "hospital" infection, is an infection occurring in a patient during the process of care in a hospital or other health care facility which was not present or incubating at the time of admission (WHO).

A death rate of 8.3% was reduced to 2.3% by introducing the **simple measure of proper hand washing** before and after any clinical examination. Unfortunately, at the same time, anti-microbial resistant pathogens have risen in number and are estimated to contribute to ~23,000 deaths in and outside of hospitals annually.

COMMON HOSPITAL INFECTIONS

1. **Urinary tract infections:** UTIs account for ~30–40% of nosocomial infections; up to 3% of bacteriuric patients develop bacteremia and most common HAI.

   Order of pathogen importance – E.coli > Enterococci > Staphylococci > Candida.
2. **Surgical wound infections:** Wound infections occur in ~500,000 patients each year, account for ~15–20% of nosocomial infections, contribute up to 7–10 extra postoperative hospital days, depending on the operative procedure and pathogen(s) and contribute to second most common HAI.

   Order of pathogen importance – Staph. aureus and CONS > Enterococci > E.coli > P. aeruginosa > other GNB to a lesser extent.
3. **Pneumonia:** Historically, pneumonia has accounted for ~10–15% of nosocomial infections; ventilator-associated pneumonia (VAP) occurred in 1 to >4 patients per 1000 ventilator-days, and these infections were reported as responsible for a mean of 10 extra hospital days. Most cases of bacterial nosocomial pneumonia are caused by aspiration of endogenous or hospital-acquired oropharyngeal (and occasionally gastric) flora. Nosocomial pneumonias are associated with more deaths than are infections at any other body site.

   Order of pathogen importance – P. aeruginosa > Staph. aureus.
4. **Intravascular device–related bacteremias:** It cause ~10–15% of nosocomial infections; central vascular catheters (CVCs) account for most of these bloodstream infections.

   Order of pathogen importance – Staph. aureus and CONS > Enterococci > Candida > E. coli > other GNB to a lesser extent.

   Note: E. coli accounts overall for more HAI than any other single organism but Staphylococci are a close second in HAI.

SOURCES OF HAI

(See Figure on the Next Page).

HAI can be *endogenous* (self-infection from another site in the body) or *exogenous* (from another person or from an environmental source).

EXAMPLES OF EVIDENCE-BASED "BUNDLED INTERVENTIONS" TO PREVENT COMMON HEALTH CARE–ASSOCIATED INFECTIONS AND OTHER ADVERSE EVENTS

Prevention of Central Venous Catheter Infections

Catheter insertion bundle:

- Educate personnel about catheter insertion and care.

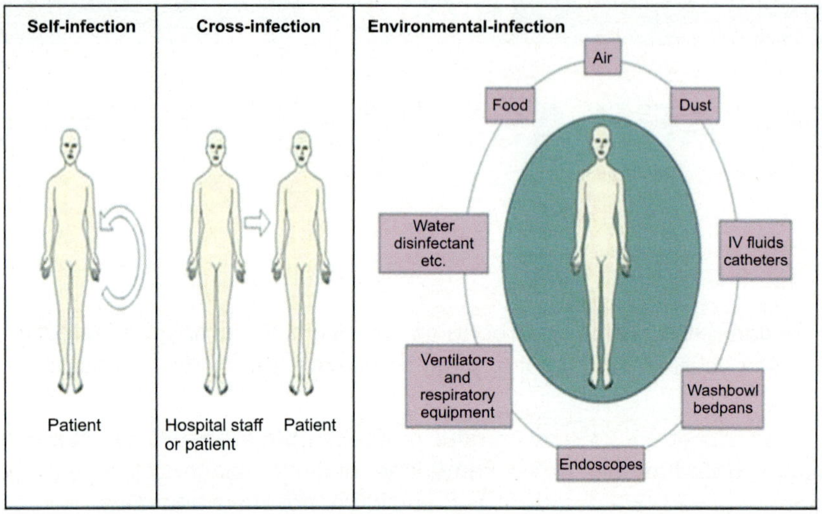

- Use chlorhexidine to prepare the insertion site.
- Use maximal barrier precautions and asepsis during catheter insertion.
- Consolidate insertion supplies (e.g., in an insertion kit or cart).
- Use a checklist to enhance adherence to the "insertion bundle".
- Empower nurses to halt insertion if asepsis is breached.

Catheter maintenance bundle:

- Cleanse patients daily with chlorhexidine.
- Maintain clean, dry dressings.
- Enforce hand hygiene among health care workers.
- *Ask daily:* Is the catheter needed? Remove catheter if not needed or used.

Prevention of Ventilator-Associated Events

- Elevate head of bed to 30–45 degrees.
- Decontaminate oropharynx regularly with chlorhexidine (controversial).
- Give "sedation vacation" and assess readiness to extubate daily.
- Use peptic ulcer disease prophylaxis.
- Use deep-vein thrombosis prophylaxis (unless contraindicated).

Prevention of Surgical-Site Infections

- Choose a surgeon wisely.
- Administer prophylactic antibiotics within 1 hour before surgery; discontinue within 24 hours.
- Limit any hair removal to the time of surgery; use clippers or do not remove hair at all.
- Prepare surgical site with chlorhexidine-alcohol.
- Maintain normal perioperative glucose levels (cardiac surgery patients).
- Maintain perioperative normothermia (colorectal surgery patients).

Prevention of Urinary Tract Infections

- Place bladder catheters only when absolutely needed (e.g., to relieve obstruction), not solely for the provider's convenience.

- Use aseptic technique for catheter insertion and urinary tract instrumentation.
- Minimize manipulation or opening of drainage systems.
- *Ask daily:* Is the bladder catheter needed? Remove catheter if not needed.

Prevention of Pathogen Cross-Transmission

Cleanse hands with alcohol hand rub before and after all contacts with patients or their environments.

These components of care are supported by clinical trials and experimental evidence in the specified populations; they may prove valuable for other surgical patients as well.

Source: Adapted from information presented at the following websites: *www.cdc.gov/hicpac/pubs.html*; *www.cdc.gov/HAI/prevent/prevention.html*; *www.ihi.org.*

MCQs

1. **Most common organism associated with Nosocomial infections is:**
   (a) Pseudomonas aeruginosa
   (b) Enterococci
   (c) E. coli
   (d) Streptococci
2. **Most common Nosocomial infection is:**
   (a) SSI
   (b) UTI
   (c) Pneumonia
   (d) Bacteriemia
3. **Most effective and common method for to prevent common health care-associated infections is:**
   (a) Cleanse hands with alcohol hand rub before and after all contacts with patients or their environments
   (b) Maintain clean, dry dressings
   (c) Prepare surgical site with chlorhexidine–alcohol
   (d) Educate personnel about HAI
4. **Most common source of HAI is:**
   (a) From an environmental source
   (b) From healthy carrier
   (c) From health care staff
   (d) Self-infection from another site in the body
5. **Most common type of health care-associated respiratory tract infection is:**
   (a) Health care-associated bacterial pneumonia
   (b) Health care-associated legionnaire's disease
   (c) Nursing home (NH)-associated pneumonia
   (d) Ventilated-associated pneumonia (VAP)
6. **All the following are true about nosocomial infections except:** *(AI 04)*
   (a) Manifest after 48 hrs of admission
   (b) UTI is most common nosocomial infection reported
   (c) Denote a new condition which is unrelated to the patient's primary conditions
   (d) May already present at the time of admission
7. **The most common pathogens responsible for nosocomial pneumonitis in the ICU are:** *(AI 05)*
   (a) Gram positive bacteria
   (b) Gram negative bacteria
   (c) Fungus
   (d) Virus

8. Which of the following causes highest risk of nosocomial infection to a patient? *(AIIMS 07)*

(a) Patient admitted for elective surgery
(b) HIV patient coming in follow up OPD
(c) Patient undergoing endoscopy
(d) Patient admitted for normal delivery

9. In a post-operative intensive care unit five patients devolved post-operative wound infections on the same wound. The best method to prevent cross infection occurring in other patients in the same ward is to: *(AIIMS 12)*

(a) Give antibiotics to all other patients in the ward
(b) Fumigate the ward
(c) Disinfect the ward with sodium hypochlorite
(d) Practice proper hand hygiene

10. Most common catheter related blood stream infections caused by: *(AIIMS 09)*

(a) Candida albicans
(b) Gram negative bacteria
(c) Staphylococcus aureus
(d) CONS

11. There is an outbreak of MRSA infections in a ward. What is the best way to control the infection? *(JIPMER 05)*

(a) Vancomycin given empirically to all the patients
(b) Fumigation of ward frequently
(c) Washing hand before and after
(d) Wearing mask before any invasive procedure in ICU

ANSWERS

1.	(c)	2.	(b)	3.	(a)
4.	(d)	5.	(d)	6.	(d)
7.	(b)	8.	(a)	9.	(d)
10.	(d)	11.	(c)		

Chapter 4

GENERAL MICROBIOLOGY

Microbiology: Study of microorganisms.

Medical microbiology is a branch of medical science concerned with the prevention, diagnosis and treatment of infectious diseases. In addition, this field of science studies various clinical applications of microbes for the improvement of health. There are four kinds of **microorganisms** that cause infectious disease: **bacteria, fungi, parasites and viruses.**

Virus	Bacteria	Fungi	Protozoa
• Smallest infections agent • Size–20-200 nm	• Prokaryotes • Size: 1-5 μm	• Eukaryotes • Size: 5-10 μm	• Eukaryotes • Size: 10-20 μm
• Smallest virus → Parvo Virus • Biggest virus → Pox Virus	• Smallest bacteria: Mycoplasma • Largest bacteria: Bacillus anthracis	–	–
• All viruses obligate intracellular	• Unicellular	• Multicellular	• Multicellular
• Contain either DNA or RNA • Never present both • Artificial media not possible	• Contains DNA + RNA • Surrounded by rigid cell wall	• DNA + RNA • Surrounded by cell wall → Chitinous	• DNA + RNA • Cell wall present
• All are non-motile	• Motile (Flagella) • Non-motile	• No-motile	• Motile
• Multiply by viral infective cycle	• Multiply by asexually – binary fission	• Sexually – Meiosis • Asexually – Mitosis	• Sexually – Meiosis • Asexually – Mitosis

Prokaryotic Cells	Eukaryotic Cells
Small cells (< 5 μm)	Larger cells (> 10 μm)
Always unicellular	Often multicellular
No nucleus or any membrane – bound organelles	Always have nucleus and other membrane – bound Organelles
Single chromosome DNA is circular, without proteins	Multiple chromosome DNA is linear and associated with proteins to form chromatin
Ribosomes are small (70S)	Ribosomes are large (80S)
No cytoskeleton	Always has a cytoskeleton
Cell division is by binary fission	Cell division is by mitosis or meiosis
Reproduction is always asexual	Reproduction is asexual or sexual
Cytoplasmic • Cytoplasmic Streaming → Absent • Pinocytosis → Absent • Membrane bound intracellular → Organelles absent	Cytoplasmic • Cytoplasmic Streaming → Present • Pinocytosis → Present • Membrane bound intracellular → Organelles present

Contd.

Contd.

Cell Envelope • Peptidoglycan cell wall present except Mycoplasma • Sterols in cell membrane absent except Mycoplasma • Diaminopimelic acid – Present in some	Cell Envelope • Peptidoglycan cell wall absent • Sterols in cell membrane – Present • Diaminopimelic acid – Absent

HISTORICAL BACKGROUND

1. **Antonie Van Leeuwenhoek** (1632-1723): Bacteria were first observed and discovered by him, a draper from Holland, whose hobby was grinding lenses; he described three major morphological forms of bacteria, findings confirmed by Robert Hook in 1678.
2. **Louis Pasteur: Father of Microbiology**
    - Established that fermentation was result of microbial activity.
    - Developed differing growth needs or bacteria.
    - Started studies on anthrax, Cholera and hydrophobia (Rabies vaccine) **(CAR).Q**
    - Coined the term vaccineQ, when he first attenuated culture of Anthrax bacillus and proved that inoculation of such cultures in animals induced specific protection against anthrax.
    - He described the method of Pasteurization.
    - **Disproved "*the theory of spontaneous generation*".Q**
    - Introduction of sterilization techniques.
3. **Robert Koch: Father of Bacteriology**
    - Studies on culture and character of Anthrax bacillus.
    - Introduction of staining technique and methods of obtaining bacteria in pure culture.
    - Bacilli of Tuberculosis (1882) and Vibrio cholera (1883).
    - Using criteria developed by his teacher, Jacob Henle (1809-1895), established the relationship between Bacillus anthracis and anthrax.
    - **Koch's phenomenon** – He observed that guinea pigs already infected with tubercle bacillus responded with an exaggerated inflammatory response when injected with the tubercle bacillus or its protein. This hypersensitivity reaction is called Koch's phenomenon.
    - His criteria became known as Koch's postulates and are still used to establish the link between a particular microorganism and a particular disease:

Koch's Postulates
• The causative (etiological) agent must be present in all affected organisms but absent in healthy individuals. • The agent must be capable of being isolated and cultured in pure form. • When the cultured agent is introduced to a healthy organism, the same disease must occur. • The same causative agent must be reisolated agent from the affected host. • Exception of Koch's Postulates: – M. Leprae: Because it can't be cultured on artificial medium however it can be grown in foot pad of mice/armadillo. – Treponema Pallidum: Grown in rabbit testis.

4. **Edward Jenner:** Used a vaccination procedure to protect individuals from smallpox.
5. **Joseph Lister** (1827-1912) – **"Father of Antiseptic Surgery"**
    - Developed a system of surgery designed to prevent microorganisms from entering wounds – phenol sprayed in air around surgical incision.
    - Decreased number of post – operative infections in patients.
    - His published findings (1867) transformed the practice of surgery.

6. **Emil von Behring** (1854-1917) and **Shibasaburo Kitasato** (1852-1931) – Induced the formation of diphtheria tetanus antitoxins in rabbits which were effectively used to treat humans thus demonstrating humoral immunity.
7. **Elie Metchnikoff** (1845-1916) and **Paul Ehrlich** – Demonstrated the existence of phagocytic cells in the blood. Selective theory of Ab formation, **Paul Ehrlich discovered SALVARSAN (Magic bullet) for Syphilis, also known as Father of Chemotherapy.**
8. **Charles Chamberland** (1851-1908) – Identified viruses as disease – causing agent – Tobacco Mosaic Virus.
9. **Laveran** – Discovery of malarial parasite in unstained preparation.
10. **Alexander Fleming** – Discovery of "Wonder Drug Penicillin" (Major medical revolution – What u think?)
11. **Karry B Mullis** – Father of PCR (Polymerase chain reaction) – Changed the future of diagnostics in Microbiology.Q

MICROSCOPY

- Microorganisms are extremely small. The size of the bacteria is expressed in micrometers (1 μ = 10^{-3} mm) whereas viruses are measured in nanometers (1nm = 10^{-3} μm).
- Properties of a Microscope – 1. Good resolution, 2. Good contrast, 3. Good magnification.

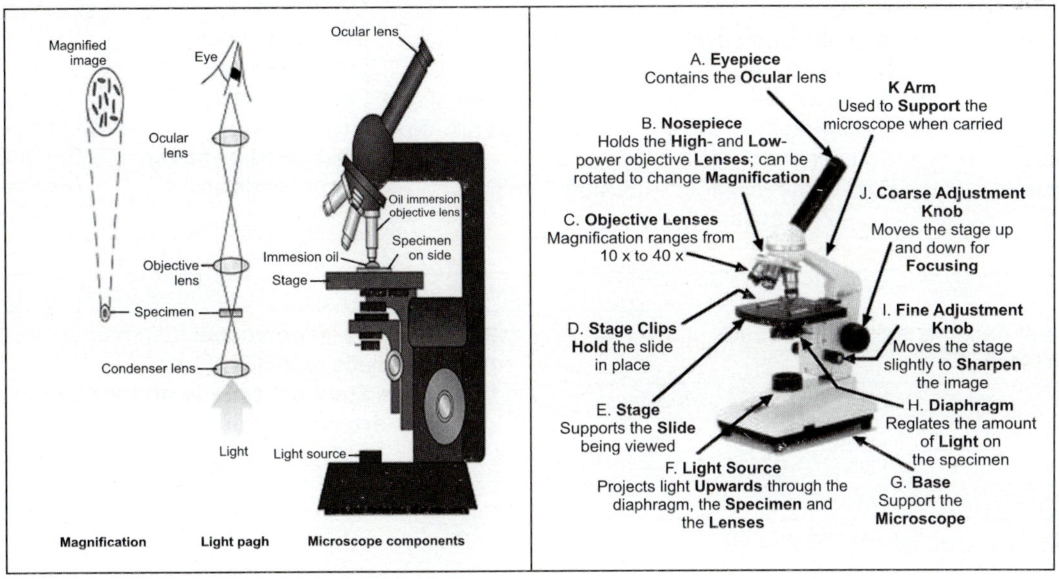

Types of Microscopes

Simple	• Similar to a magnifying glass and has only one lens.
Light microscope/ Compound microscope	Objective lens of 10X, 40X, 100X with 10X eye piece maximum achieved with oil immersion lens. • Both live and killed organism can be seen by light microscope. • Resolving power – 0.2 μm or 200 nm. • None of virus can be seen by light microscope. Except – Pox virus (200 nm).
Phase contrast microscope	Used for **internal structures of cell,** special condenser and objective lens, converts difference in phase to difference in intensity of light, producing light and dark contrast in the image.
Dark field/Ground microscope	• Object – bright, field – dark. • Reflected light.Q • Used to demonstrate – Spirochetes.
Fluorescent microscope	Specimens exposed to (UV light) of shorter wavelength results in emission of longer wavelength visible light. Fluorescent dyes like Auramine, Rhodamine are used.
Electron microscope	• Uses a magnetic field to bend beams of electrons: Instead of using lenses to bend beams of light.

Contd.

Contd.

	• Highest resolving power – 0.1 nm.Q • Only microscope can be seen are killed organism and technique of shadow casting is employed (achieved by deposition of thin layer of platinum) but now new Freeze etching can be employed to see living cells. • Two types: (a) Transmission EM -2D. (b) Scanning EM -3D and higher resolution.

Staining Techniques

- Increase contrast of microorganism so that they can be visualized easily.
- Before staining, the fixation of the smear to the slide is done.
- Classified into types of stains

Simple stain	Differential stain	Structural or special stains	Impregnation methods	Negative staining
• One dye, one step • Direct stain using basic dye • Negative stain using acidic dye, i.e., Methylene blue	• More than one dye • Gram stain, acid fast • Primary dye Decolorizing step • Counter stain E.g.– Gram stain – Z.N. stain	• Identify structures within or on cells • Different parts of cell are stained different colors • Albert stain	Too thin bacterial structures are seen under light microscope, thickened by **silver impregnation**	Background is stained dark but bacteria stained out in contrast E.g. **India ink, Nigrosin stain**

Acid fast stain	Albert stain
• Acid fastness of bacteria is due to presence of mycolic acid in the cell wall	• It is used only for corynebacterium to demonstrate metachromatic granules. • **Using this stain bacteria is stained green and the granules are stained purple.**

Organism	% of acid tolerance/Fastness
M.TB	20%
M. Leprae	5%
Nocardia	1%
Bacterial Spores	0.5-1%
Cryptosporidium	.25-1%

• In this stain bacteria is seen as Red in color and the surrounding is stained Blue.

Morphology of Bacteria

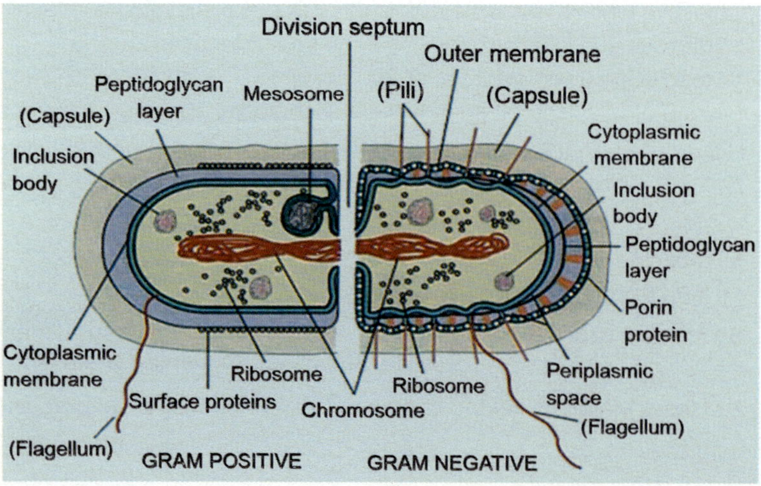

A. Cell Wall

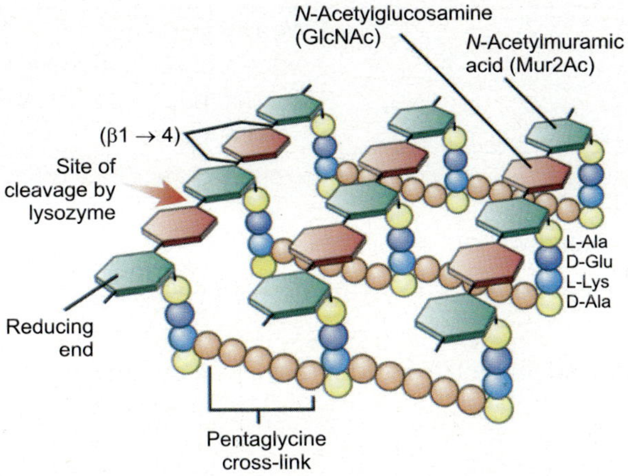

- Major function is to give shape and rigidity to the bacteria.
- It is 10-25 nm in thickness and provides protection to the bacteria against osmotic lysis.
- The basic structural unit of cell wall is called as peptidoglycan which is composed of 2 compounds, i.e., **N-acetyl glucosamine (NAG) and N-acetyl muramic acid (NAM).**
- Difference between cell walls of gram positive and gram negative bacteria.

Differences Between Gram Positive Cell and Gram Negative Cell wall

	Gram-Positive	**Gram-Negative**
Color of Gram-Stained Cell	Purple	Reddish-Pink
Representative Genera	Bacillus, Staphylococcus, Streptococcus	Escherichia, Neisseria, Pseudomonas
Distinguishing Structures/Components		
Peptidoglycan	Thick layer	Thin layer
Teichoic acids	Present	Absent
Periplasm	Absent	Present
Outer membrane	Absent	Present
Endotoxin (lipopolysaccharide)	Absent	Present
Porin proteins	Absent (unnecessary because there is no outer membrane)	Present; allow passage of molecules through outer membrane
General Characteristics		
Sensitivity to penicillin	Generally more susceptible (with notable exceptions)	Generally less susceptible (with notable exceptions)
Sensitivity to lysozyme	Yes	No (unless also treated with EDTA)
Form that results from removal of peptidoglycan	**Protoplast**	**Spheroplast**

Difference Between Exotoxin and Endotoxin

Exotoxin	**Endotoxin**
Proteinaceous	**Lipopolysaccharides**
Heat labile	Heat stable
Actively secreted by bacteria	Part of cell wall
Can be separated from cultures easily	Obtained only by cell lysis
Enzymatic action	Not enzymatic action
Specific pharmacological effect for each toxin	Nonspecific effect
Specific tissue affinity	No specific tissue affinity

Contd.

Contd.

Highly antigenic Active in very minute doses Action neutralized by specific antibody Can be toxoided	Weakly antigenic Active only in large doses Not neutralized by antibody Can be toxoided
Produced mostly by gram positive bacteria	Produced mostly by gram negative bacteria

- **Protoplast** – It is a gram +ve bacteria without a cell wall.
- **Spheroplast** – It is a gram –ve bacteria with only some parts of cell wall.
- **L-form of bacteria:**
  - These are the bacteria produced in the lab without a cell wall by growing them in a medium containing penicillin (lister institute).

B. Flagella

- 3 parts:
  (a) **Filament** – Long thin, helical structure composed of protein flagellin/H Ag.
  (b) **Hook** – Curved fixable segment.
  (c) **Basal body** – Stack of rings firmly anchored in cell wall.
- Rotates 360°.
- Some G+ and G- bacteria are motile by flagella – made of protein subunits → Flagellin **Number and Arrangement of flagella.**

- **Monotrichous:** Single polar flagella
  - Pseudomonas aeruginosa[Q]
  - Vibrio cholera
- **Lophotrichous:** Tuft at one end
  - Spirillum minus
- **Amphitrichous:** Tuft at both ends
  - Alcaligenes faecalis
- **Peritrichous:** All around bacteria
  - E.coli, Salmonella, Proteus

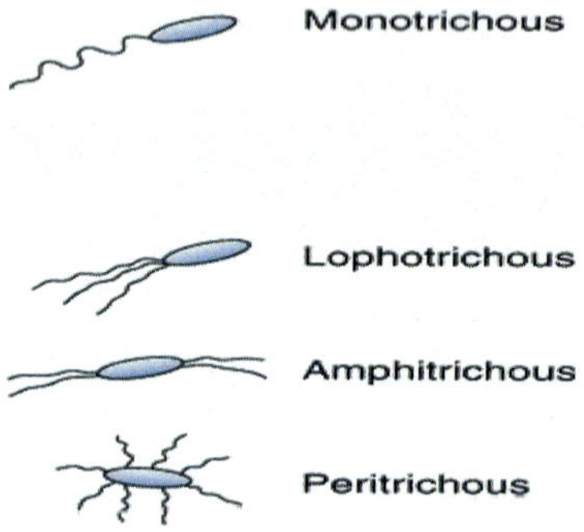

- **Peculiar Motility:**

Motility	Example
Darting	• Vibrio Cholerae, Campylobacter
Tumbling	• Listeria Monocytogenes at 20-25°C Q
Gliding	• Mycoplasma
Swarming	• Proteus, Cl. tetani, Vibrio parahaemolyticus
Stately	• Bacillus, Clostridium
Corkscrew **Flexion – Extension (Endoflagella)**	• Spirochetes
Twitching, Wobbling, Jerky	• Trichomonas vaginalis
Falling Leaf	• Giardia lambliaQ

- **Demonstration of Flagella or Motility**
  - Can be done by direct or indirect methods.
  - Motility can be seen by Dark – ground microscope and by hanging drop method.

- **Direct method by increasing the thickness of flagella using silver impregnation method.**
- Bacteria which are motile without flagella:
  - Mycoplasma.
  - Spirochaetes.

C. Fimbriae

- Fine, proteinaceous, hairlike bristles emerging from the cell surface.
- Function in adhesion to other cell and surface.

D. Pilli

- Rigid tubular structure made of pilin protein.
- Found only in gram – negative cells.
- Function to join bacterial cells for partial DNA transfer called conjugation.

E. Capsule

Found in some G+ and G- bacteria

- Polysaccharide in nature **[Except – Bacillus anthracis (Polypeptide in nature) and Yersinia].**
- Demonstration of capsule:
  - Negative staining as India ink stain.
  - **Quellung reaction/Capsular swelling reaction** – It is a type of Ag – Ab reaction in which Ab's against capsule are used to make it more prominent.

    Examples: H. influenza, Pneumococci, N. meningitis, Klebsiella.

F. Mesosomes

- These are infoldings of cell membrane into the cytoplasm of bacteria.
- They are the principle site of respiratory enzymes in bacteria, i.e., functionally they are similar to mitochondria.
- Additionally they also play a role in cell division.

G. Inclusion Body

- They are the energy stores present in cytoplasm bacteria.
- They are more developed in cases of starvation, **Examples–Metachromatic granules/polymetaphosphate/ Babeernst granules/polar bodies.**
- These are present in corynebacterium diphtheria as energy store.
- They cannot be seen by ordinary gram stain but can be seen by a special call as "Albert's stain/Neisser's stain/ ponder's stain.

Bacterial Spore/Endospore (Chemical composition–Keratin coat Calcium lipicolinate)

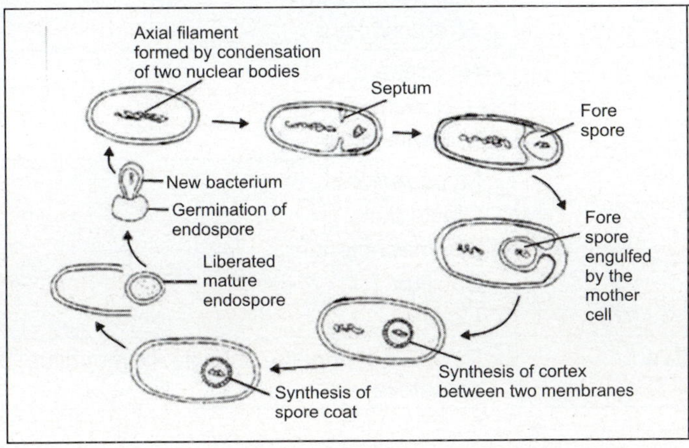

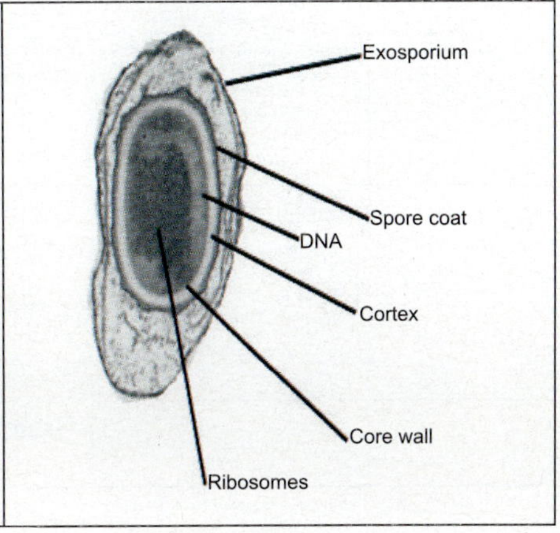

- **Highly resistant resting form:**
  - Bacillus, Clostridium, Sarcina, Coxiella.
  - Terminal, Spherical – C. tetani.Q
  - Terminal, oval – C. tertium.
  - Sub terminal – C. perfringens.
  - Central – B.cereus, C. bifermentans.
- Favours spore formation – ↑O_2, oxalate agar, 2% NaCl.
- **Sporicidal – EFGH:**
  I. Ethylene oxide.
  II. Formal dehyde.
  III. Glutaral dehyde.
  IV. Hypochlorite.
  V. H_2O_2.
  VI. Autoclave, Hot air oven, Plasma sterilization.
  VII. O Phthalic acid, Peracetic acid.

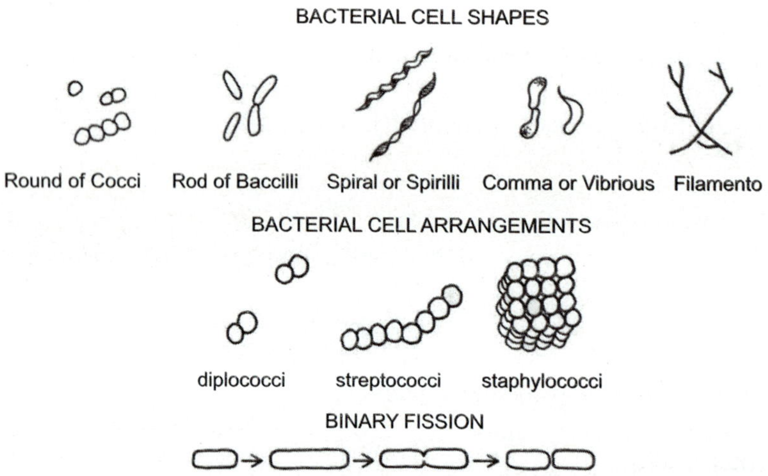

- Strepto – Chains.
- Staphylo – Grape like clusters.

Shapes:

Spherical	Coccus/Cocci	Gram +ve	• Staphylococcus • Streptococcus
		Gram -ve	• Neisseria – Gonorrheae – Meningitidis
Rod	Bacilli/ Bacillus	Gram +ve	• Mycobacteria • Clostridium • Corynebacterium • Bacillus • Listeria
		Gram -ve	• E. Coli, salmonella, shigella, hemophilus, brucella, bordetella

Contd.

Contd.

Coma Shaped		Gram +ve	• Vibrio Cholerae
Filamentous			• Nocardia • Actinomyces
Spiral/Helical bacteria		Flexible, Rigid	• Spirochaetes, Helicobacter Campylobacter

Bacterial Structures and Their Functions

Structure	Chemical composition	Function
Glycocalyx	Polysaccharide	Adherence to surfaces
Capsule	Polysaccharide	Phagocytosis
Cell wall 1,2,3	Peptidoglycan	Rigid support protection vs. osmotic pressure
Outer membrane (porin, LPS)	Lipid A Somatic O polysaccharide	Endotoxin O antigen
Cytoplasmic membrane	Lipid bilayer	Osmotic barrier Oxidative and transport enzymes
Periplasm (Only Gram –ve)	Space between inner membrane and outer membrane	Hydrolytic enzymes (phosphatases, B-lactamases etc)
Mesosome	Invagination of Cytoplasmic membrane	Division septa

Bacterial Growth Curve

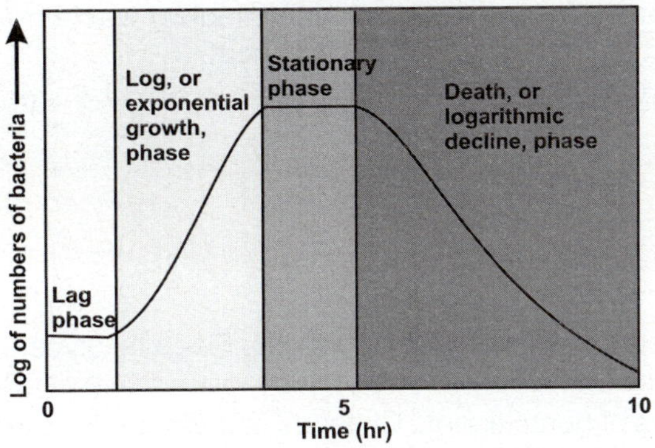

Lag phase – Bacteria increases in size, accumulate nutrients and accommodate to environment.

Log phase – Exponential increase in number of bacteria.

Stationary phase – Viable = Non viable (Dead = live organism) (S = sporulation happens in stationary phase).

Decline phase – Accumulation of toxic metabolites and there is decline in number.

STERILIZATION AND DISINFECTION

Sterilization	Disinfection	Antisepsis
• A process by which an article, surface or medium is freed off all living microorganism including spores.	Destruction and removal of all pathogenic organisms.	A process by which a living tissue is removed all pathogenic org. leaving behind non-pathogenic org. and spores.

- **Asepsis:** It is a process where the chemical agents (antiseptics) are applied on the body surfaces (skin), which kill or inhibit the microorganisms present on skin.
- **Decontamination or Sanitization:** Reduction of pathogenic microbial population to a certain level at which items are considered as safe to handle without protective attire.
- **Factors influencing efficacy of Sterilant or Disinfectant:** Organism load, Nature of the organism, concentration of the chemical, nature of the disinfectant/sterilant, duration of exposure, Temperature, pH, presence of organic matter, presence of Biofilm.Q
- **Resistance order of Microorganism to Disinfectant/Sterilizing agents – Q: Prions > Cryptosporidium oocysts > Endospores > Mycobacteria > other parasite cysts > small non-enveloped viruses > Trophozoites > GNB > Fungi > Large non-enveloped viruses > GPB > Enveloped viruses.**

DRY HEAT

- **Flaming:** The article should be sterilized on the hot flame of Bunsen burner – Inoculation wire and loop, forceps, mouth of glass wares (test tube, flask).
- **Incineration (870-1200°C):** It is used for the disposal of biomedical waste materials. It burns the anatomical waste and microbiological waste converting into ash, flue gas and heat.
- **Hot air oven:** It is also called dry heat sterilizer. The articles should be sterilized at the temperature 160°C for 2 hours.Q

  HOT–GPS (memory aid).

  G –Glasswares, glass syringes.

  P–Paraffin oil, powder.

  S–Sharps.

  - Glassware like test tube, pipette, flask and glass syringes. Fixed oil glycerin, liquid paraffin, propylene glycol and zinc oxide etc. sterilized by this method.
  - **Sterilization control** – Spores of nontoxigenic Cl. tetani and **Bacillus subtilis subsp. niger. Q**, Thermocouples, Browne's tube.

MOIST HEAT

- **Pasteurization**
  - 63°C for 30 min **(Holder method)** – Not able to kill spores.
  - 72°C for 15-20 sec **(Flash method)** followed by rapid cooling to 13°C better method.
    Coxiella burnetti resists Holders method, but killed by Flash method.Q
- **Inspissation (Fractional sterilization)**
  - 80 to 85°C for 30 min (for 3 days) by Inspissator.
  - For media containing egg or serum – (LJ media, Dorset's egg medium, Loeffler's serum slope).Q
- **Tyndallisation (Intermittent sterilization):** 100°C, 20 min, 3 consecutive days.
  - Nutrient media and media containing sugars or gelatin.Q
  - 1st day all vegetative bacteria are killed. On II and III day spores that germinate are killed.
- **Autoclave – 121°C for 15 min with 15 lbs. pressure.**
  - This type of sterilization is done by steam heat under pressure.
  - **Use:** Surgical dressing, Culture media, rubber, gloves, surgical instrument are sterilized by this method (Autoclaved).
  - **Sterilization control:** Spores of Geobacillus stearothermophilus (Bacillus stearothermophilus)Q, Thermocouples, Browne's tube, Autoclave tapes.

FILTRATION

- **Filters are used to remove microbial population from heat labile materials** like vaccines, antibiotics, toxins, chemicals, beverages, serum and sugar solutions.
- Also use in purification of water and Air purification.
- **Sterilization control** – Serratia marcescens and Brevundimonas diminuta.

Depth filters Candle filters, Asbestos filters, Sintered glass filters – They are used in industrial applications like filtration of food, chemicals and beverages.

- **Membrane filters** (Pore diameter – 0.22 μm) – Purification of water (water testing for V. cholera and S. typhi), vaccines, antibiotics, toxins, chemicals, serum and sugar solutions.
- **HEPA and ULPA** – Air purification in Biosafety cabinets and operation theaters.

RADIATION

Ionizing Radiation	Non-Ionizing Radiation
• Ionising radiations (X-rays, Gamma rays and Cosmic rays) (High penetrating power) • **MOA:** Breakage of DNA • Also known as **COLD sterilization.Q** • **Uses:** Disposable rubber or plastic syringes, infusion sets, catheters, catgut sutures, tissue grafts.Q	• UV rays and Infrared • Lethal to humans • **Uses:** For entryways of operation theatres and laboratories.

PLASMA STERILIZATION

- It is type of chemical sterilization using H_2O_2; H_2O_2 is vaporized and than it is converted into plasma.
- When H_2O_2 vapors are energized into plasma, hydroxyl, hydroperoxyl free radicals are generated.
- **MOA:** Direct erosion of cells and free radical induced damages.
- **Sterilization control:** Geobacillus stearothermophilus (Bacillus stearothermophilus).Q

CHEMICAL AGENTS (STERILIZATION/DISINFECTION)

(a) Phenol (Carbolic Acid)

- **Lister (Father of antiseptic surgery)** first used Phenol as antiseptic agent.
- Obtained from distillation of coal tar.
- Unlike other chemical agents its activity is least affected by organic waste material hence it is used to clean dirty surfaces.
- **Phenol as Disinfectant:** Cresol, xylenol, Lysol, orthophenylphenol (used in Hospitals and Labs).
- **Phenol as Antiseptics:** Dettol **(chloroxylenol)** and Savlon **(chlorhexidine + cetrimide)** – > Savlon is much better than Dettol.

(b) Alcohol

- **Ethyl alcohol:** Used in 60-70% concentration (if 100% is used it will cause dehydration of skin protein, so used in 60-70%).
- **Isopropyl alcohol:** Hand rubs and sanitizers.
- **Methyl alcohol:** It causes dehydration of bacterial cell wall:
  - Used in 60-70% conc. and used to kill fungal spores hence used to clean old wooden furniture and old books.
- **Isopropyl alcohol is better than ethyl alcohol as it is a better fat solvent, more bactericidal and less volatile.**

(c) Aldehyde

- Formaldehyde:
  - Used in 2 forms – gaseous and liquid form.
  - Gaseous form is used for fumigation of OT.
  - 10% aqueous solution of formalin is used for a preservative of anatomical specimen.

- Glutaraldehyde:Q
  - Used 2% conc. and is called as cidex, accepted as sterilant and High level disinfectant.
  - Used to sterilize endoscope including cystoscope and bronchoscope.
  - Also used to sterilize anaesthesia equipment like face mask and ET tube.

(d) Halogens

- Chlorine (Bleaching powder, sodium hypochlorite and chloramine).
- HOCl
  - Strong oxidizing agent and effective disinfectant.
  - Used for purification of water.
- Iodine
  - Used as an antiseptic.
  - Tincture iodine – 2% Iodine in a water-ethanol solution – effective antiseptic.
  - However in pure form it is toxic and irritant, hence it is used in combination with an organic carrier Providone and called as Providone iodine (Iodophore). Betadine is commonly used iodophores.

(e) Ethylene Oxide (ETO/EO)

- Gaseous sterilant.
- **EO sterilization cycles – Cold cycle at 37± 5°C and Warm cycle 54± 5°C.Q**
- **It is alkylating agent,** high penetrating power, >10% becomes Explosive.
- Used for sterilization of:Q
  - Disposable plastic material, syringes, catheter, cannulas.
  - Suture material, Dental equipment and heart, lung machines.
  - **Bacillus globigi** – Biological control for testing of Ethylene oxide sterilizers.

(f) Quaternary NH_4^+ compound

- **3 group** – cationic (Most important) cause loss of membrane permeability, cell proteins are denatured.
- **Common cationic compound** are Acetyl trimethyl ammonium bromide (Cetavalon or cetrimide) and Benzalalkonium chloride. Activity is greatest at an alkaline pH.
- **Anionic** – Common soaps, have strong detergent action but antimicrobial action.
- **Non ionic (Amphoteric)** – Tego compounds possess detergent activities of anionic and antimicrobial activity of cationic compounds. Active against Gram positive and gram negative.
- Used as antiseptic/disinfection.

(g) Aniline dyes and Acridine dyes (Activity reduced in pre-sence of Organic materials) – Used as skin and wound antiseptics Egs – Aniline dyes – Crystal violet, Gentian violet, brilliant green, Malachite green. They are more active against Gram positive bacteria, no activity against MTB. Acridine dyes like acriflavine, Proflavine.

TESTING EFFICACY OF DISINFECTANTS

- **Phenol coefficient (Rideal Walker) Test**
  - Any Phenolic disinfectant compared with phenol against S.Typhi.
- **Chick Martin Test**
  - It is a modification of Rideal and Walker test.
  - Disinfectants acts in the presence of organic contaminants (e.g., dried yeast, faeces, etc.) to simulate the natural conditions.
- **Capacity (Kelsey-Sykes) Test**
  - Capacity of a disinfectant to retain its activity when repeatedly used microbiologically in increase load.

Spaulding's Criteria of Devices

Clinical device	Definition	Example	Infectious risk
Critical device	Medical device **intended to enter a *normally sterile environment,* tissue or vasculature**	Surgical instruments, *cardiac* and urinary catheters, implants, eye and dental instruments	High (to be sterilized)
Semi-critical device	Medical device intended to come in **contact with *mucous membranes or minor skin* breaches**	Respiratory therapy and anaesthesia equipments, endoscopes, laryngoscope, tonometers, rectal/vaginal/esophageal probes etc.	High, Intermediate (Sterilized/HLD)
Non-critical devices	Medical devices that come in **contact *with intact skin***	BP cuff, ECG electrodes, bedpans, crutches. Stethoscope, thermometer	Low (ILD/LLD)
Medical equipments	Device or component of a device that does not typically come in direct contact with patient	Examination table, computers	Low (LLD)

Inoculating loop or wire, the tip of forceps and searing spatulas	Flaming
Contaminated cloth, animal carcasses and Pathological material	Incineration
Glasswares, syringes, petridishes, test tubes	Hot air ovenQ
Culture media	AutoclavingQ
Sharp instrument	5% cresol or Hot air oven
Clinical thermometer	Savlon
Cystoscope, endoscope, face masks, plastic endotracheal tubes	GlutaraldehydeQ
Milk	PasteurizationQ
Suture material except cat gut	AutoclaveQ
Catgut sutures	Ionizing radiationQ
Bacterial vaccines	Vaccine bathQ
Dressing, aprons, gloves, catheter except sharp instrument	Autoclaving
Heat sensitive catheters, ward fumigation, sick room	Fumigation
Prepacked syringes	Gamma radiationQ
Culture media containing sugar and gelatin	TyndallisationQ

CULTURE MEDIA

- **Culture media** are artificially prepared substances which provide the basis for the growth of bacteria or micro-organisms.
- **Constituents of Culture media** – Water, Electrolytes, Peptone, Agar, Meat Extracts, Yeast Extracts, Malt Extracts, Blood and Serum.

No.	**Media**	**Important Ingredients**	**Action of Important Ingredients**	**Method of Sterilization**	**Uses**
			SIMPLE MEDIA		
1.	Peptone Water	Peptone, Salt, Water	Basic requirement for growth of microorganisms	Autoclaving	1. Used as a base for other media 2. Used for the growth of non-fastidious microorganism
2.	Nutrient Broth	Peptone water and Meat extract	–Do–	–Do–	–Do–
3.	Nutrient Agar	Nutrient broth and agar agar	–Do–	–Do–	–Do–
4.	Semisolid Agar	–Do–	–Do–	–Do–	1. Used for detecting motility of bacteria
			ENRICHED MEDIA		
1.	Blood Agar	Nutrient agar and blood	Blood is for enriching the medium	Sterile blood added to Autoclaved nutrient agar at < 55° C	1. Used for the growth of staphylococci; Pneumo-cocci and Neisseria group 2. To differentiate the hemolytic properties
2.	Chocolate Agar	Blood agar heated at 56°C for 1 hour	When blood is heated factors X and V are released from RBC, which are required for microorganisms	Blood agar Plates are kept in hot air oven at 56° C for 30 minutes	1. For growth of H, influenza 2. For growth of pyogenic Streptococci 3. For growth of Neisseria group
3.	Loeffler serum agar	Nutrient broth glucose, serum	Serum and glucose for enriching the medium	Inspissation	1. For growth of C. diphtheria
4.	Dorset egg medium	Nutrient broth egg	Egg for enriching the medium	Inspissation	1. Used for growth of Mycobacterium tuberculosis
			ENRICHMENT MEDIA		
1.	Alkaline peptone water	Peptone water pH -8.6	High pH inhibits commensals other than Vibrio species	Autoclaving	Used for the growth of Vibrio cholerae
2.	Selenite F broth	Peptone water and sodium hydrogen Selenite	Selenite enriches the growth of Salmonella and inhibits growth of coliform organisms	Tyndallisation	Enriching Salmonella species from faecal specimens
			SELECTIVE MEDIA		
1.	Potassium tellurite Medium	Nutrient agar, blood and potassium tellurite	Blood is for enriching the medium. Potassium tellurite is less inhibitory to C. diphtheria compared to other throat commensals	Autoclaving	1. Used for the growth of C. diphtheriae
2.	Xylose Lysine Deoxycholate (XLD) Agar	Xylose, Lysine, Deoxycholate and Phenol red	Deoxycholate inhibits intestinal organism	Autoclaving	For growth of salmonella

Contd.

Contd.

3.	Thiosulphate Citrate Bile Salt Sucrose (TCBS) Agar	Thiosulphate, Citrate, Bile Salt, Sucrose, Bromothymol blue pH:8.6	Bile salt and alkaline pH inhibits the growth of coliform organism	Autoclaving	For the growth of Vibrio cholera from faecal sample
4.	Lowenstein Jensen Medium	Egg, Malachite green, mineral salts and glycerol	Egg to enrich the medium, Malachite green is least Inhibitory for Mycobacterium tuberculosis, Glycerol allows the growth of human variety	Inspissation	1. Used for the growth of Mycobacterium species
5.	Sabourauds Dextrose Agar	Glucose, peptone, agar pH: 5.4	Low pH and high sugar content make it selective for fungus	Autoclaving	1. For cultivation of fungus
			DIFFERENTIAL/INDICATOR MEDIA		
1.	MacConkey's Agar	Peptone water, agar agar, sodium Taurocholate, lactose, neutral red	Sodium Taurocholate is inhibitory to non-intestinal organisms. Lactose when fermented leads to change of pH to acidic which in turn cause change of colour of Neutral red to pink	Autoclaving	1. For growth of intestinal organisms 2. For differentiating lactose fermenting organisms from non-lactose fermenting organisms
			TRANSPORT MEDIA		
1.	Stuart's Media	Charcoal, inorganic phosphates, buffer, sodium thioglycolate	Charcoal absorbs the bacterial inhibitory substances Reducing agents prevents oxidation during the transportation	Autoclaving	1. Provides viability of Gonococci and aerobes
2.	V. R. Medium	Crude salt PH 8.6	High alkaline condition preserves viability of Vibrio species	Autoclaving	1. For transportation of Vibrio Cholerae
3.	Glycerol saline Medium	Glycerol, sodium and potassium hydrogen phosphate	Prevents growth of intestinal commensals	Autoclaving	1. Preserves Salmonella, shigella from faecal specimen
			ANAEROBIC MEDIA		
1.	Robertson Cooked Meat Medium (RCM)	Nutrient broth and Meat pieces	Meat pieces are for producing anaerobic condition	Autoclaving	1. For cultivation of anaerobic organisms
2.	Thioglycolate				
			BLOOD CULTURE MEDIA		
1.	Glucose broth	Nutrient broth, glucose, Sodium citrate	Enrichment of pyogenic organism	Steam Sterilization	Culture of pyogenic organism from blood
2.	Taurocholate Broth (Bile broth)	Nutrient broth and Sodium Taurocholate	Sodium Taurocholate is inhibitory to non-intestinal organism	Autoclaving	For growth of salmonella from blood

BACTERIAL GENETICS

- DNA molecule composed of two strands of supplementary nucleotides wound together in form of double helix as deduced by **Watson and Crick.**
- Double stranded DNA molecule – 1000 micron long when straightened. Each strand has deoxyribose sugar and phosphate groups (A & G) are Purines (T&C) are pyrimidines, two strands are held together by hydrogen bonds.
  - A + T = G + C constant for each species.
- **RNA** – Structurally similar but ribose sugar is present and Uracil replaced by Thymine.
- **Gene** – Segment of DNA which specifies a particular polypeptide.
- **Codon** – Genetic information in sequence of three nucleotides (Triplet code).

Central Dogma:

- DNA → RNA → protein.
- **mRNA:** Introns + exons (Prokaryote – only exon) (Introns are removed).
- **Start codon:** AUG.Q
- **Shine:** Dalgarno sequence – AGGAGG (Q Kozak sequence-Eukaryote).
- **Anti-Shine:** Dalgarno sequence – CCUCCU.
- **Stop codon:** UAG ("amber"),UAA ("ochre"), UGA ("opal").Q

Plasmid:

- **Extra chromosomal DNA substances.**
- Circular and double stranded DNA molecules that encode traits that are not essential for bacterial viability.Q
- **Plasmids are of different types:**
  - F factor (Fertility factor).
  - R factors (Resistance factor).
  - Col factor.
- Plasmids confer new properties to recipient bacteria
  - Resistance to one or several antibiotics.
  - Production of toxins.
  - Synthesis of cell surface structures required for adherence or colonization.
- Plasmids integrated with host chromosome are known as *episomes*.

Phenotypic variation – Bacterial cell may exhibit different phenotypic appearances, reversible.

1. Salmonella typhi is flagellated but grown in phenol produces without flagella.
2. Inducible enzyme like β galactosidase is produced when grown in medium containing lactose.

Gene Regulation – Operon concept by (Jacob and Monod).

Mutation

Random, undirected heritable variation caused by change in nucleotide sequence of the DNA of the cell. Frequency ranges from $10^{(-2)}$ to $10^{(-10)}$ per bacterium per division.

Condition lethal mutant – Able to live under certain permissive conditions but not under restrictive conditions.

Types of Mutation

Point mutation – Base pair substitution, Frame shift mutation.

Multisite mutation – Large number of base pairs are altered in DNA by **Addition, deletion, duplication, inversion.**

Base pair substitution – Transition, Transversion.

Transition is purine replaced by purine, Pyrimidine replaced by pyrimidine.

Transversion is purine replaced by pyrimidine, pyrimidine replaced by purine.

FRAME shift mutation – DNA replication one or few base pairs are inserted into or deleted from the DNA, it shifts the normal reading frame.

- Both substitution and frame shift mutation give rise to an altered codon which specifies different amino acid known as **missense mutation.**
- **Nonsense mutation** – **Stop codon terminates** prematurely protein synthesis and partial polypeptide is produced.
- Tests for **mutation** – Fluctuation test, Replica plating, Amies test (for mutagenicity).

1. **Transduction:** Transfer of genetic material from on bacterium to another by a bacteriophage is known as transduction. Most widespread mechanism of gene transfer among Staphylococcus aureus (MRSA).Q
2. **Transformation:** Transfer of genetic material through the agency of free DNA. (**BPH** – Bacillus, Pneumococcus and Hemophillus influenza)–Griffith (pneumococcus).Q
3. **Conjugation:** DNA is transferred through direct cell contact. Gram negative anerobes like E. coli, *Bacteroides, Porphyromonas, and Fusobacterium use this method of gene transfer.* Most widespread mechanism of gene transfer among prokaryotes. DESCRIBED BY LEDERBERG AND TATUM IN E.COLI (K12)Q
4. **Lysogenic Conversion:** Phage DNA becomes integrated with bacterial chromosome as the prophage which codes for new characteristic, e.g., Toxin production in Corynebacterium diptheriae.

Transduction

- **Generalised or restricted.**
- Lysogenic conversion.
- **Phage coded toxin:**
  - Diphtheria toxin, cholera toxin, E. coli.
  - Str pyogenes exotoxin A, C.
- Bacteriophage passes two types of life cycle – Lytic (Virulent) cycle and Lysogenic (Temperate) cycle.

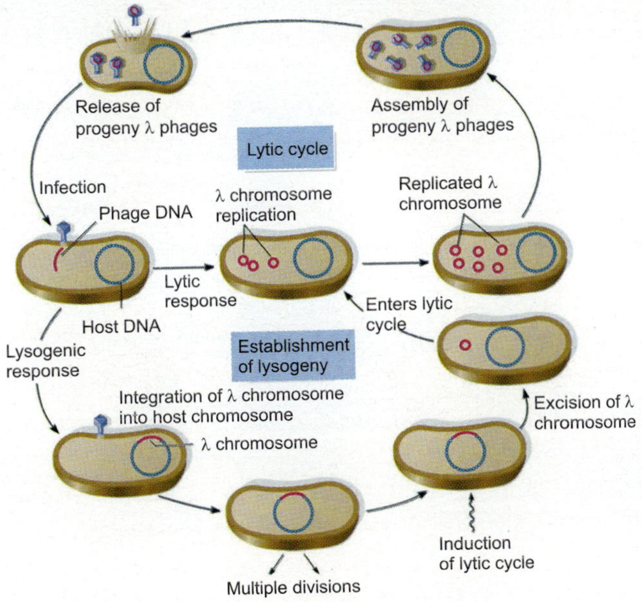

Transformation

- Agency of free DNA.
- **Griffith experiment** – Mouse dead by dead capsulated Pneumococcus + live non capsulated Pneumococcus and on autopsy he found live capsulated Pneumococcus thereby proving transforming factor plays role which was further confirmed by **Avery, Macleod and McCarty** in 1944 as free DNA.

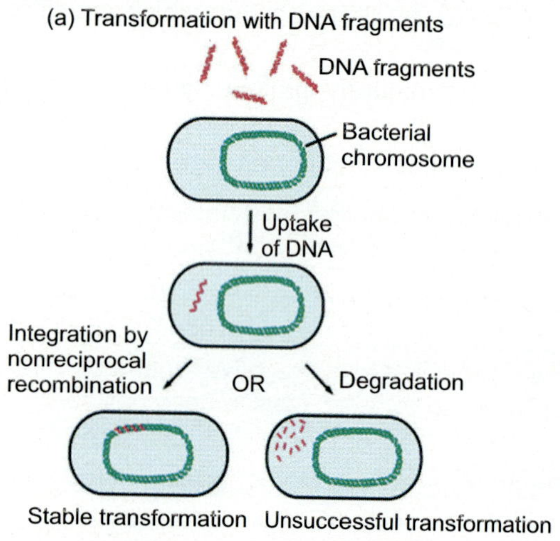

Conjugation

- **Male donor mates with female recipient, forms conjugation tube by sex pilus,** transfers the plasmid coding for sex pilus, thus making female to male bacteria.
- **F factor** – Codes for sex pilus and self transfer but doesn't carry any drug resistant gene.
- **HFr** – F factor integrated to chromosome, high frequency conjugation with F- cell, but rarely converts F- to F+ cell.
- **F′** – F factor released from chromosome carrying chromosomal gene.

R factor – (RTF + r determinants + other virulence genes).

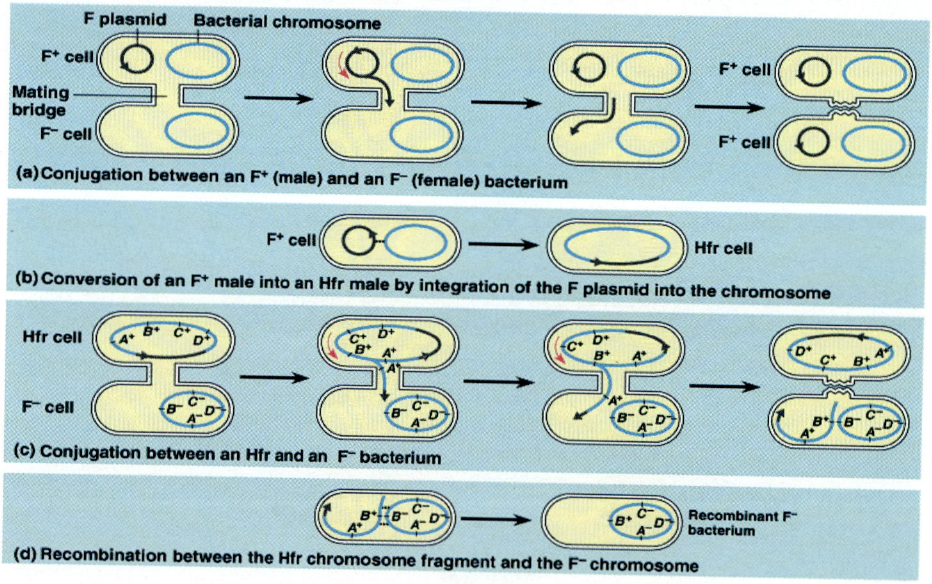

Transposon

- **Jumping gene** – Between chromosome and extra chromosomal DNA.
- Barabara McClintok–Discovered it.
- **Hair pin like** – Centre + inverted repeats on both end.
- Carry drug resistant gene.
- Non replicative.
- DNA homology not required for transfer.

PCR

- Polymerase chain reaction – Requires:
  - **Taq Polymerase enzyme.**
  - Primers.
  - Nucleotide, Mg.Q
  - Steps.
- DNA extraction.
- Amplification:
  - **Denaturation (95°C).**
  - **Primer annealing (55°C).**
  - **Extension (72°C).**
- Gel electrophoresis of amplified product or by real time PCR machine analysed.

PCR is used for rapid analysis of organisms within hours, versatile tool useful in infectious, genetic or neoplastic diseases, in forensic investigations.Q

BACTERIOLOGY OF WATER

Indicator of Fecal Contamination of Water

- Thermotolerant E.coli (recent contamination) – Most definite.
- Coliform count.
- Fecal streptococci.
- Clostridium perfringens.

Detection of Coliform Count

- Presumptive coliform count.
- Multiple tube method.
- Presmuptive coliform count–Most probable number detected by McCardy table.
- MacConkey fluid medium is used.

Differential Coliform Count

Eijkman test: To detect Thermotolerant E.coli grown at 44°C and Indole +ve.

MCQs

1. **Which is an eukaryote?** *(PGI Nov 2013)*
   (a) Mycoplasma (b) Bacteria
   (c) Fungus (d) Chlamydia
2. **Prokaryotes are characterised by:** *(AI 06)*
   (a) Absence of nuclear membrane (b) Presence of microvilli on its surface
   (c) Presence of smooth endoplasmic reticulum (d) All of the above
3. **Mesosomes in bacteria are functional unit for:** *(Recent MCQ)*
   (a) Lipid storage (b) Protein synthesis
   (c) Respiratory enzymes (d) None
4. **Which of the following is not capsulated?** *(Recent MCQ)*
   (a) Pneumococcus (b) Cryptococcus
   (c) Meningococcus (d) Proteus

5. Bacteria with tuft of flagellae at one end are called:
(a) Monotrichate
(b) Bipolar
(c) Peritrichate
(d) Lophotrichate

6. Non motile organism: *(Recent MCQ)*
(a) E. coli
(b) Vibrio cholera
(c) Proteus vulgaris
(d) Shigella dysentery

7. All are true *except*:
(a) Exotoxin has enzymatic action
(b) Endotoxin has enzymatic action
(c) Exotoxin is highly antigenic
(d) Endotoxin is weakly antigenic

8. All of the following organisms are known to survive intracellularly *except*: *(AI 05)*
(a) Neisseria meningitides
(b) Salmonella typhi
(c) Streptococcus pyogenes
(d) Legionella pneumophila

9. All the following pathogenic bacteria fulfill Kochs postulates *except*:
(a) Treponema pallidum
(b) Yersinia pestis
(c) Bacillus anthracis
(d) Helicobacter pylori

10. True regarding lag phase is all *except*:
(a) Bacteria adapts to environment
(b) Bacteria increases in size
(c) Exponential growth is there
(d) It is the first phase of bacterial growth curve

11. Which one of the following bacteria is facultative anaerobe? *(AI 07)*
(a) Pseudomonas
(b) Bacteroides
(c) Escherichia
(d) Clostridia

12. Cell wall deficient organisms are: *(Recent MCQ)*
(a) Chlamydia
(b) Mycoplasma
(c) Staphylococcus
(d) Clostridium

13. Exaltation is: *(UPPGMEE 02)*
(a) Decreased virulence
(b) Increased virulence
(c) No change
(d) None

Staining Methods and Microscopy of Bacteria

14. Dark ground microscopy is used for:
(a) TPI
(b) Kahn's test
(c) FTA-ABS
(d) VDRL

15. Dye used in fluorescent microscopy:
(a) Thioflavin T
(b) Congo red
(c) Brilliant blue
(d) Eosin
(e) Auramine

16. Wet India ink preparation is used for demonstration of: *(PGI May 14)*
(a) Flagella
(b) Capsule
(c) Slender organism
(d) Spirochetes
(e) Fimbriae
(f) Flagella, Spirochaetes

17. All organisms show bipolar staining *except*:
(a) Calymatobacter granulomatis
(b) Yersinia pestis
(c) H. influenzae
(d) Pseudomonas mallei

Sterilization and Disinfection

18. Sterilising agents include: *(PGI May 14)*

(a) Ethylene oxide
(b) Alcohol
(c) Dry heat
(d) Ether
(e) Chlorhexidine

19. The best skin disinfectant: *(Recent MCQ)*

(a) Alcohol
(b) Betadine
(c) Savlon
(d) Phenol

20. Which of the following used for skin disinfection?

(a) Isopropyl alcohol
(b) Cresol
(c) Chlorhexidine
(d) Lysol

21. Sterilisation of media containing serum: *(Recent MCQ)*

(a) Autoclaving
(b) Micropore filter
(c) Gamma radiation
(d) Centrifugation

22. Which of the following is true about pasteurization? *(AI 2K)*

(a) It kills all bacteria and spores
(b) It kills all bacteria except thermoduric bacteria
(c) It kills 95% of microorganisms
(d) All bacteria are destroyed

23. Intermittent sterilization:

(a) Pasteurisation
(b) Boiling
(c) Autoclaving
(d) Tyndallization

24. Hot air oven is used for sterilization of *except*: *(MP 2001)*

(a) Glass wares
(b) Dusting powder
(c) L.J.media
(d) Liquid paraffin

25. Autoclaving is done in: *(Recent MCQ)*

(a) Dry air at 121 degree C and 15 psi
(b) Steam at 100 degree C for 30 minutes
(c) Steam at 121 degree C for 15 minutes
(d) Dry air at 160 degree C for 30 minutes

26. Out of the following the true statement regarding sterilization is: *(AI 97)*

(a) Dry heat is the best method of sterilization of liquid paraffin
(b) All glass wares are best sterilized by boiling at 100°C
(c) Bacterial vaccines are best sterilized by ethylene oxide
(d) Pasteurization of milk by flash method is done by heating at 63 degree C for 30 minutes

27. Endoscope tube is sterilized by: *(Recent MCQ)*

(a) Glutaraldehyde
(b) Formalin
(c) Autoclaving
(d) Boiling

28. The operating temperature in an ethylene oxide sterilization during a warm cycle is: *(AIIMS 04)*

(a) 49-63°C
(b) 92-110°C
(c) 20-35°C
(d) 68-88°C

29. Which of the following is an important disinfectant on account of effectively destroying gram positive and gram negative bacteria viruses and even spores at low pH levels?

(a) Alcohol
(b) Hexachlorophene
(c) Phenol
(d) Chlorine

30. According to Spaulding classification system of sterilization, following is true *except*: *(AIIMS Nov 10)*

(a) "Non-critical devices" come into contact with intact skin

(b) Semi-critical equipment need low-level sterilization

(c) "Semi-critical devices" come into contact with non-sterile mucous membranes or non-intact skin

(d) Cardiac catheter is critical equipment

31. Which of the following is an intermediate level disinfectant?

(a) 2% glutaraldehyde
(b) Ethylene oxide
(c) Hypochlorite
(d) None

32. Plasma sterilization accuracy is assessed using:

(a) Bacillus subtilis
(b) Bacillus stereothermophilus
(c) Staphylococcus aureus
(d) Clostridium tetani

33. Sputum can be disinfected by all *except*:

(a) Autoclaving
(b) Chlorhexidine
(c) Boiling
(d) Cresol

34. Choose the correct ones for the decreasing order of resistance to sterilization: *(PGI Nov 13, Dec 07)*

(a) Prions, Bacterial spores, Bacteria
(b) Bacterial spores, Bacteria, Prions
(c) Bacteria, Prions, Bacterial spores
(d) Prions, Bacteria, Bacterial spores
(e) Bacterial spores, Prions, Bacteria

35. Which of the following statements regarding disinfectant is not true?

(a) Hypochlorites are bactericidal and inactivated by organic matter

(b) Glutaraldehyde is sporicidal and not inactivated by organic matter

(c) Formaldehyde is bactericidal, sporicidal and virucidal

(d) Phenol is bactericidal and readily inactivated by organic matter

36. Phenol coefficient indicates: *(JIPMER 2014)*

(a) Efficacy of a disinfectant
(b) Dilution of a disinfectant
(c) Quantity of a disinfectant
(d) Purity of a disinfectant

37. Swarming growth on culture is characteristic of which Gram-negative organism?

(a) Clostridium welchii
(b) Clostridium tetani
(c) Bacillus cereus
(d) Proteus mirabilis

38. Specific reason to disallow the sample for culture: *(Recent MCQ)*

(a) Sample brought within 2 hours of collection

(b) Sample brought in sterile plastic container

(c) Sample brought in formalin

(d) Sample obtained after cleaning the collection site

Culture Methods and Culture Media

39. Which anticoagulant is used when blood is sent for blood culture?

(a) Sodium citrate
(b) EDTA
(c) Oxalate
(d) SPS

40. Robert Koch assistant advised him to use agar instead of gelatine for solidifying culture media for cultivation of bacteria as:

(a) Agar has more nutrition pattern
(b) Gelatin melts at 37°C
(c) Gelatin is not easily available
(d) Agar is cheaper

41. pH of Sabourauds agar is:

(a) 12 (b) 8-10 (c) 4-6 (d) 6-8

42. Blood agar is:

(a) Enriched media
(b) Indicator media
(c) Enrichment media
(d) Selective media

Bacterial Genetics

43. Jumping gene is: (*PGI 98*)

(a) Transposon
(b) Cosmid
(c) Episome
(d) Plasmid

44. The segment of DNA between chromosomal and extrachromosomal DNA molecules within the cells are: (*UP 06, 07, 09*)

(a) Transposons
(b) Cosmid
(c) Plasmid
(d) EPisomes

45. False regarding bacterial plasmids is: (*Manipal 06, 09*)

(a) Extrachromosomal
(b) Eliminated by treating with radiation
(c) Transmission of different species
(d) Can cause lysogenic conversion

46. Bacteria may acquire characteristics by all of the following *except*: (*Kerala 09*)

(a) Taking up soluble DNA fragments across their cell wall from other species
(b) Incorporating part of host DNA
(c) Through bacteriophages
(d) Through conjugation
(e) Mutation

47. Genetic information is transferred by phage is called: (*Recent MCQ*)

(a) Transformation
(b) Transduction
(c) Lysogenic conversion
(d) Transcription

48. F factor integrates with bacterial chromosome to form: (*PGI 93*)

(a) HFr
(b) F-ve
(c) RTF+r
(d) RTF

49. Horizontal transmission of 'R' factor is by:

(a) Transduction
(b) Transformation
(c) Conjugation
(d) Fusion

50. F plasmid of high frequency recombination is a: (*APPG 09*)

(a) Extrachromosomal
(b) Chromosomal
(c) Mesosomes
(d) Ribosomes

51. Property of acquiring antibiotic resistance from viral colony is by: (*PGI 96*)

(a) Transference
(b) Conjugation
(c) Transduction
(d) Mutation

52. The following phenomenon is responsible for antibiotic resistance in bacteria due to slime production:

(a) Co-aggregation
(b) Biofilm formation
(c) Mutation evolving in altered target site TB antibiotics
(d) Mutation evolving a target bypass mechanism

53. The role of plasmids in conjugation was first described by Lederberg and Tatum (46) in: (*AIIMS Nov 02*)

(a) H. influenzae
(b) Corynebacterium
(c) Pseudomonas
(d) E.Coli

ANSWERS AND EXPLANATIONS

1. **Ans. is 'c'** i.e., Fungus (***Ref:*** *Ananthanarayan, 9th/e, p. 10 and 8th/e, p. 10, 13*)

   Prokaryotes – Bacteria and blue green algae.

   Eukaryotes – Fungi, parasites, plants and animals.

2. **Ans. is 'a'** i.e., Absence of nuclear membrane (***Ref:*** *Ananthanarayan, 9th/e, p. 10 and 8th/e, p. 10, 13*)

Prokaryotes	Eukaryotes
Nuclear membrane absent	**Nuclear membrane well defined**
Cytoplasmic structures absent, e.g., Mitochondria, Lysosomes, Golgi apparatus, and endoplasmic reticulum are absent.	**All these cell organelles are present**
In cell wall muramic acid and diaminopimelic acids (DAPA) present	**Both absent in cell wall**
No sterols in cell membrane	**Sterols present in cell membrane**
E.g.: Bacteria, blue-green algae	**Fungi, protozoa, slime moulds**
Site of respiration – Mesosomes	**Mitochondria**

3. **Ans. is 'c'** i.e., Respiratory (***Ref:*** *Ananthanarayan, 9th/e, p. 16, 17 and 8th/e, p. 18*)

   Mesosomes are the principle site of respiratory enzymes in bacteria, i.e., functionally they are similar to mitochondria.

4. **Ans. is 'd'** i.e., Proteus (***Ref:*** *Ananthanarayan, 9th/e, p. 280, 613 and 8th/e, p. 279-280*)

   Most of Bacterial Capsule is made up of polysaccharide but Bacillus anthracis capsule is polypeptide in nature.

   Proteus is non-capsulated and motile (produce swarming on blood agar).

5. **Ans. is 'd'** i.e., Lophotrichate (***Ref:*** *Ananthanarayan, 9th/e, p. 19 and 8th/e, p. 21*)

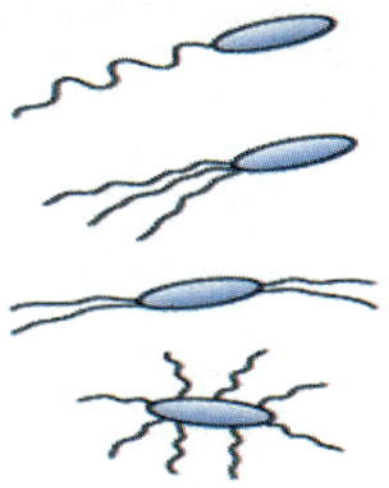

6. **Ans. is 'd'** i.e., Shigella dysentery (*Explained in book text*)

   Entire Enterobacteriaceae family is motile except Shigella and Klebsiella.

7. **Ans. is 'b'** i.e., Endotoxin has enyzmatic action (***Ref:*** *Ananthanarayan, 8th/e, p. 78, 79, 9th/e, p. 80-81*)

   Highly enzymatic activity is present in Exotoxin not endotoxin. (*Rest explained in book text*).

8. **Ans. is 'c'** i.e., Streptococcus pyogenes (*Explained in book text*)

   Streptococcus pyogenes grows extracellular and causes pyogenic infection.

   Intracellular bacteria are Listeria monocytogenes, Legionella, Yersinia, Salmonella typhi, Shigella, Neisseria, Mycobacterium, Francisella tularensis, Pneumococci.

9. **Ans. is 'a'** i.e., Treponema pallidum (***Ref:*** *Ananthanarayan, 9th/e, p. 405 and 8th/e, p. 271*)

   There are some bacteria which do not satisfy that Koch's postulates as they cannot be isolated on culture media like T. pallidum and M. leprae.

10. **Ans. is 'c'** i.e., Exponential growth is there (*Explained in book text*)

    Exponential growth occurs in Lag phase not in log phase.

11. **Ans. is 'c'** i.e., Dry heat (***Ref:*** *Ananthanarayan, 8th/e, p. 271*)

    All member of Enterobacteriaceae family are facultative anaerobes.

    Pseudomonas – strict aerobe.

    Clostridium and Bacteroids – Anaerobes.

12. **Ans. is 'b'** i.e., Mycoplasma (***Ref:*** *Ananthanarayan, 9th/e, p. 386 and 8th/e, p. 16*)

Mycoplasma is bacteria that are cell wall deficient and hence don't possess a stable morphology.

Mycoplasma represents Stable L-forms.

- L-forms named after Lister INSTITUTE, London.
- Streptobacillus moniliformis, Mycoplamsa.
- Resistant to cell wall acting drug.

Protoplast (Gm+ve), Spheroplast (Gm -ve).

13. **Ans. is 'b'** i.e., Increased virulence (***Ref:*** *Ananthanarayan, 9th/e, p. 74 and 8th/e, p. 78*)

Increased virulence – Exaltation.

Decreased virulence – Attenuation.

14. **Ans. is 'a'** i.e., TPI (***Ref:*** *Ananthanarayan, 9th/e, p. 11 and 8th/e, p. 13, 376*)

In TPI test, the serum of patient with complement and T. pallidum maintained in a complex medium anaerobically. If the antibodies are present, the treponemes are immobilized, that is rendered the no motility, when examined under dark ground illumination.

15. **Ans. is 'e'** i.e., Auramine (***Ref:*** *Ananthanarayan, 9th/e, p. 10, 11 and research articles*)

Auramine, Rhodamine, Lissamine, Fluoresceine, isothiocynate.

16. **Ans. is 'b'** i.e., Capsule (*Explained in book text*)

India ink staining is Negative staining – used for capsule demonstration.

17. **Ans. is 'c'** i.e., H. influenzae (***Ref:*** *Ananthanarayan, 9th/e, p. 331 and 8th/e, p. 333, 397*)

Safety pin like appearance – Bipolar staining – Y. pestis, Burkholderia, H. ducreyi, Calymatobacter granulomatis, Vibrio parahemolyticus.

18. **Ans. are 'a, c'** i.e., Ethylene oxide and Dry heat (***Ref:*** *Ananthanarayan, 9th/e*)

Important methods of sterilization are – Heat, Ionizing radiation, Ethylene oxide gas, Plasma, Formaldehyde, Glutaraldehyde.

19. **Ans. is 'b'** i.e., Betadine (***Ref:*** *Ananthanarayan, 9th/e*)

Best skin disinfectant is Povidone iodine, Aqueous and alcohol based povidone iodine preparations are widely used in skin disinfection and skin preparation of the skin.

Savlon and Dettol are more active against gram positive bacteria than gram negative bacteria.

20. **Ans. are 'a, c'** i.e., Isopropyl alcohol and Chlorhexidine (***Ref:*** *Ananthanarayan, 9th/e*)

Skin disinfectant – Chlorhexidine (Savlon), Isopropyl alcohol, Povidone iodine-Betadine (best skin disinfectant).

21. **Ans. is 'b'** i.e., Micropore filter (*Explained in book text*)

Serum, trypsin, growth factors, proteins, amino acids, vitamins and hormones are thermolabile and may decompose during autoclaving, so must be sterilized by Membrane filters.

Membrane filters has less pore size than bacteria size and made up with cellulose acetate, cellulose nitrate, polycarbonate etc.

22. **Ans. is 'b'** i.e., It kills all bacteria except thermoduric bacteria (***Ref:*** *Ananthanarayan, 9th/e, p. 31, 8th/e, p. 31-32*)

Thermoduric bacteria – Bacteria which can survive, to varying extents, the pasteurization process.

Pasteurization kills nearly 90% of bacteria in milk except certain bacteria like Coxiella burnetti which is resistant to Holders method of sterilization but killed by Flash method of Sterilization.

23. **Ans. is 'd'** i.e., Tyndallization (***Ref:*** *Ananthanarayan, 9th/e, p. 31 and 8th/e, p. 31-32*)

Sugar and Gelatin containing media are sterilized by heating at 100°C for 20 mins on three successive days. First day all vegetative forms are killed. Second day germinating spores and remaining if present killed on final day.

24. Ans. is 'c' i.e., L.J. media (***Ref:*** *Ananthanarayan, 9th/e, p. 30 and 8th/e, p. 31, 32*)

L.J. media is sterilized by Inspissator.

Hot air oven is used to sterilize – Glassware, Glass syringes, Swabs, Forceps, Scissors, scalpels, Liquid paraffin, Dusting powder, Fat and grease.

25. Ans. is 'c' i.e., Steam at 121 degree C for 15 minutes (***Ref:*** *Ananthanarayan, 9th/e, p. 32 and Baveja, 4th/e, p. 33*)

Steaming at 121°C for 15 mins at 15 lbs pressure.

26. Ans. is 'a' i.e., Dry heat is the best method of sterilization of liquid paraffin

(***Ref:*** *Ananthanarayan, 9th/e, p. 30 and 8th/e, p. 31, 32, 33; Baveja, 4th/e, p. 30*)

Liquid paraffin is sterilized by Hot air oven (dry heat).

27. Ans. is 'a' i.e., Glutaraldehyde (***Ref:*** *Baveja, 4th/e, p. 35*)

Effective against Mycobacterium species, fungi and virucidal, less toxic and irritant to eyes and skin than Formaldehyde, Accepted as sterilant and high level disinfectant can be used in presence of organic matter used as 2% buffered solution (CIDEX) for 20 min used for cystoscopes, endoscopes, bronchoscope, Sterilize plastic endotracheal tubes, face masks.

28. Ans. is 'a' i.e, 49-63°C (***Ref:*** *Ananthanarayan, 9th/e, p. 35, 36; Baveja, 4th/e, p. 38*)

EO sterilization cycles – Cold cycle at 37± 5 and Warm cycle 54 ± 5°C.

29. Ans. is 'd' i.e., Chlorine (***Ref:*** *Baveja, 4th/e, p. 36*)

Disinfection action of chlorine compounds is by release of free chlorine, when hypochlorites are added to water forms hypochlorous acid which is strong oxidizing agent and effective disinfectant, action is influenced by organic matter. Hypochlorite (1%) used for routine serological disinfection, should not be used in presence of formaldehyde as it is carcinogenic.

30. Ans. is 'b' i.e., Semicritical equipment need low-level sterilization (***Ref:*** *Ananthanarayan, 9th/e, p. 37*)

Semicritical equipments need high level disinfection.

31. Ans. is 'c' i.e., Hypochlorite (*Explained in book text*)

Level of disinfectant	**Examples**
High	2% glutaraldehyde (cidex), 8% formaldehyde, H_2O_2, Ethylene oxide
Intermediate	0.5% iodine, hypochlorite, 70-90% ethanol, isopropanol
Low	Quarternary ammonium compounds, mercurials, iodophores

- **High-level disinfection:** Can be expected to destroy all microorganisms, with the exception of large numbers of of bacterial spores.
- **Intermediate disinfection:** Inactivates Mycobacterium tuberculosis, vegetative bacteria, most viruses, and most fungi; does not not necessarily kill bacterial spores.
- **Low-level disinfection:** Can kill most bacteria, some viruses, and some fungi; cannot be relied on to kill resistant microorganisms such as tubercle bacilli or bacterial spores.

32. Ans. is 'b' i.e., Bacillus stereothermophilus (*Research articles*)

Hot air oven	Clostridium tetani non-toxigenic strain, B.subtilis subsp niger
Autoclave	B.stearothermophillus, B.subtilis subsp niger
Filtration	Brivundimonas dimunata, Serratia
Ionizing radiation	B.pumilus
Ethylene oxide	B.Globigi
Plasma sterilization	B.stearothermophillus, B.subtilis subsp niger

33. Ans. is 'b' i.e., Chlorhexidine (***Ref:*** *Baveja, 4th/e, p. 34*)

Autoclaving is the safest and most effective method for sputum disinfection, incineration or buring is an effective alternative. Boiling used after an initial disinfection by 5% phenol (carbolic acid) or its derivatives like Lysol and cresol.

34. Ans. is 'a' i.e., Prions, Bacterial spores, Bacteria (*Explained in book text*)

Prions

↓

Bacterial Spores (*Bacillus atrophaeus*)

↓

Coccidia (*Cryptosporidium*)

↓

Mycobacteria (*M. tuberculosis, M. terrae*)

↓

Non-lipid or small virus (polio, *coxsackie*)

↓

Fungi (*Aspergillus, Candida spp.*)

↓

Vegetative bacteria (*S. aureus, P. aeruginosa*)

↓

Lipid or medium-sized viruses (HIV, herpes, HBV)

35. Ans. is 'd' i.e., Phenol is bactericidal and readily inactivated by organic matter (*Explained in book text*)

Phenolic act by denaturing proteins and disrupting cell membranes and effective in the presence of organic materials.

36. Ans. is 'a' i.e., Efficacy of a disinfectant (*Explained in book text*)

$$\text{Phenolic coefficient of a test disinfectant} = \frac{\text{Disinfectant (Highest dilution) that kills S.typhi in agiven time}}{\text{Phenol (Highest dilution) that kills S.typhi in a given same time}}$$

37. Ans. is 'd' i.e., Proteus mirabilis (*Explained in book text*)

Proteus (Gram negative bacilli), Clostridium tetani (Anaerobic Gram positive bacilli).

38. Ans. is 'c' i.e., Sample brought in formalin (Formalin is used for stool samples for parasitic investigations and it is anti-bacterial so cannot use for sample collection for bacterial isolation).

Guidelines for proper specimen collection:

1. Collect specimen before giving antibiotics or antivirals.
2. Collect specimen with as little skin contamination.
3. Use sterilized equipment, aseptic technique to collect specimens.
4. Clearly label the specimen with patients name, hospital ID number, Date and time of collection.
5. Collect adequate amount of specimen.
6. Clean the skin with best disinfectant like povidone iodine before taking sample.
7. Collect fluid specimens in screw capped, leak proof containers.
8. Proper transport vial should be used to carry samples.
9. Microbiology and Virology culture should not be collected in Formalin.

39. Ans. is 'd' i.e., SPS (*Book—Bailey and Scott Microbiology*)

These media contain 0.03% SPS (Sodium polyenathol sulfonate), a polyanionic anticoagulant which additionally inhibits complement and lysozyme activity.

40. Ans. is 'b' i.e., Gelatin melts at 37°C (*Explained in book text*)

Gelatin melts at relatively low temperature (<35°C) while agar melts at around 90°C, so normal bacterial cultures are preferred over agar rather than Gelatin which melts at normal incubation temperature of 37°C.

41. Ans. is 'c' i.e., 4–6 (***Ref:*** *Ananthnarayan, 9th/e, p. 592 and 8th/e, p. 601*)

Sabourauds dextrose agar (Selective media) is maintained at PH of 5.4 and same is used for fungal culture.

42. Ans. is 'a' i.e., Enriched media (*Explained in book text*)

Blood agar-enriched media – use for demonstration of Hemolysis and swarming.

43. Ans. is 'a' i.e., Transposon (***Ref:*** *Ananthanarayan, 9th/e, p. 63 and 8th/e, p. 64*)

Transposons are also known as jumping genes.

Transposons are also known as jumping genes. They move between chromosomal DNA and extra chromosomal DNA within cell. They take part in drug resistance mechanism.

44. Ans. is 'a' i.e., Transposons (*Already explained*)

45. Ans. is 'd' i.e., Can cause lysogenic conversion (***Ref:*** *Ananthanarayan, 9th/e, p. 60 and 8th/e, p. 60*)

- Lysogenic conversion is due to phage (viral) genome, not due to bacterial plasmid.
- Plasmid is extrachromosomal DNA and Radiation can damage Plasmid.
- Plasmid can be transferred to different species, e.g., multi-drug resistance transfer between shigella and E. coli factor.

46. Ans. is 'b' i.e., Incorporating part of host DNA (***Ref:*** *Ananthanarayan, 9th/e, p. 59, 60 and 8th/e, p. 64*)

Mutation can bring changes like drug resistance.

Gene transfer in bacteria:

(a) Transformation – Transfer of genetic material through the agency of free DNA.

(b) Transduction – Transfer of a portion of DNA by bacteriophage.

(c) Conjugation – Transfer of genetic material by physical contact.

(d) Lysogenic conversion – Incorporation of phage DNA into host DNA.

47. Ans. is 'b' i.e., Transduction (*Already explained*)

48. Ans. is 'a' i.e., HFr (Explained in book text)

Cells in which f factor is integrated into chromosome is known as HFr cells.

49. Ans. is 'c' i.e., Conjugation (***Ref:*** *Ananthanarayan, 9th/e, p. 62 and 8th/e, p. 64*)

50. Ans. is 'a' i.e., Extrachromosomal (***Ref:*** *Ananthanarayan, 9th/e, p. 60, 8th/e, p. 60*)

F factor being a plasmid, it may integrate with bacterial chromosome.

51. Ans. is 'c' i.e., Transduction (***Ref:*** *Ananthanarayan, 9th/e, p. 59 and 8th/e, p. 63, 67, 681*)

Acquiring antibiotic resistance by viral colony (bacteriophage) is by transduction.

52. Ans. is 'b' i.e., Biofilm formation (***Ref:*** *Greenwood's Medical Microbiology, 16th/e, p. 16, 38, 86*)

Slime is an amorphous, viscid colloidal material that is secreted extracellularly by some bacteria (e.g., Staph epidermidis). The slime remains around the bacteria and provides a matrix in which biofilm formation can take place. In biofilm formation the bacterial colony is spread very thinly (300-400 nm thick) for e.g., formation of biofilms on catheters and prosthetic devices. This biofilm formation in the slime provides antibiotic resistance by restricting access of drugs to the bacterium.

53. Ans. is 'd' i.e., E.coli (***Ref:*** *Ananthanarayan, 9th/e, p. 651*)

Bacterial conjugation was first observed by Lederberg and Tatum in strain of E.coli K-12.

RED ALERT POINTS

1. **Protoscope, Endoscope is sterilized by: Cidex (2% Glutaraldehyde).**
2. Ethylene oxide is used for gaseous sterilization, used to sterilize disposable plastic petridishes, sutures, syringes, heart lung machines, respirators and dental equipments, materials are sterilized for 4 hours at 55 degree C.
3. **Multiple drug resistance spreads by: Conjugation, in TB by mutation and S. aureus by transduction.**
4. **Louis Pasteur is associated with liquid culture concept, coined term vaccine, Vaccine – Cholera, anthrax, rabies (CAR).** Mycobacterium tuberculosis was discovered by: Robert Koch, given solid media concept, hanging drop method. **Microscope was invented by: Antony Van Leeuwenhoek and called organisms as little animalcules.**
5. **Cytoplasmic membrane of bacteria is responsible for:** Selective permeability, contain enzymes necessary for cell wall synthesis. **Mesosomes are vesicular, convoluted structures formed as invaginations of plasma membrane into the cytoplasm, principal centre of respiratory enzymes.**
6. **Peptidoglycans are present in:** Cell wall of gram positive bacteria (thick peptidoglycan layer and muramic acid), gram negative cell wall have periplasmic space, lipids and thin layer of peptidoglycan.
7. **Bacterial cell wall is composed by:** Mucopeptide (peptidoglycan or murein) **scaffoldings of N-acetylglucosamine and N-acetyl muramic acid,** cell wall possesses target sites for antibiotics, lysosomes and bacteriophages. It confers rigidity upon bacteria, takes part in cell division.
8. **Important features of exotoxin:** Protein, enzymatic action, highly antigenic, can be toxoided, produced by both gram (+)ve and gram (-)ve bacteria.

   Important features of endotoxin: Lipopolysaccharide, no enzymatic action, weakly antigenic, produced by gram (-) ve bacteria only.
9. **Order of gram staining:** Gentian violet → Iodine → Ethanol → Safranin.
10. **Special staining methods for T. pallidum:** Fontana's method (for staining films), Levaditi method (for tissue sections).
11. **Schaeffer Fulton test:** Stains bacterial endospores. Kinyoun stain – Modification of acid fast stain.

PRACTICE QUESTIONS

History

1. **Pasteur credited with discovery of:**
   (a) Anthrax vaccine
   (b) Rabies vaccine
   (c) Autoclave
   (d) All of the above
2. **Principles of asepsis in surgery was introduced by:**
   (a) Lister
   (b) Semmelweis
   (c) Pasteur
   (d) Koch
3. **The first human disease proved to have a viral etiology was:**
   (a) Small pox
   (b) Chicken pox
   (c) Rabies
   (d) Yellow fever
4. **Electron microscope was invented by:**
   (a) Ruska
   (b) Ivanisevic
   (c) Goodpasture
   (d) Rous
5. **Which of the following is a recent addition to the Koch's postulates?**
   (a) DNA of isolated bacteria should be identified
   (b) It should be possible to maintain a bacterial cell line
   (c) Specific antibodies to the bacteria should be demonstrated
   (d) All of the above
6. **PCR discovered by:**
   (a) Von Behring
   (b) Pfeiffer
   (c) Metchinkoff
   (d) Kary B Mullis
7. **Koch postulates are all *except*:**
   (a) Organism constantly associate with the lesion
   (b) It is isolated in a pure culture
   (c) When an antigen is introduced in the body, antibodies are formed
   (d) Mycobacterium tuberculosis is an exception to Kochs postulate

Morphology

8. **The resolving power of light microscope is limited by:**
   (a) Lens power
   (b) Length of column
   (c) Wavelength of light
   (d) Colour of light
9. **The resolving power of an electron microscope is:**
   (a) 0.1 nm
   (b) 1 nm
   (c) 100 micron metres
   (d) 200 nm
10. **In supravital staining:**
   (a) Cells are dead
   (b) Cells are alive
   (c) Molecular activity is preserved
   (d) Cell metabolism continues
11. **Bacterial capsules are best demonstrated by:**
   (a) Methylene blue stain
   (b) Grams-II stain
   (c) Negative staining
   (d) Impregnation technique

12. Which of the following is used for impregnation technique?

(a) Silver salts
(b) India Ink
(c) Fluorescein blue
(d) Any of the above

13. When lysosomes act on a gram positive bacterial cell wall it leads to formation of:

(a) Protoplast
(b) Spheroplast
(c) L-forms
(d) All of the above

14. Spheroplast differ from protoplast in:

(a) They are formed from Gram positive bacteria
(b) They are motile
(c) Some cell wall material present
(d) All of the above

15. Following are true of Gram negative bacterial cell wall compared to Gram positive bacteria *except*:

(a) Presence of lipopolysaccharide
(b) Presence of Teichoic acid
(c) Presence of sulphur containing amino acids
(d) Thinner

16. Following are true of Gram positive cell wall *except*:

(a) Variety of amino acids
(b) Absence of LPS
(c) Presence of Teichoic acid
(d) Absence of periplasmic space

17. Volutin granules are believed to be:

(a) Clumps of DNA
(b) Store house of ATP
(c) Mitotic spindle proteins
(d) Clumps of RNA

18. Volutin granules appear when C. diphtheriae is cultured in:

(a) Nutritionally deficient medium
(b) Presence of antibiotics
(c) Symbiosis with pneumococci
(d) All of the above

19. Gram positive bacteria which secrete a strong exotoxin is:

(a) *C.diphtheriae*
(b) *G.renale*
(c) *Morganella*
(d) *B.subtilitis*

20. A nephlometer is used to measure:

(a) Rate for bacterial multiplication
(b) Count of bacteria
(c) Metabolic rate of bacteria
(d) Motility of bacteria

21. During the lag phase of bacterial growth curve there is:

(a) Increase in number
(b) Increase in size
(c) Increased metabolic rate
(d) Decreased metabolic rate

22. Sporulation occurs in:

(a) Lag phase
(b) Log phase
(c) Stationary phase
(d) Decline phase

23. Uniformly staining small sized bacteria are seen in:

(a) Lag phase
(b) Log phase
(c) Stationary phase
(d) Decline phase

24. Which of the following enzyme is absent in anaerobes?

(a) Catalase
(b) Cytochrome peroxidase
(c) Pyruvate carboxylase
(d) All of the above

25. Which of the following bacteria can grow in very wide range of temperatures?

(a) *Pseudomonas*
(b) *Gonococcus*
(c) *Pneumococcus*
(d) *Spirochaetes*

26. Which of the following bacteria grows at very high temperature?

(a) *H.influenzae* (b) *B. stearothermophilus*
(c) *Cl. tetani* (d) *Cl. perfringenes*

27. Thermal death point of most bacteria is between:

(a) 40°C and 55°C (b) 50°C and 60°C
(c) 70°C and 80°C (d) 80°C and 100°C

28. What is lyophilisation?

(a) Means of destroying bacteria (b) A method of sterilization
(c) Freeze drying of bacteria (d) Powdering of bacteria

Sterilization and Disinfection

29. Following are sterilized by hot air oven *except*:

(a) Glassware (b) Swabs
(c) Liquid paraffin (d) Vaccines

30. In pasteurization by holder method the temperature used is:

(a) 63°C for 30 min (b) 72°C for 15 seconds
(c) 100°C for 20 minutes (d) 120°C for 15 minutes

31. The temperature used in tyndallization is:

(a) 62°C (b) 80°C
(c) 100°C (d) 120°C

32. Ultraviolet rays are used for sterilizing:

(a) Operation rooms (b) Beds
(c) Hospital waste (d) All of the above

33. Disposable syringes are best sterilized by:

(a) Autoclaving (b) Hot air oven
(c) Chemicals (d) Gamma ray

34. To be effective as an antiseptic alcohol concentration used is:

(a) 100% (b) 95%
(c) 70% (d) 50%

35. Heart lung machines and respirators are sterilized by:

(a) Formaldehyde (b) Ethylene oxide
(c) Glutaraldehyde (d) Gamma rays

36. Rideal Walker test is used to test the efficacy of a:

(a) Autoclave (b) Hot air oven
(c) Fitters (d) Chemical disinfectants

Culture Media and Culture Methods

37. Which of the following is used as a carrier media for enteric bacilli?

(a) Wilson-Blair medium (b) Buffered glycerol saline
(c) Stuart's medium (d) Mc Conkey agar

38. Craiges tube is used to differentiate bacteria with different:

(a) Growth rate (b) Oxygen requirements
(c) Sizes (d) Motility

39. Kovac's reagent is used to look for:

(a) Indole production
(b) Sugar fermentation
(c) Citrate utilization
(d) None of the above

Bacterial Genetics

40. Operon concept of gene function was introduced by:

(a) Khoranna
(b) Watson and Crick
(c) Jacob and Monad
(d) Mendel

41. Which of the following is the most widespread method of genetic transfer among bacteria?

(a) Transformation
(b) Transduction
(c) Lysogenic conversion
(d) Conjugation

42. Lysogenic conversion refers to:

(a) Lysis of bacteria
(b) Inclusion of prophage of DNA in bacteria
(c) Conversion of one bacterial strain to other
(d) Any of the above

43. Bacterial conjugation was first discovered by:

(a) Lederberg and tatum
(b) Avery McLeod
(c) Griffith
(d) Leeuwenhoek

44. The col factories responsible for synthesis of:

(a) Conjugation tube
(b) Bacteriocins
(c) Colony identifying protein
(d) None of the above

45. The resistance transfer factor was first demonstrated in:

(a) Pseudomonas
(b) Shigella
(c) Salmonella
(d) E.Coli

46. Following are true of transferable drug resistance *except*:

(a) Multiple drug resistance simultaneously
(b) Virulence of bacteria same
(c) Prevent by drug combinations
(d) Very high degree of resistance

47. Genetic engineering by nature is carried out by:

(a) Operans
(b) Transposons
(c) Colfactor
(d) Codons

48. Which of the following is the most important enzyme tool used in genetic engineering?

(a) DNA transcriptase
(b) DNA directed RNA polymerase
(c) Restriction endo nucleases
(d) Reverse transcriptase

Miscellaneous

49. Exaltation refers to:

(a) Enhancement of virulence
(b) Removal for cell wall
(c) Increasing rate of replication
(d) All of the above

50. Following are true of endotoxins *except*:

(a) Heat stable
(b) Cannot be toxoided
(c) Active in very small doses
(d) No specific tissue affinity

51. The condition where bacteria circulate and multiply in the blood is called:

(a) Bacteremia
(b) Pyaemia
(c) Septicemia
(d) All of the above

52. Acid-fast organisms include all of the following *except*:

(a) Mycobacteria tuberculosis
(b) Bacterial endospores
(c) Cryptosporidium
(d) Treponema

53. Bipolar staining is characteristic of:
(a) Yersinia pestis (b) Proteus mirabilis
(c) Pseudomonas aeruginosa (d) All of the above

54. Diene's stain is used for demonstration of:
(a) Helicobacter pylori (b) Anthrax bacilli
(c) Haemophilus (d) Mycoplasma

55. Which of the following stains can demonstrate Rickettsia?
(a) Gram stain (b) Acid fast stain
(c) Giemsa stain (d) All of the above

56. Gomori-methenamine silver stain is required for demonstration of:
(a) Toxoplasma gondii (b) Leishmani denovani
(c) Borrelia burgdorferii (d) Pneumocystis carinni

57. Which of the following bacteria is/are acid fast?
(a) *Actinomyces* (b) *Nocardia*
(c) *Streptomyces* (d) All of the above

58. Fimbriae are demonstrated by:
(a) Culture (b) Gram stain
(c) Biochemical reactions (d) Haemagglutination test

59. False about mesosomes:
(a) Sites of respiratory enzymes in bacteria
(b) Analogous to mitochondria of eukaryotes
(c) Seen in relation to the nuclear body
(d) Coordinate nuclear and cytoplasmic division during binary fission
(e) Not related to protoplasmic membrane

60. False about bacterial capsule:
(a) Protect bacteria
(b) Contribute to virulence
(c) Loss of capsule by mutation also retain the virulence character of bacteria
(d) Repeated subculture my result in the loss of capsule
(e) Demonstrated by serological methods, i.e., Quellung reaction

61. Largest pathogenic Bacillus species is: *(JIPMER 2010)*
(a) Bacillus subtilis (b) Bacillus cereus
(c) Bacillus anthracis (d) Bacillus megaterism

62. Metachromatic granules are found in: *(PGI 2000)*
(a) C. diphtheriae (b) Bacillus
(c) Gardenella vaginalis (d) Acinetobacter species

63. Mesophilic bacteria are those that grow best at temperature of: *(PGI 98)*
(a) -20°C to -1°C (b) -1°C to 4°C
(c) 25°C to 40°C (d) 55°C to 80°C
(e) 20°C to 90°C

64. Agents used for sterilization: *(PGI Nov 10)*
(a) Ethylene oxide (EO) (b) Ionizing radiation
(c) 2% Glutaraldehyde (d) Formaldehyde with low pressure steam
(e) Percholic acid

65. Heating and subsequent plating is a method used for isolation of: *(PGI 93)*

(a) C. diphtheriae
(b) Vibrio
(c) Salmonella
(d) Clostridium

66. Moist heat kills the following *except*: *(PGI 83, 02)*

(a) Brucella
(b) Mycobacteria
(c) Salmonella
(d) Coxiella burnetti

67. A chest physician performs bronchoscopy in the procedure room of the outpatient department to make the instrument safe for use in the next patient waiting outside, the most appropriate method to disinfect the endoscope is by:

(a) 70% Alcohol for 20 min
(b) 2% Glutaraldehyde for 20%
(c) 2% Glutaraldehyde for 10%
(d) 1% Sodium hypochlorite for 15 min

68. Heat labile instruments for use in surgical procedure can be best sterilized by: *(AI 03)*

(a) Absolute alcohol
(b) Ultraviolet rays
(c) Chlorine releasing compounds
(d) Ethylene oxide gas

69. The disposable plastic syringe are best sterilized by: *(Delhi 08)*

(a) Formaldehyde
(b) Ethylene oxide
(c) Hexachloride
(d) UV radiation

70. Sporicidal agents is/are: *(PGI 09, 11)*

(a) Glutaraldehyde
(b) Ethylene oxide
(c) Formaldehyde
(d) Benzaalkonium chloride
(e) Chlorine

71. According to Spaulding classification system of sterilization, following is true *except*: *(AIIMS 10)*

(a) Non-critical devices come into contact with intact skin
(b) Semi-critical equipment need low level sterilization
(c) Semi-critical devices come into contact with non-sterile mucous membranes or non-intact skin
(d) Cardiac catheter is critical equipment

72. Browne's tube is used for: *(NBE Based NEET 12)*

(a) Steam sterilization
(b) Radiation
(c) Chemical sterilization
(d) Filtration

73. Phenolic disinfectant are: *(PGI 05)*

(a) Dettol
(b) Cresol
(c) Lysol
(d) Carbolic acid
(e) Savlon

74. All are true regarding disinfectants *except*: *(AIIMS 11)*

(a) Glutaraldehyde is sporicidal
(b) Hypochlorites are virucidal
(c) Ethylene oxide is intermediate disinfectant
(d) Phenol usually requires organic matter to act

75. Agent which on addition to a colony inhibits its growth and on removal the colony regrow is: *(AI 99)*

(a) Bacteriostatic
(b) Bactericidal
(c) Antibiotic
(d) Antiseptic

76. Sterilization of fiber optic is done by: *(DNB 12)*

(a) Glutaraldehyde
(b) Chlorine
(c) Autoclave
(d) Phenol

77. All of the sterilization methods are properly matched *except*: *(NBE Based AI 13)*

(a) Catgut suture – Radiation
(b) Culture media – Autoclaving
(c) Bronchoscope – Autoclaving
(d) Glassware and syringes – Hot air oven

78. Which one of the following is true? *(AIIMS 06, AI 07)*

(a) Agar has nutrient properties
(b) Chocolate agar is a selective media
(c) Additional selective substances in a solid medium is called as enrichment medium
(d) Nutrient broth is basal medium

79. In nutrient agar concentration of agar is: *(NEET 13)*

(a) 1%
(b) 2%
(c) 3%
(d) 4%

80. Robert Koch assistant advised him to use agar instead of gelatin for solidifying culture media for cultivation of bacteria: *(AI 10, NEET 13)*

(a) Agar has more nutrients
(b) Gelatin melts at 37°C
(c) Gelatin is not easily available
(d) Agar is cheaper

81. Growth of cell-free artificial solid medium is possible for following *except*: *(TN 09)*

(a) Ureaplasma urealyticum
(b) Mycoplasma pneumoniae
(c) C and L form of Proteus vulgaris
(d) Chlamydia

82. Smith Noguchi's media is used for: *(AIIMS 95)*

(a) Salmonella
(b) Klebsiella
(c) Spirochetes
(d) Bacillus

83. In a patient with UTI, CLED media is preferred over MacConkey agar because: *(AIIMS 2001)*

(a) It is a differential medium
(b) It inhibits swarming of Proteus
(c) Promotes growth of Pseudomonas
(d) Promotes growth of Staph aureus and Candida

84. Which one of the following specimen is not refrigerated prior to inoculation: *(JIPMER 10)*

(a) CSF
(b) Urine
(c) Pus
(d) Sputum

85. Stain used in electron microscopy: *(DNB 12)*

(a) 2.5% FAM
(b) Phosphotungstic acid
(c) Saffranin
(d) Coomassie blue

86. Silver impregnation technique is used in the identification of: *(DNB 13)*

(a) Spirochetes
(b) Leptospira
(c) Borrelia
(d) All of the above

87. In blood culture the ratio of blood to reagent is: *(NBE Based AI 13)*

(a) 1:5
(b) 1:20
(c) 1:10
(d) 1: 100

88. Lysis of bacterial colony in culture is seen by which? *(NBE Based AI 13)*

(a) Pox
(b) HSV
(c) Bacteriophage
(d) CMV

89. Drug resistance is not transferred by: *(PGI 2005)*

(a) HFr
(b) Transposons
(c) Plasmids
(d) Chromosomes

90. Conjugation does not involve: *(PGI 2007)*

(a) Bacteriophage (b) HFr
(c) Fr (d) Plasmid

91. False regarding bacterial plasmid is: *(Manipal 12)*

(a) Extrachromosomal DNA (b) Eliminated by treating with radiation
(c) Transmission of different species (d) Can cause lysogenic conversion

92. The specialized type of microscope, which enables quantitative measurement of the chemical constituents of cells, is the: *(Comed 12)*

(a) Optical microscope (b) Interference microscope
(c) Phase contrast microscope (d) Polarized microscope

93. Secular trend in influenza is due to: *(JIPMER 10)*

(a) Antigenic shift (b) Antigenic drift
(c) Endemicity (d) Virulence

94. Recommended transport medium for stool specimen suspected to contain enteric pathogen is: *(Karnataka 11)*

(a) Amie's medium (b) Buffered glycerol saline medium
(c) MacConkey medium (d) Stuart's medium

95. Antonie van Leeuwenhoek is associated with: *(DNB 12)*

(a) Telescope (b) Microscope
(c) Staining procedure (d) Immunization

96. Arrangement of lens from eye to source of light, in light microscope: *(NBE Based 13)*

(a) Ocular lens: Subjective lens: Condensor lens (b) Subjective lens: Ocular lens: Condensor lens
(c) Condensor lens: Subjective lens: Ocular lens (d) Subjective lens: Condensor lens: Ocular lens

ANSWERS

1.	(d)	2.	(a)	3.	(d)	4.	(a)	5.	(c)	6.	(d)	7.	(d)	8.	(c)
9.	(a)	10.	(a)	11.	(c)	12.	(a)	13.	(a)	14.	(c)	15.	(b)	16.	(a)
17.	(b)	18.	(a)	19.	(a)	20.	(b)	21.	(b)	22.	(c)	23.	(b)	24.	(a)
25.	(a)	26.	(b)	27.	(b)	28.	(c)	29.	(d)	30.	(a)	31.	(c)	32.	(a)
33.	(d)	34.	(c)	35.	(b)	36.	(d)	37.	(b)	38.	(d)	39.	(a)	40.	(c)
41.	(b)	42.	(b)	43.	(a)	44.	(b)	45.	(b)	46.	(c)	47.	(b)	48.	(c)
49.	(a)	50.	(c)	51.	(c)	52.	(d)	53.	(a)	54.	(d)	55.	(c)	56.	(d)
57.	(b)	58.	(d)	59.	(e)	60.	(c)	61.	(c)	62.	(a),(c)	63.	(c)	64.	(a), (b) (c), (d)
65.	(d)	66.	(d)	67.	(b)	68.	(d)	69.	(b)	70.	(a),(b) (c),(e)	71.	(b)	72.	(a)
73.	(b),(c) (d)	74.	(c), (d)	75.	(a)	76.	(a)	77.	(c)	78.	(d)	79.	(b)	80.	(b)
81.	(d)	82.	(c)	83.	(d)	84.	(a)	85.	(b)	86.	(d)	87.	(c)	88.	(c)
89.	(a)	90.	(a)	91.	(d)	92.	(b)	93.	(a)	94.	(b)	95.	(b)	96.	(a)

Chapter 5

BACTERIOLOGY

STAPHYLOCOCCUS

- Gram positive cocci, Non fastidious and facultative anaerobes.
- Multiple and arranged in **grape like clusters,** Non motile, non-sporing and non-acid fast.
- All species are **catalase test +ve and Oxidase test is –ve.**

STAPHYLOCOCCUS AUREUS

Staphylococcal Diseases:

Toxin Mediated Infections

1. **Staphylococcal scalded skin syndrome (SSSS)**
   - C/b **Epidermolytic toxin:** Often occurs in newborn (severe form is called Ritter's disease and milder form Pemphigus neonatorum).
2. **Toxic shock syndrome** (DOC – Clindamycin)
   - Multiple system disorder associated with vaginal tampon during menstruation.
   - Fever + Shock + rash + multiple system failure + death.
   - c/b TSST/**Enterotoxin F (Superantigen).**
3. **Food Poisoning (Enterotoxin A)**

   ICP – 1-6 hours (Heat stable, preformed toxin, Vagal stimulation is mechanism of action) and it mimics Bacillus cereus (Emetic strain) in incubation period.

Other Infections:

- **Folliculitis** – Superficial infection of hair follicle.
- **Furuncle (boil)** – Deep infection of hair follicle.
- **Carbuncle** – Multiple furuncles.
- **Breast abscess** – In lactating mother.
- **Cellulitis** – In skin when spreads to subcutaneous tissue.

Acute osteomyelitis, Acute endocarditis, Hospital acquired pneumonia, **Botryomycosis.Q**

Pyomyositis – MCC – Skeletal muscle infection.

Pathogenesis and Virulence Factors:

Cell Wall Associated:

- Peptidoglycan (Endotoxin like activity).
- Teichoic acid (helps in adhesion to mucosal surfaces).
- Protein A – binds to Fc part of IgG and involve up in a reaction called **Coagglutination.Q**

Contd.

Contd.

- Bound coagulase enzyme (which brings about clotting or coagulation of plasma).

Enzymes:

Free coagulase, Hyaluronidase, Phosphatase, Lipase, DNAse, Staphylokinase/fibrinolysin (Helps in spreading infection).

Toxins:

- **Hemolysins** – Damaged RBC – α β γ δ.
- **Leukocidin (Panton Valentine toxin)**–It acts synergistically with γ-hemolysin to damage leucocytes, RBC and macrophages.
- **Epidermolytic/Exfoliative toxin** – Responsible for SSSS.
- **Enterotoxins** – Food poisoning due to preformed toxin (1-6 hours), stimulates the vagus nerve and the vomiting center of the brain, i.e., Type A (most common), Other types B, C1-3, D, E, H and I.

Synergohymenotropic toxins are γ-hemolysin and Panton Valentine toxin because they are not active individually, but in combination they are hemolytic and leucocidal.Q

Lab Diagnosis:

Sample collection:

Pus, Wound swab, Wound Aspirate, Blood etc (According to the site of infection).

Direct Microscopy:

Gram staining of sample – GPC in Clusters with numerous pus cells.

Culture:

- **Blood agar** – β hemolysis (exhibits **Hot-cold phenomenon**-hemolysis starts with 37°C but becomes evident only after chilling).
- **Selective medium – Mannitol Salt agar and Ludlam's medium.Q**
- **Pigmentation (Non-diffusible) – Golden yellow and Pigmentation** enhanced by prolonged aerobic incubation at 22-25°C or by Tween agar.

Identification tests:

- Catalase test +ve.
- Coagulase (Slide and Tube) test:
  Positive – Staph. aureus.
  Negative – CONS (i.e., S. Epidermidis, S. Saprophyticus).
  Note – Both tube (Free) and Slide (Bound) Coagulase positive for S. aureus, S. hyicus and S. intermedius.

Antibiotic Susceptibility Testing (AST)

Done on Mueller Hinton Agar by Kirby Bauer Disc diffusion method.Q

DOC for MSSA – Penicillin G.

DOC for MRSA – Vancomycin (Alternatives-Quinupristin, dalfopristin, TMP-SMX, Daptomycin, Linezoid, Teicoplanin).

STAPH. EPIDERMIDIS

- Normal flora on skin, oropharynx and vagina.
- **Biofilm formation** is a property to cling to surface and causes prosthetic–device (IV catheters, shunts, grafts, pacemaker wires, prosthetic valves, CSF shunts etc.) related infections.
- On blood agar – γ **(Non-hemolytic) – Hemolysis**.

Diseases:

- **MCC of infective endocarditis due to prosthetic valve < 1 year** (After 1 year Streptococcus viridans).
- **Prosthetic** – Device related infections.
- **Remember** – This fellow is **Novobiocin sensitive.Q**

STAPH. SAPROPHYTICUS

- Common cause of UTI in female with child bearing age and sexually active young women.Q
- **Identification Test** – Novobiocin (5 μg) Disk test – Resistant (Sensitive to Staph epidermidis).Q

EXTRA EDGE POINTS ***

- **Superantigens – TSST-1, ET and Enterotoxins of S. aureus and S. pyogenic exotoxin (SPE A and C)** – They stimulate the T-cells non-specifically (by binding to Vβ region of T-cell receptors) causing excessive production of cytokines which leads to fatal multisystem diseases.
- **Vancomycin resistant S. aureus (VRSA)** – Resistance due to Van A gene. DOC – Quinupristin, dalfopristin, TMP-SMX, Daptomycin, Linezoid.
- **MRSA is due to Mec A gene and major change is in PBP changes to PBP2a (PBP** – Penicillin binding proteins).
- **Remember friends – Alpha hemolysin shows paradoxical action and Beta hemolysin shows Hot and Cold phenomenon.**

MCQs

1. **Which of the following is catalase +ve gram positive cocci?** *(Recent MCQ)*
   (a) Staphylococcus (b) Streptococcus
   (c) Listeria (d) Meningococci
2. **All of the following statements about staphylococcus aureus are true, *except*:** *(AI 10)*
   (a) Most common source of infection is cross infection from infected people
   (b) About 30% of general population is healthy nasal carriers
   (c) Epidermolysin and TSS toxin are superantigens
   (d) Methicillin resistance is chromosomally mediated
3. **Most common staphylococcal phage strain causing hospital infection:** *(Recent MCQ)*
   (a) 80/81 (b) 79/80
   (c) 3A/3C (d) 69/70

Virulence Factors

4. **All are true regarding staphylococcal toxin *except*:** *(AIIMS Dec 97)*
   (a) Beta haemolysin shows hot cold phenomenon
   (b) Mainly endotoxin
   (c) Enterotoxin causes food poisoning
   (d) Exfoliative toxin causes Ritter's disease
5. **Synergohymenotroic toxins of Staphylococcal consists:** *(PGI May 14)*
   (a) α toxin (b) β toxin
   (c) γ toxin (d) δ toxin
   (e) Panton-Valentine toxin
6. **Staphylococcal scalded skin syndrome is caused by:** *(Recent MCQ)*
   (a) Hemolysin (b) Coagulase
   (c) Enterotoxin (d) Epidermolytic toxin
7. **True about protein A of staph aureus:** *(Recent MCQ)*
   (a) Causes opsonization (b) Binds to Fc portion of IgG
   (c) Stimulate phagocytosis (d) T-cell mitogen

8. **Staphyloccocal pathogenicity is indicated by:** *(Recent MCQ)*
   (a) Coagulase positivity
   (b) Hemolysis
   (c) Lipoteichoic acid
   (d) Endotoxin

9. **Staph aureus virulence is due to:** *(PGI 98)*
   (a) Coagulase
   (b) Endotoxin
   (c) Hemolysis
   (d) Pigmented colonies

Food Poisoning

10. **Staphylococcal food poisoning includes the following feature:** *(AIIMS 01)*
    (a) Incubation period of 24 hours
    (b) Requires immediate antibiotics
    (c) Common with dairy products
    (d) Heat labile enterotoxin

11. **A child after consuming food in a party complains of diarrhea within 1-5 hours. The diagnosis is:** *(AIIMS 01, 96, 95)*
    (a) S. aureus
    (b) Streptococcus
    (c) Clostridium perfringens
    (d) Clostridium botulinum

12. **Incubation period of staphylococcal food poisoning is:** *(Recent MCQ)*
    (a) 4-6 hrs
    (b) 6-12 hrs
    (c) 12-18 hrs
    (d) 18-24 hrs

13. **Staph. aureus causes vomiting in 16-18 hours. The mechanism of action is:** *(AIIMS May 02)*
    (a) Stimulation of C AMP
    (b) Vagal stimulation
    (c) Stimulation of C GMP
    (d) Acts through ganglioside GM receptor

14. **Enterotoxin responsible for most of the cases of food poisoning by staphylococcus:** *(Recent MCQ)*
    (a) Type E
    (b) Type C
    (c) Type B
    (d) Type A

15. **The following are characteristic features of staphylococcus food poisoning *except*:** *(AIIMS 04)*
    (a) Optimum temperature for toxin production is 37°C
    (b) Intradietic toxin is responsible for intestinal symptoms
    (c) Toxin can be destroyed by boiling for 30 minutes
    (d) Incubation period is 1-6 hours

Infections Caused by Staph Aureus

16. **Which of the following organism is implicated in the causation of botryomycosis?** *(Recent MCQ AI 2014-15 Pattern)*
    (a) Staphylococcus aureus
    (b) Staphylococcus albus
    (c) Pseudomonas aeruginosa
    (d) Streptococcus pneumonia

17. **Which organism causes toxin shock syndrome?** *(Recent MCQ)*
    (a) Pneumococcus
    (b) E. coli
    (c) Staphylococcus aureus
    (d) Enterococcus

18. **Toxic shock syndrome is caused by:** *(PGI Nov 14)*
    (a) Streptococcus pyogenes
    (b) Staphylococcus aureus
    (c) Strept albicans
    (d) E. durans

19. **The most frequent cause of scalded skin syndrome is:** *(Recent MCQ)*
    (a) Staphylococci
    (b) Pneumococci
    (c) Enterococci
    (d) Meningococci

20. Staph aureus causes: *(Recent MCQ)*
(a) Erythrasma
(b) Chancroid
(c) Acne vulgaris
(d) Bullous impetigo

Lab, Diagnosis and Treatment

21. Which of the following is not mechanism for resistance to MRSA? *(AI 10)*
(a) Resistance is chromosomally mediated
(b) Produced mainly by alteration in PBPs
(c) MRSA resistance is absolutely beta-lactamase independent
(d) Intrinsic resistance is known

22. All of the following are true about Methicillin resistance in MRSA, *except*: *(AI 11)*
(a) Resistance is produced as a result of altered PBP's
(b) Resistance may be produced by hyperproduction of beta lactamase
(c) Resistance is primarily mediated/transmitted via plasmids
(d) Resistance may be missed at incubation temperature of 37°C during susceptibility testing

23. Which of the following statements is most correct regarding resistance to methicillin in MRSA? *(AI 11)*
(a) Resistance is produced as a result of alteration in Penicillin Binding Proteins (PBP)
(b) Resistance is produced by production of beta lactamase
(c) Resistance is mediated by plasmids
(d) Expression of resistance is enhanced by incubating at 37°C during susceptibility testing

24. Transfer of drug resistance in staphylococcus is by: *(PGI 97)*
(a) Transduction
(b) Transformation
(c) Conjugation
(d) Transfection

25. A diabetic patient developed cellulite is due to S. aureus, which was found to be methicillin resistant on the antibiotic sensitivity testing. All of the following antibiotics will be appropriate *except*: *(AI 06)*
(a) Vancomycin
(b) Imipenem
(c) Teicoplanin
(d) Linezolid

26. Drug of choice for MRSA: *(Recent MCQ)*
(a) Penicillin G
(b) Ceftriaxone
(c) Vancomycin
(d) Cefazoline

27. Staphylococcus oxacillin resistance is best detected by: *(Recent MCQ)*
(a) Cefotixin MIC
(b) Cefotixin disc diffusion
(c) Oxacillin disc diffusion
(d) Oxacillin agar

28. Blood culture is positive in which infection of staph. aureus? *(Recent MCQ)*
(a) TSS
(b) SSSS
(c) Infective endocarditis
(d) Impetigo

29. All of the following statements are true regarding Staphylococci *except*: *(AIIMS Nov 04)*
(a) A majority of infections caused by coagulase-negative Staphylococci are due to Staphylococcus epidermidis
(b) β-lactamase production in Staphylococci is under plasmid control
(c) Expression of methicillin resistance in Staphylococcus aureus increases when it is incubated at 37°C on blood agar
(d) Methicillin resistance in Staphylococcus aureus is independent of β-lactamase production

Coagulase Negative Staphylococci

30. A patient in an ICU is on a CVP line. His blood culture shows growth of gram positive cocci which are catalase positive and coagulase negative. The most likely etiological agent is: *(AIIMS May 03)*

(a) Staplylococcus aureus
(b) Staplylococcus epidermidis
(c) Streptococcus pyogenes
(d) Enterococcus faecalis

31. Staphylococcus differs from streptococcus by: *(Recent MCQ)*

(a) Coagulase test
(b) Catalase test
(c) Phosphatase
(d) Gram negative

32. Catalase positive, beta-hemolytic staphylococcus: *(Recent MCQ)*

(a) S. aureus
(b) S. epidermidis
(c) S. saprophyticus
(d) None

33. Catalase positive coagulase negative beta hemolytic bacteria: *(Recent MCQ)*

(a) Strep pyogenes
(b) Staph aureus
(c) Coagulase negative staph
(d) Enterococci

34. True statement regarding non-coagulase staphylococci is: *(AI 99)*

(a) They are non-pathogenic
(b) They commonly infect indwelling prosthesis
(c) They may cause scarlet fever
(d) They are separated by gram staining

35. Which one of the following gram positive organism is most common cause of UTI among sexually active women? *(PGI 99)*

(a) Staphylococcus epidermidis
(b) Staphylococcus aureus
(c) Staphylococcus saprophyticus
(d) Enterococcus

36. A 30-year-old female is on antibiotics with prolonged IV cannulation, has spike of fever, the likely cause is: *(AIIMS Nov 09)*

(a) Pseudomonas aeruginosa
(b) Coagulase negative Staphylococci
(c) Streptococcus agalactiae
(d) E. Coli

37. Staphylococcus aureus differs from staphylococcus epidermidis:

(a) Is coagulase positive
(b) Forms white colonies
(c) A common cause of UTI
(d) Causes endocarditis in drug addicts

38. Catalase positive novobiocin resistant bacteria is: *(Recent MCQ Pattern)*

(a) Staphylococcus aureus
(b) Staphylococcus epidermidis
(c) Staphylococcus saprophyticus
(d) None of the above

39. To differentiate between staphylococcus epidermidis and staphylococcus saprophyticus, which is used? *(Recent MCQ Pattern)*

(a) Coagulase test
(b) Catalase test
(c) Novobiocin sensitivity
(d) None of the above

40. A 25-year-old man with 3 weeks fever presented with tricuspid valve vegetation. Patient is intravenous drug abuser. Most common cause of endocarditis in this patient is: *(AIIMS Nov 09)*

(a) Staph. aureus
(b) Candida albicans
(c) Pseudomonas
(d) Strep. viridans

ANSWERS AND EXPLANATIONS

1. **Ans. is 'a'** i.e., Staphylococcus
   - Catalase +ve GPC = Staphylococcus species.
   - Catalase –ve GPC = Streptococcus species.
2. **Ans. is 'a'** i.e., Most common source of infection is cross infection from infected people
   (***Ref:*** *Harrison, 18th/e, p. 1160-1166 and 17th/e, p. 873-879; Jawetz, 24th/e, p. 224-230*)
   - **Most common source of infection of staph. aureus is endogenous infection from individuals own colonizing strains. Most individuals who develop Staph. aureus infections do so with their own colonizing strains.**
   - The chief sources of infection are shedding human lesions, fomites contaminated from such lesions, and the human respiratory tract and skin.
3. **Ans. is 'a'** i.e., 80/81
   - Staph aureus strains are further classified into subspecies level on the basis of phage typing.
   - National reference center for phage typing – **MAMC, New Delhi.**
   - Phage typing is a method used for detecting single strains of bacteria. It is used to trace the source of outbreaks of infections.
   - **Phage type 80/81** is known to cause hospital infections throughout the world so these strains are also called as epidemic strains.

Virulence Factors

4. **Ans. is 'b'** i.e., Mainly endotoxin (***Ref:*** *Ananthanarayan, 9th/e, p. 201-203 and 8th/e, p. 198-199*)
   - Endotoxins are part of the outer membrane of the cell wall of Gram-negative bacteria. E Staphylococcus does not produce endotoxin. Endotoxin is produced by gram (-) ve organisms, **the only gram (+)ve organism secreting endotoxin is listeria.**
5. **Ans. is 'c'** i.e., γ toxin; 'e' Panton-Valentine toxin (***Ref:*** *Ananthanarayan, 9th/e, p. 202 and 8th/e, p. 198*)
   - **γ-hemolysin and Panton-Valentine toxin [Panton-Valentine leukocidin (PVL)] are classified as family of Synergohymenotropic toxins** because they cannot act individually, but in combination they are leucocidal and hemolytic.
   - **PVL is an important virulence factor in CA-MRSA infections.**
6. **Ans. is 'd'** i.e., Epidermolytic toxin (***Ref:*** *Ananthanarayan, 9th/e, p. 203 and 8th/e, p. 198-199*)
   - Epidermolytic toxins of S aureus are two distinct proteins of the same molecular weight. **Exfoliative toxin A is (*ETA*) chromosomal encoded** and located on a phage and is heat stable. **Exfoliative toxin B is plasmid mediated and heat labile.**

     These epidermolytic toxins yield the generalized desquamation of the staphylococcal scalded skin syndrome by dissolving the mucopolysaccharide matrix of the epidermis. The toxins are superantigens.
7. **Ans. is 'b'** i.e., Binds to Fc part of IgG (***Ref:*** *Ananthanarayan, 9th/e, p. 197, 198*)
   - Protein A is a cell wall component of S aureus strains and is a bacterial surface protein called as **microbial surface components recognizing adhesive matrix molecules (MSCRAMMs).**

     Bacterial attachment to host cells is mediated by MSCRAMMs, and these are important virulence factors.

     Protein A of Staph aureus binds to Fc terminal of IgG (IgG 1, 2 and 4 but not IgG3) and prevents opsono-phagocytosis by PMNs.
   - Protein A has become an important reagent in immunology and diagnostic laboratory technology; for example, protein A with attached IgG molecules directed against a specific bacterial antigen agglutinates bacteria that have that antigen **("coagglutination").**
8. **Ans. is 'a'** i.e., Coagulase positivity (***Ref:*** *Ananthanarayan, 9th/e, p. 201 and 8th/e, p. 198*)
   - Most consistent association of virulence is **production of coagulase.**

- **Coagulase binds to prothrombin; together they become enzymatically active and initiate fibrin polymerization. Coagulase may deposit fibrin on the surface of staphylococci, perhaps altering their ingestion by phagocytic cells or their destruction within such cells.** Coagulase production is considered synonymous with invasive pathogenic potential.

9. **Ans. is 'a'** i.e., Coagulase (***Ref:*** *Ananthanarayan, 9th/e, p. 201-202 and 8th/e, p. 195*)
   - Already explained in Ans. 8.

Food Poisoning

10. **Ans. is 'c'** i.e., Common with dairy products (***Ref:*** *Ananthanarayan, 9th/e, p. 202 and 8th/e, p. 198*)
11. **Ans. is 'a'** i.e., S. aureus (***Ref:*** *Ananthanarayan, 9th/e, p. 202 and 8th/e, p. 198*)
12. **Ans. is 'a'** i.e., 4-6 hours (***Ref:*** *Ananthanarayan, 9th/e, p. 202 and 8th/e, p. 198*)
    - Incubation period of staphylococcal food poisoning is 1-6 hours.
    - Toxin can be detected by ELISA, Latex agglutination test and toxin gene detection by PCR.
13. **Ans. is 'b'** i.e., Vagal stimulation (***Ref:*** *Harrison, 18th/e, p. 1162 and 17th/e, p. 875*)
14. **Ans. is 'd'** i.e., Type A (***Ref:*** *Harrison, 18th/e, p. 1165, 1166; Ananthanarayan, 8th/e, p. 198*)
    - Eight antigenic types of enterotoxins are currently known A, B, C1, C2, C3, D, E and H.
    - Type A is responsible for most of the cases.
    - Type F does not cause food poisoning, but causes TS Syndrome.
15. **Ans. is 'c'** i.e., Toxin can be destroyed by boiling for 30 minutes

    (***Ref:*** *Ananthanarayan, 9th/e, p. 202 and 8th/e, p. 198*)
    - "The toxin is relatively heat stable, resisting 100°C for 10 to 40 minutes". Even if the bacteria are killed by warming, the heat stable toxin is not destroyed.

Infections Caused by Staph Aureus

16. **Ans. is 'a'** i.e., Staphylococcus aureus (***Ref:*** *Ananthanarayan, 9th/e, p. 394 and 8th/e, p. 608*)
    - Botryomycosis (bacterial pseudomycosis) (Mycetoma like lesion) is an uncommon chronic bacterial infection of skin caused by masses of colonizing bacteria.
17. **Ans. is 'c'** i.e., Staphylococcus aureus (***Ref:*** *Harrison, 18th/e, p. 1166-1176*)
    - Toxic shock syndrome is caused by:
      (i) Staphylococcus aureus.
      (ii) Streptococcus pyogenes.
18. **Ans. is 'a'** i.e., Streptococcus pyogenes **and 'b'** i.e., Staphylococcus aureus

    (***Ref:*** *Harrison, 18th/e, p. 1166, 1176 and 17th/e, p. 875, 886*)
19. **Ans. is 'a'** i.e., Straphylococci (***Ref:*** *Harrison, 18th/e, p. 1164-1167; Ananthanarayan, 9th/e, p. 199*)
    - Staphylococcal scalded skin syndrome (SSSS) is caused by an exfoliative toxin produced by roughly 5% of Staphylococcus aureus. As the syndrome evolves, an initial infection occurs, commonly at a site such as the oral or nasal cavities, throat, or umbilicus.
20. **Ans. is 'd'** i.e., Bullous impetigo

    (***Ref:*** *Harrison, 19th/e, p. 1164-1167; Ananthanarayan, 9th/e, p. 203 and 8th/e, p. 199*)
    - **Impetigo is divided into two types:**
      (i) Non-bullous impetigo (Impetigo contagiosum): Caused by staphylococcus aureus and streptococcus pyogenes.
      (ii) Bullous impetigo: Caused by staphylococcus aureus.

Lab. Diagnosis and Treatment

21. Ans. is 'c' i.e., MRSA resistance is absolutely beta-lactamase independent

Mechanism of Resistance of MRSA

- There are three known mechanisms for which staphylococcus aureus become resistant to methicillin:
  - (i) Presence of an **acquired penicillin binding protein (PBP2a,)** Most cases.
  - (ii) Modification of **normal (Intrinsic) penicillin binding proteins.**
  - (iii) **Hyperproduction of β-lactamase** → Rare.
- S. aureus strains have four intrinsic penicillin binding proteins (PBPs) which have high affinity for β-lactam antibiotics.
- **PBP2a is an inducible acquired protein that is produced only by MRSA.** It is not an intrinsic PBP.
- PBP2a has very low affinity for β-lactam antibiotics → staph. aureus strains containing PBP2a, i.e., MRSA are resistant to all β-lactam antibiotics.
- Production of PB2a is by chromosomally coded mec A gene which alters PBP to PBP-2a.
- Drug resistance can be transferred between S. aureus strain by Transduction.

Friends See other options also carefully:

- Resistance to MRSA is chromosomally mediated and involves production of an altered penicillin-binding protein (PBP2a).
- **MRSA resistance is not absolutely β-lactamase independent. Though altered penicillin binding protein is involved in most strains, β-lactamase production is also involved, rarely.**

22. Ans. is 'c' i.e., Resistance is primarily mediated via plasmids

Another beautiful question:

- **Resistance in MRSA is chromosomally mediated** (not plasmid mediated).
- Most common mechanism of antibiotic resistance in MRSA is alteration in PBP's. This is primarily mediated via chromosomal Mec-A gene which codes for altered PBP-2A.
- Rarely, resistance may be produced by hyperproduction of beta-lactamase.

  "Methicillin resistance is expressed more at 30 degree C than at 37 degree C, so susceptibility studies for methicillin are routinely performed at reduced temperature (30°-35° C for 24 hours), with increased concentration of salt in the medium to enhance the expression of resistance."
- Therefore, resistance may be missed at incubation temperature at 37°C during susceptibility testing.

23. Ans. is 'a' i.e., Resistance is produced as a result of alteration in Penicillin Binding Proteins

- Main mechanism involved in is – Resistance in MRSA is mainly produced by the presence of an altered penicillin binding protein.

24. Ans. is 'a' > 'c' i.e., Transduction > Conjugation (***Ref:** Ananthanarayan, 9th/e, p. 201 and 8th/e, p. 197*)

- Production of β-lactamase is usually controlled by plasmids which are transmitted by transduction (more common) or conjugation.

25. Ans. is 'b' i.e., Imipenem (***Ref:** Harrison, 18th/e, p. 1168 and 17th/e, p. 879*)

"The carbapenem imipenem has excellent activity against methicillin – sensitive S. aureus but not M.R.S.A." Because MRSA is resistant to all Beta-lactam antibiotics including cephalosporins and carbapenems.

26. Ans. is 'c' i.e., Vancomycin (***Ref:** Harrison, 18th/e, p. 1168*)

- Vancomycin is the DOC for MRSA.
- Other dugs – Quinupristin, dalfopristin, TMP-SMX, Daptomycin, Linezolid, Teicoplanin.

27. Ans. is 'b' i.e., Cefoxitin disc diffusion

- Oxacillin (also methicillin) resistance is detected by finding the presence of mec A gene.

  "Cefoxitin disc diffusion has been reported to more accurately predict mec A gene presence than oxacillin disc diffusion."

- **The Clinical and Laboratory Standards Institute (CLSI), recommends the cefoxitin disk screen test, the latex agglutination test for PBP2a, or a plate containing 6 µg/ml of oxacillin in Mueller-Hinton agar supplemented with 4% NaCl as alternative methods of testing for MRSA.**

28. Ans. is 'c' i.e., Infective endocarditis (***Ref:*** *Laboratory Tests in Medical Microbiology, p. 912*)

- Blood culture is positive when bacteria present in blood, i.e., when there is bacteremia.
- Infective endocarditis is a complication of staphylococcal aureus bacteremia (SAB). Thus blood culture may be positive.
- **Staphylococcal scalded skin syndrome (SSSS) and impetigo do not have bacteremia.**
- In toxic shock syndrome (TSS) due to staphylococcus aureus, bacteremia is uncommon (in contrast, bacteremia is common in streptococcal TSS).

29. Ans. is 'c' i.e., Expression of methicillin resistance in staph aureus increases when it is incubated at 37°C on blood agar (***Ref:*** *Ananthanarayan, 9th/e, p. 204 and 8th/e, p. 197; Harrison, 18th/e, p. 1168 and 17th/e, p. 879, 880*)

β-lactamase production is controlled by plasmid.

About Option 'a'

"Approximately 75% of the infections caused by coagulase negative staphylococci are due to staphylococcus epidermidis."

Coagulase Negative Staphylococci

30. Ans. is 'b' i.e., Staphylococcus epidermidis

(***Ref:*** *Ananthanarayan, 9th/e, p. 206 and 8th/e, p. 202; Harrison, 18th/e, p. 1167 and 17th/e, p. 878*)

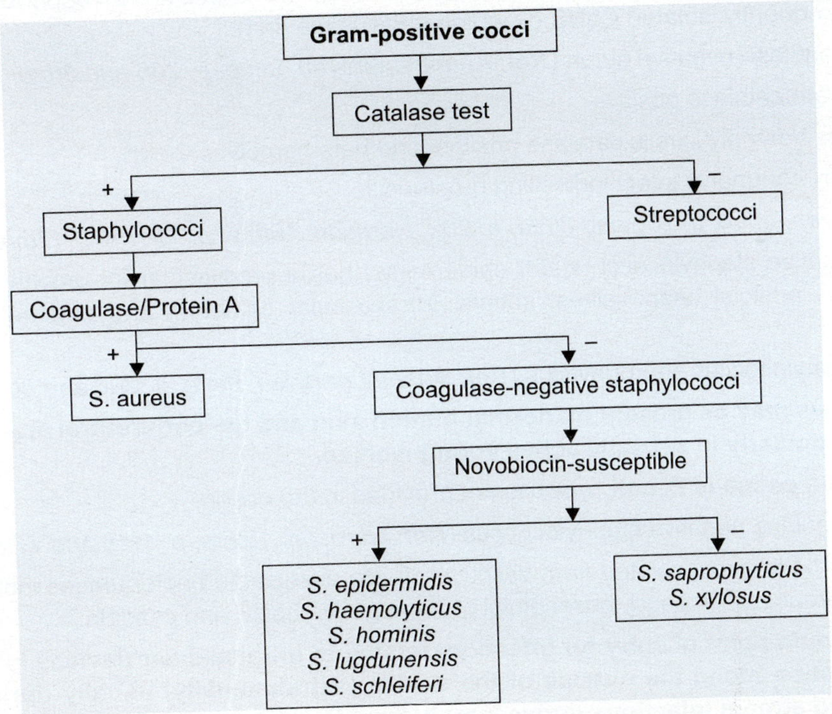

- The isolated organism is catalase (+)ve → option (c) and (d) can be ruled out – Streptococci (Str. pyogenes, enterococci) are catalase (-)ve.
- The isolated organism is coagulase negative → option (a) (staph. aureus) can be ruled out as it is coagulase (+)ve.
- Now we are left with staphylococcus epidermidis which is catalase (+)ve and coagulase (-)ve.

- Following fact also support our diagnosis of Staph. epidermidis in this patient:

  "Staph. epidermidis is a coagulase negative staphylococcus, which has predilection for growth on implanted foreign bodies such as intravascular catheters, shunts, artificial heart valves and prosthetic appliances, leading to bacteremia."

Also Know:

- Staphylococcus aureus can be distinguished from coagulase negative staphylococci also by **phosphatase→** Staph. aureus is phosphatase positive, while coagulase negative staphylococci are phosphatase negative.

31. **Ans. is 'b'** i.e., Catalase test (***Ref:** Ananthanarayan, 9th/e, p. 200 and 8th/e, p. 196*)
    - Coagulase test is used to differentiate the different species of staphylococci (staph. aureus, staph. epidermidis).
    - Catalase test is used to differentiate staphylococci from streptococci.
    - Coagulase test cannot be used to differentiate streptococci from staphylococci because certain species of staphylococci are coagulase negative (coagulase negative staphylococci) as streptococci.
32. **Ans. is 'a'** i.e., S. aureus (***Ref:** Essentials of Medical Microbiology, p. 779*)
    - All staphylococci are catalase positive.
    - Amongst staphylococci, Staph. aureus and Staph. haemolyticus (CONS) are beta hemolytic.
    - **Most species of coagulase negative staphylococcus species are non-hemolytic except Staph. haemolyticus.**
    - Staphylococcus haemolyticus is a member of the coagulase-negative staphylococci (CoNS). It is part of the skin flora of humans, and its largest populations are usually found at the axillae, perineum, and inguinal areas. S. haemolyticus also colonizes primates and domestic animals. It is a well-known opportunistic pathogen, and is the second-most frequently isolated CoNS (S. epidermidis is the first).
33. **Ans. is 'c'** i.e., Coagulase negative staph (***Ref:** Ananthanarayan, 9th/e, p. 206 and 8th/e, p. 202*)
    - Staphylococci are catalase positive.
    - Staphylococcus haemolyticus is catalase positive and beta hemolytic CoNS.
34. **Ans. is 'b'** i.e., They commonly infect indwelling prosthesis

    (***Ref:** Ananthanarayan, 9th/e, p. 206 and 8th/e, p. 202; Harrison, 18th/e, p. 1167 and 17th/e, p. 878*)
    - Coagulase negative staphylococci (staph epidermidis) has a predilection for growth on the implanted foreign bodies such as artificial heart valves, shunts, intravascular catheters and prosthetic appliances leading to bacteremia.
35. **Ans. is 'c'** i.e., Staphylococcus saprophyticus (***Ref:** Ananthanarayan, 9th/e, p. 206 and 8th/e, p. 202*)

    Staph saprophyticus may be present on normal human skin and the periurethral area and can cause urinary tract infection, particularly in sexually active young women.

    Note: Most common cause is E. coli, which is not provided in the option.
36. **Ans. is 'b'** i.e., Coagulase negative staphylococcus (***Ref:** Harrison, 18th/e, p. 1116 and 17th/e, p. 839*)

    "The most common pathogens isolated from vascular device-associated bacteraemias include coagulase negative staphylococci, S. aureus, enterococci, nosocomial gram negative bacilli and candida."
    - **The most common point of entry for infection, related to intravascular devices is the insertion site, with spread of infection along the outside of the device (extraluminally) usually during the first week after insertion. Blood stream infections derive largely from the cutaneous microflora of the insertion site.**
37. **Ans. is 'a'** i.e., Coagulase positive (***Ref:** Ananthanarayan, 9th/e, p. 206 and 8th/e, p. 202*)
    - Already explained.
38. **Ans. is 'c'** i.e., Staphylococcus saprophyticus (***Ref:** Ananthanarayan, 9th/e, p. 202*)
    - All staphylococcus are catalase positive.
    - Staphylococcus saprophyticus is resistant to novobiocin.

39. Ans. is 'c' i.e., Novobiocin sensitivity

- Already explained.

40. Ans. is 'a' i.e., Staph. aureus (***Ref:*** *Harrison, 18th/e, p. 1052, 1053 and 17th/e, p. 789, 790*)

- Infective endocarditis in intravenous drug abusers commonly involves the tricuspid valve and are caused by Staphylococcus aureus.
- Most common cause of native value endocarditis → Staph. aureus.
- Most common cause of early onset prosthetic valve endocarditis (< 2 months and 2-12 months) → Coagulase - negative staphylococci.
- Most common cause of late onset prosthetic valve endocarditis (> 12 months) → Streptococci (e.g., streptococcus viridans).
- Most common cause of endocarditis in I.V. drug abusers → Staph. aureus.

STREPTOCOCCUS

- Gram positive cocci, arranged in chains, Facultative anaerobes.
- Non motile, non sporing and nonacid fast and they are part of the normal flora.
- Catalase test –ve, oxidase test –ve.
- Catalase test is used to differentiate staphylococcus from streptococcus.
- Categorized on basis of hemolytic pattern, surrounding the colonies on 5% sheep blood agar.

Classification:

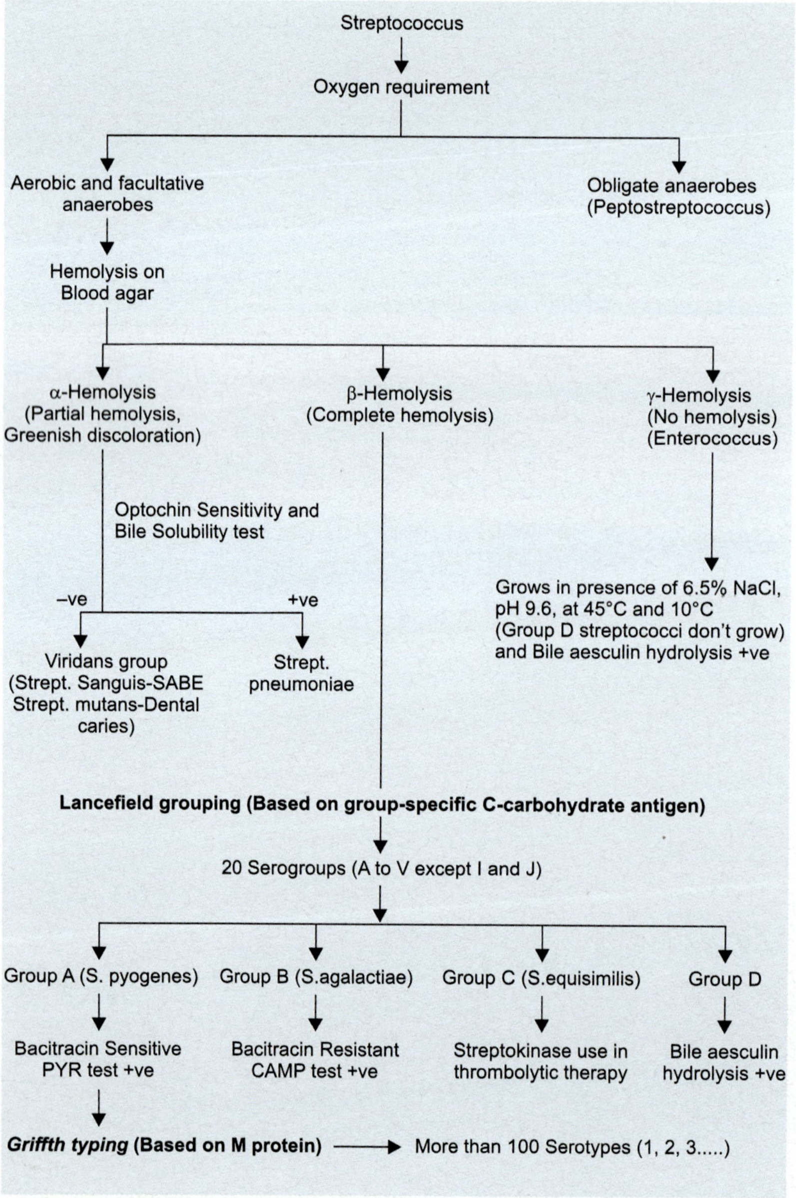

STREPTOCOCCUS PYOGENES

Streptococcal Diseases:

- Respiratory – Sore throat.
- Skin infection – Impetigo (MCC), Erysipelas Cellulitis (MCC), Necrotizing fasciitis (Flesh eating bacteria) and rarely scarlet fever.
- **Non suppurative complications** – Acute rheumatic fever and Acute glomerulonephritis.

Pathogenesis and Virulence Factors:

Cell Wall Associated:

- **Protein M – Basis of Griffith typing,** inhibits the phagocytosis and Abs to Protein M is protective.
- Lipoteichoic acid – Helps in adhesion.
- Polysaccharide Capsule – Made up with Hyaluronic acid.

Toxins:

- **Hemolysins/streptolysin:**
  1. Streptolysin O-O_2 labile, strongly antigenic, active in reduced state, cytotoxic to neutrophils, platelets and cardiac tissue.
  2. **Streptolysin S** – O_2 stable, Non Antigenic, responsible for hemolysis.
- **Erythrogenic/Pyrogenic Exotoxin/Dick/Scarlet Toxin** (A,B,C) – Responsible for scarlet fever, toxic shock syndrome, necrotizing fasciitis. A, C acts as Superantigen.

Enzymes:

- **Streptokinase/fibrinolysin** – Facilitating the spread of infection.
- **DNase** – Responsible for the serous nature of exudates.

Antigenic Cross Reactivity:

Between streptococcal Ags and the corresponding human Ags.

- Cell wall **M** protein **– M**yocardium (tropomyosin and myosin).
- Cell wall **C** carbohydrate – **Cardiac valves.**
- Cytoplasmic **membrane** – Glomerular vascular **intima.**
- **Peptidoglycan – Skin antigens.**
- **Hyaluronic acid – Synovial fluid.**

Lab Diagnosis:

Sample Collection:

Pus, Pus swab, throat swab, exudates and Blood (According to the site of infection).

Transport medium – Pike's medium.

Direct Microscopy:

Gram staining of sample – GPC in chains with numerous pus cells.

Culture:

Blood agar – β hemolysis.

Selective medium – Crystal violet blood agar and PNF (Polymyxin B, Neomycin, Fusidic acid) media.

Identification tests:

- Catalase – Negative.
- Sensitive to Bacitracin (0.04 U). Q
- **PYR test – Positive (Confirmatory test).**
- **Serology:**
  1. **Anti streptolysin–O (ASO)** Abs are raised (>200 IU/ml) in most of the streptococcal infections and used as standard marker for retrospective diagnosis of streptococcal infections.

Contd.

Contd.

2. **Anti-DNase B Abs** (300-350 units/ml) can be used for retrospective diagnosis of pyoderma and acute glomerulonephritis where ASO titer is low.
3. **Streptokinase and DNase** are used in thrombolytic therapy (in empyema cases) to liquefy the thick exudates.

Antibiotic Susceptibility Testing

Done on Blood agar by Kirby Bauer Disc diffusion method.

Treatment of Group A

- Pharyngitis, impetigo, erysipelas, cellulitis – Penicillin G.
- Pneumonia/empyema – Penicillin G + drainage.
- Necrotizing fascitis – Sx debridement + Penicillin G + clindamycin.
- Streptococcal TSS – Penicillin G + clindamycin +Iv Ig.

Streptococcus Agalactiae (Group B)

- Regularly resides in human vagina, pharynx and large intestine.
- **Can be transferred to infant during delivery and cause severe infection so Pregnant woman should be screened and treated.**
- Most prevalent cause of neonatal pneumonia, sepsis and meningitis.
- In India MCC of meningitis in neonates – E. Coli.
- In world MCC of meningitis in neonates – S agalactiae.
- Wound and skin infections and endocarditis in debilitated people.
- CAMP test +ve, Bacitracin resistant.
- DOC – Penicillin G.

Streptococcus Viridans/Viridans Streptococci

- Commensals of mouth and URT.
- **S. sanguis** – Most common viridans causing SABE (sab acute bacterial endocarditis).
- **S. mutans** – **Dental caries**, dental plaques.
- **S. salivarius** – **Longest chain** having Streptococci.

Group D Streptococci and Enterococci

- **Group D Streptococci – Includes fecal Streptococci and non-enterococci.**
- **Enterococcus faecalis, E faecium, E. durans.**
- Normal colonists of human large intestine.
- Cause opportunistic urinary, wound and skin infections, particularly in debilitated persons.
- Cultured on **Bile aesculin agar.Q**
- VRE (Vancomycin resistant Enterococci) are reported now-a-days. Mechanism involved is due to **(D alanyl D lactate variation results in the loss of one hydrogen bonding interaction from five to four).Q**
- **DOC – Combination of Penicillins and aminoglycosides.Q** (Enterococci-intrinsic resistant to cotrimoxazole and cephalosporins).

Streptococcus Pneumoniae/Pneumococcus

- Lanceolate diplococci with polysaccharide capsule.
- **On blood agar they are Alpha hemolytic and show Carrom coin or draughtsman appearance.**
- **Quellung reaction** – Capsular swelling by type-specific anti-serum.
- **Bile solubility test** – Positive because of autolytic amidase which is activated by bile salts.
- **Sensitivity to Optochin.**
- **MCC of acute meningitis in adults.**
  MCC of community acquired pneumonia.
  MCC acute otitis media in children.

Contd.

Contd.

MCC bacterial cause of sinusitis.

DOC – Penicillin.

- **Marker** – CRP by latex agglutination test.
- **Capsular Ag detection test in CSF (Pneumococcal meningitis) by latex agglutination test.**
- **Vaccines:**
  1. **Polyvalent polysaccharide vaccine/23-valent Pneumococcal polysaccharide (PPV23) vaccine** – Contains capsular polysaccharide of most prevalent 23 serotypes and Contradiction in children of <2-3 years.
  2. **Polysaccharide protein conjugate vaccine/7** – Valent polysaccharide conjugate (PCV-7) vaccine – Contains capsular polysaccharide of 7 serotypes added to protein conjugate like CRM 197 protein of C. diphtheria. It can be given to children of <2-3 years.

MCQs

STREPTOCOCCI

Classification

1. **Lancefield grouping of streptococci is done by using:** *(AIIMS Nov 07)*
   (a) M Protein
   (b) Group C peptidoglycan cell wall
   (c) Group C carbohydrate antigen
   (d) Staining properties
2. **A child presents with sepsis. Bacteria isolated showed beta hemolysis on blood agar, resistance to bacitracin and a positive CAMP test. The most probable organism causing infection is:** *(AI 10)*
   (a) S. Pyogenes
   (b) S. Agalactiae
   (c) Enterococcus
   (d) S. Pneumoniae
3. **Catalase negative beta hemolytic streptococci is:** *(Recent MCQ)*
   (a) Str. pneumoniae
   (b) Str. pyogenes
   (c) Str. aglactiae
   (d) Enterococcus
4. **All are medically important streptococci *except*:** *(DNB Nov 13 Pattern)*
   (a) Strep. pyogenes
   (b) Strep. agalactiae
   (c) Strep. equisimilus
   (d) Strep. salivarius

Group 'A' Streptococci

5. **Streptococcal Toxic shock syndrome is due to the following virulence factor:** *(Recent MCQ)*
   (a) M protein
   (b) Pyrogenic exotoxin
   (c) Streptolysin O
   (d) Carbohydrate cell wall
6. **Which of the following streptococcal antigen cross reacts with synovial fluid?** *(AI 08)*
   (a) Carbohydrate (group A)
   (b) Cell wall protein
   (c) Capsular hyaluronic acid
   (d) Peptidoglycan
7. **Which toxin of streptococcus causes hemolysis?** *(PGI Nov 14)*
   (a) Streptolysin O
   (b) Streptolysin S
   (c) Streptodornase
   (d) Hyaluronidase
8. **Streptolysin O functionally and structurally related to:** *(PGI Nov 14)*
   (a) Tetanolysin
   (b) Pneumolysin
   (c) Streptolysin S
   (d) Clostridium perfringens 0 toxin
   (e) Listeriolysin

9. Streptococcus all are true *except*: (*AIIMS May 11, 10*)
(a) Streptodornase cleaves DNA
(b) Streptolysis O is active in reduced state
(c) Streptokinase is produced from serotype A, C, K
(d) Pyrogenic toxin A is plasmid mediated

10. Virulence factor of group A beta hemolytic streptococci: (*Recent MCQ*)
(a) Prt. M
(b) Prt. T
(c) Prt. R
(d) Lipotechoic acid

11. All are true about streptococcus *except*: (*AI 01*)
(a) M protein is responsible for production of mucoid colonies
(b) M protein is responsible for virulence
(c) Mucoid colonies are virulent
(d) No resistance to penicillin has been reported

Infections Caused by Str. Pyogenes

12. A child presents with infective skin lesion of the leg culture was done which showed gram +ve cocci in chains which where hemolytic colonies. The test to confirm the organism is: (*AIIMS Nov 11, May 07, Nov 06, AI 07*)
(a) Bile solubility
(b) Optochin sensitivity
(c) Bacitracin sensitivity
(d) Catalase positive

13. In a school child had abscess on lower leg. Swab taken revealed gram positive beta-hemolytic streptococci, and these were bacitracin sensitive. School physician observed that similar organism was isolated from throats of many other children. Which of the following is true statement with regards to this patient? (*AIIMS Nov 10*)
(a) Difference in surface protein can differentiate the pathogenic bacteria from the pharyngeal culture bacteria
(b) Component C carbohydrate can differentiate the pathogenic bacteria from the throat culture bacteria
(c) MEG 3 positive are throat culture streptococci
(d) Depending on M protein the cutaneous pathogenic bacteria can be differentiated from the pharyngeal culture bacteria

14. A boy with skin ulcer on leg, culture reveals beta hemolysis. Cultures from school children with sore throat some days back also revealed beta hemolysis. What is the similarity between both? (*AIIMS Nov 10*)
(a) Mec A gene is related to it
(b) M protein is same
(c) C carbohydrate antigen is same
(d) Strains causing both are same
(e) Streptozyme test is an active haemagglutination test

15. Streptococcal GN is best diagnosed by: (*PGI 99*)
(a) ASO titre
(b) Anti DNAse
(c) Antihyaluronidase
(d) Culture

16. 11-year-old child presented with sore throat since 3 days, which medium is used to culture the throat swab? (*Recent MCQ*)
(a) Blood agar
(b) L. J. medium
(c) Stewart medium
(d) Chocolate agar

17. Streptococcal skin disease is diagnosed by antibody against: (*Recent MCQ*)
(a) DNAase A
(b) DNAase B
(c) DNAase C
(d) DNAase D

18. An outbreak of streptococcal pharyngitis has occurred in a remote village. In order to carry out the epidemiological investigations of the outbreak it is necessary to perform the culture of the throat swab of the patients suffering from the disease. The transport media of choice would be: *(AIIMS Nov 04)*

(a) Salt mannitol media
(b) Pike's media
(c) Stuart's media
(d) Cary Blair media

19. Regarding ASO titre all are seen *except*: *(AIIMS Nov 09)*

(a) ASO can be increased in school children
(b) May be negative in post streptococcal glomerulonephritis
(c) ASO titre included in major criteria in Jones criteria
(d) May not be elevated in 20% cases of carditis

Streptococci Other than Group 'A'

20. 45 years old Ramlal has intraabdominal sepsis. The causative organism was found to be vancomycin, gentamycin and ampicillin resistant. It grows well in presence of 6.5% NaCl and arginine. Bile esculin hydrolysis is positive. Which of the following is this organism? *(AIIMS Nov 01)*

(a) Streptococcus agalactae
(b) Enterococcus fecalis
(c) Streptococcus bovis
(d) Streptococcus pneumonia

21. Which group of streptococcus grow at > 60°C? *(Recent MCQ)*

(a) A
(b) B
(c) C
(d) D

22. Which of the following organisms, when isolated in the blood, requires the synergistic activity of penicillin plus an aminoglycoside for appropriate therapy? *(AIIMS Nov 04)*

(a) Enterococcus faecalis
(b) Staphylococcus aureus
(c) Str. pneumoniae
(d) Bacteroides fragilis

23. False about gram positive cocci is: *(AI 08)*

(a) Staph. saprophyticus causes UTI in females
(b) Most enterococci are sensitive to penicillin
(c) Non pathogenic strains are coagulase negative
(d) Neonatal meningitis causing streptococci hydrolyses hippurate

24. A patient admitted to an ICU is on central venous line for the last one week. He is on ceftazidime and amikacin. After 7 days of antibiotics he develops a spike of fever and his blood culture is positive for gram positive cocci in chains, which are catalase negative. Following this, vancomycin was started but the culture remained positive for the same organism even after 2 weeks of therapy. The most likely organism causing infection is: *(AIIMS Nov 11, May 06, Nov 06, AI 07)*

(a) Staphylococcus aureus
(b) Viridans streptococci
(c) Enterococcus faecalis
(d) Coagulase negative Staphylococcus

25. True statement regarding Pneumococcus is:

(a) Virulence is due to polysaccharide capsule
(b) Capsule is protein in nature
(c) Antibodies against capsule are not protective
(d) Resistance to penicillin has not yet been reported

26. In a patient of orbital cellulitis, microorganism on culture show greenish colonies and optochin sensitivity. The most likely organism is: *(AI 00)*

(a) *Strep, viridans*
(b) *Staphylococcus*
(c) *Pseudomonas*
(d) *Pneumococcus*

27. Most common causative organism for lobar pneumonia is: *(AIIMS 04)*

(a) Staphylococcus aureus
(b) Streptococcus pyogenes
(c) Streptococcus pneumoniae
(d) Haemophilus influenzae

28. An infant had high grade fever and respiratory distress at the time of presentation to the emergency room. The sample collected for blood culture was subsequently positive showing growth of α-hemolytic colonies. On Gram staining these were Gram-positive cocci. In the screening test for identification, the suspected pathogen is likely to be susceptible to the following agent: *(AI 07, AIIMS May 2012)*

(a) Bacitracin
(b) Novobiocin
(c) Optochin
(d) Cloxacillin

29. After Splenectomy, most common infection: *(PGI 00)*

(a) Pneumococcal
(b) *E.coli*
(c) *Klebsiella*
(d) *Streptococcus*

30. All are true about streptococcus pneumoniae *except*: *(AI 2011)*

(a) Capsule aids in infection
(b) Common infection is otitis media
(c) Respiratory tract of carriers is most important source of infection
(d) Meningitis caused by S. pneumoniae is milder than others

31. Quellung phenomenon is seen in:

(a) *Pneumococcus*
(b) *Streptococcus*
(c) *Staphylococcus*
(d) *Hemophilus*

32. C reactive protein is:

(a) Produced by pneumococcus
(b) A marker of septicemia
(c) Raised in acute inflammation
(d) Low in rheumatoid arthritis

33. Streptococcus pneumoniae, true is: *(SGPGI 05)*

(a) Vaccine is made from capsular polysaccharide
(b) Vaccine is routinely given to Indian children
(c) Catalase and oxidase positive
(d) Bile insoluble and optochin sensitive

34. Risk of Pneumococcal meningitis is seen in: *(AIIMS 99)*

(a) Post-splenectomy patient
(b) Patient undergone neurosurgical intervention
(c) Patient following cardiac surgery
(d) Patient with hypoplasia of lung

35. False statement regarding pneumococci includes all *except*: *(DNB 2012)*

(a) Pneumolysin is the most important virulence factor
(b) Quellung reaction is due to C substance
(c) IgA protease is an important virulence factor
(d) Type I strain is most virulent

36. True statements about pneumococcus are all *except*: *(AI 99)*

(a) Pneumolysin a thiolactivated toxin, exerts a variety of effects on ciliary and PMN's action
(b) Autolysin may contribute to the pathogenesis of pneumococcal disease by lysing bacteria
(c) Anticapsular antibodies are serotype specific
(d) The virulence of pneumococci is dependent only on the production of the capsular polysaccharide

37. Necrotizing fasciitis is caused by, all *except*:

(a) Staphylococcus aureus
(b) Beta haemolytic streptococci
(c) Clostridium perfringens
(d) Pneumococcus

ANSWERS AND EXPLANATIONS

STREPTOCOCCI

Classification

1. **Ans. is 'c'** i.e., Group C carbohydrate antigen (***Ref:*** *Ananthanarayan, 9th/e, p. 209 and 8th/e, p. 205*)
   - Hemolytic streptococci were further classified by Lancefield serological classification into groups based on nature of 'C' carbohydrate antigen on the cell wall.
2. **Ans. is 'b'** i.e., S. Agalactiae (***Ref:*** *Ananthanarayan, 9th/e, p. 210 and 8th/e, p. 206, 215*)
   - CAMP reaction is given by S. agalactiae.
   - Positive for Hippurate hydrolysis and resistant to Bacitracin.
3. **Ans. is 'b'** i.e., Str. pyogenes **and 'c'** i.e., Str. agalactiae (***Ref:*** *Ananthanarayan, 9th/e, p. 210 and 8th/e, p. 206*)
   - Streptococcus pyogenes after growth overnight on a 10 cm plate with 5% sheep blood agar.
   - Group B streptococci are β-hemolytic and produce zones of hemolysis that are only slightly larger than the colonies (1–2 mm in diameter).
4. **Ans. is 'd'** i.e., Strep. salivarius (***Ref:*** *Ananthanarayan, 9th/e, p. 210 and 8th/e, p. 206*)
   - Streptococcus salivarus is normal flora of oral cavity and rarely causes disease to human. Other three streptococci (in options) are pathogenic to man.

Group 'A' Streptococci

5. **Ans. is 'b'** i.e., Pyrogenic exotoxin

   (***Ref:*** *Ananthanarayan, 9th/e, p. 213 and 8th/e, p. 208; Harrison, 18th/e, p. 1177 and 17th/e, p. 886*)
   - Fulminant, invasive S pyogenes infections with streptococcal toxic shock syndrome are characterized by shock, bacteremia, respiratory failure, and multiorgan failure. Death occurs in about 30% of patients.
   - Streptococcal T.S.S. is associated with the production of pyrogenic exotoxin 'A' (SPE-A).
   - **SPE-A and SPE- C are superantigens.**
   - Another name is erythrogenic toxin A, B, C.
6. **Ans. is 'c'** i.e., Capsular hyaluronic acid (***Ref:*** *Ananthanarayan, 9th/e, p. 212 and 8th/e, p. 207-208*)

   Refer Text.
7. **Ans. is 'a'** i.e., Streptolysin O; **'b'** i.e., Streptolysin S

   (***Ref:*** *Ananthanarayan, 9th/e, p. 212 and 8th/e, p. 208; Greenwood, 16th/e, p. 177*)
   - **Remember that streptolysin S and streptolysin 'O' both can cause hemolysis.**
   - **But Streptolysin 'S' is responsible for hemolysis seen around streptococcal colonies on the surface of blood agar.**
   - Now the question arises, if both are hemolytic then why only streptolysin S is responsible for hemolysis around streptococcal colonies on the surface of blood agar. The answer is:

     Streptolysin 'O' is **oxygen labile ('O' for oxygen labile), it is inactive in the presence of oxygen.** So, it can cause hemolysis in reduced state only. That is why streptolysin 'O' cannot cause hemolysis on the surface of blood agar.
   - Streptolysin 'S' is **oxygen stable ('S' for stable)** → can cause hemolysis in the presence of oxygen and is responsible for hemolysis around streptococcal colonies.
8. **Ans. is 'a'** i.e., Tetanolysin; **'b'** i.e., Pneumolysin; **'d'** i.e., Clostridium perfringens toxin **and 'e'** i.e., Listeriolysin
   - Its biological action resembles the oxygen labile hemolysin of clostridium perfringens (perfringolysin O or θ toxin), clostridium tetani (tetanolysin), S. pneumoniae (pneumolysin), L. monocytogenes (Listeriolysin 'O'), Bacillus cereus (Cereolysin 'O'), and B. thuringiensis (Thuringolysin 'O').
9. **Ans. is 'd'** i.e., Pyrogenic toxin A is plasmid mediated

   (***Ref:*** *Ananthanarayan, 9th/e, p. 213 and 8th/e, p. 208; Greenwood, 16th/e, p. 177-78; Harrison, 18th/e, p. 1176, 1177 and 17th/e, p. 881-883*)

- Three toxin types of streptococcal pyro exotoxin have been identified: A, B and C. **Type A and C are bacteriophage coded, while type B gene is chromosomally mediated**.
- **Streptolysin 'O' is oxygen labile;** therefore, it is active in reduced state only.
- **Streptokinase (fibrinolysin)** is expressed on all strains of streptococcus pyogenes (including A, C, K). It activates plasminogen to plasmin so breakdown the fibrin barrier around the infection site and facilitates the spread of infection.
- **Deoxyribonucleases/DNase (streptodornases)** hydrolyze nucleic acids (e.g., DNA).

10. Ans. is 'a' i.e., Prt. M (***Ref:*** *Ananthanarayan, 9th/e, p. 212 and 8th/e, p. 207*)

- M protein is a major virulence factor of S pyogenes. **When M protein is present, the streptococci are virulent, and in the absence of M type-specific antibodies, they are able to resist phagocytosis by polymorphonuclear leukocytes by inhibiting activation of the alternate complement pathway.**

11. Ans. is 'a' i.e., M protein is responsible for the production of mucoid colonies

(***Ref:*** *Ananthanarayan, 9th/e, p. 212 and 8th/e, p. 207*)

- **Capsule is responsible for the production of mucoid colonies (not M protein).**

Let's talk about other options.

Option 'c':

Virulent strains, on fresh isolation form lesions, **produce a matt (finely granular) colony,** while **avirulent strains from 'glossy' colonies.**

Option 'd':

"All beta hemolytic group 'A' streptococci are sensitive to penicillin G." (*Ananthanarayan, 7th/e, p. 211*)

Infections Caused by Str. Pyogenes

12. Ans. is 'c' i.e., Bacitracin sensitivity (***Ref:*** *Ananthanarayan, 9th/e, p. 215 and 8th/e, p. 211-212*)

- Infective skin lesion with gram positive cocci in chains and hemolytic colonies suggest infection of streptococcus pyogenes.
- A **convenient method for the identification of Str. pyogenes is their sensitivity to bacitracin → Maxted's observation.Q**

Gram positive cocci (causing skin lesions)

↓

Arranged in grape like clusters
Catalase (+) ve, Beta hemolytic
From golden yellow pigment

↓

Staphylococcus aureus
- Furunculosis
- Bullous impetigo

↓

Arranged in chains
Catalase (-) ve, Beta hemolytic
No golden yellow pigment

↓

Streptococcus pyogenes
Impetigo contagiosa

13. Ans. is 'd' i.e., Depending on M protein the cutaneous pathogenic bacteria can be differentiated from the pharyngeal culture bacteria (***Ref:*** *Sherris Medical Microbiology, p. 716*)

- Bacitracin sensitive gram positive beta hemolytic cocci is streptococcus pyogenes.
- Two most common sites of infection with streptococci are the upper respiratory tract (pharyngitis, tonsillitis) and the skin (impetigo).
- S. pyogenes causing skin infection (impetigo) tend to belong to different 'M' serotypes than those associated with respiratory infection (pharyngitis).

  "The M protein types of a S. pyogenes most commonly associated with skin infection (impetigo) are different from those causing respiratory infection (pharyngitis).

14. Ans. is 'c' i.e., C carbohydrate antigen is same (***Ref:*** *Ananthanarayan, 9th/e, p. 211-216 and 8th/e, p. 205-210*)

- The carbohydrate 'C' antigen is group specific, i.e., beta-hemolytic group A Streptococci (Str. pyogenes) have same 'C' antigen.
- It has already been explained that strains causing skin infection and throat infection are different and belong to different 'M' serotypes (option 'b', and 'd' are incorrect).

15. Ans. is 'b' i.e., Anti DNAse; **'c'** Antihyaluronidase (***Ref:*** *API, 7th/e, p. 663*)

"Anti-streptolysin: O (ASO), anti-DNAase B, anti-hyaluronidase, anti-NADase are elevated in more than 95% cases of PSGN (Post-streptococcal glomerulonephritis) secondary to Pharyngitis." – API

Anti DNAase B and anti-hyaluronidase are elevated in more than 85% cases of PSGN following skin infection." – API

16. Ans. is 'a' i.e., Blood agar (***Ref:*** *Essential of Pediatric Microbiology, p. 486*)

- Most common bacterial cause of sore throat (pharyngitis) in children is Streptococcal pyogenes.
- The culture medium of choice for throat swab sample is **sheep blood agar plate.**

Remember Friends:

Most common cause of sore throat (acute pharyngitis) in children is–**Rhinovirus being the most common organism (Viral pharyngitis).Q**

17. Ans. is 'b' i.e., DNAase B

18. Ans. is 'b' i.e., Pike's media (***Ref:*** *Ananthanarayan, 9th/e, p. 215 and 8th/e, p. 211*)

"For cultures, swabs should be collected under vision from the affected site and either plated immediately or sent to the laboratory in Pike's medium (**blood agar containing crystal violet and sodium azide**)."

- This medium is also used to preserve Streptococcus pyogenes, pneumococci and Haemophilus influenzae from nose and throat swabs.
- Crystal violet inhibits gram positive bacteria and sodium azide inhibits gram-negative rods and non-haemolytic streptococci.

19. Ans. is 'c' i.e., ASO titre included in major criteria in Jones criteria

Streptococci Other than Group A

20. Ans. is 'b' i.e., Enterococcus fecalis

(***Ref:*** *Ananthanarayan, 9th/e, p. 217-218 and 8th/e, p. 216; Jawet'z, 23rd/e, p. 235*)

- Enterococci grow in the presence of bile and hydrolyze esculin → bile esculin positive.
- It also grow in presence of 6.5% NaCl, pH 9.4.

21. Ans. is 'd' i.e., D (***Ref:*** *Ananthanarayan, 9th/e, p. 217 and 8th/e, p. 216; Jawetz, 23rd/e, p. 235*)

- Among streptococci, Enterococcus (group D streptococcus) is heat resistant.

22. Ans. is 'a' i.e., Enterococcus faecalis (***Ref:*** *Harrison, 18th/e, p. 1186, 1187 and 17th/e, p. 888, 889*)

"Most strains of enterococci are resistant to penicillins, aminoglycosides and sulfonamides. They show **intrinsic resistance to cephalosporins and cotrimoxazole.** Synergistic action of Penicillin and aminoglycoside against enterococci combination therapy is recommended."

23. Ans. is 'b' i.e., Most enterococci are sensitive to penicillin (***Ref:*** *Jawetz, 24th/e, p. 243*)

24. Ans. is 'c' i.e., Enterococcus fecalis (***Ref:*** *Ananthanarayan, 9th/e, p. 211, 215-218 and 8th/e, p. 206, 216; Harrison, 18th/e, p. 1180-1183 and 17th/e, p. 888*)

- Option 'a' and 'd' can be excluded by following information in question:
  1. The isolated cocci are arranged in chains while staphylococci are arranged in grape like clusters.
  2. The isolated organism is catalase negative while staphylococci are catalase positive.
- Now two options are left:
  Option 'b' – Viridans streptococci.
  Option 'c' – Enterococcus fecalis.

These two can be differentiated by following points:

1. Enterococci are a frequent cause of nosocomial bacteremia in patients with intravascular catheters, while viridans streptococcal bacteremia occurs in neutropenic patients, particularly after bone marrow transplantation or high dose chemotherapy for cancer.
2. Enterococci are intrinsically resistant to all cephalosporins and also show high level of resistance to aminoglycosides. Resistance to vancomycin has also become quite common with enterococci, while viridans streptococci are sensitive to vancomycin and vancomycin is the drug of choice for presumptive treatment of viridans grp bacteremia.

- Friends, it is obvious that the infecting organism in this patient is Enterococcus as patient has developed bacteremia on central venous line and he is not responding to cephalosporin, aminoglycoside and vancomycin.

25. Ans. is 'a' i.e., Virulence is due to polysaccharide capsule

- **Capsular polysaccharide is the principal virulence factor, protects it from phagocytosis. Other virulence factors are** toxins (pneumolysin and autolysin).

26. Ans. is 'd' i.e., Pneumococcus

Gram-positive cocci which form α-hemolytic colonies (Greenish colonies) and is optochin sensitive is pneumococcus.

The characteristic features of pneumococcus are: (BIO) (Memory Aid)

(a) **Bile solubility.**

(b) **Optochin sensitivity.**

(c) **Inulin fermentation.**

(d) **Shows quellung reaction (capsular delineation).**

(e) **Forms draughtsman or carrom coin colonies (Colonies with central umbonation).**

27. Ans. is 'c' i.e., Streptococcus pneumoniae

- **Most common cause of lobar pneumonia: Pneumococcus.**
- **Most common cause of acute sinusitis: Pneumococcus.**
- **Most common cause of adult meningitis: Pneumococcus.**
- **Most common cause of atypical pneumonia: Mycoplasma pneumoniae.**
- **Most common infection of pneumococcus: Otitis media.**

28. Ans. is 'c' i.e., Optochin

Gram-positive cocci with α-hemolytic bacterium causing respiratory infection are most probably pneumococcus. It is differentiated from other streptococci by optochin sensitivity.

29. Ans. is 'a' i.e., Pneumococcus

Splenectomy increases the risk of following infections:

Bacterial: *Pneumococcus, H influenzae, Gram negative enteric organism.*

Parasitic: *Babesia.*

Viral: *Risk of viral infection is not increased.*

30. Ans. is 'd' i.e., Pneumococcus

Meningitis caused by S. pneumoniae is milder than others.

Mortality due to meningitis: E.coli > Pneumococcus > Listeria monocytogenes > H influenzae > Meningococci > Gp B Streptococci.

31. Ans. is 'a' i.e., Pneumococcus (***Ref:*** *Ananthanarayan, 8th/e, p. 220, 9th/e, p. 223*)

- **A positive reaction shows clumping because of cross-linking of the antibodies and pneumococci. The halo effect around the pneumococci is apparent capsular swelling.** A negative control would show no clumping or capsular swelling.

32. Ans. is 'c' i.e., Raised in acute inflammation (***Ref:*** *Ananthanarayan, 8th/e, p. 221, 9th/e, p. 223*)

- C-reactive protein (CRP) is an annular (ring-shaped), pentameric protein found in blood plasma, whose levels rise in response to inflammation and disappears once the inflammation subsides. It is an **acute-phase protein** (nonspecific) of **hepatic origin** that increases following interleukin-6 secretion by macrophages and T cells.

33. Ans. is 'a' i.e., Vaccine is made from capsular polysaccharide

(***Ref:*** *Ananthanarayan, 8th/e, p. 223, 9th/e, p. 221*)

- There are currently two types of pneumococcal vaccines: pneumococcal conjugate vaccine (PCV13) and pneumococcal polysaccharide vaccine (PPSV23).
- There are more than 90 types of pneumococcal bacteria.
- PCV13 protects against 13 types which is better than previous 7 types.
- PPSV23 protects against 23 types.
- Both vaccines provide protection against illnesses like meningitis (infection of the covering of the brain and spinal cord) and bacteremia (blood infection). PCV13 also provides protection against pneumonia (lung infection).
- **PCV13:** Pneumococcal conjugate vaccine for all infants and children, and adults 19 years and older at high risk for disease.
- **PPSV23:** Pneumococcal polysaccharide vaccine for all adults 65 years and older and those 2 years of age and older at high risk for disease.

34. Ans. is 'a' i.e., Post-splenectomy patient (***Ref:*** *Harrison, 18th/e, p. 1155*)

Indications: It is recommended for people with:

- Sickle cell disease.
- A damaged spleen or no spleen.
- **Cochlear implant.**
- Cerebrospinal fluid (CSF) leaks.
- HIV/AIDS or other diseases that affect the immune system (such as diabetes, cancer, or liver disease).
- Chronic heart or lung disease.
- Children who take medications that affect the immune system, such as chemotherapy or steroids.

35. Ans. is 'c' i.e., IgA protease is an important virulence factor (***Ref:*** *Greenwood, 8th/e, p. 192*)

- Most important virulence factor is capsule and **serotype 3 followed by 7 are most virulent strains.**

36. Ans. is 'd' i.e., The virulence of pneumococci is dependent only on the production of the capsular polysaccharide

37. Ans. is 'd' i.e., Pneumococcus

Necrotizing fascitis may be caused by:

- Group A streptococcus or mixed aerobic anaerobic bacteria.
- Cl. perferingens.
- Strains of MRSA that produce panton valentine leukocidin (PVL) toxin.

NEISSERIA

- Gram negative diplococci, Non-motile, non-sporing, non-acid fast.
- Strict aerobes, Fastidious, Catalase and oxidase +ve.

N. Gonorrhoeae (Gonococci)

Gonococci is a Gram negative cocci which is classified on the basis of **Pili arrangement and auxotyping.**

Pathogenesis and Virulence Factors:

- **Pili or fimbriae** – Helps in adhesion and prevent phagocytosis.
- **IgA1 proteases** – Cleave mucosal IgA and protect the organisms from the action of mucosal IgA Abs.
- **Lipooligosaccharide/LOS (endotoxin)** – Shock, DIC, Myocardial dysfunction. Morbidity and Mortality of Meningococcal infection directly proportional to endotoxin amount.
- **Outer membrane Proteins** – Protein 1, Protein 2.

Mode of Infection:

- It is exclusively veneral except Ophthalmia neonatorum (Transmission occurs during birth from colonized maternal genital flora).

Lab Diagnosis:

- Samples – Urethral swab (Men) and Cervical swab (Women).
- Transport medium – **Stuart's medium and Amies medium.**
- Microscopy – Gram staining of sample reveals Gram negative Kidney shaped Non-capsulated diplococci.
- Culture – Selective media – **Thayer Martin media and Modified New York City medium.Q**
- **RCUT (Rapid carbohydrate utilization test) – Ferment only Glucose.**
- Vaccine is not available.

Gonococcal Diseases:

- **Acute urethritis (Most common in males).**
- **Water-can perineum (Periurethral tissues causing abscess with sinus formation in male).**
- **Mucopurulent cervicitis (Most common in females).**
- **Adult vagina is resistant to gonococcal infection so Vulvovaginitis is not seen in adult females.**
- **Gonococcal vaginitis (Prepubertal girls and Post-menopausal women).**
- In pregnant women (Salpingitis, PID, Premature delivery, chorioamnionitis and sepsis in the infant).
- **Ophthalmia neonatorum** (most common in neonates).
- Septic arthritis is most common manifestation of systemic infection.

Prophylaxis:

- Early detection of cases, treatment of both partner, tracing of contacts, Heath education and use of condoms.
- **DOC** – Ceftriaxone and Cefixime.

N. Meningitidis (Meningococci)

Meningococci is classified into 13 serotypes on basis of capsular polysaccharides (A,B,C,Y,W,E) are the main ones.

Mode of infection – Droplet inhalation.

Lab Diagnosis:

- Transport medium – Stuart's medium and Amies medium.

CSF Examination:

- **Gram staining** – Meningococci appears as diplococci (lens-shaped) predominantly within the polymorphs and possess polysaccharide capsule.

Contd.

Contd.

- Biochemical analysis – ↑CSF pressure, ↑Protein and ↓ glucose.
- Culture – Thayer Martin media, Blood culture, Chocolate agar.
- Serology – Abs to capsular Ags by ELISA.
- PCR.

Meningococcal Diseases:

- **Fulminant meningococcemia** (Most rapid lethal form of septic shock, differs from other septic shock by prominence of hemorrhagic skin lesion 'petechiae purpura' and development of DIC).
- **Waterhouse Friderichsen syndrome (Severe form of Fulminant meningococcemia).**

Pathogenesis and Virulence Factors:

- **Capsular polysaccharide** – Principal virulence factor and Protects from complement mediated phagocytosis. On the basis of capsule meningococci are typed into 13 serogroups, only 5 are responsible for diseases (A, B, C, Y and WI35)
  - Most common and epidemics caused by type A.
  - Type B-prevalent in developed world.
- **Outer membrane proteins** – show antigenic variability.
- **Lipooligosaccharide/LOS (endotoxin)** – Marked endotoxic activity.
- **IgA proteases** – Cleave mucosal IgA.

DOC: Ceftriaxone and Cefotaxime given for 7 days.

Vaccine Prophylaxis of Meningococci:

- Polysaccharide bivalent (serogroups A and C) vaccine Or Quadrivalent (serogroups A, C, Y and WI35) and ineffective in age <2 years so given after 2 years.
- Conjugate capsular vaccine can be given to young children (Carrier protein – Tetanus toxoid or Diphtheria toxoid).
- **No vaccine is available for Serogroup B because Serogroup B capsule is less immunogenic and also found to be encephalitogenic.Q**

EXTRA EDGE POINTS****

- Deficiency of complement C5-C9 in alternative or classical complement pathway, increase risk of Meningococcal infection.
- Skin lesion in meningococci is due to Endotoxin, Important source is carriers.
- NGU (Non-Gonococcal Urethritis)/Nonspecific Urethritis – Caused by Chlamydia trachomatis (Most common), Ureaplasma urealyticum, Mycoplasma hominis, Candida albicans, Trichomonas vaginalis, HSV and CMV.
- Gonococci is Intracytoplasmic gram negative, doesn't involve testis and incubation period is 2-15 days.Q
- Metastatic **complications of Gonococcus** is endocarditis, meningitis, arthritis, Water can perineum, Fitz Hugh Curtis syndrome and Polyarthritis.
- Meningococci and gonococci grow best on media containing complex organic substances such as heated blood, hemin, and animal proteins and in an atmosphere containing 5% CO_2 (e.g., candle jar).

MCQs

Meningococci

1. **The following bacteria are most often associated with acute neonatal meningitis *except*:**
   (a) Escherichia coli (b) Streptococcus agalactiae
   (c) Neisseria meningitidis (d) Listeria monocytogenes
2. **Young female with 3 days fever presents with headache, BP 90/60 mmHg, Heart rate of 114/min, and pin point spots developed distal to BP cuff. Most likely organism is:** (*AIIMS May 2013*)

(a) Brucella abortus
(b) Brucella suis
(c) N. meningitidis
(d) Staphylococcus aureus

3. **The following statements about Meningococcal meningitis are true *except*:** *(AI 03)*
(a) The source of infection is mainly clinical cases
(b) The disease is more common in dry and cold months of the year
(c) Chemoprophylaxis of close contacts of cases is recommended
(d) The vaccines are not affective in children below 2 years of age

4. **Xavier and Yogender stay in the same hostel of same university, Xavier develops infection due to group B meningococcus. After few days Yogender develops infection due to Group – C meningococcus. All the following are true statement *except*:** *(AI 02)*
(a) Educate students about meningococcal transmission and take preventive measures
(b) Chemoprophylaxis to all against both group B and group C
(c) Vaccine prophylaxis of contacts of Xavier
(d) Vaccine prophylaxis of contacts of Yogendra

5. **Neisserial infection are associated with:**
(a) Deficiency of early complements
(b) Deficiency of late complements
(c) There is not such association
(d) Any deficiency can be associated

6. **Meningococci differ from gonococci in that they:**
(a) Are intracellular
(b) Possess a capsule
(c) Causes fermentation of glucose
(d) Are oxidase positive

7. **Differentiation of Neisseria gonorrhoeae and Neisseria meningitidis is by:** *(AI 90)*
(a) Glucose fermentation
(b) Maltose fermentation
(c) V.P. reaction
(d) Indole test

8. **The vaccine against N. meningitidis contains:** *(ICS 00)*
(a) Whole bacteria
(b) Capsular polysaccharide
(c) Somatic '0' antigen
(d) Lipopolysaccharide protein complex

Gonococci

9. **The best site to obtain a swab in asymptomatic gonorrhea is:** *(AI 95, 02)*
(a) Endocervix
(b) Urethra
(c) Lateral vaginal wall
(d) Posterior fornix

10. **The virulence factor of Neisseria gonorrhoeae includes all of the following *except*:** *(AIIMS 03)*
(a) Outer membrane proteins
(b) IgA protease
(c) M protein
(d) Pilli

11. **Which of the following literally means flow of seeds?**
(a) Anthrax
(b) Clostridia
(c) Gonorrhoea
(d) Proteus

12. **Which of the following is culture media for Neisseria gonorrhea?**
(a) Blood agar
(b) Bile aesculin agar
(c) Mannitol salt agar
(d) Modified New York agar

13. **Incubation period of gonorrhoea is:** *(AIIMS 04)*
(a) 1-2 days
(b) 2-8 days
(c) 8-10 days
(d) 10-15 days

14. **Virulence of gonococci is due to:**
(a) Pili (b) Endotoxin (c) Exotoxin (d) None

15. Selective media for meningococcus is:

(a) Blood sugar
(b) Deoxycholate agar
(c) Thayer Martin media
(d) Mcleod media

16. Virulence factor for meningococci: *(PGI Dec 2007)*

(a) Capsule
(b) Pilli
(c) Endotoxin
(d) Coagulase
(e) M protein

17. Which of the following is not found in meningococci?

(a) Peptidoglycan
(b) Plasmid
(c) Mitochondria
(d) Capsule

18. All are true about Neisseria gonorrhoea *except*:

(a) Gram positive cocci
(b) Cause stricture of urethra
(c) Involves seminal vesicles and spreads to epididymis
(d) Drug of choice is ceftriaxone

19. Least suspectible to gonococcal infection:

(a) Anterior urethra
(b) Testis
(c) Prostrate
(d) Epididymis

20. Which of the following statements best characterize Moraxella catarrhalis?

(a) A gram negative pleomorphic rod that can cause endocarditis
(b) A gram negative rod, fusiform shaped, that is associated with periodontal disease but may cause sepsis
(c) The causative agent of rat bite fever
(d) The causative agent of sinusitis, bronchitis and pneumonia

ANSWERS AND EXPLANATIONS

1. **Ans. is 'c'** i.e., Neisseria meningitidis (***Ref:*** *Harrison, 19th/e, p. 996*)

Causes of Meningitis are:

(a) **Neonatal < 1 Month:**

- Bacterial causes: E Coli > Group B Streptococci > Other Gram negative bacilli > Listeria monocytogenes.
- Viral and Protozoal Infection: TORCH, Varicella Zoster and HIV.
- Spirochetal and fungal infections.

(b) **1-11 Months:** N. meningitidis > Strep pneumoniae > H. influenzae.

(c) **1-20 Years:** N. meningitidis > Strep pneumoniae > H. influenzae.

(d) **More than 20 Years:** Strep pneumoniae.

2. **Ans. is 'c'** i.e., N. meningitidis (***Ref:*** *Harrison, 19th/e, p. 998*)

- The patient has low blood pressure, tachycardia (a state of shock) along with meningitis. Meningococcal meningitis is the most common meningitis complicated by shock.
- Meningitis is the most common complication of meningococcemia. It usually begins suddenly with an intense headache, vomiting, and stiff neck and progresses to coma within a few hours.
- **The Glasgow Meningococcal Septicaemia Prognostic Score (GMSPS) is probably the best-performing scoring system studied so far and may be clinically useful for severity assessment in meningococcal disease.**

3. **Ans. is 'a'** i.e., The source of infection is mainly clinical cases

- The sources of infection are carriers not cases. Meningococcal meningitis occurs in epidemic waves (e.g., in military encampments, in religious pilgrims, and in sub-Saharan Africa, the so-called "meningitis belt"); and a smaller number of sporadic interepidemic cases.
- **Serogroup A is responsible for the majority of outbreaks in sub-Saharan Africa**, whereas **serogroup B is most often the cause of sporadic infections.**
- About 5–30% of the normal population may harbor meningococci in the nasopharynx during interepidemic periods. During epidemics, the carrier rate goes up to 70–80%. A rise in the number of cases is preceded by an increased number of respiratory carriers. **More important is the reduction of personal contacts in a population with a high carrier rate. This is accomplished by avoidance of crowding or administration of vaccines.**

4. **Ans. is 'c'** i.e., Vaccine prophylaxis of contacts of Xavier

   For Group B Meningococci no vaccine is available as polysacchride capsule of Group B is poorly immunogenic and it is also encephalitogenic due to cross reactive antigen on neural cells.

   - But recently FDA has approved Serogroup B meningococcal vaccines (Recombinant) – (Bexsero→ and Trumenba→). These two, newly licensed serogroup B meningococcal vaccines are an important step forward for controlling serogroup B meningococcal disease, especially in outbreak settings. For outbreaks caused by serogroup B meningococcal disease, vaccination with a serogroup B meningococcal vaccine is recommended for those 10 years or older identified as being at increased risk because of the outbreak.

   Source – *http://www.cdc.gov/meningococcal/outbreaks/index.html*

5. **Ans. is 'b'** i.e., Deficiency of late complements – C5 to C9
   - Other risk factors – Hyposplenism and Hypogammaglobulinemia.
6. **Ans. is 'b'** i.e., Possess a capsule
7. **Ans is 'b'** i.e., Maltose fermentation
   - Neisseria meningitidis ferment maltose and glucose both but gonococci only glucose (G for g).
8. **Ans is 'b'** i.e., Capsular polysaccharide

Gonococci

9. **Ans is 'a'** i.e., Endocervix

   Diagnosis of Gonococcal Infection

   In Acute Gonorrhea

   (a) Endocervical Culture 80-90% sensitivity is taken.

   Note: High Vaginal swab is not to be taken.

   (b) Urethral Discharge – 50% Sensitivity.

   (c) Rectal swab (If there is history of rectal sex).

   In Chronic Gonorrhea

   (a) Morning drop secretion.

   (b) Exudate after prostatic massage.

   (c) Centrifuged deposit of urine when no urethral discharge.

10. **Ans. is 'c'** i.e., M protein is virulence factor of Streptococcus pyogenes, not Gonococci.

    Already explained in book text.

11. **Ans. is 'c'** i.e., Gonorrhoea

    Gonorrhoea is a Greek word which means – **flow of seed** (from the mistaken belief that the discharge contained semen).

12. **Ans. is 'd'** i.e., Modified New York agar, other than this Thayer martin is also used for culture of Gonococci.
13. **Ans. is 'b'** i.e., ICP – 2 to 8 days and remember two types of typing is done Auxotyping and Pili Based typing.

14. Ans. are 'a' and 'b' i.e., Pili and lipooligosacchride plays a role in virulence with additional iron factors like Transferrin and Lactoferrin.

Already explained in book text.

15. Ans. is 'c' i.e., Thayer Martin media (Chocolate agar with antibiotics like Nystatin, Colistin, Vancomycin and Trimethoprim).

16. Ans. is 'a,b,c' i.e., Remember Pilli also plays role of virulence in meningococci.

17. Ans. is 'c' i.e., Its logical mitochondria but plasmid is also rarely seen as a feature of meningococci.

18. Ans. is 'a' i.e., Gram positive cocci.

19. Ans. is 'b' i.e., Testis, least suspectible to gonococci.

20. Ans. is 'd' i.e., Moraxella catarrhalis is a gram negative diplococcus arranged as pair with adjacent flattened. Obligate aerobe, catalase, oxidase positive, nonfermenters, DNAase +, cause of bronchitis, bronchopneumonia, conjunctivitis, sinusitis and otitis media. More than 95% produce betalactamases.

CLOSTRIDIUM

- Gram positive spore forming bacilli, strict anaerobes.
- **Mostly motile except: Cl. perfringens, Cl. Tetani (type 6).**
- Non-capsulated except Cl. perfringens and Cl. butyricum.
- Medically important – Cl. perfringens, Cl. tetani, Cl. botulinum, Cl. difficile.
- Cl. perfringens, Cl. tetani – Normal flora of Human intestine.
- Spores of Clostridium are present in soil, dust and air.
- Industrial Importance – Cl. butyricum and Cl. acetobutylicum are used in preparation Butanol and Acetone.

Spores Types of Various Clostridia Species

- **Spherical and Terminal** (Drumstick appearance) – Cl. tetani, Cl. Tetanomorphum.
- **Oval and Terminal** (Tennis racket appearance) – Cl. difficile, Cl. tertium.
- **Subterminal** – Cl. perfringens (Boxcar appearance), Cl. botulinum.
- **Oval and Central** – Cl. bifermentans.

Clostridium as Human Pathogen

1. *The Gas gangrene group:*
   - Established pathogens – Cl. perfringens (60%), **Cl. septicum (Citron bodies),** Cl. novyi.
   - Less pathogenic – Cl. histolyticum, Cl. tertium.
   - Doubtful pathogens – Cl. bifermentans, Cl. sporogenes.
2. *Tetanus:* Cl. tetani.
3. *Acute colitis* (Antibiotic associated diarrhea): Cl. difficile.
4. *Food poisoning:*
   - Gastroenteritis – Cl. perfringens (type A).
   - **Necrotising enteritis – Cl. perfringens (type C) beta toxin.**
   - Botulism – Cl. botulinum.

Cultivation

- Clostridium species grows well in anaerobic medium like RCM Broth and Thioglycollate broth.
- Subculture is done on Blood agar from RCM Broth or Thioglycollate broth by using MacIntosh flides jar or Gas pack.

Cl. Perfringens (Cl. Welchii)

- 80% of cases are caused by Cl. perfringens.
- Capsulated, non-motile, shows stormy fermentation, Sub-terminal spores but does not produce spores in tissues or in Culture media.

CL. PERFRINGENS DISEASES

1. **Gas gangrene**
   - MCC of gas gangrene by Type A.
   - Occurs in severely crushed injury.
   - Involves necrosis of muscles.
   - **Most important toxin for gas gangrene is Alpha toxin Lethal, Lecithinase (phospholipase C). Which is responsible for (Nagler's reaction).Q**
   - Spores are usually destroyed within 5 minutes by boiling but **those of food poisoning strains of Type A and certain C strain resist boiling for several hours.**
   - Rx-Sx debridement
     - If excessive injury – amputation of limb.

Contd.

Contd.

2. **Gastroenteritis (Food poisoning)**
   - Meat/milk products.
   - 2nd or 3rd MCC of food poisoning.
   - IP – 8-24 hours.
   - Due to heat labile enterotoxin type A.
3. **Enteritis necroticans (Pigbel)**
   (Ischemic necrosis of the jejunum and gas in the tissue).
   - **Caused by β toxin of type C strain.Q**

Virulence Factors:

- Four major toxins– α, β, ε and iota.
- Eight minor toxins – Gamma, Delta, Lambda, Kappa, Theta, Eta, Mu and Nu.
- Other toxins – Neuraminidase and Enterotoxin.

Alpha toxin is the most important toxin and it is lethal, Lecithinase (phospholipase C).

- Cl. perfringens is found in faeces and contaminates the skin or perineum, buttocks, thigh.
  - **Typically, gas gangrene begins with the sudden onset of pains in the region of the wound, which helps differentiate it from spreading cellulitis.**
  - Crepitus in a wound is produced by Cl. Welchii.
- Rx-Sx debridement
  - If excessive injury – amputation of limb.

Lab Diagnosis

- **Specimens:** Necrotic tissues, Muscle fragments, exudates from deeper parts of the wound and left over food.
- **Direct Microscopy:** Boxcar shaped GPB without spores in Gram staining are suggestive of Cl. perfringens.
- **Culture:** Robertson cooked meat (RCM) broth turns into pink color due to saccharolytic nature of Cl. perfringens, Egg yolk agar and Thioglycollate broth.
- **Identification tests:** Target hemolysis (double zone hemolysis), Nagler's reaction, Reverse CAMP test +ve, stormy fermentation in litmus milk.Q

Cl. Tetani

Gram Positive, Anaerobic spore forming bacilli and Motile with swarming tendency (except type 6). **Swarming** is also shown by **Bacillius cereus – Gram +ve bacilli and Proteus mirabilis and Proteus vulgaris – Gram –ve bacilli.**

Cl. Tetani Diseases:

- Bacteria multiply in local wound, produce tetanus toxin reach CNS and **disease occurs:**
  - Lock jaw/Trismus (first symptom).
  - Arching of back – opisthotonus.
  - Death respiratory muscle paralysis/due to convulsions.

Virulence factors: Cl. tetani produces 2 exotoxins (Tetanolysin and Tetanospasmin):

1. **Tetanolysin:** Heat labile, oxygen labile hemolysin.
2. **Tetanospasmin (Tetanus toxin):** Oxygen stable but heat labile and Neurotoxin (toxin is plasmid coded).

Mechanism: Blocks release of inhibitory neurotransmitters glycine/GABA and leads to spastic descending paralysis.

Mode of Transmission (Spores are present in soil, dust and air)

1. Injury (superficial abrasions, punctured wounds, road traffic accidents).
2. Surgery done without proper asepsis.
3. Neonates following abortion/delivery, due to unhygienic practices.
4. Otogenic tetanus.

Note: It is non-infectious so there is no person to person spread.

Lab Diagnosis:

- Specimen: Excised tissue bits from the necrotic depths of wounds (wound swabs are not acceptable).
- Direct Microscopy: In gram staining – GPB with terminal spores (Drumstick appearance).
- Culture: RCM broth turns into Black due to proteolytic nature of Cl. tetani.
- Swarming on Blood agar.
- Toxigenicity tests:
  1. In vitro hemolysis inhibition test (Detects only tetanolysin) – Hemolysis on blood agar is inhibited by adding anti-toxin.
  2. In vivo mouse inoculation test – Black RCM broth injected into root of the tail of a test mouse and Death occurs within two days.

Prevention:

- Active Immunization (Vaccine) – Tetanus toxoid (TT) in form of Monovalent or Combined vaccine (DPT).
  Site: TT is given by deep intramuscular route at anterolateral aspect of thigh (Children) and in deltoid (adults).
- Protective titer – Persons are said to be protected if tetanus antitoxin titre is equal or more than 0.01 unit/ml.
- Surgical debridement is vitally important because it removes the necrotic tissue that is essential for proliferation of the organisms and Penicillin strongly inhibits the growth of C tetani and stops further toxin production. Antibiotics may also control associated pyogenic infection.

Recommendation for prevention of tetanus after injury

Immunity category	Wound < 6 hrs, clean, non-penetrating, negligible tissue damage	Other wounds
A	Nothing required	Nothing required
B	1 Dose of toxoid	1 Dose of toxoid
C	1 Dose of toxoid	1 Dose of toxoid + HTIG
D	Toxoid complete dose	Toxoid complete dose + HTIG

A – Taken complete course of TT/Booster within past 5 years.
B – Taken complete course of TT/Booster within past > 5 years to < 10 years.
C – Taken complete course of TT/Booster within past > 10 years.
D – **Not** taken complete course of TT/Booster or immunity status is not known.

Cl. Botulinum

- Anaerobic GPB with sub-terminal spores.
- Widely distributed as saprophytes in soil, animal manure, vegetables and sea mud.
- It is an agent of Bioterrorism.
- Cl. botulinum is non-invasive and pathogenicity is due to neurotoxin 'Botulinum Toxin' (BT).
- Serotypes (8 serotypes) – A, B, C1, C2, D, E, F and G.
- A, B, E causes human disease and most severe being serotype A.
- All serotypes produce neurotoxin, except C2 which produces an enterotoxin.
- CNS is not affected by the BT.

CL. BOTULINUM DISEASES

1. **Food Borne Botulism (Due to preformed BT)**
   - Most common source – Homemade canned food.
   - Most cases are sporadic and IP – 18-36 hours.
   - **Diplopia, Dysphagia, Dysarthria, Ptosis and Constipation (But No Diarrhoea).Q**
   - Flaccid descending paralysis and Respiratory muscle paralysis leads to death.
2. **Infant Botulism (Due to Ingestion of Spores)**
   - Most common source – Honey.
   - Spores produce toxin in gut.
   - **Floppy child syndrome** – Most common type (can't feed milk, can't sit due to muscle paralysis).
   - Occurs in below 1 year of age.
3. **Wound Botulism**
   - Contamination of wounds with spores.
   - It presents like food borne botulism except absence of gastrointestinal symptoms.

Therapeutic Uses:

- BT (BOTOX) – In Strabismus, Blepharospasm, myoclonus and prevent wrinkles.

Pathogenesis and Virulence Factors:

Its pathogenesis is due to production of powerful neurotoxin (Botulinum toxin/BT) and it is one of the most potent neurotoxins on the planet.

Mechanism of Action

- **BT binds to Ach receptors on the nerves terminals (NMJ, post ganglionic parasympathetic nerve endings and peripheral ganglia) which result in Blockage of release of the Ach.** Leading to Flaccid descending paralysis (Parasympathetic system).
- Presynaptic action on motor nerve ending.

Lab Diagnosis:

- Specimens: Faeces and Food
- Direct Microscopy: In gram staining: GPB with Sub-terminal spores or without spores.
- Culture: RCM broth turns into pink due to saccharolytic nature of serotypes C, D, E and Black due to proteolytic nature of serotypes A, B, F.
- Serotyping with type specific antisera.
- Toxin demonstration (Mouse Bioassay).
- Food borne botulism is confirmed by demonstration of the bacillus or the toxin in food or feces.

Treatment:

- Ventilator support.
- Anti botulinum serum.
- Sx debridement of wound.
- Penicillin/Metronidazole.

Clostridium Difficile

- It is a normal gut commensal.
- **Causes:**
  Pseudomembranous colitis and Antibiotic associated diarrhea.

Risk Factors:

- Prolonged hospital stay and prolonged antibiotic uses.
- Old age, severe illness, antacid treatment and GIT surgery.
- Almost all antibiotics even the ones used in treatment of pseudomembranous colitis can cause the disease due to:
  - Clindamycin (MC).
  - Ampicillin/Amoxicillin.
  - Cephalosporins.

Lab Diagnosis:

- Isolation of bacilli followed by Toxigenicity testing.
- **Culture – CCFA (cefoxitin cycloserine fructose agar), CCYA (cefoxitin cycloserine egg yolk agar).**
- Toxin demonstration:
  - **Cell culture cytotoxin assay in stools is the best test. (Demonstration of enterotoxin and cytotoxin on Hep 2 cell lines is done).**
  - By ELISA for Toxin A and B.
  - PCR – Detection of toxin B gene in stool.
  - Colonoscopy and histopathology.

DOC:

- Oral Metronidazole (Mild to moderate cases).
- Oral Vancomycin (Recurrent or severe cases).
  (Only condition in which oral vancomycin is given).

EXTRA EDGE POINTS****

- Clostridia which show Proteolytic activity (convert meat into black color) are Cl. tetani, Cl. botulinum A, B and F.
- Clostridia which show Saccharolytic activity (convert meat into pink color) are Cl. perfringens, Cl. difficle and Cl. botulinum C, D and E.
- Gas gangrene is caused by alpha and theta toxin.
- Tetanus affects primarily presynaptic terminals and incubation period is about 6-10 days.
- Non-neurotoxic toxin is C2, gene for botulinum toxin is encoded by a bacteriophage, Clostridium baratti may cause botulism.
- Blood is not present in Pseudomembranous colitis.

MCQs

Clostridium

1. **Saccharolytic species of clostridia:** *(Recent MCQ)*
   (a) C. tetani (b) Cl. cochlearum
   (c) Cl. septicum (d) None
2. **Which of the following species of clostridium species does not break carbohydrate and protein?** *(Recent MCQ)*
   (a) Sporogenes (b) Septicum
   (c) Cochlearum (d) Novyi
3. **Drumstick appearance is seen in:** *(Recent MCQ)*
   (a) Cl. tetani (b) Cl. Tetanomorphum
   (c) Cl. Sphenoids (d) All

Clostridium Perfringens (WELCHII)

4. **Regarding gas gangrene one of the following is correct:** *(AI 04)*
   (a) It is due to clostridium botulinum infection
   (b) Clostridial species are gram-negative spore forming anerobes
   (c) The clinical features are due to the release of protein endotoxin
   (d) Gas is invariably present in the muscle compartments

5. The following statements are true regarding Clostridium perfrigens *except*: *(AI 05)*

(a) It is the most common cause of gas gangrene
(b) It is normally present in human faces
(c) The principal toxin of C. perfringens is the alpha toxin
(d) Gas gangrene producing strains of C. perfringens produce heat resistant spores

6. Most common organism responsible for gas gangrene is: *(Recent MCQ)*

(a) Clostridium perfringens
(b) Clostridium difficile
(c) Clostridium tetani
(d) Clostridium septicum

Toxins and Pathogenicity

7. Gas gangrene is due to: *(PGI Nov 14)*

(a) Alpha toxin
(b) Theta toxin
(c) Beta toxin
(d) Delta toxin
(e) Epsilon toxin

8. Opacity around colonies of clostridium perfringens is due to: *(Recent MCQ)*

(a) Theta toxin
(b) Lecithinase
(c) Desmolase
(d) Cytokinin

9. Each of the following statements concerning clostridium perfringens is correct *except*: *(Recent MCQ)*

(a) It cause gas gangrene
(b) It cause food poisoning
(c) It produces exotoxin
(d) It is a gram negative rod that does not ferment lactose

10. Gastrointestinal enteritis necroticans is caused by: *(PGI Dec 07)*

(a) Clostridium difficile
(b) Clostridium perfringens
(c) Botulinum
(d) C. Jejuni
(e) Pseudomonas

11. Regarding Clostridium perfringens gas gangrene, false is: *(AIIMS Nov 09, 10)*

(a) Common cause of gas gangrene
(b) Nagler reaction positive
(c) Most common toxin is hyaluronidase
(d) Food poisoning strain of Cl. perfringens produces heat resistant spores

12. Incubation period of gas gangrene is: *(PGI 94)*

(a) 1-3 days
(b) 4-6 days
(c) 7-10 days
(d) 10-15 days

13. Gas gangrene is caused by all *except*: *(AIIMS May 09)*

(a) Cl. histolyticum
(b) Cl. novyi
(c) Cl. septicum
(d) Cl. sporogenes

Lab Diagnosis and Treatment

14. "Citron bodies" boat of leaf shaped pleomorphic organism in an exudate is: *(Recent MCQ)*

(a) Cl. welchii
(b) Cl. edematiens
(c) Cl. septicum
(d) Cl. tetani

15. Naegle's reaction detects: *(PGI 86)*

(a) Coagulase
(b) Hyaluronidase
(c) Lecithinase
(d) None of the above

16. Naegler's reaction is shown by: *(DNB Pattern)*

(a) Clostridium tetani
(b) Clostridium welchii
(c) Mycobacterium tuberculosis
(d) Mycobacterium leprae

CLOSTRIDIUM TETANI

Morphology and Characteristics

17. Clostridium tetani is: *(PGI 94)*

(a) Gram positive bacilli
(b) Gram negative bacilli
(c) Gram positive cocci
(d) Gram negative cocci

18. True about clostridium tetani: *(PGI Dec 03)*

(a) It is gram +ve
(b) Drum stick appearance
(c) Grows in aerobic environment
(d) It is gram –ve

19. Swarming growth on culture is characteristic of which Gram positive organism? *(Recent MCQ)*

(a) Clostridium welchii
(b) Clostridium tetani
(c) Bacillus cercus
(d) Proteus mirabilis

20. All are true regarding tetanus *except*: *(AIIMS Nov 10)*

(a) Transmission through contaminated wounds and injuries
(b) More common in winters and dry weather
(c) Reservoir in soil and intestines of humans and animals
(d) No herd immunity of life long immunity

Toxins and Pathogenicity

21. Tetanus affects primarily: *(Recent MCQ)*

(a) Presynaptic terminal of spinal cord
(b) Post synaptic terminal of spinal cord
(c) Neuromuscular junction
(d) Muscle fibres

22. Mechanism of action of tetanospasmin: *(Recent MCQ)*

(a) Inhibition of GABA release
(b) Inhibition cAMP
(c) Inactivation of Ach receptors
(d) Inhibition of cGMP

Diagnosis, Treatment and Prevention of Tetanus

23. Toxigenicity of tetanus is done on: *(DNB Aug 13 Pattern)*

(a) Rabbit
(b) Horse
(c) Mouse
(d) Guinea pig

24. A person has received complete immunization against tetanus 10 years ago. Now he presents with a clean wound without any lacerations from an injury sustained 2.5 hours ago. He should now be given: *(AI 01)*

(a) Full course of tetanus toxoid
(b) Single dose of tetanus toxoid
(c) Human tet globulin
(d) Human tet globulin and single dose of toxoid

25. A 10-year-old boy following a road traffic accident presents to the casuality with contaminated wound over the left leg. He has received his complete primary immunization before preschool age and received a booster of DT at school entry age. All of the following can be done *except*: *(AIIMS 01)*

(a) Injection TT
(b) Injection of human antiserum
(c) Broad spectrum antibodies
(d) Wound debridement and cleaning

26. The most effective way of preventing tetanus is: *(AIIMS 01)*

(a) Surgical debridement and toilet
(b) Hyperbaric oxygen
(c) Antibiotics
(d) Tetanus toxoid

27. All of the following statements regarding Clostridium tetani are true, *except*: *(AI 11)*

(a) Spores are resistant to heat
(b) Primary immunization consists of three doses
(c) Incubation period is 6-10 days
(d) Person to person transmission does not occur

Clostridium Botulinum

28. Botulism is a disease of: *(Recent MCQ)*

(a) Neural transmission caused by the toxin of the bacterium clostridium botulinum
(b) Muscular transmission caused by the toxin of the bacterium clostridium botulinum
(c) Neuromuscular transmission caused by the toxin of the bacterium clostridium botulinum
(d) Non neuromuscular transmission caused by the toxin of the bacterium clostridium botulinum

29. Among the toxin produced by clostridium botulinum, the non-neurotoxic one is: *(Recent MCQ)*

(a) A
(b) B
(c) C1
(d) C2

30. Botulinum toxin acts on: *(Recent MCQ)*

(a) Sympathetic system
(b) Parasympathetic system
(c) Amygdala
(d) Motor cortex

31. Botulinum affects all *except*: *(AI 07)*

(a) Neuromuscular junction
(b) Preganglionic junction
(c) Post ganglionic nerves
(d) CNS

Pathogenicity and Clinical Features

32. The following statements are true regarding botulism *except*: *(AIIMS May 03)*

(a) Infant botulism is caused by ingestion of preformed toxin
(b) Clostridium botulinum A, B, C and F cause human disease
(c) The gene for botulinum toxin is encoded by a bacteriophage
(d) Clostridium baratti may cause botulism

33. Botulism is most commonly due to: *(Recent MCQ)*

(a) Egg
(b) Milk
(c) Meat
(d) Pulses

34. All occurs in botulism *except*: *(AIIMS Dec 97)*

(a) Diplopia
(b) Diarrhea
(c) Dysphagia
(d) Dysarthria

35. An 18-year-old male presented with acute onset descending paralysis of 3 days duration. There is also history of blurring of vision for the same duration. On examination, the patient has quadriparesis with areflexia. Both the pupils are non-reactive. The most probably diagnosis is: *(AIIMS 06)*

(a) Poliomyelitis
(b) Botulism
(c) Diphtheria
(d) Porphyria

36. All of the following statements about Botulism are true *except*: *(AI 97)*

(a) Botulism is caused by endotoxin
(b) Honey ingestion causes infant botulism

(c) Constipation is seen
(d) Detection of antitoxin in the serum can aid in diagnosis

37. Botulism causes: *(Recent MCQ)*
(a) Descending flaccid paralysis
(b) Descending spastic paralysis
(c) Ascending paralysis
(d) Ascending spastic paralysis

CLOSTRIDIUM DIFFICILE

Clostridium Difficile – Associated Disease

38. Most common organism responsible for, pseudomembranous colitis is: *(Recent MCQ)*
(a) Clostridium difficile
(b) Clostridium botulism
(c) Clostridium histolyticum
(d) Clostridium butyricum

39. A patient of acute lymphocytic leukemia with fever and neutropenia develops diarrhea after administration of amoxicillin therapy, which of the following organism is most likely to the causative agent? *(AIIMS Nov 05)*
(a) Salmonella typhi
(b) Clostridium difficile
(c) Clostridium perfringenes
(d) Shigella flexneri

40. Cause of clostridium difficile associated diarrhea: *(Recent MCQ)*
(a) Trauma
(b) Dairy products
(c) Fried rice
(d) Antibiotic use

Pathogenicity, Diagnosis and Treatment

41. Pseudomembranous colitis, all are true *except*: *(AIIMS May 07)*
(a) Toxin A is responsible for clinical manifestation
(b) Toxin B is responsible for clinical manifestation
(c) Blood in stools is a common feature
(d) Summit lesions is early histopathological finding

42. True regarding pseudomembranous colitis are all *except*: *(AI 2000)*
(a) It is caused by clostridium difficile
(b) The organism is a normal commensal of gut
(c) It is due to production of phospholipase A
(d) It is treated by vancomycin

43. Patient present with abdominal pain, diarrhea takingclindamycin for 5 days. Treated with metronidazole symptoms subsided. What is the causative agent? *(Recent MCQ)*
(a) Clostridium difficile
(b) Clostridium perfringens
(c) Clostridium welchi
(d) Clostridium marneffi

ANSWERS AND EXPLANATIONS

Clostridium

1. **Ans. is 'c'** i.e., Cl. septicum (***Ref:*** *See above explanation*)
   - Cl. septicum is predominating saccharolytic. Cl tetani is only proteolytic and Cl cochlearum neither proteolytic nor saccharolytic.
2. **Ans. is 'c'** i.e., Cochlearum (***Ref:*** *Ananthanarayan, 8th/e, p. 250*)
   - Neither proteolytic nor saccharolytic → Cl. cochlearum.

3. **Ans. is 'a'** i.e., Cl. tetani (***Ref:*** *Ananthanarayan, 9th/e p. 252 and 8th/e, p. 256*)

Position	Shape of the bacillus	Example
Central	Spindle shaped	Cl. bifermentans
Subterminal	Club shaped	Cl. perfringens
Oval and terminal	Tennis racket	Cl. tertium
Spherical and terminal	Drum stick	Cl. tetani

Clostridium Perfringens (CLOSTRIDIUM WELCHII)

4. **Ans. is 'd'** i.e., Gas is invariably present in the muscle compartments.

(***Ref:*** *Ananthanarayan, 9th/e, p. 253-254; Harrison, 18th/e, p. 1206, 1207 and 17th/e, p. 906*)

- Gas gangrene is characterized by rapid and extensive necrosis of muscle accompanied by gas formation and systemic toxicity.
- It is caused by C1 perfringens (not C1 botulinum) and is due to alpha exotoxin (not endotoxin).
- Clostridial species are gram (+) ve spore forming.

5. **Ans. is 'd'** i.e., Gas gangrene producing strains of C. perfringens produce heat resistant spores.

(***Ref:*** *Harrisons 17th/e, p. 906 and 16th/e, p. 847, Ananthanarayan, 9th/e, p. 253-254 and 8th/e, p. 251, 252, 253; Greenwood, 16th/e, p. 231*)

"Heat-resistant spores produced by food poisoning strains that can survive boiling for several hours, whereas the spores of the type 'A' strains that cause gas gangrene are inactivated within a few minutes by boiling." – *Greenwood, 16th/e, p. 231*

- Cl. perfringens is a normal inhabitant of the large intestines of human beings and animals. It is found in the feces and contaminates the skin of the perineum, buttocks and thighs. Type A predominates in fecal flora of humans as well as in soil.
- The alpha toxin is produced by all types of C1. perfringens and most abundantly by type 'A' strains. This is the most important toxin biologically and is responsible for profound toxemia of gas gangrene.
- **Some 80% of the cases of gas gangrene is usually caused by C. perfringens**, while C. novyi, C. septicum and histolyticum cause most of the remaining cases.

6. **Ans. is 'a'** i.e., Clostridium perfringens (***Ref:*** *Harrison, 18th/e, p. 1206, 1207 and 17th/e, p. 906*)

Toxins and Pathogenicity

7. **Ans. is 'a'** i.e., Alpha toxin **and 'b'** i.e., Theta toxin (***Ref:*** *Ananthanarayan, 9th/e, p. 254 and 8th/e, p. 252, 253*)

- Alpha toxin is most important toxin biologically and is responsible for the profound toxemia of gas gangrene. The alpha toxin of **C perfringens type A is a lecithinase, and its lethal action is proportionate to the rate at which it splits lecithin (an important constituent of cell membranes) to phosphorylcholine and diglyceride.**
- Along with alpha-toxin, theta-toxin plays an important role in the pathogenesis of gas gangrene. The theta toxin has similar hemolytic and necrotizing effects but is not a lecithinase. It is a member of the cholesterol-dependent cytolysins that act by forming pores in cell membranes.

8. **Ans. is 'b'** i.e., Lecithinase (***Ref:*** *Ananthanarayan, 9th/e, p. 251-255 and 8th/e, p. 252-253*)

Naegler's reaction: This reaction is produced by C. perfringens as opalescence in 20% human serum or egg yolk media due to Lecithinase (phospholipase) activity of alpha toxin, it splits lecithin into phosphorylcholine and diacylglycerol in the presence of Ca^{++} and Mg^{++} ions.

9. **Ans. is 'd'** i.e., It is a gram negative rod that does not ferment lactose

(***Ref:*** *Ananthanarayan, 9th/e, p. 253-255 and 8th/e, p. 252-254*)

- Clostridium perfringens is gram positive, spore forming anaerobic bacteria that ferments lactose.

10. **Ans is 'b'** i.e., Cl. perfringens (***Ref:*** *Previous explanations*)

- Necrotising enteritis (enteritis necroticans or Pigbel) is caused by Cl. perfringens.

11. Ans. is. 'c' i.e., Most common toxin is hyaluronidase (***Ref:*** *Previous explanation*)

- The most common and most important toxin produced by Cl. perfringens is α-toxin (lecithinase).

12. Ans. is 'a' i.e., 1-3 days; **'b'** i.e., 4-6 days (***Ref:*** *Ananthanarayan, 9th/e, p. 257 and 8th/e, p. 255*)

- The incubation period of gas gangrene depends upon the causative organism:

Cl. perfringens	→	10-48 hrs (1 to 2 days)
Cl. septicum	→	2-3 days
Cl. novyi	→	5-6 days

If you will have to choose one option, go ahead with 10-48 hours, as 80% of the gas gangrene cases are caused by Cl. perfringens (Cl. welchii).

13. Ans. is 'd' i.e., Cl. sporogenes

(***Ref:*** *Ananthanarayan, 9th/e, p. 257; Harrison, 18th/e, p. 1206, 1207 and 17th/e, p. 903*)

- Some 80% of the cases of gas gangrene is usually caused by C. perfringens, while C. novyi, C. septicum and C. histolyticum cause most of the remaining cases.

Lab. Diagnosis and Treatment

14. Ans. is 'c' i.e., Clostridium septicum (***Ref:*** *Ananthanarayan, 8th/e, p. 256 and 7th/e, p. 256*)

"Citron bodies and boat or leaf shaped pleomorphic bacilli with irregular staining suggest Cl. septicum."

15. Ans. is 'c' i.e., Lecithinase (***Ref:*** *Ananthanarayan, 9th/e, p. 254 and 8th/e, p. 252*)

- It detects alpha toxin which is a phospholipase (lecithinase C).
- Explained in Ans No. 8.

16. Ans. is 'b' i.e., Clostridium welchii (***Ref:*** *Ananthanarayan, 9th/e, p. 252-254*)

CLOSTRIDIUM TETANI

Morphology and Characteristics

17. Ans. is 'a' i.e., Gram positive bacilli (***Ref:*** *Ananthanarayan, 9th/e, p. 259 and 8th/e, p. 256*)

- All clostridia are anaerobic, spore forming, gram positive bacilli.

18. Ans. is 'a' i.e., It is gram +ve; **'b'** i.e., Drum stick appearance

(***Ref:*** *Ananthanarayan, 9th/e, p. 259 and 8th/e, p. 256-257*)

- C. tetani is a gram (+) ve bacillus.
- The spores are spherical terminal and bulging, giving the bacillus characteristic 'drum stick' appearance.
- It is an obligatory anaerobe that grows only in the absence of oxygen.

Remember:

- There is no person to person transmission in tetanus → tetanus patient is not infectious.

19. Ans. is 'b' i.e., Clostridium tetani (***Ref:*** *Ananthanarayan, 9th/e, p. 259 and 8th/e, p. 257, 280*)

Swarming Growth

- Swarming growth is due to motility of bacteria. In young culture discrete colonies are seen but thereafter actively motile cells spread on the surface of the plate in successive waves to form a thin filmy layer in concentric circles.
- Gram positive organism showing swarming growth → C. tetani and Bacillus cereus.
- Gram negative organism showing swarming growth → Proteus mirabilis, Proteus vulgaris and Vibrio parahaemolyticus.

20. Ans. is 'b' i.e., More common in winters and dry weather

(***Ref:*** *Ananthanarayan, 9th/e, p. 261; Harrison, 19th/e, p. 1197 and 17th/e, p. 898; Park, 20th/e, p. 272, 273*)

- Tetanus is common in areas where soil is cultivated, in rural areas, in warm climates, during summer months, and among males.
- Infection is acquired by contamination of wounds with tetanus spores.

- **Reservoir of infection:** The natural habitat of organism is soil and dust. The bacilli may be found in the intestine many herbivorous animals, e.g., cattle, horses, goat and sheep and are excreted in their feces. The bacilli may be found in the intestine of man without causing ill effects.
- Tetanus is one disease in which herd immunity does not protect the individual.

Toxins and Pathogenicity

21. Ans. is 'a' i.e., Presynaptic terminal of spinal cord

- Tetanus toxin (tetanospasmin) blocks release of glycine and GABA from presynaptic terminals in brainstem spinal cord which leads to spastic muscle contraction.

22. Ans. is 'a' i.e., Inhibition of GABA release

(***Ref:*** *Harrison, 19th/e, p. 1197, 1198; Ananthanarayan, 9th/e, p. 260 and 8th/e, p. 259, 260*)

- Tetanospasmin blocks the release of inhibitory neurotransmitters (GABA and glycine) in brainstem spinal cord.

Diagnosis, Treatment and Prevention of Tetanus

23. Ans. is 'c' i.e., Mouse (***Ref:*** *Textbook of Microbiology and Immunology by Parija, p. 249*)

- Strains of clostridium tetani are tested by production of toxins by following methods:
  - (i) In vitro neutralization of toxin on blood agar for only tetanolysin not for tetanospasmin.
  - (ii) In vivo neutralization test on mice.

24. Ans. is 'b' i.e., Single dose of tetanus toxoid

(***Ref:*** *Park, 19th/e, p. 263; Ananthanarayan, 9th/e, p. 262, 263 and 8th/e, p. 261*)

All wounds receive surgical toilet

- Wounds less than 6 hours old, clean, non-penetrating And with negligible tissue damage
  - Immunity category → Treatment
    - A — Nothing more required
    - B — Toxoid 1 dose
    - C — Toxoid 1 dose
    - D — Toxoid complete course
- Other wounds
  - Immunity category → Treatment
    - A — Nothing more required
    - B — Toxoid 1 dose
    - C — Toxoid 1 dose + Human Tet. Ig.
    - D — Toxoid complete Course + Human Tet. Ig

A = Has had a complete course of toxoid or a booster dose within the past 5 years.

B = Has had a complete course of toxoid or a booster dose more than 5 years ago and less than 10 years ago.

C = Has had a complete course of toxoid or a booster dose more than 10 years ago.

D = Has not had a complete course of toxoid or immunity status is unknown.

- The person in this question belongs to category B, so should receive one dose of tetanus toxoid.

25. Ans. is 'b' i.e., Injection of human antiserum

(***Ref:*** *PSM Park, 19th/e, p. 263*)

- See above Question.
- Boy in this question comes under category B.

26. Ans. is 'd' i.e., Tetanus toxoid (***Ref:*** *Ananthanarayan, 9th/e, p. 262-263 and 8th/e, p. 259*)

- The obvious and most dependable method of prevention is to build up antitoxic immunity by active immunization (administration of tetanus toxoid) by routine immunization of children and booster doses where appropriate.
- Tetanus is best prevented by active immunization with tetanus toxoid. – *PSM Park*

Remember

- The most effective way of preventing tetanus → Tetanus toxoid
- The most effective way of preventing gas gangrene → Surgical debridement

27. Ans. is None (All the above are true) (***Ref:*** *Harrison, 17th/e, p. 898-900; Park, 21st/e, p. 286, 284, 285*)

CLOSTRIDIUM BOTULINUM

Botulinum Toxin

28. Ans. is 'c' i.e., Neuromuscular transmission caused by the toxin of the bacterium clostridium botulinum (***Ref:*** *Ananthanarayan, 8th/e, p. 261*)

- Botulinum toxin is absorbed from the gut, enters the blood circulation, and binds to receptors of presynaptic membranes of motor neurons of the peripheral nervous system and cranial nerves. The toxin does not cross the blood brain barrier or affect the central nervous system.
- Botulinum toxins act by blocking the release of acetylcholine at synapses and neuromuscular junction. Resulting in lack of muscle contraction and flaccid paralysis.

29. Ans. is 'd' i.e., C_2 (***Ref:*** *Ananthanarayan, 9th/e, p. 264 and 8th/e, p. 261*)

All serotypes (A, B, C1, D, E, F, G) produce neurotoxin except C2 which produces cytotoxic (enterotoxin).

30. Ans. is 'b' i.e., Parasympathetic system

(***Ref:*** *Harrison, 18th/e, p. 1200 and 17th/e, p. 901; Ananthanarayan, 9th/e, p. 264 and 8th/e, p. 262*)

- Botulinum neurotoxin, whether ingested, inhaled or produced in the intestine or a wound, enters the vascular system and is transported to peripheral cholinergic nerve terminals, including neuromuscular junctions, post-ganglionic parasympathetic nerve endings, and peripheral ganglia. The central nervous system is not involved.

31. Ans. is 'd' i.e., CNS (***Ref:*** *Harrison, 18th/e, p. 1200 and 17th/e, p. 901*)

- The central nervous system is not involved because the toxin does not cross the blood brain barrier.

Pathogenicity and Clinical Features

32. Ans. is 'a' i.e., Infant botulism is caused by ingestion of preformed toxin

(***Ref:*** *Ananthanarayan, 9th/e, p. 264-265 and 8th/e, p. 261-262; Harrison, 18th/e, p. 1200 and 17th/e, p. 901; Greenwood, 16th/e, p. 239*)

- Infant botulism is caused by ingestion of spores. Spores are ingested in food, get established in the gut and there produce the toxin.
- "Seven main types of C. botulinum, designated A-G, produce antigenically distinct toxins with pharmacologically identical action. All types can cause human disease, but type A, B and E are most common."

  – *Greenwood, 16th/e, p. 239*

  (In Harrison and Ananthanarayan, eight types of C. botulinum A, B, C_1, C_2, D, E, F, G have been mentioned).

33. Ans. is 'c' i.e., Meat (***Ref:*** *Harrison, 18th/e, p. 1200; Ananthanarayan, 9th/e, p. 264 and 8th/e, p. 261-262*)

- Food borne botulism is due to usually preserved food, meat and meat products, canned vegetables and fish.
- The most common offenders are spiced, smoked, vacuum packed, or canned alkaline foods that are eaten without cooking. In such foods, spores of C botulinum germinate; that is, under anaerobic conditions, vegetative forms grow and produce toxin.

34. Ans. is 'b' i.e., Diarrhoea (***Ref:*** *Harrison, 18th/e, p. 1201 and 17th/e, p. 901*)

- Paralytic ileus or severe constipation is seen in Botulism poisoning (not diarrhoea).

35. Ans. is 'b' i.e., Botulism (***Ref:*** *Harrison, 18th/e, p. 1201 and 17th/e, p. 901*)

- Acute descending paralysis, are areflexia, blurring of vision and non-reactive pupils suggest the diagnosis of botulism.
- Diphtheria, polio and porphyria do not present with non-reactive pupil.

36. Ans. is 'a' i.e., Botulism is caused by endotoxin

(***Ref:*** *Ananthanarayan, 9th/e, p. 264 and 8th/e, p. 262 and Harrison, 18th/e, p. 1200, 1201 and 17th/e, p. 901*)

- Cl. botulinum produces a powerful exotoxin (not endotoxin) that is responsible for the pathogenesis.
- Source of infection for infant botulism is contaminated honey.
- Symmetric descending paralysis with parasympatholytic symptoms like constipation and urinary retention are characteristic.
- A retrospective diagnosis may be made by detection of antitoxin in the patient's serum but it may not be seen in all cases.

37. Ans. is 'a' i.e., Descending flaccid paralysis (***Ref:*** *Harrison, 18th/e, p. 1201*)

- Botulism causes acute descending paralysis of flaccid type (Areflexia).

CLOSTRIDIUM DIFFICILE

Clostridium Difficile-Associated Disease

38. Ans. is 'a' i.e., Clostridium difficile

(***Ref:*** *Harrison, 19th/e, p. 1091, 1092 and 17th/e, p. 819, 820; Ananthanarayan, 9th/e, p. 265 and 8th/e, p. 263*)

- Pseudomembranous colitis is the advanced form of clostridium difficile-associated disease (CDAD).
- Pseudomembranous colitis is diagnosed by detection of one or both C difficile toxins in stool and by endoscopic observation of pseudomembranes or microabscesses in patients who have diarrhea and have been given antibiotics.

39. Ans. is 'b' i.e., Clostridium difficile (***Ref:*** *Harrison, 18th/e, p. 1091, 1092 and 17th/e, p. 819, 820*)

- It is a case of clostridium difficile-induced diarrhoea.
- Clostridium difficile should always be considered as a possible cause of diarrhoea in cancer patients who have received antibiotics.

40. Ans. is 'd' i.e., Antibiotic use (***Ref:*** *Harrison, 19th/e, p. 1091, 1092; Ananthanarayan, 9th/e, p. 265 and 8th/e, p. 263*)

- CDAD is almost exclusively associated with prolonged antibiotic use.

Pathogeniciy, Diagnosis and Treatment

41. Ans. is 'c' i.e., Blood in stools is a common feature.

"Frank blood in stool is not common." (*Topley's, 10th/e, p. 1121*)

ABOUT OTHER OPTIONS

Option (a) and option (b)

- Toxin A and B both are responsible for clinical manifestation.

"Once C. difficile is established in the bowel, disease is a consequence of the production of two large protein toxins, Toxin A and B." (*Topley's, 10th/e, p. 1120*)

- Toxin A has both histotoxic and enterotoxic activity and is of major importance in causation of tissue damage and luminal fluid accumulation.
- Toxin B may independently cause tissue damage.

Option (d)

"In the earliest stage of disease 'summit-lesions', tiny superficial intercryptal erosions, may be found."

42. Ans. is 'c' i.e., It is due to production of phospholipase A

(***Ref:*** *Harrison, 18th/e, p. 1091 and 17th/e, p. 819; Ananthanarayan, 9th/e, p. 265 and 8th/e, p. 263*)

- Asymptomatic fecal carriage of C. difficile is very common during first 6 months that means it is a normal commensal of gut during first 6 months, but it is not regarded as a normal commensal of adults.
- DOC – Mild to moderate cases – oral metronidazole, Severe or recurrent cases – Vancomycin.

43. Ans. is 'a' i.e., Clostridium difficile (***Ref:*** *Previous explanations*)

Abdominal pain and diarrhea after taking clindamycin for 5 days suggest the diagnosis of CDAD.

Patient responding to metronidazole, further confirms the diagnosis (Metronidazole is the DOC for CDAD).

CORYNEBACTERIUM DIPHTHERIAE

- Gram +ve: nonacid fast, non-sporing: non-capsulated, non-motile bacilli.
- Arrangement: V.L, cuneiform, Chinese letter pattern.
  - Also known **as KLB (Kleb Loeffler's Bacillus).**
  - **Metachromatic granules:** They are present at ends or poles of the bacilli (also called as polar bodies/volutin granules/Babes-Ernest bodies) and they are storage granules of bacteria, composed of polymetaphosphates.
  - Special stains for demonstration of granules, Neisser's and Ponder's stains. **Memory Aid (PAN).**

C. Diphtheria Diseases (Diphtheria is toxemia but not a Bacteremia)

1. **Respiratory Diphtheria:**
   - Faucial (Tonsillopharyngeal) diphtheria (MC) leads to formation of pseudomembrane coat (tough, greyish-white, leathery layer).
   - **Most severe form** of respiratory diphtheria – Laryngeal and bronchial airways due to extension of pseudomembrane. Which may result in fatal airway obstruction leading to asphyxia, mandates Tracheostomy.
   - **Bull-neck appearance.Q**
2. **Cutaneous Diphtheria:**
   - It is due to organism itself and is **Not toxin mediated** so skin lesion may also be caused by non-toxigenic strain and Most commonly occurs in extremities.
3. **Systemic Complication:**
   - **Polyneuropathy and myocarditis** are the late toxin manifestations.
   - Other complications include renal failure, encephalitis, and cerebral infarction.

Virulence Factors (Diphtheria toxin/DT)

- Heat labile polypeptide exotoxin.
- **DT is coded by a Bacteriophage (Betacorynephage), carrying tox gene, through Lysogenic conversion.**
- **Mechanism of action:**

  DT has 2 parts, Part A (Active) and Part B (Binding). Part B Binds to the cell receptors and facilitates the entry of **Part A which causes ADP ribosylation of EF-2** this step leads to inhibition of translation (Protein synthesis) and cell death.

Lab Diagnosis

- **Specimen:** Throat swab or portion of pseudomembrane.
- **Direct Microscopy:**

  Gram staining: Gram positive bacilli arranged in V.L. cuneiform, Chinese letter pattern.

  Albert's staining: Green color bacilli with bluish black metachromatic granules.
- **Culture:**

  Loeffler's serum slope (Enriched media) – Rapid growth (6-8 hrs) with Enhanced the granules production and Blood agar.

Selective Media:

- Potassium tellurite blood agar (PTA).Q
- Cysteine Potassium tellurite blood agar (Tinsdale medium).
- Hiss's serum sugar media for testing sugar fermentation properties.
- Toxin demonstration:
  - **In vivo:** Done on guinea pigs or rabbits can be intracutaneous or subcutaneous.
  - **In vitro:** Elek's gel precipitation test, Toxin detection by ELISA, Detection of tox gene by PCR, MALDI-TOF and Immunochromatographic strip assay.

Prophylaxis

- Single vaccine: Diphtheria toxoid.
- Combined vaccine: DPT, Diphtheria and Tetanus toxoid and dT (TT and adult dose Diphtheria toxoid).
- Administration of DPT:

  Doses: Three doses at 6, 10, 14 weeks of birth followed by two booster doses at 16-24 months and 5 years.

Site: IM at anterolateral aspect of thigh.

- **Schick test:** It is an intradermal toxin-antitoxin neutralization test, obsolete now-a-days since toxoid preparations are safe. Test determines suspectibility of an individual to diphtheria.

  This test provides information regarding immune status and hypersensitivity to toxin.

  Vaccine was given only to those who are susceptible to this test.

Treatment

- Diphtheria antitoxin or antidiphtheria serum (ADS) along with erythromycin.
- Asphyxia – tracheostomy is done in emergency.

EXTRA EDGE POINTS****

- Leather term is used for diphtheria, **IP – 2-6 days,** diphtheria carrier is best diagnosed by throat swab culture.
  - **For toxoid vaccine preparation Park William 8 strain (Q) is used.**
  - Toxin production depends on optimum iron concentration (0.1 mg/lt).
- One unit of diphtheria antitoxin was defined as the smallest amount of antitoxin required to neutralise – 100 MLD of toxin.
- Diphtheroid or Coryneforms are the non-diphtherial corynebacteria, that usually exist as normal commensals in the throat, skin, conjunctiva and other areas.
- Clinically resembling diphtheria: C. ulcerans and C. pseudotuberculosis produces Diph. Toxin and causes localized ulceration in throat.
- Biotyping (McLeod's classification) of Corynebacterium diphtheriae – Based upon colony appearance on potassium tellurite agar.

  Gravis – Daisy head colony.

  Intermedius – Frog's egg colony.

  Mitis – Poached eggs colony.
- **Ehrlich phenomenon:** It is about presence of varying amount of toxin in toxoid preparation.
- **Erythrasma** is a skin disease that causes brown, scaly skin patches. It is caused by the Gram-positive bacterium **Corynebacterium minutissimum.**
- IOC for carriers – throat and nose swab culture.

MCQs

1. C. diphtheriae is also called as: (*Recent MCQ*)

(a) Pfeffiers bacilli
(b) Whitmore bacilli
(c) Robert Koch bacilli
(d) Kleb-Loeffler's bacilli

Morphology

2. True about Corynebacterium diphtheriae is: (*Recent MCQ*)

(a) Loeffler's serum is highly selective media for C. diphtheriae
(b) Elek gel is a precipitation test
(c) Gram negative bacilli, nonmotile, noncapsulate
(d) Metachromatic granules is produced on stain only by one strain of C. diphtheriae

3. Daisy head colonies are seen in which biotype? *(Recent MCQ)*
(a) Gravis (b) Intermedius
(c) Mitis (d) Stutzeri

Toxigenicity and Pathogenicity

4. Diphtheria toxin acts by: *(Recent MCQ)*
(a) Inhibiting acetyl choline release (b) Inhibiting glucose transport
(c) Increasing levels of cyclic AMP (d) Inhibiting protein synthesis

5. All are true regarding diphtheria toxin *except*: *(AIIMS Sept 96, AI 98)*
(a) Toxin blocks elongation of protein
(b) Beta lysogenic strain produces toxin
(c) Iron is critical for toxin production
(d) Toxin is necessary for local wound production

6. Lysogenic conversion is seen in: *(Recent MCQ)*
(a) C. diphtheriae (b) Salmonella
(c) Staphylococcus (d) E.coli

Laboratory Diagnosis

7. A child presented with fever and lymphadenopathy. Oral examination shows a grey membrane over right tonsil. Which of the following medium will be used for early diagnosis of pathogen? *(AIIMS 02)*
(a) Nutrient agar (b) Blood agar
(c) Loeffler's serum slope (d) Lowenstein Jensen medium

8. Investigation of choice of diphtheria carrier is: *(AIIMS June 97)*
(a) Throat Swab Culture (b) Gram's stain
(c) Albert stain (d) Zeil Neelsen stain

9. Most definitive media to grow C.diphtheriae for culture: *(AIIMS Nov 99)*
(a) L.J. Media (b) Blood Tellurite media
(c) Cary Blair media (d) Loeffler's serum slope

Treatment and Prophylaxis

10. Most important element in treatment of diphtheria: *(Recent MCQ)*
(a) Antitoxin (b) Tetracycline
(c) Erythromycin (d) Penicillin

11. Ehrlich phenomenon seen in: *(Recent MCQ)*
(a) Proteus (b) Mycobacterium TB
(c) Corynebacterium (d) Staphylococcus

12. True statement regarding diphtheria is: *(AI 97)*
(a) It can be diagnosed by demonstration of antibodies by ELISA
(b) Immunisation prevents carrier state
(c) Treatment of contacts is not indicated
(d) Iron has critical value in the production of toxin.

Neutralization test

13. Regarding Shick's test which of the following is false? *(AIIMS 2000)*

(a) Erythematous reaction in both arm indicates hypersensitivity

(b) Positive test means that person is immune to Diphtheria

(c) Diphtheria antitoxin is given intradermally

(d) Test done to find out immune status against diphtheria

Non-Diphtheria corynebacterium

14. Toxin is produced by all *except*: *(Latest Q)*

(a) C. diphtheriae (b) C. ulcerans

(c) C. hofmanni (d) C. pseudotuberculosis

15. Which non-diphtheria corynebacterium is used as immunomodulator?

(a) C. diphtheriae (b) C. parvum

(c) C. hofmanni (d) C. pseudotuberculosis

16. Erythrasma is caused by:

(a) C.diphtheriae (b) C. minutissimum

(c) C. hofmanni (d) C. pseudotuberculosis

ANSWERS AND EXPLANATIONS

1. **Ans. is 'd'** i.e., Klebs-Loeffler bacillus (***Ref:*** *Ananthanarayan, 9th/e, p. 236 and 8th/e, p. 232*)

   The diphtheria bacillus was first observed and described by Klebs but was first cultivated by Loeffler (1884). Therefore, it is known as Klebs-Loeffler Bacillus (KLB).

2. **Ans. is 'b'** i.e., Elek's Gel is a precipitation test (***Ref:*** *Ananthanarayan, 9th/e, p. 237, 240 and 8th/e, p. 232, 233*)

   - Elek's is a precipitation test. It is an in vitro test for toxigenicity of the diphtheria bacillus.
   - Selective medium for C. diphtheriae is tellurite blood agar (e.g., Mc Leod's, Hoyle's Media and Tinsdale Medium).
     - All strains of C. diphtheriae show metachromatic granules on staining.
     - C. diphtheriae is gram (+) ve, non-motile and non-capsulated.

3. **Ans. is 'a'** i.e., Gravis

   Biotypes of Diphtheria Bacilli

   Based on colony morphology on the tellurite medium and other properties, McLeod classified diphtheria bacilli into three types:

Features	1. Gravis	2. Intermedius	3. Mitis
Case fatality rate	High	High	Low
Complications	Paralytic, hemorrhagic	Hemorrhagic	Obstructive
Predominance	In epidemic areas	Epidemic areas	Endemic areas
Spread	Rapid	Rapidly than mitis	Less rapid
Colony on TBA	'Daisy head' colony	'Frog's egg' colony	'Poached egg' colony
Hemolysis	Variable	Non-hemolytic	Usually hemolytic

4. **Ans. is 'd'** i.e., Inhibiting protein synthesis (***Ref:*** *Ananthanarayan, 9th/e, p. 238 and 8th/e, p. 234*)

   An exotoxin with a similar mode of action can be produced by strains of Pseudomonas aeruginosa.

5. **Ans. is 'd'** i.e., Toxin is necessary for local wound production

"Corynebacterium diphtheriae does not need to be toxigenic to establish localized infection. In the nasopharynx or skin, for example, but non-toxigenic strains also not yield the localized or systemic effect. C diphtheriae does not typically invade deep tissues and practically never enters the bloodstream.

6. **Ans. is 'a'** i.e., C. diphtheriae

The toxigenicity of the diphtheria bacilli depends on the presence in it of corynephages (tox +). **Nontoxigenic strains may be rendered toxigenic by infecting them with beta phage or some other larger phage. This is known as lysogenic conversion or phage conversion.**

C. diphtheriae does not need to be toxigenic to establish localized infection. – *Jawetz latest e/p. 274*

7. **Ans. is 'c'** i.e., Loeffler's serum slope (***Ref:*** *Ananthanarayan, 9th/e, p. 240 and 8th/e, p. 235-236*)

Fever, cervical lymphadenopathy and grey membrane on the tonsil extending to anterior pillar is suggestive of diphtherial infection. For rapid growth the specimen is inoculated on Loeffler's serum slope which shows the growth in 6 hours.

8. **Ans. is 'a'** i.e., Throat Swab Culture

Carriers are detected by cultural methods – swabs are taken from nose and throat and it is examined by culture methods for diphtheria bacilli. (*Park, 24th/e, p. 536*)

Asymptomatic Carriers and Contacts: All carriers and contacts of persons carrying a toxigenic strain should receive antibiotic prophylaxis: Benzathine penicillin G (600,000 units for persons younger than 6 years old and 1,200,000 units for those 6 years old and older). Or

A 7- to 10-day course of oral erythromycin (40 mg/kg/day for children and 1 g/day for adults). The immunization history of all exposed individuals should be established and updated. Immunized individuals receive a single reinforcing dose according to age. Patients should be kept under surveillance and antitoxin treatment should be given at first signs of illness.

9. **Ans. is 'b'** i.e., Blood Tellurite media

Already explained in book text.

10. **Ans. is 'a'** i.e., Antitoxin (***Ref:*** *Ananthanarayan, 9th/e, p. 242, 8th/e, p. 239*)

- Erythromycin is more active than penicillin in treatment of carriers.
- Diphtheria is a serious illness. Doctors treat it immediately and aggressively with these medications:
  - **An antitoxin:** If doctors suspect diphtheria, the infected child or adult receives an antitoxin after proper Allergy testing.
  - **Antibiotics:** Diphtheria is also treated with antibiotics, such as penicillin or erythromycin. It reduces duration of infectivity.

11. **Ans. is 'c'** i.e., Corynebacterium

(It is due to presence in toxin preparation of varying amounts of toxoid and antitoxin to combine in varying proportions and is called **Ehrlich phenomenon**).

Ehrlich defined the minimum lethal dose (MLD) of the diphtheria toxin as the least amount of toxin required to kill a guinea pig weighing 250 g within 96 hours after subcutaneous inoculation.

12. **Ans. is 'd'** i.e., Iron has critical value in the production of toxin

Optimum level of iron needed is 0.1 mg/litre for toxin production but higher concentration (0.5 mg/litre) inhibits the production of toxin by upregulating toxin gene in the chromosome. (*Ananthanarayan, 9th/e, p. 238*)

13. **Ans. is 'b'** i.e., Positive test means that person is immune to Diphtheria

Schick Test

Type – Neutralization test (Toxin – antitoxin).

Use – It is used for susceptibility for diphtheria, Intradermal test readings are at 1-2 days and 5-7 days but not in use because safer toxoid preparations are available.

Interpretation of the test Reaction in control arm indicates hypersensitivity (erythema and induration).

Schick Test Positive means that person is susceptible to Diphtheria so vaccine was administered.

Schick Test Negative means that person is immune to Diphtheria.

14. Ans. is 'c' i.e., Corynebacterium hofmannii

(***Ref:*** *Ananthanarayan, 9th/e, p. 242 and 8th/e, p. 239; Harrison, 17th/e, p. 893-941*)

Among the Corynebacterium species, three Corynebacterium produce diphtheria toxin: C. diphtheriae, C. pseudotuberculosis and C. ulcerans. "Like C. diphtheriae, C. pseudotuberculosis and C. ulcerans can produce toxin and cause clinically resembling Diphtheria." – *Greenwood*

15. Ans. is 'b' i.e., C. parvum

The immunomodulator Corynebacterium parvum stimulates the reticuloendothelial system and causes splenic hypertrophy. The ability of C parvum to stimulate splenic regeneration in hemisplenectomized mice and decrease susceptibility to intranasal pneumococcal challenge was studied.

16. Ans. is 'b' i.e., Corynebacterium minutissimum (***Ref:*** *Ananthanarayan, 9th/e, p. 212 and 8th/e, p. 239*)

Erythrasma is a localized infection of the stratum corneum usually affecting the axilla and groin, is caused by C. minutissimum. **Erythrasma lesions emit coral red color in Wood's lamp examination.**

BACILLUS

BACILLUS ANTHRACIS

• Causative agent of Anthrax (Zoonotic). • Gram +ve, long rectangular rods arranged in chains (Bamboo stick appearance) and Aerobes/facultative anaerobes. • Non-motile, Spore forming, capsulated (Polypeptide). • Largest bacterium causing disease. • Ist bacteria to be isolated by Robert Koch in pure culture and Koch postulates were made. • First bacterium spores were identified. • First bacterial disease of human live attenuated vaccine was developed by L. Pastuer. • First disease of human for serological test – Ascolis Thermopreciptin test.	**Virulence Factors** • **Anthrax toxin** (Tripartile toxin) and plasmid (pX01) coded. **Edema factor (EF)/Factor 1** – It's an active fragment and increases host cell cAMP. **Protective factor (PF/PA)/Factor 2** – It is the binding fragment and provides attachment sites for EF and LF. **Lethal factor (LF)/Factor 3** – Cause cell death. • **Polypeptide Capsule:** It is plasmid (pX02) coded. It inhibits the complement mediated phagocytosis.
Lab Diagnosis • Specimens – Pus, sputum, CSF. • Direct demonstration: Gram staining – GPB with Bamboo stick appearance. McFadyean's reaction – Show purple capsule with blue bacilli (Polychrome methylene blue stain). • Culture: Nutrient agar – Medusa head colonies. Gelatin stab agar – Inverted fir tree appearance.	**Selective Media** Solid medium with penicillin-colonies gives String of pearl appearance. PLET (Polymyxin, lysozyme, EDTA and thallous) medium. • Ab detection by ELISA. • Gene detection by PCR. **DOC** – Penicillin In Penicillin allergy – Ciprofloxacin, Erythromycin, Doxycyline, Tetracycline.

Diseases

1. Cutaneous Anthrax (Hide Porter's diseases/**Malignant pustule**) – **Most common** and least dangerous, occurs in Dock workers, Butcher, abattoir and farmer.
2. Pulmonary Anthrax (Inhalational anthrax/Wool sorter's disease) – Typically causes hemorrhagic pneumonia and hemorrhagic mediastinitis.
3. Intestinal Anthrax – Rare form and causes bloody diarrhea.
   - Charbon is another name for Malignant pustule.

   Agent of Bioterrorism – Spores of B. anthracis are most common agents of Bioterrorism and Pulmonary Anthrax is the most common form to cause Bioterrorism (Category A) outbreaks.

BACILLUS CEREUS

• Gram Positive Bacilli, spore forming, Motile (swarming), non-capsulated and not show String of pearl appearance.
• It is a normal habitant of soil, also widely isolated from food items.

DOC: Clindamycin, Erythromycin, Vancomycin, Aminoglycosides and Tetracycline.

Note: It is resistant to Penicillins (By producing Beta-lactamase) and Trimethoprim.

• Characteristic of Bacillus cereus food poisoning is pain in abdomen.
• Anthrax bacilli differ from anthracoid bacilli by being nonmotile.

Food poisoning	
Emetic Type	**Diarrheal Type**
IP –<6 hours	IP 8 – 16 hours
By performed Heat stable emetic toxin (Resembling S.aureus enterotoxin)	By Heat labile enterotoxin, secreted in intestine (Similar to C. perfringens enterotoxin)
Chinese fried rice is etiology. • Vomiting, abdominal Cramps.	Occurs in many food products. • Diarrhea, fever, abdominal cramps.

MCQs

1. **An abattoir worker developed pustule which later progress to necrotic ulcer. Which of the following stain is useful for demonstration of organism from smear made from pustule?** *(Recent MCQ)*
   (a) Polychrome methylene blue (b) Calcofluor white
   (c) Giemsa (d) Modified kinyoun stain
2. **Characteristic of Bacillus cereus food poisoning is:** *(AIIMS Nov 10)*
   (a) Presence of fever (b) Presence of abdominal pain
   (c) Absence of vomiting (d) Absence of diarrhoea
3. **Which of the following is true regarding anthrax?** *(PGI 01)*
   (a) McFadyean reaction shows capsule
   (b) Humans are usually resistant to infection
   (c) Less than 100 spores can cause pulmonary infection
   (d) Gram stain shows organism with bulging spores
4. **A man, after skinning a dead animal, developed a pustule on his hand. A smear prepared from the lesion showed the presence of gram-positive bacilli in long chains which were positive for McFadyean's reaction. The most likely etiological agent is:** *(AI-04)*
   (a) Clostridium tetani (b) Listeria monocytogenes
   (c) Bacillus anthracis (d) Actinomyces species
5. **A malignant pustule is a term used for:**
   (a) An infected malignant melanoma (b) A carbuncle
   (c) A rapidly spreading rodent ulcer (d) Anthrax of skin
6. **Noninvasive diarrhea can be caused by the following *except*:** *(AI 09)*
   (a) Shigella (b) B. cereus
   (c) Salmonella (d) Y. enterocolitica
7. **All are true about cutaneous anthrax *except*:** *(UP 02)*
   (a) Extremely painful lesions (b) The whole area is congested and edematous
   (c) Central crustation with black eschar (d) Satellite nodule around inguinal region
8. **String of pearl appearance seen in:**
   (a) Clostridium (b) Bacillus anthracis
   (c) Pneumococcus (d) Staph. aureus
9. **All are true about Bacillus *except*:**
   (a) Mc Fadyean's reaction is used in presumptive diagnosis of anthrax infection
   (b) Medusa head appearance of colonies in gelatin stab culture
   (c) PLET is the selective medium
   (d) Ascoli's thermoprecipitation test is used for laboratory diagnosis
10. **All true about anthrax *except*:**
    (a) Mc Fadyean's reaction shows capsule
    (b) Less than 100 spores can cause pulmonary disease
    (c) Gram stain shows organism with bulging spores
    (d) Sputum microscopy can aid in diagnosis

ANSWERS AND EXPLANATIONS

(Ananthanarayan, 8th/e, p. 245; 9th/e, p. 247)

1. **Ans. is 'a'** i.e., Polychrome methylene blue

   It is a case of cutaneous anthrax (a pustule developing into a necrotic ulcer) as Soil is contaminated with anthrax spores from the carcasses of dead animals. These spores remain viable for decades. Perhaps, spores can germinate in soil at a pH of 6.5 at proper temperature. Grazing animals infected through injured mucous membranes serve to perpetuate the chain of infection. Contact with infected animals or with their hides, hair and bristles is the source of infection in humans and polypeptide capsule is demonstrated by Gurr's polychrome methylene blue (McFadyean's reaction).

2. **Ans. is 'b'** i.e., Presence of abdominal pain

   Bacillus cereus food poisoning is of two types. Emetic type and Diarrheal type abdominal cramps are common feature in both. Other features are:

   (a) **Emetic Type:** History of intake of fried rice from Chinese restaurant 6 hours earlier. Mediated by enterotoxin resembling Staphylococcal Enterotoxin.

   (b) **Diarrhoeal Type:** History of intake of cooked meat and vegetables 8-16 hours earlier. Mediated by enterotoxin resembling E. coli.

3. **Ans. is 'a'** i.e., McFadyean reaction shows capsule, Humans are usually resistant to infection and Sputum microscopy helps in diagnosis in case of pulmonary anthrax.

   Stained smears from the local lesion or of blood from clinical samples of human or dead animals often show chains of large gram-positive rods (spores are not in clinical samples). Anthrax can be identified in dried smears by direct immunofluorescence staining techniques.

4. **Ans. is 'c'** i.e., Bacillus anthracis

   It is a typical presentation of cutaneous anthrax. When a blood film from an animal suspected to die of or suffering from anthrax is stained with Polychromic methylene blue and examined under microscope the chains of bacilli are seen surrounded by an amorphous purplish material representing the capsular material. It is the McFadyean's reaction.

5. **Ans. is 'd'** i.e., Anthrax of skin

   Cutaneous anthrax also known as hides porter disease or malignant pustule. There is formation of Eschar which later changes to pustule common in workers of Dockyard and shipyard.

6. **Ans. is 'b'** i.e., Bacillus cereus

   Invasive diarrhea is caused by Salmonella, Shigella, Enteroinvasive E.coli and Campylobacter jejuni.

7. **Ans. is 'a'** i.e., Extremely painful lesions

   The lesions begin as a papule that evolves into a painless vesicle. The lesions typically are 1–3 cm in diameter and have a characteristic central black eschar.

8. **Ans. is 'c'** i.e., Bacillus anthracis

   On penicillin agar-string of pearl appearance is seen and in Gelatin stab culture inverted fir tree appearance is seen.

9. **Ans. is 'b'** i.e., Medusa head appearance of colonies in gelatin stab culture

   Medusa head appearance is seen on agar microscopy, Bamboo stick appearance seen on gram staining.

   PLET – stands for Polymyxin , Lysozyme, EDTA and Thallous acetate

10. **Ans. is 'c'** i.e., Less than 100 spores can cause disease

    The infectious dose varies greatly from species to species and is route dependent. The inhalation anthrax infectious dose (ID) for humans primarily has been extrapolated from inhalation challenges of nonhuman primates (NHP) or studies done in contaminated mills. Estimates vary greatly but the medium lethal dose (LD50) is likely within the range of 2,500-55,000 spores. It is believed that very few spores (10 or less) are required for cutaneous anthrax.

    Source – https://www.cdc.gov/biosafety/publications/bmbl5/bmbl5_sect_viii_a.pdf

    Spores of B. anthracis are as broad as the bacterium and do not swell the bacterium. Blood or sputum smears can demonstrate the gram positive rods for diagnosis of pulmonary anthrax also called Wool sorter disease.

NOCARDIA AND ACTINOMYCES

NOCARDIA

- Gram positive branching filamentous bacilli.
- Aerobic, weak/partially acid fast (0.5-1% H_2SO_4).
- Found in soil and vegetables.
- N. asteroids and N. brasiliensis are most common pathogens.

Mode of Transmission

- **Inhalation** of fragmented bacterial mycelia.
- **Transcutaneous inoculation** of the bacteria.
- **Person to person transmission is not known.**

Clinical Manifestations

- **Pneumonia/pulmonary nocardiosis** – **Most common.**
- **Extra pulmonary nocardiosis –** Most common is **Brain abscess** then skin, kidney, bone and muscle.
- **Actinomycetoma.**

Lab Diagnosis

- Specimens – Sputum, pus from abscess and granules.
- **Direct Microscopy.**

Gram staining (Brown-Brenn modification) – Gram positive branching filamentous bacilli.

Modified Acid-Fast staining – (0.5-1% H_2SO_4) – Appear as branching filamentous red colored bacilli.

Histopathology – H and E stain for the granules.

- **Culture** (Slow grower 2-2 weeks)
  - SDA, BHI agar.
  - Selective media – **Paraffin bait technique,** LJ medium, Buffered yeast extract containing Polymyxin and vancomycin.

DOC – Sulfonamides and Cotrimoxazole.

ACTINOMYCES

- **Gram positive branching filamentous bacilli.**
- Anaerobic, non-acid fast.
- Found in soil and Normal flora of mouth, intestine and vagina.
- **A. israelii** is most common pathogen to human.

Mode of Transmission

- **Infection is Mostly Endogenous and may results from Trauma, e.g., Dental extraction.**

Clinical Manifestations

- **Cervicofacial actinomycosis –** Most common Lumpy jaw.Q
- **Pelvic form – IUCD insertion.**Q
- Disseminated form – Lungs and Liver, where multiple nodules are formed.

(Multiple sinuses towards skin with discharge of **Sulfur** granules.)

Lab Diagnosis

- **Specimens** – Discharge from the sinuses or fistula, rarely sputum or tissue section.
- Direct Microscopy.

Gram staining (Brown-Brenn modification) – Gram positive branching filamentous bacilli with club shaped ends.

Histopathological stain – H and E staining (sun-rays appearance).

- **Culture (Pus containing sulfur granules are cultured Anaerobically).**
  - Thioglycollate broth – A. israelii, Resembles Fluffy balls at the bottom of the tube.
  - BHI agar.

DOC – Penicillin.

MCQs

Nocardia

1. **Characteristic infection of Nocardia asteroides is:** (*AI 2012*)
   (a) Diarrhea
   (b) Secondary dissemination to liver
   (c) Brain abscess
   (d) Colonic diverticula
2. **The causative organism of Mycetoma is:** (*PGI 02*)
   (a) Nocardia
   (b) Dimorphic fungus
   (c) Aspergillus
   (d) Dermatophytes
3. **A clinical specimen was obtained from the wound of a patient diagnosed as nocardiosis. For the selective isolation of Nocardia sp. which one of the following would be the best method?** (*AIIMS 04*)
   (a) Paraffin bait technique
   (b) Castaneda's culture method
   (c) Craige's culture method
   (d) Hair bait technique
4. **Nocardia is differentiated from Actinomyces by:** (*PGI 02*)
   (a) Gram stain
   (b) ZN stain
   (c) Nocardia causes mycetoma, Actinomyces do not
   (d) Nocardia is facultative anaerobe
5. **True about Madura foot:**
   (a) Can erode bones
   (b) Spread to lymph nodes
   (c) Most commonly occur in hand
   (d) Slow growing
   (e) Antibiotic has no role
6. **A patient comes with history of unresponsive fever and cough. X-ray revealed pneumonia. Sputum examination showed gram positive, partially acid fast bacteria with branching filaments that grows on sheep blood agar. The most likely etiologic agents is:** (*AI 2011*)
   (a) Actinomycetes
   (b) Nocardia
   (c) Aspergillosis
   (d) Pneumococci
7. **A person 6 hours after consuming rice pudding in restaurant develops vomiting. True statements regarding food poisoning:** (*AIIMS 2011*)
   (a) Caused by Staphylococcus aureus
   (b) Preformed toxin
   (c) Caused by vibrio parahaemolyticus
   (d) Heat labile toxin
   (e) Culture of food is more useful than stool
8. **Which of the following is not true of Actinomycosis?**
   (a) Demonstration of filaments
   (b) Caused by Actinomyces israelii
   (c) Organism cannot be cultured
   (d) Sulphur granules in pus
9. **Most common cause of actinomycetoma in India:**
   (a) Nocardia braziliensis
   (b) Actinomadura madure
   (c) Piedra
   (d) Tinea crurin
10. **Which of the following is false about mycetoma?**
   (a) Can affect lower and upper extremities
   (b) Caused by actinomycetes and filamentous fungi
   (c) Diagnosis is by examination of pus
   (d) Uncommon in India

ANSWERS AND EXPLANATIONS

(Ananthanarayan, 8th/e, p. 393; 9th/e, p. 394; Harrison, 18th/e, p. 1324; Jawetz, 24th/e, p. 182)

1. **Ans. is 'c'** i.e., Brain abscess

   Subcutaneous abscess is the typical extrapulmonary manifestation of nocardia. The most common site of dissemination is brain.

2. **Ans. is 'a'** i.e., Nocardia

   It is a chronic, slowly progressive granulomatous infection of the skin and subcutaneous tissues. Also known as Maduramycosis or Madura foot as it was first seen in Madurai, South India.

   It can be of two types:

   Eumycetoma: Fungal agents (Madurella, Exophiala, Curvularia, Aspergillus nidulens, Fusarium, Acremonium).

   Actinomycetoma: Bacterial agents (Nocardia, Actinomadura, Streptomyces).

3. **Ans. is 'a'** i.e., Paraffin bait technique. It is a technique for isolation of Nocardia.

   Other options:

   (b) **Castaneda's culture method:** It is a method of blood culture.

   (c) **Craige's culture method:** It is a method of separation of motile bacteria from non-motile bacteria in a mixed culture.

   (d) **Hair bait technique:** It is a specific method for isolation of the keratinases producing microbes (fungi and bacteria) from soil.

4. **Ans. is 'b'** i.e., Ziehl Neelsen stain

   Nocardia – Partially acid fast, obligate aerobe, habitat is soil and infections occur exogenously.

   Actinomyces – Nonacid fast, facultative anaerobe, habitat is oral flora so infections occur endogenously.

5. **Ans. are 'a and d'** i.e., Can erode bones and slow growing

   Mode of infection is **thorn prick.** So, therefore, it commonly occurs in lower limbs. Antibiotics have a role in bacterial mycetoma. The term Madura foot is used for Mycotic (fungal) mycetoma.

6. **Ans. is 'b'** i.e., Nocardia

   The typical morphology of Nocardia is Acid Fast filamentous bacteria with right angle branching.

7. **Ans. are 'b and e'** i.e., Preformed toxin and culture of food is more useful than stool

8. **Ans. is 'c'** i.e., Organism cannot be cultured

   Pus containing sulfur granules are washed and cultured anaerobically in thioglycollate broth or Brain heart infusion (BHI) agar.

9. **Ans. is 'a'** i.e., Nocardia brasiliensis

   Most common cause of mycetoma is fungi. (***Ref:*** *Jawetz, 24th/e, p. 220*)

   Most common cause of Actinomycetoma are:

   (a) Nocardia brasiliensis.

   (b) Streptomyces somaelinsis, and

   (c) Actinomadura madurae.

10. **Ans. is 'd'** i.e., Uncommon in India

Actinomycosis

1. Which of the following statements regarding Actinomyces and Nocardia is true?

(a) Both organisms have branching growth but are prokaryotes

(b) Neither stains with Gram stain

(c) Nocardia infections are endogenous and often initiated by trauma

(d) Actinomyces causes infections in systemically compromised patients

2. Which of the following is the most predominant constituent of sulfur granules of Actinomycosis? (*AIIMS 04, Recent MCQ*)

(a) Organisms (b) Neutrophils and monocytes

(c) Monocytes and lymphocytes (d) Eosinophils

3. A farmer present with multiple discharging sinuses in the leg not responding to antibiotics. Most likely diagnosis is: (*AIIMS 02*)

(a) Madurella (b) Actinomycetoma

(c) Nocardia (d) Sporothrix

4. Anthrax bacilli differs from anthracoid bacilli by being: (*Recent MCQ*)

(a) Non-capsulated (b) Strict aerobe

(c) Non-motile (d) Hemolytic colonies on blood

5. Nocardia infection is associated most commonly with:

(a) Liver abscess (b) Lung abscess

(c) Brain abscess (d) Subcutaneous abscess

6. All of the following are true about anthrax *except*:

(a) Plasmid is responsible for toxin production

(b) Cutaneous anthrax generally resolves spontaneously

(c) Capsular polypeptide aids virulence by inhibiting phagocytosis

(d) Toxin is a complex of two fractions

7. Nocardia is stained by: (*AIIMS 08*)

(a) Acid fast stain (b) Kiram's stain

(c) Alcian blue (d) Mucin stain

ANSWERS AND EXPLANATIONS

(Ananthanarayan, 8th/e, p. 393; 9th/e, p. 390-91)

1. **Ans. is 'a'** i.e., Both organisms have branching growth but are prokaryotes.

   Option (a) – True – Both are Gram positive varying from coccoid and pleomorphic forms to branched filaments.

   Option (c) – False – Nocardia are saprophytes while actinomycetes are endogenous and infection is initiated by trauma.

   Option (d) – Also False – Nocardia causes infections in systemically compromised patients.

2. **Ans. is 'a'** i.e., Organism

   A typical presentation of Actinomycosis is subcutaneous swelling with discharging sinus called mycetoma. The pus from the sinus consists of granular material (sulpher granules) which on microscopic examination reveals filaments of actinomycetes.

3. **Ans. is 'a'** i.e., Madurella

   Apart from actinomycetes certain bacteria and fungi also cause subcutaneous swelling with discharging sinus. Madurella is such a condition caused by fungi and hence not responding to antibiotics.

4. **Ans. is 'c'** i.e., Non motile

Differentiating features between anthrax and anthracoid bacilli

Anthrax Bacilli	Anthracoid Bacilli
• Nonmotile	• Generally motile
• Capsulated	• Noncapsulated
• Grow in long chains	• Grow in short chains
• Medusa head colony	• Not present
• No growth in penicillin agar (10 units/ml)	• Grow usually
• Hemolysis absent or weak	• Usually well marked
• Inverted fir tree growth and slow gelatin liquefaction	• Rapid liquefaction
• No turbidity in broth	• Turbidity usual

5. **Ans. is 'b'** i.e., Lung abscess

   Pneumonia, the most common form of nocardial disease in the respiratory tract, is typically subacute; symptoms have usually been present for days or weeks at presentation. The onset is occasionally more acute in immunosuppressed patients. Cough is prominent and produces small amounts of thick, purulent sputum that is not malodorous and infiltrates and nodules tend to cavitate. Empyema is present in one-quarter of cases.

6. **Ans. is 'd'** i.e., Toxin is a complex of two fractions

   Toxin is tripartite having 3 fractions (E P L): Edema factor, protective factor and lethal factor which acts in synergy to cause action, other bacterial toxins are mostly bipartite.

7. **Ans. is 'a'** i.e., Acid fast stain

   The first step in diagnosis is examination of sputum or pus for crooked, branching, beaded, gram-positive filaments 1 μm wide and up to 50 μm long. Most nocardiae are acid-fast in direct smears if a weak acid is used for decolorization (e.g., in the modified Kinyoun, Ziehl-Neelsen, and Fite-Faraco methods). The organisms often take up silver stains.

LISTERIA MONOCYTOGENES

- Gram +ve bacilli, non-sporing.
- It is the agent of listeriosis, a serious infection caused by eating food contaminated with the bacteria.
- The disease affects primarily pregnant women, newborns, and adults with weakened immune systems.
- **Motile (Tumbling motility) at 25°C only, non-motile at 37°C.Q**

L. Monocytogenes Diseases

- Neonatal listeriosis:
  Early onset disease-occurs within 7 days of birth.
  Late onset disease-occurs between 7-21 days of birth, mostly present as *Meningitis*.
- In pregnant women – Fetal complications such as abortion, preterm delivery leads to Early onset disease and Maternal complications such as flu-like symptoms, Bacteremia.

Mode of Transmission

- Contaminated food followed by vertical transmission (mother to fetus).
- Due to its ability to survive refrigeration at 4°C, it is commonly found in stored foods.

Lab Diagnosis

- Specimens – CSF, blood and amniotic fluid.
- Gram staining – Gram +ve short bacilli, often confused with diphtheroid.
- Motility – Motile (Tumbling motility) at 25°C only, non-motile at 37°C.
- CSF examination – ↑ Pressure and ↑ lymphocyte count.
- **Culture:** Blood agar- β- hemolytic colonies.
  Trypticase soy broth with Cold enrichment method.
- Identification tests.

Anton's test, CAMP test positive, Catalase test positive.

DOC – Ampicillin Q

MCQs

1. **A major step in the pathogenesis of listeriosis is:** *(AIIMS 05)*
   (a) The formation of antigen antibody complexes with resultant complements activation and tissue damage
   (b) The release of hyaluronidase by L. monocytogenes which contribute to dissemination from local sites
   (c) The antiphagocytic activity of the L. monocytogenes capsule
   (d) The survival and multiplication of L. monocytogenes within mononuclear phagocytes and host epithelial cells
2. **A 3-week-old child presented to the pediatrician with meningitis. A presumptive diagnosis of late onset perinatal meningitis was made. The CSF culture was positive for gram positive bacilli. Which of the following characteristic of this bacteria would be helpful in differentiating it from other bacterial agents:** *(AIIMS May 05)*
   (a) Ability to grow on blood agar
   (b) Ability to produce catalase
   (c) Fermentative attack on sugars
   (d) Motility at 25 degree Celsius
3. **Microorganism motile at 25 degree Celsius but non-motile at 37 degree Celsius and shows actin binding polymerization to escape is:** *(PGI Nov 09)*
   (a) Listeria monocytogenes
   (b) Campylobacter
   (c) Yersinia pestis
   (d) Streptococcus agalactiae

4. All of the following conditions are caused by listeria *except*:

(a) Granulomatosis infantiseptica
(b) Premature birth
(c) Sepsis in immunocompromised individuals
(d) Uveitis

5. Listeria is positive for all *except*:

(a) Anton test
(b) Catalase positive
(c) Oxidase positive
(d) CAMP positive

ANSWERS AND EXPLANATIONS

1. **Ans. is 'd'** i.e., The survival and multiplication of L. monocytogenes within mononuclear phagocytes and host epithelial cells

   L. monocytogenes induces its own internalization by cells that are not normally phagocytic. Its **entry into cells** is mediated by host surface proteins classified as **internalins.** Internalin-mediated entry is important in the crossing of intestinal, blood brain, and fetoplacental barriers, an essential determinant of the pathogenesis of L. monocytogenes is its beta hemolysin, listeriolysin O (LLO). **LLO is largely responsible for mediating the rupture of the phagosomal membrane that forms after phagocytosis of L. monocytogenes. LLO probably acts by inserting into an acidifying phagosome, which prevents the vesicles maturation.**

2. **Ans. is 'd'** i.e., Motility at 25 degree Celsius

   L. monocytogenes is a short, gram positive, non-spore forming rod.The motility test rapidly differentiates listeria from diphtheroids that are members of the normal microbiota of the skin. The organism has several adhesion proteins **(Ami, Fbp A, and flagellin proteins)** that facilitate bacterial binding to the host cells and that contribute to virulence.

   It has cell wall surface proteins called internalins A and B that interact with E-cadherin, a receptor on epithelial cells, promoting phagocytosis into the epithelial cells. After phagocytosis, the bacterium is enclosed in a phagolysosome, where the low pH activates the bacterium to produce listeriolysin.

   This enzyme, along with two phospholipases, lyses the membrane of the phagolysosome and allows the listeriae to escape into the cytoplasm of the epithelial cell. **The organism proliferates, and ActA, another listerial surface protein, induces host cell actin polymerization,** which propels them to the cell membrane. Pushing against the host cell membrane, they cause formation of elongated protrusions called filopods. **These filopods are ingested by adjacent epithelial cells, macrophages, and hepatocytes, the listeriae are released, and the cycle begins again. L monocytogenes move from cell to cell without being exposed to antibodies, complement, or polymorphonuclear cells.**

3. **Ans. is 'a'** i.e., Listeria monocytogenes

   Already explained.

4. **Ans. is 'd'** i.e., Uveitis.

5. **Ans. is 'c'** i.e., Oxidase positive

MYCOBACTERIUM (T.B., LEPRAE, ATYPICAL)

- **Mycobacterium** belongs to the family Mycobacteriaceae, order Actinomycetales.
- All the species under the genus Mycobacterium should have the following minimum properties.

  Acid fastness: They resist decolonization by dilute mineral acids. Acid fastness is due to the: 1. Presence of high content of mycolic acids in the cell wall. 2. Integrity of the cell wall.
- Non-motile, Non-sporing, Non-capsulated, Strict aerobes, straight or slightly curved rod-shaped.
- **History:** Robert Koch (1882) isolated the tubercle bacilli and proves its causative role in tuberculosis as it satisfies the Koch's postulates.

  Lepra bacillus was discovered by Hansen (1874), hence it is called Hansen's bacilli.
- **Classification**

  M. tuberculosis complex: It is responsible for tuberculosis in man (M. tuberculosis, M. bovis, M. africanum).

  M. leprae (Hansen's bacilli) – Leprosy.

  Nontuberculous mycobacteria (NTM): These diverse groups of mycobacteria are isolated from animals, soil, water and occasionally cause opportunistic human infection.

  Saprophytic mycobacteria (Nonpathogenic) are isolated from soil, water and other environmental sources [M. smegmatis (contaminant in Urine), M. butyricum (butter) and M. phlei (Grass)].

MYCOBACTERIUM TUBERCULOSIS

- They are not classified as Gram positive or Gram negative.
- Acid and Alcohol fast bacilli (due to Mycolic acid – lipid layer surrounding cell wall) – They resist decolonization by 20% H_2SO_4 and absolute alcohol for 10 mins.
- Immunity provides by CD_4 cells.

M. Tuberculosis Diseases

- **Pulmonary tuberculosis** – Accounts for 80% of all cases and Divided into two:

  Primary Disease – Usually localized in middle and lower zones, Primary complex/Ghon's focus.

  Post Primary Disease – (Adult type or reactivation or secondary tuberculosis or chronic pulmonary TB) – **Puhl's lesion, Assmann focus, Simon's focus.**

  Most common hematological finding – Mild anemia and leukocytosis.
- **Extra Pulmonary tuberculosis – Most common site is lymph nodes (Cervical and supraclavicular).**

  Pleural effusion, Genitourinary tract, Skeletal TB, TB meningitis.

Sequence of Pathogenic Events

MTB – Adhesion to macrophages → Phagocytosis by macrophages → Survival inside the macrophages → Multiplication inside the macrophages → Macrophages eventually ruptures and release its bacillary content which infect other phagocytes, the cycle continues.

- **Cord factor:** Promotes the virulence of M. tuberculosis.

Lab Diagnosis

- Specimens – 2 sputum sample, gastric aspirate (in children), CSF and depending site of infection.
  - Collection of urine sample done in early morning.
- Direct Microscopy – **Ziehl-Neelsen (ZN) staining:** M. tuberculosis appears as long slender, beaded, red colored acid fast bacilli (AFB).

Fluorescent staining – Auramine Phenol or Auramine rhodamine **(Rapid screening)**

- **Culture – Digestion and Decontamination of sputum by Petroff's method** (4% NaOH) or NALC (N-acetyl-L-Cysteine) +2% NaOH.

Contd.

Contd.

Solid culture:

Egg based: Lowenstein-Jensen (LJ) medium, Dorset egg media and Petragnani media.

Blood based: Tarshis medium.

Potato based: Pawlowsky medium.

Agar based: Middlebrook 7H11 and 7H10.

Liquid media:

Middlebrook 7H9, Dubos, Proskauer.

Automated Culture System: (With OADC supplement) – Detection in 2-3 weeks.

BACTEC MGIT, BacT/Alert

- **Biochemical identification: Niacin test** – +ve for M. tuberculosis and -ve for M. bovis, NTM.
  Catalase test – M. tuberculosis and M. bovis week positive, strongly +ve for NTM.
- **Molecular methods** (Best diagnostic procedure)
  – Nested PCR, Line probe assay.

Mode of Transmission

- **Inhalational mode** – Mainly transmitted by inhalation of droplet (<5-10 μm), generated while coughing, sneezing or speaking of patients.
- **Inoculation** – Infection through direct skin contact with an infected person is uncommon.
- Ingestion – Swallowing of sputum (in infants) or consumption of unpasteurized (infected) milk.
- **Bacillary load** – 10^4 or more bacilli/ml in sputum is required for an effective transmission and can be diagnosed on Microscopy.

Diagnosis of Latent Tuberculosis

- **Tuberculin test:**
  – **Type 4 Hypersensitivity reaction (Cell mediated/Delayed type).**
  – PPD (Purified protein derivative antigen).
  – Administration – 0.1 ml of PPD containing 1 TU is injected intradermally into flexor surface of forearm.
  – Reading (Induration) – It is taken after 48-72 hours.

  Equal or more than 10 mm – Positive

  6-9 mm – Equivocal/Doubtful reaction

  Less than 5 mm – Negative

  Interpretation – Positive test in adults only indicates present or past exposure with tubercle bacilli but does not confirm the presence of active infection. In children used as diagnostic marker.

  False positive – BCG vaccination and NTM infection.

  False negative – HIV patients.
- **IGRA (Interferon gamma release assay)**
  This uses highly specific M. tuberculosis antigens such as CFP 10 (Culture filtrate protein), ESAT6 (early secreted antigenic target-6), both coded by RD1 genes.
  – **IGRA assay that measure T cell release of INF γ response to stimulation with highly TB antigens (CFP 10, ESAT6), are available by the name of T-SPOT TB and Quanti FERON TB gold.**
  – IGRA are preferred over TST for person above 5 years of age. In children under 5 years TST is preferred.

Treatment (Anti-Tubercular Drugs)

1st line drugs: Isoniazid, Rifampicin, Pyrazinamide, Ethambutol and Streptomycin.

2nd line drugs: Ethionamide, Quinolones (ofloxacin, ciprofloxacin), Aminoglycosides (kanamycin, amikacin, capreomycin), cycloserine, macrolides (clarithromycin).

MDR-TB – Resistance to Isoniazid and Rifampicin with or without resistance to other first line anti-tubercular drugs.

Treatment – Complex regimen of 2nd line drugs.

BCG VACCINATION

- Live attenuated M. bovis strain was originally used by Calmette and Guerin.
- In India – WHO recommended **Danish 1331** strain of BCG is used.
- Administration – Dose–0.1 ml, Site–Above the insertion of left deltoid, Route–Intradermally by 26 gauge tuberculin syringe. The local lesion in BCG is maximum by 28 days.
- Contraindications – HIV +ve child, Child borne to AFB +ve mother, Pregnancy, Generalized eczema.
- Other uses of BCG – Provide some protection against leprosy, leukemia and adjuvant therapy in bladder carcinoma **(Onco TICE strain of BCG).**

MYCOBACTERIUM LEPRAE

- **Obligate intracellular AFB bacilli and causative agent of leprosy.**
- **Grow in cooler areas** – Peripheral nerves, ant. chamber of the eye, URT and Testes.
- Sparing warmer areas of skin (axilla, groin, scalp and midline of the back).
- **Generation time – 12-13 days and IP – 5-7 years.**
- It can survive outside the human body – 9-16 days.
- Transmission – Nasal droplet, contact with infected soil, insect vectors, breastfeeding and skin to skin contact is not an important route.

M. Leprae Diseases

Leprosy can be classified into various categories base on clinical, bacteriological, immunological and histological status of the patients.

- Lepromatous Leprosy (LL) – IgM against PGL-1.
- Tuberculoid Leprosy (TT) – Single skin lesion and has maximum number of TH 1 cells.

Other Categories of Leprosy:

- Borderline type.
- Indeterminate type.
- Pure neuritic type.

Complications

Complications in leprosy patients may be of two types – Deformities and allergic response (called lepra reactions).

- **Type 1 Lepra reaction/Jopling type 1:** Type 4 Hypersensitivity reaction seen in Borderline leprosy.
- **Type 2 Lepra reaction/Erythema Nodosum leproticum (ENL)/Jopling type 2:** Type 3 Hypersensitivity seen in multibacillary (BL and LL) leprosy, mainly TNF-alpha is resposible.
- **Lucio's Phenomenon: Type 3 Hypersensitivity exclusively in diffuse lepromatosis form of LL, usually in untreated patients.**

Lab Diagnosis

- Specimens – Total 6 samples, four from skin (forehead, cheek, chin and buttock), one from ear lobe and nasal mucosa by nasal blow/scraping.
- ZN staining (5% H_2SO_4) – Slit Skin smear – AFB arranged in groups (cigar like bundles) to from **globi (AFB in Histocytes).** The **globi** are present inside the foamy macrophages called **Virchow's lepra cells** or **Foamy cells.**
- Culture – *Can't grow on artificial medium or tissue culture.*

Can be grown in animals – **Foot pad of mouse (common and experimental work), Nine banded armadillo (best).**

- **Lepromin test** (Detection for CMI which is biphasic) – Type 4 Hypersensitivity and *most use for prognosis not for diagnosis.*
  - **Early reaction of Fernandez – read in 24-48 hrs** (Analogous to TST).
  - **Late reaction of Mitsuda** – Reading taken after 3 weeks and peak in 4 weeks.

Prevention – There is no effective vaccine available so far. Trials were done using BCG vaccine alone or with killer lepra bacilli, ICRC bacillus.

- In HIV +ve individuals lymph node TB biopsy reveals poorly organized or no granulomas at all.
- **IgM Abs against PGL-1** (M. leprae specific phenolic glycolipid found in the cell wall) are seen in untreated LL.
- **Scrofuloderma** is a type of cutaneous tuberculosis and most common focus is lymph nodes.

ATYPICAL MYCOBACTERIUM/NONTUBERCULOUS MYCOBACTERIA (NTM)/MYCOBACTERIA OTHER THAN TUBERCLE BACILLI (MOTT)

NTM have been classified into four groups by Runyon (1959) based on pigment production and growth rate.

Group I – Photochromogenes (Produce pigment only in light)	**Group II – Scoto chromogens** (Form pigment even in dark)	**Group III – Non Photo Chromogens** (Do not produce pigments)	**Group IV – Rapid Growers** (Grows within 1 week)
• M. Kansasii • M. marinum • M. Simiae	• M. Szulgai • M. Scrofulaceum • M. Gordanae/M. Acquae **Mn: Sunder sushil girl**	• M. Intracellulare – battey bacillus • M. xenopi • M. ulcerans • M. avium	• M. fortuitum • M. chelonae

- Some atypical bacteria (e.g., M. kansasii) produce human disease indistinguishable from tuberculosis.
- M. Africanum is acquired from human and cattles.
- Mycobacterium acquired from environment source:
  - M. avium complex.
  - M. malmoense.
  - M. ulcerans. Mn – **AMU**
- M. smegmatis is not pathogenic mycobacteria.
- M. marinum causes chronic cutaneous infection when open cutaneous infection when open cutaneous lesion exposed to colonized water source, swimming pool granuloma.
- Atypical bacteria causes lymphadenitis are: M. avium, M. intracellular, M. malmoense, M. scrofulaceum, M. Kanasasii.
- **Batteys bacillus: Mycobacterium intracellulare.Q**
- **Buruli ulcer: Mycobacterium ulcerans.Q**
- **Swimming pool granuloma: Mycobacterium marinum.Q**
- MOTT causes decreased efficacy of BCG due to cross immunity.

MCQs

Mycobacterium Tuberculosis

1. **Which of the following regarding the Interferon-gamma release assays used for the diagnosis of tuberculosis is correct?** *(AI 2012)*
   (a) 1st generation Quantiferon–TB used ESAT-6
   (b) 2nd generation Quantiferon–TB (gold) used ESAT-6 and cfp-10
   (c) These tests can distinguish between M. tuberculosis and M. bovis
   (d) None of the non-tubercular mycobacteria give a positive reaction with this test
2. **Tuberculin test denotes:** *(AI 00)*
   (a) Previous or present sensitivity to tubercle proteins
   (b) Patient is resistant to TB
   (c) Person is susceptible to TB
   (d) Protective immune status of individual against TB

3. **Collection of urine sample of a patient of TB kidney is done:** *(AIIMS 00)*
   (a) 24 hours urine
   (b) 12 hours urine
   (c) In early morning
   (d) Any time
4. **True about Mantoux test:**
   (a) < 5 mm always +ve
   (b) Usually -ve after treatment
   (c) Usually read after 48-72 hours
   (d) False +ve in post measles state
5. **True regarding Mycobacterium tuberculosis is:** *(PGI 02)*
   (a) Produces visible colonies in 1 week time on Lowenstein Jenson media
   (b) Decolorized by 20% sulphuric acid
   (c) Facultative aerobe
   (d) Niacin positive
6. **Cavitation is most often seen in:** *(AI 2011)*
   (a) Mycoplasma pneumonia
   (b) Tuberculosis pneumonia
   (c) Streptococcal pneumonia
   (d) Staphylococcal pneumonia
7. **Which of the following are acid fast positive with 20% sulphuric acid?** *(PGI 02)*
   (a) M. avium
   (b) M. leprae
   (c) M. tuberculosis
   (d) Nocardia
   (e) Rhizopus
8. **Selective media for TB bacilli is:** *(PGI 01)*
   (a) NNN media
   (b) Dorset media
   (c) LJ media
   (d) Nutrient agar
   (e) Mac'Conkey media
9. **True about tuberculin test are all *except*:** *(PGI 98, 01)*
   (a) Recent conversion in adult is an indication for ATT
   (b) INH prophylaxis is started if the test is positive
   (c) No risk in negative
   (d) May be false negative in immunocompromised patients

ANSWERS AND EXPLANATIONS

1. **Ans. is 'b'** i.e., 2nd generation Quantiferon-TB (gold) used ESAT-6 and CFP-10.
   INFγ release assay (IGRA) is an in vitro assay for diagnosis of latent tuberculosis, which measures INFγ released by T cells in response to highly specific TB antigens ESAT6 and CFP-10. Currently available such assays are:
   (a) T spot TB: An enzyme linked immunosorbant assay
   (b) Quantiferon TB Gold: Whole blood enzyme linked immunosorbant assay
   Note – Serological tests are banned in India for MTB diagnosis.
2. **Ans. is 'a'** i.e., Previous or present sensitivity to tubercle proteins
   (a) Tuberculin test denotes Type IV (delayed) hypersensitivity to tuberculoprotein 0.1 ml (Purified protein derivative) and used in diagnosis of latent tuberculosis.
   (b) Positive tuberculin test indicates exposure to Mycobacterium tuberculosis in the form of infection or immunization with or without active disease.
3. **Ans. is 'c'** i.e., In early morning
   Sampling – Collect the whole of patient early morning urine on three consecutive days (Previously it was 24 hours urine collection but now it is not recommended).
   Culture of three morning urine samples yields a definitive diagnosis in 90% cases.

4. **Ans. is 'c'** i.e., Usually read after 48-72 hours

Let's consider other choices:

(a) > 10 mm is positive and 6-9 mm is Equivocal/Doubtful reaction.

(b) It becomes positive after exposure to mycobacterium tuberculosis protein either in the form of infection or immunization and remains positive even after treatment.

Note – Tuberculin test in Adults is used as Epidemiological marker and in Children is used as diagnostic marker.

5. **Ans. is 'd'** i.e., Niacin Positive

Mycobacterium tuberculosis is Niacin Positive, Neutral red Positive and Nitrate reduction test positive.

Other Options:

(a) It produces visible colonies in 6-8 weeks time on Lowenstein Jensen media.

(b) It resist decolorised by 20% sulphuric acid.

(c) It is an obligate aerobe.

6. **Ans. is 'b'** i.e., Tuberculosis pneumonia

Tuberculosis as a primary cause of respiratory failure is an uncommon occurrence with an incidence of 1.5% in patients hospitalized with pulmonary TB.

Patients with miliary or disseminated disease are especially prone to develop respiratory failure. Tuberculous Pneumonia has rarely been identified as a cause of ARF (Acute Respiratory Failure).

Acute tuberculous pneumonia presents as parenchymal consolidation with or without endobronchial spread mimicking bacterial pneumonia.

It probably represents an exudative hypersensitivity reaction to tuberculoprotein, rather than actual inflammation caused by the Mycobacterium tuberculosis organism per se. These infiltrates can appear within a matter of days and can clinically simulate acute bacterial pneumonia.

7. **Ans. are 'a and c'** – M. avium and M. tuberculosis

Mycobacterium tuberculosis and Atypical Mycobacteria resist decolorization with up to 20% Sulphuric acid.

Mycobacterium leprae resist decolorization with up to 5% Sulphuric acid.

Nocardia resist decolorization with up to 1% Sulphuric acid.

8. **Ans. are 'b and c'** i.e., LJ Media and Dorset Media.

Media for Mycobacterium tuberculosis.

Solid media: Lowenstein Jensen Media, Dorset Egg Media, Loeffler's Media, Pawlowsky media.

Liquid media: Dubos media, Middle Brook's media, Proskauer and Beck's Media, Sula's and Sauton.

9. **Ans. is 'c'** i.e., No risk in negative.

Risk of Mycobacterium tuberculosis infection is more in Mantoux negative patient, i.e., diameter of induration 5 mm or less.

M. LEPRAE

1. **Leprosy affects all the following *except*:** *(AI 07)*

(a) Testes (b) Ovaries

(c) Eyes (d) Nerves

2. **In the management of leprosy, Lepromin test is most useful for:** *(AI 03)*

(a) Herd immunity (b) Prognosis

(c) Treatment (d) Epidemiological investigations

3. **Which of the following is true regarding globi in a patient with lepromatous leprosy?**

(a) Consist of lipid laden macrophages

(b) Consist of macrophages filled with AFB

(c) Consist of neutrophils filled with bacteria

(d) Consist of activated lymphocytes

4. **The main cytokine, involved in erythema nodosum leprosum (ENL) reaction, is:**
   (a) Interleukin-2
   (b) Interferon - gamma
   (c) Tumor necrosis factor - alpha
   (d) Macrophage colony stimulating factor

5. **The following drug is not used for the treatment of type II lepra reaction:** *(AIIMS 06)*
   (a) Chloroquin
   (b) Thalidomide
   (c) Cyclosporine
   (d) Corticosteroids

6. **The following test is not used for diagnosis of leprosy:** *(AIIMS 06)*
   (a) Lepromin test
   (b) Split skin smear
   (c) Fine needle aspiration cytology
   (d) Skin biopsy

7. **Which of the following statement about lepromin test is not true?** *(AIIMS 07, 06)*
   (a) It is negative in most children in first 6 months of life
   (b) It is a diagnostic test
   (c) It is an important aid to classify type of leprosy disease
   (d) BCG vaccination may convert lepra reaction from negative to positive

8. **Under leprosy eradication program the management of single lesion is:** *(AIIMS 02)*
   (a) Single dose of Rifampicin and Dapsone
   (b) Rifampicin and Dapsone for 6 months
   (c) Rifampicin, Ofloxacin and Minocycline single dose
   (d) Rifampicin and Minocycline for 6 months

9. **The characteristic finding in a case of leprosy is:** *(AIIMS 98, 2000)*
   (a) Culture test is positive in 2-3 months in LJ media
   (b) Long contact with tuberculoid leprosy can transmit the disease
   (c) CMI is seen in Lepromatous leprosy
   (d) Macule lesion heals spontaneously

10. **Exacerbation of lesions in patients of borderline leprosy is seen in:** *(PGI 01)*
   (a) ENL (erythema nodosum leprosum)
   (b) Lepra reaction type I
   (c) Jarisch-Herxheimer reaction
   (d) Resolving leprosy

11. **Antibodies against PGL-1 are seen in:** *(AIIMS 2013, AI 2011, DNB 2012)*
   (a) Infection with M. leprae
   (b) Infection with M tuberculosis
   (c) Infection with Borrelia
   (d) Infection with Brucella

ANSWERS AND EXPLANATIONS

1. **Ans. is 'b'** i.e., Ovaries

   Mycobacterium leprae grows best in cooler areas, e.g., peripheral nerves, anterior chamber of the eye, upper respiratory tract and testes. It spares warmer areas of the skin, e.g., axilla, groin, scalp and middle of the back.

2. **Ans. is 'b'** i.e., Prognosis

   Lepromin test: It is an intradermal test with biphasic response and demonstrates the delayed type of hypersensitivity.

   (a) **Early reaction of Fernandez:** It occurs in 24-48 hours.
   (b) **Late reaction of Mistuda:** It peaks in 4 weeks and is more meaningful. It indicates that a person is able to mount cell mediated immunity against leprosy.

   It is used to:

   (a) Classify the lesion of leprosy.

(b) To assess prognosis and response to treatment.

(c) To assess resistance of individual to leprosy.

Antigen used in Lepromin test:

(a) Lepromin A: It is standard lepromin from armadillo derived lepra bacilli.

(b) Lepromin H: Human derived lepra bacilli.

3. **Ans. is 'b'** i.e., Consist of macrophages filled with AFB

Lepra bacilli may be present in tissue extracellularly or intracellulary in histiocytes. These bacilli laden cells are called Virchow, Lepra cells or foamy cells.

Globi: These are cluster of bacilli bound together by lipid like substance the glia.

4. **Ans. is 'c'** i.e., Tumor necrosis factor – α

Type I Lepra reaction	Type II Lepra reaction
Down grading or reversal reaction	Erythema nodosum leprosum
Type IV hypersensitivity	Type III hypersensitivity
TNF Play a central role	INFγ and IL are the key cytokines
Edema is the characteristics microscopic feature	Vasculitis and panniculitis are seen
Treatment DOC: Glucocorticoid Other: Clofazimine Chloroquine Analgesics	**Treatment** DOC: Thalidomide Other: Clofazimine Chloroquine Glucocorticoid Analgesics NSAIDS and Antibiotics

5. **Ans. is 'c'** i.e., Cyclosporine: See Ans. No. 4
6. **Ans. is 'a'** i.e., Lepromin test: **Lepromin test** is not used for diagnosis: Also See Ans. No. 2
7. **Ans. is 'b'** i.e., It is a diagnostic test
8. **Ans. is 'c'** i.e., Rifampicin, Ofloxacin and Minocycline single dose
9. **Ans. is 'b'** i.e., Long contact with tuberculoid leprosy can transmit the disease

Leprosy is a disease with low rate of transmission. Prolonged contact with case is required for transmission.

Other Choices

(a) Lepra bacilli cannot be grown in LJ media or any other artificial culture media. These are grown in foot pad of mouse. Or

A milliary infection can be established in nine banded armadillo.

(c) CMI is present in tuberculoid leprosy and is absent in lepromatous leprosy.

(d) There is no such report that macule lesion heals spontaneously.

Mode of transmission of leprosy:

(a) Long contact with a case of leprosy (specially household contact with lepromatous case).

(b) Nasal droplet infection.

(c) Inoculation by insect vector or by tatooing.

10. **Ans. are 'a and b'** i.e., ENL (erythema nodosum leprosum) and Lepra reaction type I
11. **Ans. is 'a'** i.e., M. leprae

PGL1 stands for M. leprae specific phenolic glycolipid found in lepra bacilli. IgM antibodies are present in 95% patient with untreated lepromatous leprosy.

60% of patient with tuberculoid leprosy and in individuals exposed to lepra bacilli without clinical disease. There for PGL 1 serology is of little diagnostic value.

ATYPICAL MYCOBACTERIA

1. **Which one of the following statement is true regarding pathogenicity of Mycobacteria species?** *(AI 06)*
   (a) M. tuberculosis is more pathogenic than M. bovis to humans
   (b) M. kansasii can cause disease indistinguishable from tuberculosis
   (c) M. africanum infection is acquired from environmental source
   (d) M. marinum is responsible for tubercular lymphadenopathy
2. **The most common focus of Scrofuloderma is:** *(AI 96, 04)*
   (a) Lung (b) Lymph node
   (c) Larynx (d) Skin
3. **True about mycobacterium other than tuberculosis:**
   (a) Causes disseminated infection
   (b) Occurs in persons with normal immunity
   (c) Causes decreased efficacy of BCG due to cross immunity
   (d) Person to person transmission is seen
4. **Scotochromogens are:**
   (a) Mycobacterium gordonae (b) Mycobacterium marinum
   (c) Mycobacterium intracellular (d) Mycobacterium avium
   (e) Mycobacterium kansasii
5. **Which of the following are photo chromogens?** *(PGI Dec 2008)*
   (a) M. Kansasii (b) M. Scorfulaceaum
   (c) M. Marinum (d) M. TB
   (e) M. Leprae
6. **Which of the following is a slow grower:** *(AIIMS May 2013)*
   (a) M. kansasii (b) M. chelonae
   (c) M. fortuitum (d) M. abscessus
7. **Rapid growing non-tuberculous mycobacteria causing lung infection are all *except*:** *(AIIMS Nov 2013)*
   (a) M. kansasii (b) M. chelonae
   (c) M. fortuitum (d) M. abscessus

ANSWERS AND EXPLANATIONS

1. **Ans. is 'b'** i.e., M. *kansasii* can cause disease indistinguishable from tuberculosis.
   Other choices:
   (a) *M. tuberculosis and M. bovis* are equally pathogenic.
   (b) *M. africanum* infection is acquired from human and cattles.
   (d) *M.* marinum causes swimming pool granuloma.
2. **Ans. is 'b'** i.e., Lymph Node
   Scrofuloderma is a type of cutaneous tuberculosis.
3. **Ans. is 'c'** i.e., Causes decreased efficacy of BCG due to cross immunity
4. **Ans. is 'a'** i.e., Mycobacterium gordonae
   Scotochromogens are:
   (a) M. Szulgai.
   (b) M. Scrofulaceum.
   (c) M. Gordonae/M acquae.

5. **Ans. are 'a' and 'c'** i.e., M Kansasii, M Marinum

Photochromogens

(a) M. Simiae.

(b) M. Marinum.

(c) M. Asiaticum.

(d) M. Kansasii.

6. **Ans. is 'a'** i.e., M. kansasii

7. **Ans. is 'a'** i.e., M. kansasii

MISCELLANEOUS MCQ ON MTB & M.LEPRAE

Mycobacterium TB and Leprae

1. **Mycobacteria can be diagnosed on microscopy when counts are:**

(a) 10,000 or more/ml (b) 1,00,000 or more/ml

(c) 1,000 or more/ml (d) 10 or more/ml

2. **Typical mycobacterium is differentiated from atypical mycobacterium by:** (*Delhi 2006*)

(a) Acid fast staining (b) Ability to grow on LJ media

(c) Niacin test (d) Motility under microscope

3. **BCG vaccine in HIV (+) newborn is:**

(a) Contraindicated (b) Double dilution

(c) Half dilution (d) Dose double

BCG vaccine should not be given to infants and children with active HIV disease. Babies born to mother with AFB positive spectum should bot be given BCG at birth, but only after a course of preventive chemotherapy.

4. **Cutaneous lesions may be produced by the following mycobacteria *except*:** (*Delhi 2001*)

(a) M. intracellulare (b) M. leprae

(c) M. marinum (d) M. tuberculosis

(e) M. ulcerans

Mycobacterium causing skin lesion:

- M. tuberculosis
- M. leprae
- M. ulcerans
- M. marinum
- M. haemophilum

5. **Acid fastness of *tubercle bacilli* is attributed to:**

(a) Presence of mycolic acid (b) Integrity of cellwall

(c) Both of the above (d) None of the above

6. **In which type of Cutaneous Tuberculosis, caseation is most commonly seen?** (*PGI 93*)

(a) Papulonecrotic (b) Scrofuloderma

(c) Lupus vulgaris (d) Erythema nodosum

(***Ref:*** *Greenwood, 18th/e, p. 213*)

7. **Single skin lesion is seen in which type of leprosy?** (*AI 93*)

(a) LL (b) TT

(c) BL (d) BT

8. **Lepra bacilli are best cultivated in:**

(a) Guinea pig (b) Armadillos

(c) Mouse foot pad (d) Nutrient agar

9. Which of the following is not a pathogenic mycobacteria? *(AI 91)*

(a) M. kansasii (b) M. scrofulaceum
(c) M. cheoleni (d) M. smegmatis

10. Mycobacterium tuberculosis is differentiated from other atypical mycobacteria by: *(SGPGI 95; AIIMS 91)*

(a) Niacin test (b) AFB staining
(c) PAS staining (d) None

11. Leprosy bacilli are cultured in:

(a) LJ medium (b) Foot pad of mice
(c) Agar plate (d) None

12. The local lesion in BCG is maximum in:

(a) 2 days (b) 7 days
(c) 28 days (d) 1 year

13. Mitsuda reaction is read after: *(MP 98)*

(a) 3 days (b) 3 hours
(c) 3 weeks (d) 3 months

14. The factor which promotes, virulence of *M. tuberculosis:* *(TN 98)*

(a) Wax D (b) Cord factor
(c) Muramyl dipeptide (d) Mycolic acid

15. BCG differs from Mantoux test by:

(a) Less sensitive and more specific (b) More sensitive and more specific
(c) More sensitive and more specific (d) Less sensitive and more specific

16. Not a pathogenic mycobacterium to human: *(TN 99)*

(a) M. paratuberculosis (b) M. kansasii
(c) M. ulcerans (d) M. intracellular

17. Rapid diagnosis of tuberculosis is possible with:

(a) Auramine rhodamine-stain (b) Zeil-Neelsen stain
(c) Geimsa stain (d) Leishman stain

18. *Mycobacterium scrofulaceum* which cause scrofula, belongs to which groups of atypical mycobacteria? *(Kerala 2K)*

(a) Photochromogens (b) Scotochromogens
(c) Non-photochromogens (d) Rapid growers
(e) None of the above

19. Mycobacterium leprae can be grown in:

(a) Teepol agar (b) Tomato juice agar
(c) Foot pad of mouse (d) LJ media

20. Photochromogenic strain of mycobacterium species is: *(Kar 2001)*

(a) M. kansasii (b) M. scrofulaceum
(c) M. avium intracellular/lare (d) M. smegmatis

21. Mycobacterium TB can be differentiated from other Mycobacterium by: (*Kerala 01*)

(a) Production of niacin
(b) Arylsulphate test
(c) Coagulase test
(d) Bile solubility test

22. Mantoux test is an indicator of:

(a) Immediate hypersensitivity
(b) Delayed hypersensitivity
(c) Cell-mediated cytotoxicity
(d) Of no interest

23. The best diagnostic procedure of M. tuberculosis: (*SGPGI 02*)

(a) PCR
(b) Auramine rhodamine stain
(c) Sputum culture
(d) Sputum examination

24. Drug resistance in tuberculosis is due to: (***Ref:*** *Jawetz, 24th/e, p. 326*)

(a) Transformation
(b) Transduction
(c) Conjugation
(d) Mutation

25. Subtype of leprosy has maximum number of TH:1 cells: (*UP 03*)

(a) TT
(b) BB
(c) LL
(d) Borderline leprosy

26. All are rapid growers *except*:

(a) M. fortuitum
(b) M. chelonei
(c) M. avium intracellulare
(d) M. smegmatis

27. All of the following are acid fast bacteria *except*: (*SGPGI 03*)

(a) Cryptosporidia
(b) Mycoplasma
(c) Mycobacteria
(d) Nocardia

28. In a patient, the lymph nodes show necrosis with poor granuloma formation with plenty of acid fast bacilli suggests: (*SGPGI 04*)

(a) Tuberculosis in an immunocompromised patient
(b) HIV with tuberculosis
(c) Sarcoidosis
(d) Mycobacterium bovis infection

(***Ref:*** *Harrison, 18th/e, p. 1346*)

In HIV positive individuals lymph node TB biopsy reveals really organized or no granulomas at all. However bacterial: is heavier than HIV negative individual.

29. Culture of lepra bacilli done in: (*Kolkata 05*)

(a) Nine banded armadillo
(b) Tail of mouse
(c) Foot pads of mice
(d) Nutrient agar

30. Mycobacterium non-pathogenic to man:

(a) M. bovis
(b) M.kansasii
(c) M. aviun intracellulare
(d) M.phlei

M. phlei is a saprophyte

31. Swimming pool granuloma is caused by: (***Ref:*** *Ananthanarayan, 9th/e, p. 57b*)

(a) M. kansasi
(b) M. avium intracellulare
(c) M. scrofulaceum
(d) M. marinum

32. Globi is:

(a) Histocyte containing acid-fast bacillus
(b) Lymphocyte containing acid-fast bacillus
(c) Nutrophill containing acid-fast bacillus
(d) Large lymphocyte containing acid-fast bacillus

33. Which of the following mycobacteria can cause disease in HIV +ve patient with a CD4 count of 600/cu.mm? (***Ref:*** *Harrison, 18th/e, p. 1548*)

(a) M. tuberculosis
(b) MAC
(c) M. chelonei
(d) M. fortuitum

34. Niacin test is not positive in:

(a) M.tuberculosis
(b) M. chelonei
(c) M. bovis
(d) M. simiae

35. Regarding biochemical reactions to differentiate different types of mycobacteria, all are true *except*:

(a) Niacin test is positive for human tubercle bacilli
(b) Arylsulfatase test is positive in atypical mycobacteria
(c) Neutral red test is for identifying virulent strains of tubercle bacilli
(d) M.tuberculosis is strongly catalase positive

36. The only mycobacterium which produces exotoxin is:

(a) M.TB
(b) M. paratuberculosis
(c) M. ulcerans
(d) M. marinum

ANSWERS

1.	(a)	**2.**	(c)	**3.**	(a)	**4.**	(a)	**5.**	(c)	**6.**	(b)	**7.**	(b)
8.	(b)	**9.**	(d)	**10.**	(a)	**11.**	(b)	**12.**	(c)	**13.**	(c)	**14.**	(b)
15.	(b)	**16.**	(a)	**17.**	(a)	**18.**	(b)	**19.**	(c)	**20.**	(a)	**21.**	(a)
22.	(b)	**23.**	(a)	**24.**	(d)	**25.**	(a)	**26.**	(c)	**27.**	(b)	**28.**	(a) and (b)
29.	(c)	**30.**	(d)	**31.**	(d)	**32.**	(a)	**33.**	(a)	**34.**	(c)	**35.**	(d)
36.	(c)												

ENTEROBACTERIACEAE (E.COLI, KLEBSIELLA, PROTEUS, SALMONELLA, SHIGELLA)

- Normally found in intestine (coliform) as a part of flora, cause disease of intestine.
- Various genus under Enterobacteriaceae family – Escherichia, Shigella, Edwardsiella, Salmonella, Citrobacter, Klebsiella, Enterobacter, Hafnia, Serratia, Proteus, Morganella, Providencia, Yersinia, Erwinia.
- Gram negative bacilli, aerobes and facultative anaerobes, non-fastidious (can grow in basal media).
- **They produce catalase (except Shigella dysenteriae type 1)Q** and do not produce oxidase.
- Motile with peritrichous flagella, **some are non-motile such as Shigella, Salmonella gallinarum-pullorum, Klebsiella**Q and reduce Nitrate to nitrite.
- Glucose is not fermented by all members of the family.
- Classification based on Lactose fermentation on MacConkey agar.

  Lactose fermenter (LF) – E.coli, Klebsiella.

  Non-lactose fermenter (NLF) – Salmonella, Shigella, Proteus, Morgenella, Providencia and Yersinia.

  Late Lactose fermenter (LLF/Paracolon bacilli) – Shigella sonnei.

ESCHERICHIA COLI

- GNB (Gram negative bacilli), Motile with peritrichous flagella, many pathogenic isolates are capsulated.
- On blood agar shows hemolysis and grows well on ordinary media.
- **Mostly are lactose fermenter** except certain verocytotoxin E.coli.
- IMViC (Indole test, MR test, VP test, Citrate test) = +,+,-,-.
- E. coli is most common cause of Catheter associated UTI (CAUTI) and UTI, also most common cause of neonatal meningitis.
- Most common cause of Intra-abdominal abscess.
- **A variant called thermotolerant E. coli (survives at 44°C) is taken as an indicator of contamination of drinking water with human or animal feces.**

Clinical Manifestations

- **UTI:** Most common cause is E. coli.
- **Diarrhea:**

  EPEC (Enteropathogenic E. coli) – Diarrhea in infants and children. Effacing lesions are seen because of damage to intestinal villi.

  ETEC (Enterotoxigenic E. coli) – Traveller's Diarrhea.

  EIEC (Enteroinvasive E. coli) – Diarrhea to Dysentery (Similar to Shigellosis). Sereny test is positive.

  EAEC (Enteroaggregative E. coli) – Persistent Diarrhoea. It also leads to travellers diarrhoea and stacked brick appearance seen in Hep 2 cell lines.

  EHEC (Enterohemorrhagic E. coli) – Hemolytic uremic syndrome (HUS), Hemorrhagic colitis.

  [**Serotype O157:H7** which **does not ferment Sorbitol** (non O157 strains ferment Sorbitol) is associated with HUS].
- **Pyogenic infections** – Most common cause of intra-abdominal abscess, peritonitis and cholangitis.
- **Meningitis** – Most common cause of neonatal meningitis, 75% of Meningitis is caused by K1 Strain (E.coli having capsule).
- **Bacteremia** – UTI is MC source of Bacteremia leading to septic shock.

– Labile toxin of E coli can be detected by inoculating into infant rabbit bowel, adult rabbit skin test positive, tissue culture of Chinese hamster ovary cell, Y1 mouse adrenal cells.Q

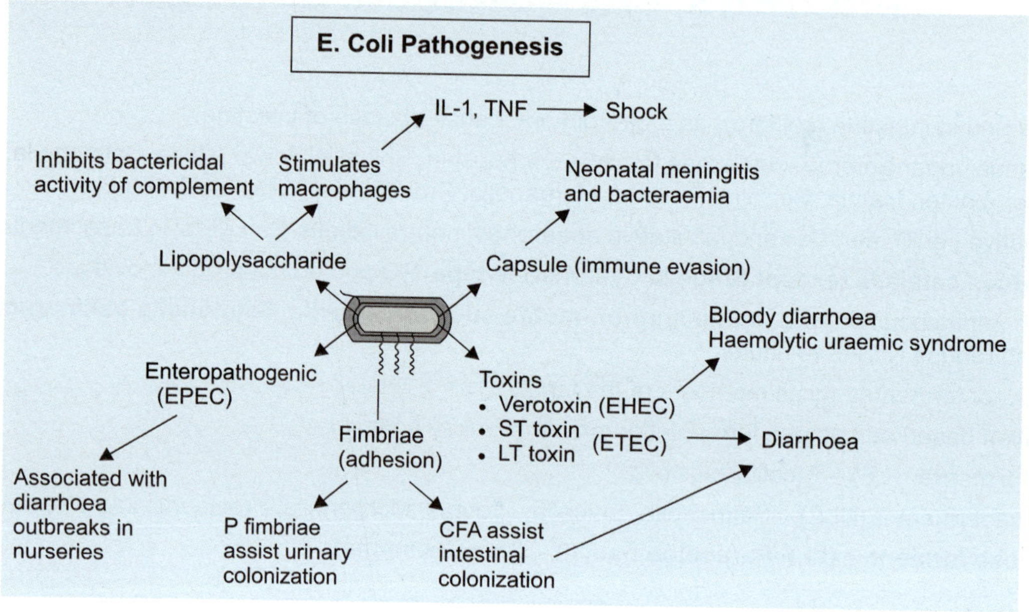

Virulence Factors

- **Surface antigens**
  - Somatic or O ag – Lipopolysaccharide (LPS), most important virulence factor and responsible for endotoxic activities.
  - Flagellar or H Ag – Makes the bacteria motile.
  - Capsular or K Ag – It is a polysaccharide capsular Ag, inhibits the phagocytosis.
  - Fimbrial antigen (Pilus) – Helps in attachment and colonization.
- **Toxins**
  - **LT (heat labile toxin)** – (Plasmid coded) – ↑cAMP so causes excessive secretion of Na/Cl/H_2O from within to outside the cell – secretory diarrhea (cells secrete water and electrolytes into lumen).
  - **ST (heat stable toxin)** – (Plasmid coded) – ↑cGMP so fluid accumulation in gut – Diarrhea.
  - **Verocytotoxin or Shiga like toxin** – (Bacteriophage coded) – It inhibits the protein synthesis by binding to 28S subunit of 60S ribosome – Cell death.

LAB DIAGNOSIS

- **Specimen** – Midstream urine and suprapubic aspiration (coma patients or infants).
- Gram staining of urine is not a reliable indicator.
- **Culture** – MacConkey agar (LF colonies) or CLED agar (inhibits the swarming of Proteus).
  Semiquantitative culture – concept was given by KASS concept.
  > 10^5 colony forming units/ml – indicative of UTI – Significant bacteriuria.
- Identification tests – IMViC test or ICUT (Indole test, Citrate test, Urease test, TSI test).

MCQs

1. **Traveller's diarrhea is caused by:** *(Manipal 08, APPG 10)*
   (a) Enteroinvasive E.coli
   (b) Enterotoxigenic E.coli
   (c) Enteropathogenic E.coli
   (d) Enteroaggregative E.coli

2. A 20-year-old male had pain in abdomen and mild fever followed by gastroenteritis. The stool examination showed presence of pus cells and RBCs on microscopy. The etiological agent responsible is most likely to be:

(a) EPEC (b) EHEC (c) ETEC (d) EIEC

3. The mechanism of action of EPEC is: *(Recent MCQ)*

(a) Adherence to enterocytes (b) Stimulates adenylcyclase
(c) Produce secretory diarrhoea (d) None of the above

4. It has been hypothesized that their exists a strong association between haemolytic uraemic syndrome: *(UPPG 11, Recent MCQ)*

(a) Salmonellae (b) Bacteriophages and corynebacteria
(c) Verocytotoxin producing E. coli (d) Clostridium difficle

5. An infant is brought to the emergency room with hemolytic uremic syndrome and thrombocytopenia. Stool sample was cultured and non-lactose fermenting colonies grown on Sorbitol MacConkey agar, which also fermented glucose with gas. Which one of the following bacteria would most likely be isolated from a stool specimen? *(APPG 05)*

(a) Shigella (b) Salmonella
(c) Aeromonas (d) E. coli 0157/H7

6. Verocytotoxin has been in individual suffering from hemolytic uraemic syndrome in their: *(AIIMS 07)*

(a) Blood (b) Tissues
(c) Faeces (d) Saliva

7. Eiken test is which type of reaction used for E. coli? *(AIIMS 10)*

(a) Precipitation (b) Agglutination
(c) Toxin antitoxin assay (d) CFT

8. Surface antigen of *E. coli* acting as virulence factors are: *(PGI 11)*

(a) LPS O Antigen (b) Enveloper K antigen
(c) Fimbriae (d) All of the above
(e) None of the above

9. True about EPEC is: *(Manipal 13)*

(a) Diarrhoea in infants (b) Least infectious
(c) Affects immunocompromised (d) Affects adults mostly

10. E. coli is an important causative agent of pyelonephritisin man. The property that helps the bacteria in this is most likely to be: *(Recent MCQ)*

(a) Adhesive property (b) Toxigenecity
(c) Haemolytic property (d) Presence of capsule

11. Most common cause of liver abscess: *(PGI 00, Recent MCQ)*

(a) Streptococcus pyogenes (b) Staph. aureus
(c) E. coli (d) Proteus

12. Most common organism causing UTI: *(PGI 10)*

(a) E.coli (b) Enterococcus
(c) Staph. saprophyticus (d) Klebsiella

13. Preformed toxin is important in food poisoning due to all *except*: *(APPG 13)*

(a) Satph. aureus (b) Cl. botulinum
(c) ETEC (d) Bacillus cereus

ANSWERS AND EXPLANATIONS

(Harrison, 19th/e, p. 1025; Ananthanarayan, 9th/e, p. 274)

1. **Ans. is 'b'** i.e., Enterotoxigenic E. coli

   Enterotoxigenic E coli (ETEC) are a common cause of "traveller's diarrhea" and a very important cause of diarrhea in children less than 5 years of age in developing countries.

   ETEC colonization factors [pili known as colonization factor antigens (CFAs)]Q specific for humans promote adherence of ETEC to epithelial cells of the small bowel. Some strains of ETEC produce a heat-labile enterotoxin (LT) that is under the genetic control of a plasmid. There is marked increase in the local concentration of cyclic adenosine monophosphate (cAMP) which leads to the end result of an intense and prolonged hypersecretion of water and chlorides and inhibition of the reabsorption of sodium.

2. **Ans. is 'c'** i.e., EIEC

   Sign of RBCs in stool – invasiveness – EIEC (Enteroinvasive E. coli) – Diarrhea to Dysentery (Similar to Shigellosis).

   Enteroinvasive E coli (EIEC) produce a disease very similar to shigellosis. The disease occurs most commonly in children in developing countries and in travellers to these countries. Similar to Shigella, EIEC strains are nonlactose or late lactose fermenters and are nonmotile. EIEC produce disease by invading intestinal mucosal epithelial cells.

3. **Ans. is 'a'** i.e., Adherence to enterocytes

   ENTEROPATHOGENIC E. COLI Pathogenesis – Attaching-and-effacing histopathology.

   Three-stage model of EPEC pathogenesis: (i) **Localized adherence** (ii) **Signal transduction** (iii) **Intimate adherence.**

   Enteropathogenic E coli (EPEC) are an important cause of diarrhea in infants, especially in developing countries. EPEC adhere to the mucosal cells of the small bowel.

   Pathogenicity requires two important factors, the bundle forming pilus encoded by a plasmid EPEC adherence factor (EAF) and the chromosomal locus of enterocyte effacement (LEE) pathogenicity island that promote the tight adherence characteristic of EPEC (attachment and effacement). After attachment, there is loss of microvilli (effacement); formation of filamentous actin pedestals or cuplike structures.

4. **Ans. is 'c'** i.e., Verocytotoxin producing E. coli

   EHEC (Enterohemorrhagic E. coli/Verocytotoxin producing E coli) – produces verotoxin (VT) whose major target is vascular endothelial cells – Hemolytic uremic syndrome (HUS), Hemorrhagic colitis – [Serotype O157:H7 which does not ferment Sorbitol (non O157 strains ferment Sorbitol)].

5. **Ans. is 'd'** i.e., E. coli 0157/H7

   Already explained in Ans. 4 and Ans 6.

6. **Ans. is 'a'** i.e., Blood

   Typical (or infection-induced) HUS is most commonly associated with Escherichia coli with somatic (O) antigen 157 and flagella (H) antigen 7 – hence the designation O157:H7. It produces a toxin called Shiga toxin or verotoxin – hence, alternative names are Shiga toxin-producing E. coli (STEC) or verotoxin-producing E. coli (VTEC).

7. **Ans. is 'a'** i.e., Precipitation

   Eiken Precipitation test is +ve for heat labile (LT) enterotoxin and –ve for heat stable (ST) enterotoxin of E.coli.

8. **Ans. is 'd'** i.e., All of the above

   Already explained in book text.

9. **Ans. is 'a'** i.e., Diarrhoea in infants

   Already explained in book text.

10. **Ans. is 'a'** i.e., Adhesive property

    Most of the urinary tract infections that involve the bladder or kidney in an otherwise healthy host are caused by a small number of O antigen types that have specifically elaborated virulence factors that facilitate colonization and subsequent clinical infections. These organisms are designated as uropathogenic E. coli.

Typically, these organisms produce hemolysin, which is cytotoxic and facilitates tissue invasion. **Strains that cause pyelonephritis express K antigen and elaborate a specific type of pilus, P fimbriae, which binds to the P blood group antigen and helps in attachment and colonization.**

11. **Ans. is 'c'** i.e., E. coli

    Polymicrobial involvement is common in pyogenic liver abscess with Escherichia coli (21%) and Klebsiella pneumoniae (16%) being the two most frequently isolated pathogens.

12. **Ans. is 'a'** i.e., E. coli (***Ref:*** *Harrison, 18th/e, p. 1249*)

    Already explained.

13. **Ans. is 'c'** i.e., ETEC (***Ref:*** *Ananthanarayan, 9th/e, p. 279*)

    ETEC first adheres with E. coli and then secretes exotoxin which causes diarrhea.

KLEBSIELLA

- GNB, Non-Motile, Capsulated, LF, Urease +ve, **IMViC = -, -, +, +.**Q
- Mucoid lactose fermenting colonies on MacConkey agar.

  K. Pneumoniae – Friedlander's Bacillus – It is important species.

Disease

- Pneumonia (characteristic sputum – **Red colored jelly like sputum**).Q
- **Ozoena (Atrophic rhinitis) – Kleb. ozaenae.**
- **Rhinoscleroma – Klebsiella rhinoscleromatis. Mikulicz cells and Russel bodies.**
- UTI, abdominal abscesses, surgical site infections.
- Soft tissue infection, Septicemia.

Interesting Fact – MDR strain of Klebsiella pneumoniae is known as Superbug (New Delhi Metallobetalactamase-1).

PROTEUS

- Gram Negative, Pleomorphic rod, Motile with peritrichous flagella, NLF, Urease test +ve.
- **Swarming on solid media.**

Inhibition of swarming of proteus – By adding bile salt – McConkey's, Hard agar – 6% agar, Chloral hydrate, Sodium azide, Boric acid, Sulphonamides.Q

- **Differs from other enterobacteria by production of enzyme Phenylalanine deaminase which is responsible for deamination of phenylalanine to phenyl pyruvic acid (PPA TEST).Q**
- Fishy odour or Seminal odour in colony.
- Proteus shows **Diene's phenomenon but remember here only Diene's method of staining is done for Mycoplasma.Q**

Diseases

1. UTI – Formation of stone – Staghorn calculus (Struvite Crystal).
2. Wound infection – Diabetic foot, Bed sores.
3. Septicemia.

DOC – Aminoglycosides and Quinolones are effective. Proteus is intrinsic resistant to Nitrofurantoin, Polymyxin and Tetracycline.

- Urease production in order – H. pylori > Proteus > Morganella morganii > Klebsiella.Q

MCQs

1. **Proteus antigen cross react with:** (*Recent MCQ*)

   (a) Klebsiella (b) Chlamydiae
   (c) Rickettsiae (d) E.coli

2. **All of the following are true *except*:** *(AI 01, Recent MCQ)*
   (a) E. coli is an aerobe and facultative anaerobes
   (b) Proteus forms uric acid stones
   (c) E. coli is motile by peritrichate flagella
   (d) Proteus causes deamination of phenylalanine to phenylpyruvic acid
3. **Dienes phenomenon is seen with:** *(PGI 02)*
   (a) Proteus mirabilis
   (b) Klebsiella
   (c) Proteus vulgaris
   (d) Providentia
   (e) Morganella
4. **Friedlanders bacillus also known as:** *(APPG 11, PGI 97)*
   (a) E. coli Pattern
   (b) Pseudomonas aeruginosa
   (c) Klebsiella pneumoniae
   (d) Vibrio parahemolyticus
5. **A newborn was admitted in an ICU for difficulty in breathing at the time of birth. On the fifth day, he became lethargic and unable to feed. The total counts increased with predominant polymorphs. Blood culture yielded growth of LF Mucoid colonies on MacConkey agar. What will be the probable cause of infection?**
   (a) E. coli
   (b) Hemophilus
   (c) Strept. pneumoniae
   (d) Klebsiella
6. **About ESBL producing bacteria, true is:**
   (a) Only seen in gram positive bacteria
   (b) Only seen in gram negative bacteria
   (c) Plasmid mediated
   (d) It is associated only with community acquired disease
7. **Klebsiella oxytoca is:**
   (a) Gram variable
   (b) Indole positive
   (c) Methyl red negative
   (d) No drug resistance reported

ANSWERS AND EXPLANATIONS

1. **Ans. 'c'** i.e., Rickettsiae (***Ref:*** *Ananthanarayan, 9th/e, p. 410*)

   Proteus antigens (OX19, OX2, OXK Strains) cross reacts with group specific alkali stable lipopolysaccharide rickettsial antigens. The application of this property is done in the Weil Felix (heterophile agglutination) test.
2. **Ans. is 'b'** i.e., Proteus forms uric acid stones

   (***Ref:*** *Surgical Pathology by Ackermann, p. 1124; Ananthanarayan, 9th/e, p. 274, 282 and 8th/e, p. 270*)

   Uric acid stone formation takes place in acidic urine, in the presence of hyperuricemia which may result from inborn errors of metabolism such as gout or the Lesch-Nyhan Syndrome.

   Proteus produces ammonia and contributes to alkalinity. It does not thus lead to formation of uric acid stones. The alkalinity leads to necrosis of renal tubular epithelium and precipitation of phosphate stones.

   The distinctive character of proteus genus is deamination of phenyl alanine to phenyl pyruvic acid (PPA +ve).

   E. coli are motile by peritrichous flagella.

   E. coli is an aerobe and facultative anaerobe.
3. **Ans. are 'a, c'** – Dienes phenomenon is used to detect swarming of Proteus

   Swarming Proteus strains exhibit the Dienes phenomenon (the mutual inhibition of swarming), and this forms the precise basis of differentiation among strains.

   When a pair of swarming Proteus mirabilis strains meets to form a Dienes line (the visible demarcation line between the two strains), a dominant strain induces cell death in the other strain at the contact point.

   Dienes method is used for the study of **Mycoplasma** colony.
4. **Ans. is 'c'** i.e., Klebsiella pneumoniae (***Ref:*** *Ananthanarayan, 9th/e, p. 280 and 8th/e, p. 278*)

"Klebsiella pneumoniae is also known as Friedlander's bacillus or Bacillus mucosus capsulatus."

(Karl Friedlander, 1847–1887, German bacteriologist) – who helped discover the bacterial cause of pneumonia in 1882.

5. **Ans. is 'd'** i.e., Klebsiella

   Klebsiella pneumoniae produces LF mucoid colonies on MacConkey agar.

6. **Ans. is 'c'** i.e., Plasmid mediated

   Extended spectrum beta lactamases (ESBL) are plasmid coded, produced by gram positive and gram negative bacteria, mainly expressed by hospital strains and also by community strains.

7. **Ans. is 'b'** i.e., Indole positive

   It is Indole positive whereas all other klebsiella are indole negative but methyl red and voges Proskauer positive.

SALMONELLA

SALMONELLA TYPHI

- Gram negative bacilli, Motile (except Salmonella **gallinarum-pullorum), noncapsulated, non sporing.Q**
- **Classical Classification (older)**

  Typhoidal Salmonella – S. typhi.

  Paratyphoidal Salmonella – S. paratyphi A and B.

  Non-typhoidal Salmonella (NTS) – They causes food borne gastroenteritis and septicemia.
- **Antigenic classification – Kauffmann White scheme.**Q
- **Molecular classification – Based on DNA hybridization,** the genus Salmonella consists of two species Sal. enterica and Sal. bongori.

Antigenic Structure

- Flagella antigen (H) – Strongly immunogenic. When mixed with antisera, it rapidly produces fluffy clumps.
- Somatic antigen (O/Biovin) – When mixed with antisera, forms chalky, granular clumps.
- Vi Ag – It is a surface polysaccharide covering the O Ag, **Agglutination with O ag of S. typhi is inhibited by Vi Ag** and it also used in vaccination. **Vi abs is used for detecting the carrier.Q**

CLINICAL MANIFESTATIONS

Enteric Fever:

- Fever **(Step ladder pattern type of remittent fever).**
- Rashes (Called **Rose spot** on the chest and trunk).
- Other symptoms: Headache, chills, cough, sweating, myalgia and arthralgia.

Gastroenteritis (Food poisoning):

- Causative agents – **S. typhimurium (MC) and S. enteritidis.**
- Abdominal pain, Nausea, vomiting, abdominal cramps and fever.
- **Sources – Poultry, meat, milk and milk production.**
- Blood culture is negative.
- **Salmonella can enter into freshly laid eggs.**

Pathogenesis

Incubation period – 10-14 days.

Infective dose – 10^3-10^6 bacilli.Q

Mode of Transmission – Faeco-oral route.

Bacteria reach small intestine **(Peyer's patches)** → Macrophages (eaten up S. typhi but not able to kill it → bacteria multiplies in it) → reaches portal blood – primary bacteremia → liver, spleen, bone marrow (organs rich in Macrophages) → multiply in large number and spills in blood – 2° Bacteremia → CI/F appear → Gallbladder → feces **(Pea-soup stool)** → next person infected by faeco-oral route.

Lab Diagnosis

- **Specimens** – Blood, Bone marrow, Stool and Urine.

- **Culture isolation** (Grows well on Basal media)
  Blood and bone marrow – BHI broth, automated BACTEC (in 1st week of illness).
  Stool Culture
  Enrichment broth – **Selenite F broth, Tetrathionate broth and Gram-negative broth.**
  Selective media – **DCA, XLD agar,** Salmonella Shigella agar, Wilson Blair's agar.
  MacConkey agar – NLF colonies.
  Identification Tests:
  Catalase +ve, Oxidase –ve, IMViC = -, +, -, +
  H_2S production – Except S. typhi A, S. paratyphi B (abundant), S. typhi (tiny) produce H_2S.
- **Salmonella ferment sugar producing acid and gas except S. typhi which is anerogenic.**
- **Widal test – Tube/Slide Agglutination Test**
  Agglutinins usually appear by end of 1st week. Titre increases steadily till the 3rd or 4th week after which it declines gradually.
  Significant Titer:
  - **H agglutination titre more than 200.**
  - **O agglutination titre more than 100.**

Antigens used: (S. typhi 901 strain)	**Interpretations:**
• O Ag of S. typhi (TO) • H Ag of S. typhi (TH) • H Ag of S. paratyphi A (AH) • H Ag of S. paratyphi B (BH)	Agglutination in TO and TH = S. typhi Agglutination in TO and AH = S. paratyphi A Agglutination in TO and BH = S. paratyphi B

- **O Agglutinin** – It has better diagnostic value than H, O Abs disappear after infection.
- **H Agglutinin** – Persist longer than O agglutinins, remains +ve after several months of infection, reaction is rapid, may be present due to prior infection.
- **Fourfold rise** in Ab titer by testing paired sera at 1 week interval is more diagnostic and indicates the true infection.
- **False positive** – Previous infection, Post TAB vaccination, Anamnestic response (malaria, dengue).
- **False negative** – 1st week of disease, carriers, due to Ab excess **(Prozone phenomenon).**
- **Diagnosis of carriers** (Rate of carriers – 5%).
- **Tests done are** – Urine/stool culture, Sewer swab culture.
- **Antibody to a particular Ag → Vi Ab (ViAg) if absent indicates poor prognosis and Remember Vi Abs are not seen in normal population.**
- **DT 104 strain** is a multidrug resistant strain of Salmonella typhimurium which emerged in early 1990.
- **Vaccines**
  1. **TAB parenteral vaccine.**
  2. Vi polysaccharide parental vaccine/**Typhim Vi (S. typhi Ty21a strain).**
  3. Typhioral/oral live attenuated S. typhi Ty21a vaccine.

SHIGELLA

- **GNB, non-motile, noncapsulated, produces NLF colonies except S. sonnei (Late LF) on MacConkey agar.**
- Catalase is produced by all except S. dysentriae.
- Classified on the basis of somatic O Ag (LPS) and Carbohydrate fermentation **(Mannitol)** pattern.
- Mannitol is fermented by all except S. dysentriae A1.

Contd.

Contd.

Species:
- S. dysentriae.
- S. flexneri (Most common Shigellosis in India).
- S. boydii.
- S. sonnei – LLF (Most common Shigellosis in World).

Lab Diagnosis
- **Specimen** – Fresh stool or mucus flakes of stool.
- **Transport media** – Sach's buffered glycerol saline.
- **Enrichment broth** – Selenite F broth, Tetrathionate broth.
- **Selective media** – DCA, XLD agar, SS agar.
- **Identification test** – IMViC = -, +, -, -.

DOC – Ampicillin or Co-trimoxazole with oral rehydration therapy.

PATHOGENESIS

Mode of transmission – Faeco-oral route.
Incubation period – 1-4 days.
Infectious dose – 10-100 bacteria.
Invasiveness is seen.

TOXINS

Endotoxin: LPS, induces intestinal ulceration and irritation.

Exotoxins:
Shigella Enterotoxin 1 and 2 – Structurally similar to Cholera toxin and found in S. flexneri.
Shiga toxin (Plasmid coded) produced by S. dysentriae, cytotoxic, similar to toxin of EHEC. Inhibits the protein synthesis to causes cell death.

Complications:
- MCC of **Bacillary dysentery in India is Shigella flexneri and most common cause of dysentery in world is Shigella sonnei**

- **Sereny test** +ve in case of EIEC or Shigella, installation of suspension of freshly isolated EIEC or Shigella into the eyes of guinea pig leads to mucopurulent conjunctivitis.

MCQs

SALMONELLA AND SHIGELLA

Morphology Characteristics and Classification

1. Shigella are divided into subgroup on the basis of ability to ferment: *(Recent MCQ)*

(a) Lactose (b) Maltose
(c) Fructose (d) Mannitol

2. Most virulent variety of shigellosis is caused by: *(UPPG 12)*

(a) S. dysentriae (b) S. sonnei
(c) S. flexneri (d) S. boydii

Shigella Toxin

3. Which of the following toxins acts by inhibiting protein synthesis? *(AI 04, Recent MCQ)*

(a) Cholera toxin (b) Shiga toxin
(b) Pertussis toxin (d) LT of enterotoxigenic E.coli

4. All are true about Shigella *except*: *(AIIMS 10, Recent MCQ)*
(a) Large dose is required for infection
(b) Associated with hemolytic uremic syndrome
(c) Causes bloody diarrhea with mucus
(d) Gut pathology is due to toxin

5. Which of the following is true about Shigella dysentriae? *(APPG 13)*
(a) It can lead to haemolytic uremic syndrome
(b) It produces an invasive enterotoxin
(c) It is an facultative aerobe
(d) It is MR negative

Lab Diagnosis

6. Shigellosis is best diagnosed by: *(Recent MCQ)*
(a) Stool examination
(b) Stool culture
(c) Sigmoidoscopy
(d) Enzyme

7. A person returns to Delhi from Bangladesh after 2 days and has diarrhea. Stool examination shows RBCs in stool. The likely organism causing is: *(AIIMS Nov 09)*
(a) Enteropathogenic E. coli
(b) Enterotoxigenic E. coli
(c) Salmonella typhi
(d) Shigella dysentriae

8. The following are gas producing salmonella *except*: *(APPG 03)*
(a) S. typhi
(b) S. enteritidis
(c) S. typhimurium
(d) S. cholera

9. Agglutination with 'O' antigen of S. typhi is inhibited by: *(Recent MCQ)*
(a) Vi Ag
(b) Flageller
(c) F antigen
(d) All the above

10. There has been an outbreak of food born salmonella gastroenteritis in the community and the stool samples have been received in the laboratory. Which is the enrichment medium of choice? *(UPPG 11)*
(a) Cary Blair medium
(b) VR medium
(c) Selenite "F" medium
(d) Thioglycollate medium

11. Salmonella typhi is the causative agent of typhoid fever. The infective dose of Salmonella typhi: *(AIIMS 06)*
(a) One bacillus
(b) 10^8-10^9 bacilli
(c) 1-10 bacilli
(d) 10^2-10^5 bacilli

12. Incubation period of salmonella typhi: *(PGI June 05, Recent MCQ)*
(a) 3-21 days
(b) 0-60 days
(c) 2-5 days
(d) 14-25 days
(e) > 60 days

13. Pea-soup stool is characteristically seen in: *(APPG 09)*
(a) Cholera
(b) Botulism
(c) Typhoid
(d) Polio

14. All of the following are true regarding typhoid *except*: *(AIIMS June 99)*
(a) Urinary carriers are more dangerous
(b) Vi ab is used for detecting carrier
(c) Vi is seen in normal population
(d) Urine carrier is associated with anomalies

15. In a patient with typhoid, diagnosis after 15 days of onset of fever is test done by: *(RJ 09, Recent MCQ)*
(a) Blood culture
(b) Widal
(c) Stool culture
(d) Urine culture

16. Diagnosis of typhoid in the first week is by: *(APPG 10)*
(a) Widal test
(b) Stock cultue
(c) Blood culture
(d) Urine culture

17. Which of the following is true regarding Salmonella infection? *(AI 96)*

(a) Urine culture is + ve in 1st week
(b) Stool culture is + ve in 1st week
(c) Blood culture is + ve in 3-7 days
(d) Widal test is +ve in 1st week

18. A 24-year-old cook in a hostel mess suffered from enteric fever 2 years back. The chronic carrier state in this patient can be diagnosed by: *(AIIMS Nov 02)*

(a) Vi agglutination test
(b) Blood culture in brain heart infusion broth
(c) Widal test
(d) Typhoid test

19. True statement about Widal test in typhoid is: *(Manipal 11)*

(a) O-antigen titre remains positive for several months and reaction to it is rapid
(b) H-antigen titre remains positive for several months and reaction to it is rapid
(c) Both remain positive for several months and reaction to both is rapid
(d) None

20. Which is true about Widal reaction? *(AI 93)*

(a) Antibody to H Ag appears first and persists
(b) Antibody to O Ag appears first and persists
(c) Antibodies to H and O Ag appears simultaneously and persists
(d) None of the above

21. All are correct regarding widal test, *except*: *(AIIMS Nov 091)*

(a) Baseline titres differ depending on the endemicity of the disease
(b) High titre value is a single widal test is not confirmative
(c) Antibodies last longer and hence is not indicative of recent infection
(d) H antibody cannot differentiate between types

22. True statement about widal test in typhoid is: *(AI 99)*

(a) Widal test is confirmative in endemic areas
(b) Antibiotic treatment does not alter widal test results
(c) Previous infection alters widal test
(d) Widal test does not alter with prior vaccination

23. Most immunogenic in Typhoid: *(UPPG 13)*

(a) Vi antigen
(b) H antigen
(c) Somatic antigen
(d) O antigen

24. Drug commonly used against enteric fever are all *except*: *(UPPG 04, Recent MCQ)*

(a) Amikacin
(b) Ceftriaxone
(c) Ciprofloxacin
(d) Azithromycin

25. Resistance of Salmonella typhi to the following antibiotics is not reported as yet in India: *(AIIMS 09)*

(a) Chloramphenicol
(b) Ampicillin
(c) Ciprofloxacin
(d) Ceftriaxone

26. Temporary carrier of typhoid is infective for: *(Recent MCQ)*

(a) < 3 weeks
(b) 3 weeks-3 months
(c) 3 months-1 year
(d) >1 year

27. Vi antigen found in: *(PGI 11)*

(a) Salmonella paratyphi A
(b) Salmonella paratyphi C
(c) Salmonella dublin
(d) Klebsiella pneumoniae
(e) Citrobacter fragilis

28. All of the following statements about non-typhoid salmonella are true, *except*: *(AI 09)*

(a) Humans are the only reservoirs
(b) Transmission is most commonly associated with eggs, poultry and undercooked meat
(c) Common in immunocompromised individuals
(d) Resistance to fluoroquinolones has emerged

29. All are true about non-typhoid salmonella *except*: *(AIIMS Mar 2012)*

(a) Poultry is source
(b) Can cause invasive disease in neonates
(c) Blood culture is more sensitive than stool culture in gastroenteritrs in adults
(d) Resistance to fluoroquinolone has emerged

30. Which is true about salmonella gastroenteritis? *(AIIMS 12)*

(a) Always associated with blood and mucus in stools
(b) Is due to exotoxin
(c) Mainly diagnosed by serological testing
(d) Does not cause fever
(e) None of these

31. DT 104 strain belongs to which of the following bacteria? *(PGI 12)*

(a) Salmonella Gallinarum
(b) Salmonella Typhi
(c) Salmonella Enteritidis
(d) Salmonella Paratyphi A
(e) Salmonella Typhimurium

ANSWERS AND EXPLANATIONS

1. **Ans. is 'd'** i.e., Mannitol (***Ref:*** *Ananthanarayan, 9th/e, p. 286 and 8th/e, p. 284*)

   Mannitol fermenting – Shigella flexneri (group B), S. boydii (group C), S. sonnei (group D). **(FaceBook Soni)**

   Mannitol non-fermenting – Shigella dysentriae (group A).

   - Based on Somatic O polysaccharide antigen, Shigella species are further divided into four groups (A, B, C, D).

2. **Ans. is 'a'** i.e., Shigella dysenteriae (***Ref:*** *Ananthanarayan, 8th/e, p. 286 and 9th/e, p. 2851*)

   Complications are most often seen in infection with Sh. dysenteriae type I and include arthritis, toxic neuritis, conjunctivitis, parotitis and in children, intussusception. HUS may occur in severe cases.

3. **Ans. is 'b'** i.e., Shiga toxin (***Ref:*** *Ananthanarayan, 8th/e, p. 286, 276 and 9th/e, p. 2841*)

   Shiga toxin (Plasmid coded) produced by S. dysentriae A1, cytotoxic, similar to toxin of EHEC. Inhibits the protein synthesis to causes cell death by inactivating 60 S ribosome.Q

   Cholera toxin and L.T. of enterotoxigenic E.coli act by cAMP.

   Pertussis toxin acts by ADP-ribosylation guanine nucleotide-binding regulatory protein (G protein in target cells).

   Toxins that act by inhibiting protein synthesis (Memory aid–DSP) – Diphtheria toxin, Shiga toxin, Pseudomonas toxin and Shiga like toxin or verotoxin of EHEC.

4. **Ans. is 'a'** i.e., Large dose is required for infection

   (***Ref:*** *Ananthanarayan, 9th/e, p. 287, 288; Paniker, 6th/e, p. 261; Jawetz, 22th/e, p. 2241*)

   Shigella is highly communicable as the infective dose for shigella is very less **(10-100 bacilli).** Essential process in the pathogenesis is invasion of the mucosal epithelial cells by the organism through phagocytosis.

   The production of toxin is also of importance for virulence but main factor is invasion of the epithelial cells of gut by the organism.

5. **Ans. is 'a'** i.e., It can lead to hemolytic uremic syndrome

(***Ref:*** *Harrison, 18th/e, p. 1283 and 17th/e, p. 963; Ananthanarayan, 9th/e, p. 282-283, 286*)

- Invasive property of shigella does not depend on enterotoxin because it is not invasive in nature and functionally resembles Cholera toxin.
- **Invasive property of Shigella dysenteriae depends on IPA protein and type 3 secretive system which are encoded by large virulence plasmids.**
- Shigella is aerobe and facultative anaerobe and Shigella is MR positive.

Lab Diagnosis

6. **Ans. is 'b'** i.e., Stool culture (***Ref:*** *Ananthanarayan, 9th/e, p. 88 and 8th/e, p. 286*)

"Diagnosis is made by isolating the bacillus from faeces."

7. **Ans. is 'd'** i.e., Shigella dysentriae

(***Ref:*** *Ananthanarayan, 9th/e, p. 79 and 8th/e, p. 285; Harrison, 18th/e, p. 1283 and 17th/e, p. 963*)

The person is suspected to have traveller's diarrhoea and Shigella dysentriae causes dysentery (RBCs in stool). The most common cause of **traveller's diarrhoea is Enterotoxigenic E.coli.**

8. **Ans. is 'a'** i.e., S. typhi (***Ref:*** *Ananthanarayan, 9th/e, p. 291 and 8th/e, p. 289*)

Salmonella ferment sugar producing acid and gas except S. typhi which is anaerogenic.

9. **Ans. is 'a'** i.e., Vi antigen

Vi antigen envelops the 'O' antigen and prevents its agglutination with O antiserum.

Vi antigen: A heat-labile somatic antigen thought to be associated with virulence in some bacteria (as of the genus Salmonella) and its abs are used for **Epidemiological typing.**

10. **Ans. is 'c'** i.e., Selenite 'F' medium (***Ref:*** *Ananthanarayan, 9th/e, p. 291 and 8th/e, p. 2881*)

Selenite F-broth and Tetrathionate broth are commonly employed as Enrichment media for Salmonella.

11. **Ans. is 'd'** i.e., 10^2-10^5 bacilli (***Ref:*** *Ananthanarayan, 9th/e, p. 295 and 8th/e, p. 293*)

- In human volunteer experiments the infective dose was found to be **10^3-10^6 bacilli.**

12. **Ans. is 'a'** i.e., 3-21 days

Incubation period – 10-14 days (*already explained in text*).

13. **Ans. is 'c'** i.e., Typhoid (*already explained in text*).

Pea-soup stool – **It is khaki-green, slimy stools typically occurs in a week of typhoid fever, at which point the patients are in toxic state and at greatest risk for the intestinal perforation and hemorrhage.**

Extra edge point – **Similar stools occur in Enteropathogenic E. coli infection of infants.**

14. **Ans. is 'c'** i.e., Vi seen in normal population (***Ref:*** *Ananthanarayan, 9th/e, p. 295 and 8th/e, p. 287, 290, 295*)

Vi ab is used for detecting carrier so it is present in carriers only not in normal population.

15. **Ans. is 'a'** i.e., Blood culture (***Ref:*** *Harrison, 18th/e, p. 1276 and 17th/e, p. 958; Jawetz, 23rd/e, p. 259*)

- **Other than a positive culture, no specific laboratory test is diagnostic for enteric fever.** – *Jawetz, p. 259*
- The diagnostic gold standard is a culture positive for S. typhi or S. paratyphi. – *Harrison, p. 958*

Widal agglutination test has been largely replaced by sensitive and specific methods such as ELISA and Immunoblotting. – *Greenwood Book, p. 255*

16. **Ans. is 'c'** i.e., Blood culture (*Explained in Ans. 22*)

17. **Ans. is 'c'** i.e., Blood culture (***Ref:*** *Harrison, 18th/e, p. 1276 and 17th/e, p. 958; Greenwood, 16th/e, p. 255*)

Blood culture is positive in approximately 90% of cases in the first week, 75% in the second week, 60% in the third week and 25% thereafter till the subsidence of pyrexia.

Blood cultures rapidly become negative on treatment with antibiotics.

A positive blood culture is diagnostic while the same significance cannot be attached to isolation from faeces or urine.

18. **Ans. is 'a'** Vi agglutination test (***Ref:*** *Ananthanarayan, 9th/e, p. 299 and 8th/e, p. 291*)

Diagnosis of Carrier:

The demonstration of Vi agglutinins indicate the carrier state. While this is useful as a screening test confirmation should be made blood culture.

Diagnosis of carriers – Screening test – Demonstration of Vi agglutinins.

Definitive diagnosis – Positive Culture.Q

In fecal carriers from feces or by duodenal aspiration.

In urinary carriers from urine.

19. **Ans. is 'b'** i.e., H-antigen titre remains positive for several months and reaction to it is rapid

(***Ref:*** *Ananthanarayan, 9th/e, p. 298 and 8th/e, p. 296-297*)

- The H-antigen is strongly immunogenic and induces antibody formation rapidly and in high titres following infection or immunization. H agglutinins persist longer than 'o' agglutinins.
- O agglutinins appear early and disappear early and indicate recent infection.

20. **Ans. is 'a'** i.e., Antibody to H Ag appears first and persists (*already explained in Ans. 24*)

21. **Ans. is 'd'** i.e., H antibody cannot differentiate between types (***Ref:*** *Ananthanarayan, 9th/e, p. 298*)

Option 'c'

In widal test 'O'antigen of S. typhi is used. As paratyphoid 'O' antigen cross reacts with S. typhi O antigen, it is not employed in widal test.

On the other hand H antigens of S. typhi, S. paratyphi 'A' and 'B' are used as they don't cross react with each other. So, H antigen can differentiate between the two types as each type has different H antigen (not cross reacting with the other).

Option 'd'

H agglutinins last longer (not 'O' antigen) as it is more immunogenic than 'O' antigen.

About other options 'a' and 'b' – Base line titres are **affected by the endemicity of disease and antibody may be present due to inapparent infection,** immunization or prior infection especially in high endemic areas. So, distribution of agglutinin is 'normal sera' in different areas is different.

So, a four-fold increase in titer in two tests done 2 weeks apart is diagnostic in Widal test.

22. **Ans. is 'c'** i.e., Previous infection alters widal test (***Ref:*** *Ananthanarayan, 9th/e, p. 298 and 9th/e, p. 296-297*)

People who have had prior infection or immunization may develop an anamnestic response during unrelated fever and may show **false positive reaction.** This may be differentiated by repetition of test after a week. The anamnestic response shows only a transient rise, while in enteric fever the rise is sustained.

About Other Options:

Antibiotic (Chloramphenicol) treated cases may show a poor agglutinin response.

Other than a positive culture, no specific laboratory test is diagnostic.Q

Both prior vaccination (immunization) or infection can alter the widal test.

23. **Ans. is 'b'** i.e., H-Antigen

H Ag is made up with flagellin protein – heat labile protein which is strongly immunogenic.

24. **Ans. is 'a'** i.e., Amikacin (***Ref:*** *Harrison, 18th/e, p. 1277 and 17th/e, p. 591*)

- Amikacin may cause live bacterial vaccines (such as typhoid vaccine) not to work as well.

  Treatment of Typhoid fever.

  Empirical treatment – Ceftriaxone, Azithromycin.

25. **Ans. is 'd'** i.e., Ceftriaxone

(***Ref:*** *Ananthanarayan, 9th/e, p. 300 and 8th/e, p. 299; Harrison, 19th/e, p. 1276, 1277 and 17th/e, p. 958, 959*)

26. **Ans. is 'c'** i.e., 3 months – 1 year (***Ref:*** *Ananthanarayan, 9th/e, p. 290, 295*)

Convalescent carriers – Shed bacilli for 3 weeks - 3 months after cure.

Temporary carriers – Shed bacilli for 3 months after cure.

Chronic carriers – Shed bacilli for > 1 year.

27. Ans. are 'a,b,c,e' (***Ref:*** *Ananthanarayan, 9th/e, p. 290, 293*)

Vi antigen was originally observed in S.typhi.

The **Vi antigen with similar antigenic specificity** is also present in **– Salmonella paratyphi, Salmonella dublin, Citrobacter.**

28. Ans. is 'a' i.e., Humans are the only reservoir (***Ref:*** *Harrison, 18th/e, p. 1278, 1279 and 17th/e, p. 959-960*)

Unlike typhoid salmonella (S. typhi and S. paratyphi), where only reservoir is humans non-typhoidal salmonella can be acquired from multiple animal reservoirs.

Transmission is most commonly associated with animal food products especially eggs, poultry, undercooked meat and dairy products.

29. Ans. is 'c' i.e., Blood culture is more sensitive than stool culture in gastroenteritis in adults

(***Ref:*** *Harrison, 17th/e, p. 958-961; Ananthanarayan, 9th/e, p. 298-301*)

Most common clinical manifestation of **non-typhoidal salmonellosis is gastroenteritis.** Diagnosis is confirmed by **isolation of the organism in stool culture.**

The risk factors for invasive infection or bacteremia are: **Extremes of age – infants, old age.**

Immunocompromised state – HIV chemotherapy, steroid therapy.

30. Ans. is 'e' i.e., None of these

Diarrhea is nonbloody (option 'a' is incorrect).

It is due to invasion of bowel mucosa, not toxin mediated (option 'b' is incorrect).

It is diagnosed by isolation of organism from stools (option 'c' is incorrect).

Fever is one of the commoner symptom (option 'd' is incorrect).

31. Ans. is 'e' i.e., Salmonella typhimurium (***Ref:*** *Harrison, 19th/e, p. 1278*)

DT 104 is a strain of Salmonella Typhimurium which emerged in early 1990s. It is multidrug resistant strain and associated with an increased risk of bloodstream infection and hospitalization.

VIBRIO (HELICOBACTER PYLORI, CAMPYLOBACTER JEJUNI)

- **Gram negative curved (Comma shaped), Motile (Darting) by single polar flagellum.**
- **Fermentative, Oxidase +ve, non-sporing, non-capsulated (Except V. parahaemolyticus, V. vulnificus) and Isolated by R. Koch.**
- All are halophilic Except V. cholera, V. mimicus.
- Grows well in presence of salt and alkalinity.
- Habitat – Sea water, sea food, surface water, river and sewage.
- **Classification based on salt requirement**
  - Nonhalophilic Vibrio – 1% salt concentration is optimum but can grow without salt, e.g., V. cholera, V. mimicus.
  - Halophilic Vibrio – 7-10% salt concentration is tolerable but cannot grow in absence of salt, e.g., V. parahaemolyticus, V. vulnificus, **V. alginolyticus (Most Halophilic/Most salt tolerant/ >10%).Q**

Vibrio Cholerae

- Arranged as fish in stream appearance, shows darting motility (Single polar flagellum).
- Facultative anaerobic, catalase +ve, oxidase +ve and Man is the only reservoir of Cholera.
- V. cholerae also possess the LPS endotoxin which apparently plays no role in pathogenesis, **pathogenesis is due to Cholera toxin.**
- V. cholerae is able to stay in GIT because of motility and binds to specific receptors.
- 7th pandemic of cholera is caused by El Tor and first six by Classical vibrios.
- **Gardner and Venkatraman Classification**

  (Based on serogrouping, biotyping, serotyping and phase typing)

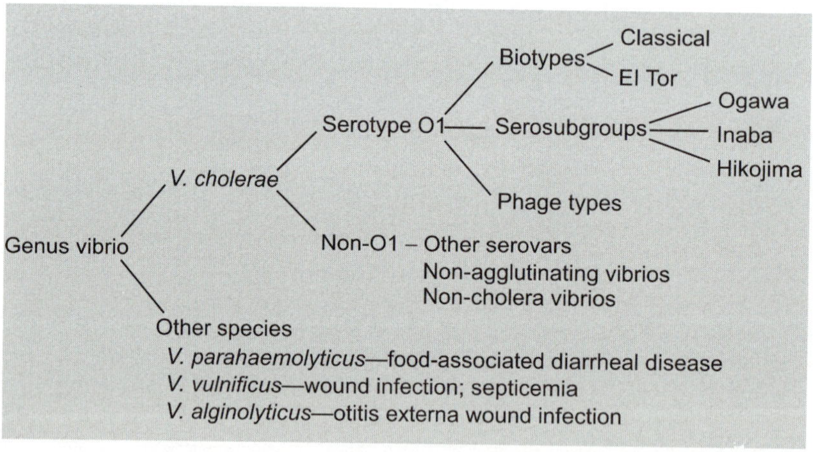

- **V. Cholerae O139**
  (1) Clinical manifestation and epidemiological features are similar to O1.
  (2) It is also called as Bengal V. cholera (Isolated in Bengal 1992).
  (3) O139 is identical to El Tor except:
  Produces O139 Lipopolysaccharide (LPS).
  Pathogenicity of O139 is due to O Ag (polysaccharide capsule).
  (4) Abs to V. cholerae is not protective against O139.
- **Enzymes** – Chitinase, Elastase, Lipase, Mucinase and Neuraminidase.

- **Cholera** [Caused by O1 (El Tor and Classical) and O139]
  - Rice watery stool, Dehydration, Painless Diarrhea with pus cells, Neutrophilia, occurrence of many cases in the same locality, Vibriocidal Ab titer measures prevalence.
  - **Shortest incubation period (1-2 days), Infective dose – 10^{6-8} bacilli.**
  - **Transmission – Fecally contaminated water, food, direct contact.**

Pathogenesis (due to cholera toxin) – Same as Heat labile ETEC (100-1000 time more potent) → ↑cAMP (ADP ribosylation of G protein and Activation of adenyl cyclase).

- B subunit of Toxin is bind to GM1 gangliosides receptor on the surface of epithelial cells and provides a channel allowing A subunit to enter the host cell → A subunit (Peptide A1) has activity of ADP-ribosylation to transfer ADP from NAD onto protein G which activates the protein G → Activates protein G induces cAMP overproduction → A large number of cAMP induces electrolyte and water hypersecretions of cells.

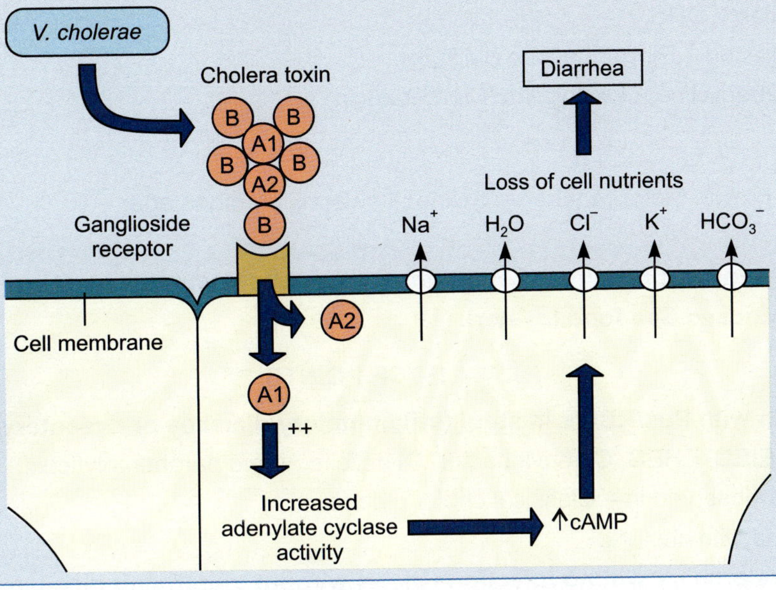

Lab Diagnosis

- **Specimens**
  Rice watery stool and Rectal swab (for carrier and convalescent patients)
- Transport medium
  - Alkaline peptone water (APW)
  - Cary Blair medium
  - Venkatraman Ramakrishna (VR) medium
  - Autoclaved sea water
- **Direct Microscopy**
  - **Hanging drop preparation for Darting Motility**
  - **Gram Staining – Gram Negative comma shaped bacilli (Fish in stream)**
- **Enriched medium**
  - APW
  - Monsur's taurocholate tellurite peptone water
- **Selective media**
  - **TCBS (Thio sulphate citrate Bile salt sucrose agar)**
  - Monsur's gelatin taurocholate trypticase tellurite
  - Alkaline bile salt agar

Contd.

Contd.

- **Identification tests (COINS – positive)**
  - C = Catalase
  - O = oxidase
  - I = Indole
  - N = Nitrate
  - S = Sucrose fermentation
    - **Cholera red reaction +ve** = (Indole and Nitrate reduction properties can be tested together.
    - **String test +ve** with 0.5% Sodium Deoxycholate.

Treatment:

- **Rehydration therapy**
  - For mild dehydration – ORS.
  - For severe dehydration – Ringer Lactate (IV fluid).
- **DOC** – Single dose Tetracycline, Doxycycline, Ciprofloxacin.

V. Parahaemolyticus

- Halophilic Vibrio, The growth factor required – Saline, it swarms on blood agar.
- I.P. – 16-18 hours.
- **Kanagawa PhenomenonQ – It produces beta hemolysis on Wagatsuma agar.Q**
- **Gastroenteritis – Uncooked Sea food (oyster).**

EXTRA EDGE POINTS****

- **Causes of Diarrhea in with Pus/RBC's in stool (Inflammatory diarrhea or dysentery)**
  Shigella, Salmonella, EIEC, EHEC, Campylobacter, Cl difficile, Vibrio parahemolyticus.
- Highest case fatality is observed in – Classical cholera vibrio.
- HUS is NOT associated with cholera.
- **V. Vulnificus – causes primary wound infection (Ulcer) without underlying disease.**

MCQs

1. The endotoxin of the following gram negative bacteria does not play any part in the pathogenesis of the natural diseases: *(APPG 15)*

(a) Escherichia coli (b) Klebsiella species
(c) Vibrio cholerae (d) Pseudomonas aeruginosa

2. Selective media for Vibrio: *(Recent MCQ)*

(a) TCBS (b) Stuart
(c) Skirrows (d) MYPA

3. All the following Vibrio species are halophilic *except*: *(UPPG 14)*

(a) V. cholerae (b) V. parahemolytics
(c) V. alginolytics (d) V. flovialis

4. All of the following are true about V. cholerae 0139 *except*: *(Manipal 14, Recent MCQ)*

(a) Clinical manifestations are similar to 01 E1 tor
(b) First discovered in Chennai
(c) Produces O139 lipopolysaccharide
(d) Epidemiologically indistinguishable from O1 E1 tor

5. Which of the following bacteria acts by increasing cAMP? *(AI 07; AIIMS 06)*
(a) Vibrio cholerae
(b) Staphylococcus aureus
(c) E. coli heat stable toxin
(d) Salmonella

6. In the small intestine, cholera toxin acts by: *(APPG 11)*
(a) ADP ribosylation of G regulatory protein
(b) Inhibition of adenyl cyclase
(c) Activation of GTPase
(d) Active absorption of NaCl

7. The effect of cholera toxin is mediated via the stimulation of following second messenger: *(UPPG 14)*
(a) cAMP
(b) cGMP
(c) Calcium-calmodulin
(d) Acetylcholine

8. About V. cholerae all statements are true *except*: *(Recent MCQ)*
(a) Nonhalophilic
(b) Cannot grow in ordinary media
(c) Can survive outside the intestine
(d) Man is the only reservoir of cholera

9. Antibiotic treatment of choice for treating cholera in an adult is a single dose of: *(UPPG 12)*
(a) Tetracycline
(b) Cotrimoxazole
(c) Doxycycline
(d) Furazolidone

10. Which of the following is the drug of choice for chemoprophylaxis of cholera? *(AIIMS 05, APPG 13)*
(a) Tetracycline
(b) Cotrimoxazole
(c) Doxycycline
(d) Furazolidone

11. A 32 years old male, Kallu, who recently visited a sea coast presented with ulcer over the left leg. The probable cause is: *(Manipal 10)*
(a) Pasteurella multocida
(b) Micrococcus halophillus
(c) Vibrio vulnificus
(d) Neisseria gonorrhea

12. All of the following statements about El-Tor Vibrios are true, *except*: *(AI 2010)*
(a) Human are the only reservoir
(b) Can survive in ice cold water for 2-4 weeks
(c) Killed by boiling for 30 seconds
(d) Enterotoxin can have direct effects on other tissues besides intestinal epithelial cells.

13. V. Cholerae able to stay in GIT because of: *(PGI 09)*
(a) Acid resistance
(b) Bile resistance
(c) Motility
(d) Binds to specific receptors
(e) Anaerobic potential

14. In patient presenting with diarrhea due to vibrio cholera, which of the following will be present? *(PGI 01, 05)*
(a) Abdominal pain
(b) Presence of leukocytes in stool
(c) Fever
(d) Neutrophilia
(e) Occurrence of many cases in the same locality

15. True about epidemiology of cholera: *(PGI 03)*
(a) Chemoprophylaxis is not effective
(b) Boiling of water cannot destroy the organism
(c) Food can transmit the disease
(d) Vaccination gives 90% protection

16. Strains of V. cholerae in Bengal: *(PGI 04)*
(a) 0: 037
(b) 0: 139
(c) 0:17
(d) 0:40
(e) 0:149

17. In a patient presenting with diarrhea and pus cells in stool, the causative organism can be all *except*: (*PGI 04*)

(a) Non-vibrio cholerae 01
(b) Enterotoxigenic E. coli
(c) Enteroinvasive E. coli
(d) Shigella dysenteriae 1
(e) Vibrio cholerae

18. Cholera is caused by: (*PGI 09*)

(a) Vibrio cholerae 01
(b) Vibrio cholerae 0139
(c) V. parahemolyticus
(d) E. coli
(e) NAG vibrio

19. A stool examination was carried out which showed organism with darting motility. Which of the following organism may be in stool? (*PGI 07*)

(a) Shigella
(b) E. coli
(c) Salmonella
(d) Campylobacter jejuni
(e) Vibrio cholerae

20. True about Vibrio alginolyticus: (*PGI 04*)

(a) Non-Haplophilic
(b) Voges Proskauer (VP) positive
(c) Swarming
(d) Cause sea borne auricular infections
(e) Does not grow in 10% NaCl

21. Which of the following has shortest incubation period? (*APPG 07*)

(a) Plague
(b) Cholera
(c) Measles
(d) Typhoid

22. Which of the following statement is true about Vibrio cholerae? (*Recent MCQ*)

(a) There is no natural reservoir
(b) Transport in alkaline peptone water medium
(c) Halophilic
(d) Oxidase negative

23. True about cholera vibrios is: (*AIIMS 12*)

(a) Can tolerate wild range of alkaline pH
(b) Nonmotile bacilli
(c) Cannot be grown in media
(d) NaCL stimulates growth

24. 7th pandemic of cholera is caused by: (*AIIMS 11*)

(a) El tor
(b) 0139 Vibrio cholerae
(c) Classical Vibrio cholerae
(d) V. mimicus

25. Ogawa, Inaba, Hikojima are the serotypes of: (*APPG 15*)

(a) Yersinia
(b) Vibrio cholerae
(c) E. coli
(d) Salmonella typhi

26. Which of the following about cholera is true? (*UPPG 15*)

(a) Invasive
(b) Endotoxin is released
(c) Recent infection in India is of classical type
(d) Vibriocidal antibody titer measures prevalence

27. The function of B subunit of cholera toxin is: (*AIIMS 10, Manipal 12*)

(a) ADP ribosylation of G protein
(b) To bind GM1 ganglioside receptor
(c) To stabilize cholera toxin
(d) To increase cGMP

ANSWERS AND EXPLANATIONS

(Harrison, 19th/e, p. 1062; Ananthanarayan, 9th/e, p. 303)

1. **Ans. is 'c'** i.e., Vibrio cholerae

   The lipopolysachharide (LPS) present in the cell wall apparently play no role in the pathogenesis of cholera but it is responsible for the immunity induced by killed vaccine. **The pathogenicity of Vibrio cholerae is mediated by its toxin.**

2. **Ans. is 'a'** i.e., TCBS

   Holding or Transport Media: Venkatraman Ramakrishnan medium, Caryblair medium, Alkaline peptone water, Monsur taurocholate tellurite water **(Mnemonic: Vicky carry water to Mansorpur).**

   Enrichment Media: Alkaline peptone water, Monsur taurocholate tellurite water.

   Selective media: Alkaline bile salt agar, GTTA (Monsur's gelatin-taurocholate trypticase-tellurite agar) TCBS (Thiosulfate-citrate-bile salts-sucrose agar).

3. **Ans. is 'a'** i.e., V. cholerae

   Classification Based on Salt Requirement

   - **Nonhalophilic Vibrio** – 1% salt concentration is optimum but can grow without salt, e.g., V. cholera, V. mimicus.
   - **Halophilic Vibrio** – 7-10% salt concentration is tolerable but cannot grow in absence of salt, e.g., V. parahaemolyticus, V. vulnificus, **V. alginolyticus (Most Halophilic/Most salt tolerant/ >10%).Q**

4. **Ans. is 'b'** i.e., First discovered in Chennai

   O139 Vibrio was isolated first in Chennai because it was not agglutinated by any of the antisera available at that time (O1-O138) and identified as Bengal strain (O139) in Bengal in 1992 and Clinical manifestation and epidemiological features are similar to O1.

   O139 is identical to El Tor except – Produces O139 Lipopolysaccharide (LPS) and Pathogenicity of O139 is due to O Ag (polysaccharide capsule).

   Abs to V. cholerae is not protective against O139.

5. **Ans. is 'a'** i.e., Vibrio cholerae

   Cholera toxin consists of two subunits:

   (a) Subunit A (Active monomeric moiety).

   (b) Subunit B (Pentameric binding moiety) – bind to GM1 gangliosides receptor.

   * Same as Heat labile ETEC (100-1000 time more potent) → ↑cAMP (ADP ribosylation of G protein and Activation of adenyl cyclase) – Increased cAMP inhibits absorptive Sodium transport system in the villus and activates the secretory chloride system in the crypts cells. As a result there is accumulation of Sodium Chloride in the lumen. They maintain osmolarity water moves passively to lumen leading to diarrhea state.

   Important Table – Remember this !!

Mechanism of Action of Some Important Bacterial Toxin	
Heat labile toxin of E.coli	Increase cAMP
Heat stable toxin of E.coli	Increase cGMP
Botulism toxin	Inhibit release of acetylcholine from peripheral nerves
Tetanus toxin	Inhibit release of glycine and GABA at presynaptic terminals
Diphtheria toxin	Inhibit protein synthesis by inactivatong EF 2

6. **Ans. is 'a'** i.e., ADP ribosylation of G regulatory protein.

   Already explained in Ans. 5 and book text.

7. **Ans. is 'a'** i.e., cAMP

   Already explained.

8. **Ans. is 'b'** i.e., Cannot grow in ordinary media. (***Ref:*** *Ananthanarayan, 9th/e, p. 304*)

   Vibrio can grow very well on ordinary media as it is non-fastidious.

   Man is the only reservoir of Cholera infection. He may be the case or carrier.

9. **Ans. is 'c'** i.e., Doxycycline (***Ref:*** *Harrison, 18th/e, p. 1293*)
   - DOC in adult – Doxycycline excepting pregnant women (if resistant, then ciprofloxacin).
   - DOC in children – Cotrimoxazole, Erythromycin and Azithromycin.
   - DOC in pregnancy – Furazolidone, Erythromycin and Azithromycin.
   - DOC for chemoprophylaxis – Tetracycline.

10. **Ans. is 'a'** i.e., Tetracycline

    Already explained.

11. **Ans. is 'c'** i.e., Vibrio vulnificus (***Ref:*** *Ananthanarayan, 9th/e, p. 312*)

    V. Vulnificus – Causes primary wound infection (Ulcer) without underlying disease (contact of open wound with sea water). It also causes sepsis in immunocompromised host.

12. **Ans. is 'd'** i.e., Enterotoxin can have direct effects on other tissues besides intestinal epithelial cells.

    (***Ref:*** *Ananthanarayan, 9th/e, p. 310*)

    V. cholera enterotoxin do not have any effects on extraintestinal tissues.

13. **Ans. are 'c and d'**

    Vibrio is aerobic.

    Already explained in book text.

14. **Ans. are 'd and e'** (***Ref:*** *Harrison, 18th/e, p. 1292*)

    V. cholerae causes non-inflammatory (no WBC, no RBC) painless watery diarrhea.

    Cholera can be transmitted by contaminated food or water so we can see many cases in the same locality.

15. **Ans. is 'c'** i.e., Food can transmit the disease

    Other choices:

    (a) Chemoprophylaxis with tetracycline is effective.

    (b) V. cholera are killed in 30 minutes at 56°C and in few seconds in boiling water.

    (c) Protection with killed vaccine is 50% and with live vaccine 80%.

16. **Ans. is ' b'** i.e., 0: 139

    O-139 strain is called Bengal V. cholerae which came from El Tor by horizontal gene transfer.

17. **Ans. are 'a, b, e'** i.e., Non-vibrio cholerae 01, Enterotoxigenic E. coli, Vibrio cholerae

    Causes of diarrhoea with RBC/Pus cells in stool (Inflammatory diarrhoea) – Shigella, Salmonella, Vibrio parahemolyticus, Enterohaemorrhagic E. coli, Yersinia, Campylobacter, Cl. difficile.

18. **Ans. are 'a, b'** i.e., Vibrio cholerae 01, Vibrio cholerae 0139

    Already explained.

19. **Ans. are 'd, e'** i.e., Campylobacter jejuni, Vibrio cholerae

    Darting motility is shown by Vibrio and Campylobacter (single polar flagellum).

20. **Ans. are 'b, c and d'** i.e., Voges Proskauer (VP) positive, Swarming, Cause sea borne auricular infections.

    V. alginolyticus – High salt tolerant, VP positive, produce swarming on non-selective solid media. It has been associated with infections of eyes, ears and wounds being exposed to sea water.

21. **Ans. is 'b'** i.e., Cholera

    IP of cholera – 1-2 days.

    Infectious dose – 10^6 bacilli.

22. **Ans. is 'b'** i.e., Transport in alkaline peptone water medium.

    Already explained.

23. Ans. are 'a and d' i.e., Can tolerate wild range of alkaline pH, NaCL stimulates growth.

Grows well in presence of salt (0.1-1%) and alkalinity (pH 8.5-9.5).

24. Ans. is 'a' i.e., El tor

7th pandemic of cholera is caused by El Tor and 8th pandemic is proposed by O139.

25. Ans. is 'b' i.e., Vibrio cholerae

Already explained in book text.

26. Ans. is 'd' i.e., Vibriocidal antibody titer measures prevalence

Vibriocidal antibody titer has been used as an epidemiological marker for the determination of recent cholera infection.

27. Ans. is 'b' i.e., To bind GM1 ganglioside receptor

Already explained.

HELICOBACTOR PYLORI

- Gram negative curved spiral bacilli, motile with lophotrichous flagella, Microaerophilic.
- Transmission – From man to man, Feco-orally by orogastric route.
- **Pathogenesis**
  - Grows optimally at pH 6-7 and are likely to be killed at gastric low pH.
  - Highly motile therefore it can survive under low gastric pH and found deep in mucus layer overlying the gastric mucosa.
  - **Massive production of Urease enzyme**, which produces ammonia and buffers the gastric pH.
  - **Vacuolating cytotoxin (VacA) is the major virulence factor – formed vacuoles in the cytoplasm of the Epithelial cells.Q**
  - **Cytotoxin associated Gene A (CagA) – responsible for formation of Type 4 Secretory system and interferes with the metabolism of Epithelial cells.**
- **Clinical manifestations** (H. pylori infection remains lifelong if untreated)
  - **Duodenal ulcer (80%) and Gastric ulcer (60%)** are associated with H. pylori.
  - **Gastric adenocarcinoma, gastric MALT lymphoma, Autoimmune gastritis, Hyperacidity.**
  - Chronic gastritis in adults due to the reinfection and Treatment prevents the gastric lymphoma.
  - Approximately 50% of world population and 85% of developing countries are affected by H. pylori.
- **Lab Diagnosis**
  - Invasive tests (Multiple biopsy by Endoscopy)

    Gram staining – Gram negative curved spiral bacilli.

    Histopathology – Warthin starry silver stain is used.

    Culture – Campylobacter media can be used like **Skirrow's media, Chocolate agar and should be incubated under Microaerophilic conditions at 37°C.**

    Identification tests – Urease, catalase and oxidase are positive.

    Rapid Urease test (Biopsy urease test) – (Most sensitive test) – If bacteria is present in Gastric.Q

    Biopsy, it will give +ve test.
  - **Noninvasive tests**

    Urea breath test – Most accurate test.

    Stool Ag test – Monitoring of therapy and screening of children.

    ELISA/Immunoblot – Detection of IgG level, simplest test.

CAMPYLOBACTER JEJUNI

- Gram negative curved bacilli/S-shaped **(Gull wing Appearance),** Motile (Darting) by polar flagellum, non-sporing, Microaerophilic (5% O_2, 10% CO_2).

- Found in the intestine of the animals and transmitted by raw or undercooked meat or food products (poultry), direct contact with infected animals.
- **Clinical manifestations – Inflammatory diarrhea (Bloody), abdominal pain, fever, GB syndrome, Bacteremia, vascular infections, meningitis.**
- **Lab Diagnosis**
  - Specimen – Feces or rectal swab.
  - Transport media – Cary Blair medium.
  - **Selective media – Skirrow's medium, CVA (Cefoperazone vancomycin amphotericin B) medium, Campy BAP media, Campylobacter blood agar, Butzler media.**
  - **Incubation at 42°C under Microaerophilic condition.Q**
- **DOC**

  In Diarrheal disease – Erythromycin or Azithromycin.

  In Systemic infection – Parenteral Gentamycin or imipenem.

MCQs

1. **The most sensitive test for H. pylori is:** *(PGI 99)*
   (a) Breath test (b) Rapid urease test
   (c) Culture of biopsy (d) Microscopy of biopsy
2. **All of the following are true about Helicobacter pylori *except*:** *(AI 98)*
   (a) About 50% of world population affected
   (b) 85% of population is affected, in some developing countries
   (c) All children in developing countries have immunity by five years of age
   (d) Infection is common in low socio-economic status
3. **Helicobacter pylori is not associated with:** *(AIIMS 03)*
   (a) Gastrointestinal lymphoma (b) Gastric cancer
   (c) Gastric leiomyoma (d) Peptic ulcer
4. **Which of following is false regarding H. pylori?** *(Recent MCQ)*
   (a) With chronic infection urease breath test become negative
   (b) H. pylori infection remains lifelong if untreated
   (c) Endoscopy is diagnostic
   (d) Toxigenic strains usually cause ulcer
5. **Which of the following correctly describe H. pylori?** *(PGI 05)*
   (a) Gram-negative cocci curved (b) Gram-positive cocci straight
   (c) Gram-positive bacilli curved (d) Gram-negative bacilli straight
   (e) Gram-negative bacilli curved rod
6. **H. pylori true about:** *(PGI 04)*
   (a) Gram (+)ve spiral organism
   (b) It is a protozoa
   (c) Causes chronic gastritis in adults due reinfection
   (d) Treatment prevents gastric lymphoma
   (e) Duodenal mucosa normal
7. **True about H. pylori:** *(Recent MCQ)*
   (a) It is flagellated (b) Involved in causation of peptic ulcer disease
   (c) Hypergastrinemia caused by it (d) It is a Gram (-)ve organism

8. Regarding H. pylori, all are true *except*: *(PGI 05]*

(a) Gram-negative bacillus
(b) Strongly associated with duodenal ulcer
(c) Associated with lymphoma
(d) C-14 urea breath test is used in diagnosis
(e) It should be eradicated in all cases whenever detected

9. True about H. pylori: *(Recent MCQ)*

(a) Seen in 85 to 90% cases of gastric ulcer
(b) Seen in 20 to 25% cases of duodenal ulcer
(c) Transmitted from man to man, feco-orally and by orogastric route
(d) Common in adults of developing countries

10. Microaerophilic bacteria is: *(AIIMS May 09)*

(a) Campylobacter
(b) Vibrio cholera
(c) Pseudomonas
(d) Salmonella

11. True statement about H. Pylori: *(PGI 02, APPG 10)*

(a) 75% of ulcers are associated with H. Pylori
(b) Medical therapy is Tx of choice
(c) 90% cases of duodenal ulcer associated with H. Pylori
(d) 60% of H. Pylori colonization develop ulcer

12. Gastric ulcers of H. Pylori, true: *(PGI 09)*

(a) Gm+ve aerobes
(b) Invade mucosa and muscularis layers
(c) Rapid urease test on endoscopy is diagnostic
(d) Culture confirm eradication
(e) Causes MALT of stomach

13. About Helicobacter pylori, all are true *except*: *(AIIMS 96)*

(a) Is a Gram -ve spiral bacteria
(b) Uncommon in undeveloping Asian countries
(c) Urea breath test +ve
(d) Associated with duodenal ulcer

14. Which of the following has potent urease activity? *(Recent MCQ)*

(a) Proteus mirabilis
(b) Brucella melitensis
(c) Helicobacter Pylori
(d) Ureaplasma urealyticum

15. Which of the following organism is strongly urease positive? *(Recent MCQ)*

(a) H. Pylori
(b) Proteus
(c) Bordetella pertussis
(d) Brucella

16. True about Helicobacter pylori is: *(AI 98, UPPG 08)*

(a) Culture and gram staining of biopsy is the gold standard investigation
(b) Controlled urea breath is negative with massive infection
(c) Anti urease antibody are produced only by invasive strains
(d) Urease activity provides protective environment to the bacilli

17. True about Helicobacter pylori are all *except*: *(APPG 10, Recent MCQ)*

(a) Urea, breath test is diagnostic
(b) Gram negative, flagellated bacilli

(c) Risk factor for development of adenocarcinoma of stomach

(d) It provides life-long immunity

18. A 35 years old patient complains of abdominal cramps along with profuse diarrhea. The treating physician wants to process the stool culture for isolation of Campylobacter jejuni. Which of the method of choice for stool culture? (*AIIMS 04*)

(a) Culture on TCBS medium and incubated at 37°C under aerobic conditions

(b) Culture on Skirrow medium and incubated at 42°C under microaerobic conditions

(c) Culture on MacConkey medium and incubated at 42°C under aerobic conditions

(d) Culture on Wilson and Blair medium and incubated at 37°C under microaerobic conditions

19. Regarding Campylobacter jejuni which is not true? (*AIIMS 09*)

(a) Most common cause of Campylobacteriosis

(b) Poultry is the cause of the disease

(c) Human is the only reservoir

(d) Causes Guillain-Barré syndrome

ANSWERS AND EXPLANATIONS

(Harrison, 19th/e, p. 1038; Ananthanarayan, 9th/e, p. 400)

1. **Ans. is 'b'** i.e., Rapid urease test (***Ref:*** *Harrison, 17th/e, p. 947*)

   Rapid urease test/Biopsy urease test – **Most sensitive,** simple and quick.

   Culture of biopsy obtained by upper GI endoscopy – **Most specific test.**

2. **Ans. is 'c'** i.e., All children in developing countries have immunity by five years of age (***Ref:*** *Harrison, 16th/e, p. 886*)
   - Duodenal ulcer (80%) and Gastric ulcer (60%) are associated with H. pylori.
   - Gastric adenocarcinoma, gastric MALT lymphoma, Autoimmune gastritis, Hyperacidity.
   - Chronic gastritis in adults due to the reinfection and Treatment prevents the gastric lymphoma.
   - Approximately 50% of world population and 85% of developing countries are affected by H. pylori.

3. **Ans. is 'c'** i.e., Gastric leiomyoma

   Gastric leiomyoma is the most common benign tumour of the stomach occurring in middle age. Most leiomyomas of stomach are asymptomatic but ulceration may cause pain and signs of gastrointestinal bleeding and causative agent is not H. pylori.

4. **Ans. is 'a'** i.e., With chronic infection urease breath test become negative

   It becomes negative only after treatment and is used to access outcome of treatment.

5. **Ans. is 'e'** i.e., Gram-negative bacilli curved rod

   Already explained.

6. **Ans. are 'c, d'**

   Already explained in Book text.

7. **Ans. are 'a, b, c, d'**

   H. pylori is associated with hyperacidity.

8. **Ans. is 'e'** i.e., It should be eradicated in all cases whenever detected.

   In asymptomatic cases no treatment is given.

9. **Ans. are 'c, d'**

   Transmission – From man to man, Feco-orally by orogastric route.

10. **Ans. is 'a'** i.e., Campylobacter

    Microaerophilic bacteria – H. pylori, campylobacter, B. burgdoferi and T. pallidum.

11. **Ans. are 'a, b'**

    Already explained.

12. Ans. are 'c, e'

Rapid urease test on endoscopy is diagnostic and Causes MALT of stomach. Under normal circumstances H. pylori do not invade the gastric mucosa. It is found deep in the mucosal layer near the epithelial surface where physiologic pH is present.

13. Ans is 'b' i.e., Uncommon in undeveloping Asian countries (***Ref:*** *Harrison, 17th/e, p. 946*)

Approximately 85% of developing countries are affected by H. pylori.

14. Ans. is 'c' i.e., Helicobacter Pylori (***Ref:*** *Ananthanarayan, 8th/e, p. 399, 7th/e, p. 408*)

Already explained book text.

15. Ans. is 'a' i.e., H. Pylori (***Ref:*** *Ananthanarayan, 8th/e, p. 399, 7th/e, p. 408*)

Already explained.

16. Ans. is 'd' i.e., Urease activity provides protective environment to the bacilli (***Ref:*** *Harrison, 17th/e, p. 947*)

Gram staining is not gold standard.

17. Ans. is 'd' i.e., It provides life-long immunity (***Ref:*** *Harrison, 17th/e, p. 946*)

Helicobacter pylori infection doesn't provide life-long immunity.

18. Ans. is 'b' i.e., Culture on Skirrow medium and incubated at 42°C under microaerobic conditions

The culture characteristics are most important in the isolation and identification of C jejuni. Selective media are needed, and incubation must be in an atmosphere with reduced O_2 (5% O_2) with added CO_2 (10% CO_2). Incubation of primary plates for isolation of C jejuni should be at 42°C. **Although C jejuni grows well at 36–37°C, incubation at 42°C prevents growth of most of the other bacteria present in feces, thus simplifying the identification of C jejuni.** Several selective media are in widespread use. **Skirrow's medium contains vancomycin, polymyxin B, and trimethoprim to inhibit growth of other bacteria.**

19. Ans. is 'c' i.e., Human is the only reservoir

Campylobacter enteritis resembles other acute bacterial diarrheas, particularly shigella dysentery. The source of infection may be food (e.g., milk, undercooked fowl) or contact with infected animals or humans and their excreta. Outbreaks arising from a common source, such as unpasteurized milk. **C jejuni serotype O19 have been associated with Guillain-Barré syndrome and Alpha chain disease.**

PSEUDOMONAS AERUGINOSA, YERSINIA PESTIS

PSEUDOMONAS AERUGINOSA

- **Gram Negative bacilli, Motile, Obligate Aerobic, Non-fermenter, Pigment producing, Oxidase +ve.Q**
- Also known as P. pyocyanea.
- Non-capsulated but some strains possess capsule (Slim layer) in Cystic fibrosis patients.
- Grows well at 37°C-42°C on ordinary media.
- **Selective media – Cetrimide agar.Q**
- Pigments (Diffusible).Q
  Pyocyanin – Bluish-green.
  Pyoverdin – Yellowish-green.
  Pyorubin – Bright red.
  Pyomelanin – Brown-black.

Diseases
- It is MCC and most serious cause of infection in burns.Q
- Causes malignant otitis externa.Q
- Also cause **Shanghai fever and Intravenous catheter related infection.Q**
- Produces **Blue pus with characteristic Fruity odour.Q**
- **Pigments grow better on Kings media.Q**

BURKHOLDERIA

BURKHOLDERIA PSEUDOMALLEI
- **Gram Negative bacilli, Aerobic**
  Also known as **Pseudomonas pseudomallei/Whitmore's Bacilli.Q**
- **Agent of bioterrorism (Category B).**
- **Motile and Oxidase +ve.Q**
- Transmission – Inoculation, inhalation or ingestion.
  Man to Man transmission is rare.
- Causative agent of **Melioidosis (Vietnam time bomb disease) Most common form of Melioidosis is pulmonary infection.Q**
- **Gram staining – Bipolar/Safety pin like appearance and can be better appreciated with Methylene blue.**
- **Selective media – Ashdown media.**

BURKHOLDERIA MALLEI
- **Gram Negative bacilli, Aerobic.**
- It is strict Zoonotic.
- Also known as Pseudomonas mallei.
- Non-Motile and Oxidase -ve.Q

CAUSATIVE AGENT OF GLANDERS DISEASEQ
- Transmission – From Horse to man by direct inoculation or inhalation.
- Diagnosis by Mallein test (analogous to tuberculin test).

DOC (pseudomallei and mallei) – Ceftazidime or Carbepenems.

YERSINIA PESTIS

- Gram negative coccobacilli, Non-motile, Capsulated, Exhibits Bipolar staining.

Agent of bioterrorism and causative agent of Plague

- Natural reservoir – Field mice (Tatera indica).
- Source of infection – Infected rodents and fleas (In case or pneumonic plague but not for bubonic plague).
- **Vector – Rat flea (X. cheopsis).**
- Transmission – From bite of infected Flea.
- Clinical manifestations – Bubonic plague (Most common formQ) Pneumonic plague (Rare but most infectious) and Septicemic plague (rare).
- **Lab Diagnosis**
  - **Specimens** – Blood for culture Aspirates of enlarged lymph node for smear and culture.
  - **Microscopy** – Bipolar/Safety pin like appearance with **Wayson's stain** Q, Giemsa stain, Methylene blue, Wright's satin.
  - **Culture** – Shows **stalactite growth in Nutrient broth with oil or Ghee.Q**
  - **Selective media** – CIN (Cefsulodin, irgasan, novobiocin) agar.

DOC – Streptomycin and Tetracycline.

MCQs

1. **Which species of Pseudomonas is the most common cause of intravenous catheter related infection?** *(AIIMS 08, Manipal 12)*
   (a) Pseudomonas cepacia (b) P. aeruginosa
   (c) P. maltophilia (d) Burkholderia Pseudomallei
2. **Which one of the following drugs is an antipseudomonal penicillin?** *(Recent MCQ)*
   (a) Cephalexin (b) Cloxacillin (c) Piperacillin (d) Dicloxacillin
3. **The following statements are true regarding meliodosis *except*:** *(AI 05, APPG 14)*
   (a) It is caused by Burkholderia mallei
   (b) The agent is a gram-negative aerobic bacteria
   (c) Bipolar staining of etiological agent is seen with methylene blue
   (d) The most common form of meliodosis is pulmonary infection
4. **An organism grown on agar shows green colored colonies; likely organism is:** *(AI 01, Recent MCQ)*
   (a) Staphylococcus (b) E. coli
   (c) Pseudomonas (d) Peptostreptococcus
5. **A girl from Shimla presented with fever, malaise and axillary/inguinal lymphadenopathy and organism shows stalactite growth on culture. Which of the following is the causative organism?** *(AIIMS 08)*
   (a) Yersinia pestis (b) Francisella
   (c) Burkholderia pseudomallei (d) Pasturella
6. **All of the following statement about plague are wrong *except*:** *(AIIMS 04)*
   (a) Domestic rat is main reservoir
   (b) Bubonic is the most common variety
   (c) The causative bacillus can survive upto 10 years in the soil of rodent burrows
   (d) Incubation period for pneumonic plague is one to two weeks
7. **A 50-year-old chronic alcoholic male agriculture worker presented with high grade fever of one week with spells of chills and rigor. Examination of the respiratory system reveals bilateral crepitation with scattered rhonchi. Multiple subcutaneous nodules were found on extensor surface of left forearm and left leg. Direct microscopy of the pus aspirate from the nodules reveals plenty of grams (-) ve bacilli with bipolar staining.**

Culture reveals distinct rough corrugated grey white colonies on blood agar. The organisms were motile and oxidase – positive. The most likely diagnosis is: *(AIIMS 03)*

(a) Plague (b) Melioidosis (c) Bartonellosis (d) Actinomycosis

8. **The drug of choice for chemoprophylaxis in contacts of a patient of pneumonic plague is:** *(Recent MCQ)*

(a) Penicillin (b) Rifampicin
(c) Erythromycin (d) Tetracycline

9. **True about Y. pestis:** *(PGI 06, 03)*

(a) Gram +ve (b) Gram –ve (c) Motile (d) Non-motile
(e) It is coccobacilli

10. **True statement(s) about Y. pestis is/are:** *(PGI 04)*

(a) Gram-positive
(b) Non-motile
(c) Benzyl penicillin is given in prophylaxis
(d) Patients are kept isolated till 48 hours of treatment
(e) Repeated blood culture is diagnostic

11. **A farmer from Himachal Pradesh present with inguinal lymphadenopathy. On examination multiple small ulcers are seen in leg. Which of the following stain would you prefer for bipolar staining of etiologic agents of this case?** *(AIIMS 2010)*

(a) KOH (b) Gram stain (c) Wayson's (d) Nigrosin

12. **A farmer presents to the emergency department with painful inguinal lymphadenopathy and history of fever and flu like symptoms. Clinical examination reveals on ulcer in the leg. Which of the following stain should be used to detect suspected bipolar stained organism?** *(AI 2011)*

(a) Alberts stain (b) Ziehl-Neelsen stain
(c) Wayson's stain (d) McFayden's stain

13. **The mode of infection of Pasturella multocida:** *(AI 09)*

(a) Endogenous infection (b) Animal bites or scratches
(c) Human beings (d) Aersols and dust

14. **A young boy had a flea bite while working in a wheat grain godown. After 5 days he developed fever and had axillary lymphadenopathy. A smear was sent to the laboratory to perform a specific staining. Which one of the following staining method would help in the identification of the suspected pathogen?** *(AI 06)*

(a) Albert staining (b) Ziehl-Neelsen staining
(c) McFayden's staining (d) Wayson's staining

15. **A 17-year-old girl with cystic fibrosis has a slight increase in her frequent cough and production of mucoid sputum. A sputum specimen is obtained and plated on routine culture media. The predominant growths are Gram-negative bacilli that form very mucoid colonies after 48 hours of incubation. These bacilli are oxidase positive, grow at 42°C, and have a grapelike odor. These Gram-negative bacilli are which of the following?** *(Recent MCQ)*

(a) Klebsiella pneumoniae (b) Pseudomonas aeruginosa
(c) Staphylococcus aureus (d) Streptococcus pneumoniae

ANSWERS AND EXPLANATIONS

(Harrison, 19th/e, p. 1042, 1070; Ananthanarayan, 9th/e, p. 314, 319)

1. **Ans. is 'b'** i.e., P. aeruginosa

Etiology of bacteremia associated with IV catheters – Staphylococcus epidermidis > Staphylococcus aureus > Candida albicans > Enterococcus > (E. coli, Klebsiella, P. aeruginosa, Viridans streptococci).

2. **Ans. is 'c'** i.e., Piperacillin (***Ref:*** *Harrison, 18th/e, p. 1269*)

   Penicillin active against Pseudomonas: Piperacillin, Piperacillin – Tazobactum, Mezlocillin, Ticarcillin, Ticarcillin-Clavulanate.

3. **Ans. is 'a'** i.e., It is caused by Burkholderia mallei (***Ref:*** *Jawetz, 24th/e, p. 265*)

   Causative agent of Melioidosis (Vietnam time bomb disease) is Burkholderia pseudomallei and most common form of Melioidosis is pulmonary infection. It is also known as Pseudomonas pseudomallei/Whitmore's bacilli.

4. **Ans. is 'c'** i.e., Pseudomonas (***Ref:*** *Ananthanarayan, 9th/e, p. 314*)

   Pigments (Diffusible) – Pyocyanin – Bluish-green, Pyoverdin – Yellowish-green (Fluoroescin), Pyorubrin – Bright red, Pyomelanin – Brown-black.

5. **Ans. is 'a'** i.e., Yersinia pestis (***Ref:*** *Ananthanarayan, 9th/e, p. 372*)

   YERSINIA PESTIS – Shows stalactite growth in Nutrient broth with oil or Ghee.

6. **Ans. is 'b'** i.e., Bubonic is the most common variety (***Ref:*** *Ananthanarayan, 9th/e, p. 322*)

   Clinical manifestations – Bubonic plague (Most common form) Pneumonic plague (Rare but most infectious) and Septicemic plague (rare).

   Natural reservoir – Field mice (Tatera indica) not Domestic rat.

   SOI – Infected rodents and fleas (In case or pneumonic plague but not for bubonic plague).

7. **Ans. is 'b'** i.e., Melioidosis (***Ref:*** *Harrison, 18th/e, p. 1272*)

   Clinical history suggesting – Meliodosis.

   Bipolar staining shows by – Calymatobacterium granulomatis, Yersinia, Pasteurella, H ducreyi, Vibrio parahemolyticus, Pseudomonas pseudomallei.

8. **Ans. is 'd'** i.e., Tetracycline (***Ref:*** *Ananthanarayan, 9th/e, p. 324*)

   Tetracycline (500 mg 6 hourly) or Doxycycline (100 mg twice a day) should be given to all contacts of pneumonic plague.

9. **Ans. are 'b, d, e'** (***Ref:*** *Ananthanarayan, 9th/e, p. 319*)

   Gram negative coccobacilli, Non-motile, Capsulated, Exhibits Bipolar staining, agent of bioterrorism and causative agent of Plague.

10. **Ans. are 'b, e'** (***Ref:*** *Ananthanarayan, 9th/e, p. 320*)

    Blood is taken for culture and aspirates of enlarged lymph nodes for smear and culture. In pneumonia, sputum is cultured; in possible meningitis, cerebrospinal fluid is taken for smear and culture. All materials are cultured on blood agar, chocolate, and MacConkey agar plates and in brain-heart infusion broth. Growth on solid media may be slow, requiring more than 48 hours, but blood culture results are often positive in 24 hours.

11. **Ans. is 'c'** i.e., Wayson's (***Ref:*** *Ananthanarayan, 9th/e, p. 323*)

    Y. pestis – Bipolar/Safety pin like appearance with Wayson's stain.

    Clinical presentation of patient indicating that it is case of Bubonic plague.

12. **Ans. is 'c'** i.e., Wayson's stain (***Ref:*** *Ananthanarayan, 9th/e, p. 323*)

    Already explained.

13. **Ans. is 'b'** i.e., Animal bites or scratches (***Ref:*** *Ananthanarayan, 9th/e, p. 325*)

    P. multocida – Nonmotile, gram negative bacilli, resembling Yersinia but oxidase positive, Indole positive.

14. **Ans. is 'd'** i.e., Wayson staining (***Ref:*** *Ananthanarayan, 9th/e, p. 321-323*)

    Already explained.

15. **Ans. is 'b'** i.e., Pseudomonas aeruginosa

    Mucoid strain of Pseudomonas aeruginosa causes chronic respiratory tract infection in cystic fibrosis patients. Pseudomonas aeruginosa colonies have a characteristic sweet fruit like odor.

HAEMOPHILUS

- Haemophilus species are Gram negative bacilli, Oxidase +ve, capsulated, pleomorphic, nonsporing.
- Based on growth requirements [X factor (Hemin), V factor (NAD) and CO_2] and Hemolytic property on blood agar, Haemophilus species are classified into H. influenzae, H. ducreyi, H. aegyptius, H. haemolyticus, H. parahaemolyticus, H. aphrophilus, H. paraphrophilus and H. parainfluenzae.
- H. influenzae, H. aegyptius and H. haemolyticus – require both X factor and V factor for growth but other species requires either X factor or V factor for growth.Q

Haemophilus Influenzae

- Also called **Pfeiffer's bacillus.Q**
- Capsulated, Coccobacilli, Non motile, non sporing, Nonacid fast and Nutritionally fastidious.
- It can be part of normal flora of some persons.Q
- Non capsulated strains are nontypeable.
- First free living bacteria whose complete genome is sequenced.

Virulence Factor

- **Capsular polysaccharide** – Most Imp. Virulence factor, Inhibits phagocytosis.
  - **Based on Capsular polysaccharide H. influenzae has 6 serotypes–(a,b,c,d,e,f) b subtype is Most Dangerous.**
- Endotoxin – LPS.
- IgA 1 protease – cleaves the IgA 1 Abs present on the mucosal surface.
- Adhesion proteins and pili – helps in attachment.

Hib Conjugate VaccineQ

- **PRP (Polyribosyl ribitol phosphate) Ag from type B capsule is used for vaccine.**
- Capsular Ags are less immunogenic to children, so they are conjugated with adjuvants like Toxoids (Tetanus, Diphtheria).

Clinical Manifestations

Invasive (Type B)	Non invasive
Always by capsulated Hematogenous spread	Non capsulated Contiguous spread
MCC of Epiglotittis, Pneumonia, bacteremia	2nd MCC of CAP (Community acquired pneumonia in adults)
Meningitis	Otitis media in children

Lab Diagnosis

- **Specimen** – CSF, blood, sputum, pus, aspirates.
- **Gram staining** – Gram negative coccobacilli.
- **Culture:**
  - Grows only on Chocolate agar (Provides X and V factors).Q
  - **Fildes agar and Levinthal's agar** are alternative of Chocolate agar.
  - Show **Satellitism on Blood agar with Staph. aureus.Q**

DOC – Type B → Ceftriaxone and Cefotaxime.

Non capsulated → Levofloxacin and Azithromycin.

H. Ducreyi

- Required **only X factor** for growth.
- Etiologic agent of **Chancroid/Soft Chancre.Q**
  - **Painful genital ulceration,** bleeds easily, STD.
  - Enlarged Inguinal Lymphadenopathy (bubo).
- **IP – 4-7 days.**
- Transmission – Heterosexually (Most common).

DOC – Azithromycin (single dose)

Lab Diagnosis

- **Specimen** – Exudate or swab from the edge of ulcer.
- **Gram staining** – Gram negative coccobacilli with Appearance of – **Rail road track, School of fish appearance, safety pin appearance.**
- **Culture** – Chocolate agar.

  Guys these fellows love chocolate as Neisseria sps. also loves the same.

MCQs

1. **Satellitism is seen in culture of:** *(APPG 14, Recent MCQ)*
   (a) Hemophilus influenzae (b) Streptococcus
   (c) Klebsiella (d) Proteus
2. **Disease caused by Hemophilus species:** *(PGI June 09)*
   (a) Chancroid (b) Influenza
   (c) Acute epiglotitis (d) Brain abscess
   (e) Brazillian purpuric fever
3. **False about H. influenzae:** *(AIIMS Nov 10)*
   (a) It needs X and V factor for growth
   (b) Protein capsule plays an important role in pathogenecity
   (c) It is a rare cause of meningitis in the first 2 months of life
   (d) Most common invasive manifestation is meningitis
4. **True about H. influenzae:** *(PGI Nov 10)*
   (a) Also called as Pfeiffer's bacilli
   (b) In acute infections capsulated strains are often isolated
   (c) Gram negative motile bacilli
   (d) Easily stainable
   (e) VP test positive
5. **Hemophilus ducreyi is the causative agent of:** *(Recent MCQ)*
   (a) Soft sore (b) Hard chancre
   (c) Urethritis (d) Granuloma inguinale
6. **True about H. influenzae:** *(AIIMS Nov 10)*
   (a) Grown on sheep blood agar and CO_2 (b) It is not capsulated
   (c) Invasive strain is most common (d) Gram positive
7. **All the following are true about H. influenza *except*:** *(AIIMS 03, Recent MCQ)*
   (a) It can be part of normal flora of some persons
   (b) The serotyping is based on bacterial outer membrane protein

(c) It requires Hemin and NAD for growth in culture medium

(d) Type b is responsible for invasive disease

8. **A 2 years old child is brought to the emergency with history of fever and vomiting. On examination he has neck rigidity. CSF examination shows polymorhphs more that 200/ml; protein 100 mg/dl and glucose 10 mg/dl. The Gram's stain shows the presence of Gram-negative coccobacilli. The culture shows of bacteria only on chocolate, agar and not on blood agar. The causative agent is:** *(AIIMS 02)*

(a) Neisseria meningitidis
(b) Haemophilus influenzae
(c) Branhamella catarrhalis
(d) Legionella Pneumophila

ANSWERS AND EXPLANATIONS

(Harrison, 19th/e, p. 1010; Ananthanarayan, 9th/e, p. 327)

1. **Ans. is 'a'** i.e., Hemophilus influenzae

Show Satellitism on Blood agar with Staph. aureus.

2. **Ans. are 'a, c, e'**

Disease caused by H influenzae	
Species	**Disease**
H. influenzae	Meningitis, Epiglottitis, Pneumonia, Bronchitis Arthritis, Pericarditis, Endocarditis
H. aegypticus	**Brazillian purpuric fever** **Pink conjunctivitis**
H. ducreyi	Chancroid or soft sore

3. **Ans. is 'b'** i.e., Protein capsule plays an important role in pathogenecity

Capsular of H. influenzae is made up of polysaccharides and not protein.

4. **Ans. are 'a, b'**

Also called Pfeiffer's bacillus. Capsulated, Coccobacilli, Non-motile, non-sporing.

5. **Ans. is 'a'** i.e., Soft sore

Already explained as Chancroid.

6. **Ans. is 'c'** i.e., Invasive strain is most common

Already explained (Hib is the most common and most invasive serotype of H. influenzae which causes serious clinical manifestations).

Cannot grow on Blood agar as they require V (NAD) factor which is not present in Blood agar.

7. **Ans. is 'b'** i.e., The serotyping is based on bacterial outer membrane protein

Based on Capsular polysaccharide H. influenzae has 6 serotypes (a,b,c,d,e,f) b subtype is Most Dangerous.

8. **Ans. is 'b'** i.e., Hemophilus influenzae

Gram negative coccobacilli that grows on chocolate agar not on Blood agar that is Haemophilus influenzae only.

BRUCELLA AND BORDETELLA

BRUCELLA

- Gram negative coccobacilli, fastidious, nonmotile, noncapsulated, aerobic, nonsporing, Oxidase +ve.Q
- Causative agent of Brucellosis (Undulant fever/Malta fever/Mediterranean fever) a zoonotic disease and PUO.Q
- Agent of Biological warfare.

Virulence factors – LPS major virulence factors.

TransmissionQ

- Contact with infected animals (Camel, sheep, goat, pigs) – Placenta, urine milk and other discharges.
- Inhalation of infected dust or aerosols.
- Contaminated food products and ingestion of raw vegetables form infected farms.
- People at risk–Farmers, shepherds, goatherd, butters and abattoir workers.

NOTE – Man to man transmission does not occur.

- **Diagnosis of infect animal** – Milk ring test, Rose Bengal test, rapid plate agglutination test.Q

DOC:

Gold standard treatment – Streptomycin + Doxycycline.

Alternative treatment (WHO) – Rifampin + Doxycycline.

B. Melitensis (MCC of brucellosis) → in sheep and goat, most severe infection.

B. abortus → Capnophilic (Extra CO_2 for growth) cattle abortion.

B. Suis → Pigs.

B. Canis → Dogs.

- Most common focal feature of brucellosis is musculoskeletal pain.
- Classic triad of fever – Profuse night sweating, arthralgia/arthritis and Hepatosplenomegaly are present in most patients.

Lab Diagnosis

- **Specimens** – Blood, bone marrow.
- **Blood CultureQ**
  - Biphasic medium (Castanada's).
  - Automated techniques – BacT Alert and BACTEC.
- **Serological TestQ**
  1. Acute infection – Standard agglutination test (SAT) – detects IgM.
  2. Chronic infection – 2-mercaptoethanol test – detects IgG, Complement fixation test – detects both IgM and IgG, ELISA – detects Abs to LPS Ag.

MCQs

1. Malta fever is caused by: *(AIIMS 08, Recent MCQ)*

(a) Legionella (b) Borrelia burgdorferi

(c) Brucella melitensis (d) Pseudomonas

2. A farmer presenting with fever off and on for the past 4 years was diagnosed to be suffering from chronic Brucellosis. All of the following serological tests would be helpful in the diagnosis at this state *except*: *(AI 04)*

(a) Standard agglutination test (b) 2-mercaptoethanol test

(c) Complement fixation test (d) Coomb's test

3. **Brucellosis can be transmitted by all of the following modes, *except*:** (*Recent MCQ*)
   (a) Contact with infected placenta
   (b) Ingestion of raw vegetables from infected farms
   (c) Person to person transmission
   (d) Inhalation of infected dust or aerosol
4. **A farmer rearing sheep, presented with complaints of fever and weakness for the last one month. There is generalised lymphadenopathy. There was also associated hepatomegaly. Biopsy of liver showed non-caseating granuloma. There are most likely due to infection with:** (*AIIMS 00*)
   (a) Yersinia pestis
   (b) Brucella canis
   (c) Francisella tularensis
   (d) Brucella melitensis
5. **All are true about Brucella *except*:** (*AIIMS May 11*)
   (a) B. abortus is capnophilic
   (b) Transmitted by aerosol can occur occasionally
   (c) Pasteurization destroys it
   (d) 2 ME is used to detect IgA
6. **Brucella melitensis is commonly found in (animal):** (*PGI 2011*)
   (a) Pig
   (b) Camel
   (c) Sheep
   (d) Goat
   (e) Reindeer
7. **Milk ring test is done for:** (*APPG 14, Recent MCQ*)
   (a) Brucellosis
   (b) Bacteriodes
   (c) Tuberculosis
   (d) Salmonellosis
8. **A veterinary doctor had pyrexia of unknown origin. His blood culture in special laboratory media was positive for gram-negative short bacilli which was oxidase positive. Which one of the following is the likely organism grown in culture?** (*AI 06*)
   (a) Pasturella spp.
   (b) Francisella spp.
   (c) Bartonella spp.
   (d) Brucella spp

ANSWERS AND EXPLANATIONS

(Harrison, 19th/e, p. 1066 and Ananthanarayan, 9th/e, p. 339)

1. **Ans. is 'c'** i.e, Brucella melitensis

   B. Melitensis is Causative agent of Brucellosis (Undulant fever/Malta fever/Mediterranean fever) a zoonotic disease and PUO.
2. **Ans. is 'a'** i.e., Standard agglutination test

   Acute infection – Standard agglutination test (SAT) – This test detects mainly IgM antibodies which are absent in chronic brucellosis.

   SAT performed with 2-mercaptoethanol treated with serum will detects only IgG because mercaptoethanol destroys the agglutinability of IgM but does not have any effects on IgG.

   Blocking antibodies—These are IgA antibodies that interfere with agglutination by IgG and IgM and cause a serologic test result to be negative in low serum dilutions (prozone), although positive in higher dilutions. These antibodies appear during the subacute stage of infection, tend to persist for many years independently of activity of infection, and are detected by the Coombs antiglobulin method.
3. **Ans. is 'c'** i.e., Person to person transmission

   Transmission – Contact with infected animals (Camel, sheep, goat, pigs) – Placenta, urine milk and other discharges. Inhalation of infected dust or aerosols. Contaminated food products and ingestion of raw vegetables form infected farms. People at risk – Farmers, shepherds, goatherd, butters and abattoir workers. Man to man transmission does not occur.

4. **Ans. is 'd'** i.e., Brucella melitensis

   Most common focal feature of brucellosis is musculoskeletal pain.

   Classic triad of fever – Profuse night sweating, arthralgia/arthritis and Hepatosplenomegaly are present in most patients.

   History of contact with animal followed by fever, lymphadenopathy and formation of non-caseating granuloma are features of brucellosis.

5. **Ans. is 'd'** i.e., 2 ME is used to detect IgA

   2-mercaptoethanol test detects IgG in chronic infection because mercaptoethanol destroys the agglutinability of IgM but does not have any effects on IgG.

6. **Ans. are 'a, b, c, d'**

   B. Melitensis (MCC of brucellosis) → in sheep and goat, most severe infection

   B. abortus → Capnophilic (Extra CO_2 for growth) cattle abortion

   B. Suis → Pigs

   B. Canis → Dogs

   Animal that commonly act as a source of infection of human brucellosis are Swine, Camel, Sheep and Goat, Cattle and Buffaloes. In some parts of the world dog, reindeer, caribou, camels and yaks are also infected.

7. **Ans. is 'a'** i.e., Brucellosis

   Diagnosis of infect animal by Milk ring test –> In this a sample of whole milk is mixed with a drop of stained brucella antigen. (A concentrated suspension of killed brucella abortus stained with hematoxylin) and incubated in water bath at 70°C for 40 to 50 minutes. If antibodies are present in the milk the bacilli are agglutinated and rise with the cream to form a blue ring at the top, leaving the milk unstained. If the antibodies are absent no ring is formed and the milk remains uniformly blue.

8. **Ans. is 'd'** i.e.,Brucella spp

   It is a typical presentation of brucellosis and already explained in book text.

BORDETELLA

- Gram negative coccobacilli, nonmotile, strict aerobes, highly fastidious, **capsulated, fimbriated,** Non-fermenter.
- B. pertussis – causative agent of Pertussis (Whooping cough/100 days fever).
- B. parapertussis – causes milder form of pertussis by silent copy of pertussis toxin gene.
- Obligate human parasite.

Virulence Factors

- Pertussis toxin (PT) – Most imp. Virulence factor, composed of 2 subunits (A and B) like cholera toxin, A subunit having ADP ribosylating activity of G protein – ↑ cAMP – responsible for several biological effects like T cell mitogenicity, Hemagglutination, Adhesion to respiratory ciliated cells, induction of leukocytosis, histamine sensitizer.
- Endotoxin – Activities of LPS like other GNB.
- Tracheal cytotoxin – Destruction of ciliated respiratory epithelial cells by inhibits DNA synthesis.
- Filamentous hemagglutinin (FHA) secreted protein.
- Adhesins – Fimbriae or Pili, BrkA protein.

Clinical Manifestation (IP – 7-14 days)Q

1. Catarrhal stage (Maximum infectious).
2. Paroxysmal stage (Less infectious, Whooping cough).
3. Convalescent stage (Severity of cough decreases).

Lab Diagnosis

- Specimen – Nasopharyngeal Aspirate (best).

Contd.

Contd.

- Gold standard – Culture of Nasopharyngeal secretion on Regan and Lowe medium.Q
- Most sensitive – PCR.
- **DOC –** Macrolide (Erythromycin 7-14 days).
  - Erythromycin should be given to contact person.Q

Vaccine

- Whole-cell vaccine – Efficacy is good (85%).
- DPT – (Diphtheria toxoid, killed Pertussis bacteria, Tetanus toxoid), pertussis components acts as an adjuvant and increases immunogenicity of DT and TT.

Dose – 6, 10, 14 weeks, followed by 2 booster dose at 1.5 and 5 years.

- Acellular vaccine – It is composed of pertussis toxoid and 2 or more other bacterial components (FHA, PT pertactin or fimbriae).Q
- Less reactogenic and recommended for routine immunization.

EXTRA EDGE POINTS****

- Capsule of B. pertussis is not virulence factor of pertussis.Q
- Pertussis can affect people of any age.Q
- Secondary attack rate average 90% in unimmunized contacts.Q
- Sources of pertussis infection is always a case, a chronic carrier state does not exist.
- Regan-Lowe Agar is a selective medium recommended for the isolation and cultivation of *Bordetella* spp.
- Mercury drop like appearance of B. pertussis on Regan-Lowe Agar.
- Other selective media for B. pertussis is Bordet-Gengou medium (potato-blood-glycerol agar).

MCQs

1. **In which of the following organism the capsule does not act as a virulence factor?** (*AI 2011, Recent MCQ*)
   (a) H. influenzae
   (b) Strept pneumoniae
   (c) N. meningitidis
   (d) Bordetella pertussis
2. **True regarding pertussis vaccine is:** (*Recent MCQ*)
   (a) 95% of vaccinated are protected
   (b) Erythromycin should be given to contacts
   (c) Neuroparalytic complication is seen in 1 in 15000
   (d) Leukocytosis is diagnostic
3. **Mechanism of action of pertussis toxin is all *except*:** (*APPG 10, Recent MCQ*)
   (a) Act by ADP ribosylation of GI subunit
   (b) Increase in calcium
   (c) Act by decreasing GTP
   (e) B subunit having ADP ribosylating activity
4. **A 7-month-old, partially immunized child presented with cough ending in characteristic whoop. Which of the following is considered the best type of specimen to isolate the organism and confirm the diagnosis?** (*AI 11, AIIMS May 11*)
   (a) Nasopharyngeal swab
   (b) Cough plate culture
   (c) Tracheal-aspirates
   (d) Sputum

5. **Acellular pertussis vaccine contains:** *(AIIMS 2011, UPPG 13)*
   (a) Pertactin, flagillary hemagglutinin, cytotoxin, endotoxin
   (b) Pertactin, flagillary hemagglutinin, fimbriae endotoxin
   (c) Pertactin cytotoxin, fimbriae
   (d) Flagillary hemagglutinin, pertussis toxin, fimbriae
6. **All are true statement regarding pertussis *except*:** *(PGI 2012)*
   (a) Secondary attack rate averages 90% in unimmunised contacts
   (b) Incubation period is around 14 days
   (c) Erythromycin is drug of choice
   (d) Can affect people of any age
   (e) Main source of infection is chronic carriers
7. **All of the following are virulence factors of pertussis *except*:** *(APPG 12, Recent MCQ)*
   (a) Tracheal cytotoxin (b) Pertussis toxin
   (c) Capsule (d) Pertactin
8. **100 days fever is caused by:** *(RJ 07, UPPG 10)*
   (a) B. pertussis (b) Haemaphilus influenzae
   (c) Pneumococcus (d) Meningococcus
9. **The following are true for Bordetella pertussis *except*:** *(AI 03)*
   (a) It is a strict human Pathogen
   (b) It can be cultured from the patient during catarrahal stage
   (c) It leads to invasion of the respiratory mucosa
   (d) Infection can be prevented by a acellular vaccine
10. **The usual incubation period of pertussis is:** *(Recent MCQ)*
   (a) 7-14 days (b) 3-5 days
   (c) 21-25 days (d) Less then 3 days

ANSWERS AND EXPLANATIONS

(Harrison, 19th/e, p. 1021 and Ananthanarayan, 9th/e, p. 333)

1. **Ans. is 'd'** i.e., Bordetella pertussis
   Capsule of B. pertussis is not virulence factor of pertussis as Pertussis toxin (PT) – Most imp. Virulence factor.
2. **Ans. is 'b'** i.e., Erythromycin should be given to contacts
   Contact of pertussis (whooping cough) should be given prophylactic Erythromycin or Ampicillin for 10 days.
   Protection rate in vaccinated persons – 70-90%. In pertussis lymphocytosis is diagnostic.
3. **Ans. is 'a'** i.e., Act by ADP ribosylation of GI subunit
   Pertussis toxin (PT) – Most imp. Virulence factor, composed of 2 subunits (A and B) like cholera toxin. A subunit having ADP ribosylating activity of G protein – ↑ cAMP – responsible for several biological effects like T cell mitogenicity, Hemagglutination, Adhesion to respiratory ciliated cells, induction of leukocytosis, histamine sensitizer.
4. **Ans. is 'a'** i.e., Nasopharyngeal swab
   Nasopharyngeal (NP) swabs or NP aspirates (best) using saline are the preferred specimens and it is cultured on Regan and Lowe medium (selective media). Swabs should be either dacron or rayon tipped and not calcium alginate, as it inhibits the polymerase chain reaction (PCR), nor cotton, as cotton kills the organisms.

5. **Ans. is 'd'** i.e., Flagillary hemagglutinin, pertussis toxin, fimbriae

   Acellular vaccine – It is composed of pertussis toxoid and 2 or more other bacterial components (FHA, PT pertactin or fimbriae).

6. **Ans. is 'e'** i.e., Main source of infection is chronic carriers

   Sources of Pertussis infection is always a case, a chronic carrier state does not exist.

7. **Ans. is 'c'** i.e., Capsule

   Already explained.

8. **Ans. is 'a'** i.e., B. pertussis

   Already explained in book text.

9. **Ans. is 'd'** i.e., Infection can be prevented by a acellular vaccine

   Vaccine prevents disease not infection.

10. **Ans. is 'a'** i.e., 7-14 days

    Already explained.

LEGIONELLA

- Gram negative short bacilli, noncapsulated, fastidious, motile, aerobic.
- Catalase +ve, Oxidase +ve.
- **Most common species associated with human infection is L. pneumophilia (serotype 1).Q**
- Other imp. Species is **L. micdadei (Pittsburgh pneumonia agent), it is partial acid fast.**
- Natural habitat – River, lakes and streams.

TransmissionQ

- **Aspiration is predominant mode of transmission. Other modes include aerosolization, direct instillation into lungs.**
- No man to man transmission occurs.
- Aerosolization by AC, nebulizer, humidifier, overhead showers and direct installation into lungs are other modes.
- Aerosol spread leading to epidemics.

Pathogenesis

- Attachment to respiratory mucosa with the help of pili, heat shock proteins, outer membrane proteins.
- Evades intracellular killing by inhibiting phagosome-lysosome fusion.

DOC – Azithromycin and respiratory tract quinolones (Levofloxacin etc.).

Clinical Manifestations

Pontiac feverQ – flu like illness characterized by malaise, fever, headache, fatigue and myalgia with high attack rate but self limiting.

Legionnaires disease (dyspnoea, chest pain, high fever, diarrhea, unproductive cough) – 4th major cause of community acquired pneumonia (Most common – S. pneumoniae, 2nd most common – H. influenzae, 3rd most common – chlamydia pneumoniae).

- Cause atypical pneumonia which is more serious than atypical pneumonia of other agents. **Serogroup 6 is more commonly involved in hospital (water systems with 10-50% cases) outbreaks.**

Lab Diagnosis

- **Specimens** – BAL, Sputum, Bronchial wash.
- **Gram Staining** – Shows numerous neutrophils but no organism (poorly stain).
- **Cuture – BCYE (Buffered charcoal yeast extract) agar.**
- **Identification tests** – Motile, catalase +ve, Oxidase -ve, Hippurate hydrolysis test +ve.
- Ab detection – Epidemiological purpose.
- **Urinary Ag – By ELISA (Serogroup 1 specific soluble Ag) – Cheap, rapid, easy to do.**

MCQs

1. **A 70 years old patient presents with high grade fever, dry cough and abdominal pain. Sputum sample collected from patient, shows gram negative organisms that are able to grow only on charcoal yeast extract medium. The most likely organism is:** (*AI 07, AIIMS 06*)
   (a) H. influenza
   (b) Legionella
   (c) Listeria monocytogenes
   (d) M. catarrhalis
2. **All of the following are true regarding Legionella *except*:** (*AIIMS 04*)
   (a) Legionella can be grown on complex media
   (b) L. pneumophila serogroup 1 is the most common serogroup isolated from humans
   (c) Legionella are communicable from infected patients to others
   (d) L. pneumophila is not effectively killed by polymorphonuclear leukocyte

3. **A 60-year-old man is diagnosed to be suffering from Legionnaires disease after he returns home from attending a convention. He could have acquired it:** *(AI 03)*
   (a) From a person suffering from the infection while travelling in the aeroplane
   (b) From a chronic carrier in the convention center
   (c) From inhalation of the aerosol in the air conditioned room at convention center
   (d) By sharing an infected towel with a fellow delegate at the convention
4. **Anju, a 28 years female, has diarrhea, confusion, high grade fever with bilateral pneumonitis. Organism causing this:** *(Recent MCQ)*
   (a) Legionella
   (b) Neisseria meningitidis
   (c) Streptococcus pneumoniae
   (d) H. influenza
5. **Which of the following is a good media to use for diagnosis of legionnaires disease?** *(AIIMS 01, Recent MCQ)*
   (a) Theyer Martin media
   (b) BCYE agar
   (c) Bordet Gengu media
   (d) Chocolate agar
6. **Pontiac fever is caused by:** *(PGI Dec 07)*
   (a) Legionella pneumophilia
   (b) Listeria
   (c) Scrub typhus
   (d) Leptospira
   (e) Rickettsia
7. **BCYE medium is used to culture:** *(APPG 12, Recent MCQ)*
   (a) Mycoplasma
   (b) T pallidum
   (c) H. pylori
   (d) Legionella
8. **An elderly patient presented with fever, chest pain and dry cough. Sputum cultured on charcoal yeast medium, the most likely organism is:** *(APPG 14)*
   (a) H. influenzae
   (b) Moraxella catarrhalis
   (c) Legionella
   (d) Burkholderiacepacia
9. **Aerosol spread leading to epidemics is seen in infection with:** *(Recent MCQ)*
   (a) Legionella
   (b) Hemophilus
   (c) Influenza virus
   (d) Mycoplasma
10. **Methods of transmission of legionella includes all *except*:** *(Manipal 10, Recent MCQ)*
   (a) Patients to contact
   (b) Aerosol from air conditioner
   (c) From contaminated food
   (d) Through contaminated tracheal tubes

ANSWERS AND EXPLANATIONS

(Harrison, 19th/e, p. 1014; Ananthanarayan, 9th/e, p. 401)

1. **Ans. is 'b'** i.e., Legionella

   Hint – Organisms that are able to grow only on charcoal yeast extract medium.

   BCYE (Buffered charcoal yeast extract) agar is a selective media and used for isolation of Legionella.

2. **Ans. is 'c'** i.e., Legionella are communicable from infected patients to others
   - No man to man transmission occurs.
   - **Aspiration is predominant mode of transmission. Other modes include aerosolization, direct instillation into lungs.**
   - **Aerosolization by AC, nebulizer, humidifier, overhead showers and direct installation into lungs are other modes.**
   - Aerosol spread leading to epidemics.

3. **Ans. is 'c'** i.e., From inhalation of the aerosol in the air conditioned room at convention center

   Legionella can multiply in free-living amoebas and can coexist with them in biofilms. Infection of debilitated or immunocompromised humans commonly follows inhalation of the bacteria from aerosols generated from contaminated air-conditioning systems, shower heads, and similar water sources.

4. **Ans. is 'a'** i.e., Legionella

   Clinical features of legionella infection (Legionnaire disease) is very similar to other types of pneumonia (lung infection), with symptoms that include – Diarrhea, High grade fever, Cough, Shortness of breath, Muscle aches, Headaches.

   It's a triad of **Pneumonia, diarrhea and encephalitis.**

5. **Ans. is 'b'** i.e., BCYE agar

   Already explained in Book text.

6. **Ans. is 'a'** i.e., Legionella pneumophilia

   Pontiac fever – Flu like illness characterized by malaise, fever, headache, fatigue and myalgia with high attack rate.

7. **Ans. is 'd'** i.e., Legionella

   Already explained.

8. **Ans. is 'c'** i.e., Legionella

   Already explained in Ans. 4.

9. **Ans. is 'a'** i.e., Legionella

   Aerosol spread leading to epidemics.

10. **Ans. is 'a'** i.e., Patients to contact

    Already explained in Ans. 2.

MYCOPLASMA, CHLAMYDIA, RICKETTSIAE

- **Poorly gram negative so better stained by Giemsa stain and may be commensal in throat.Q**
- Lack cell wall so Pleomorphic and resistant to cell wall active antimicrobials (Beta-lactams).Q
- **Shows gliding motility, Requires sterol for growth** reproduces by binary fission and Budding, also known as PPLO (Stable L forms).Q
- Smallest prokaryotic organisms (150-350 nm) that can grow in cell free culture media and have affinity to mammalian cell membranes.Q

DOC – Oral Azithromycin

- **Primary Atypical pneumonia/Walking pneumonia – caused by M. Pneumoniae (Eaton agent).**
- **Colonies of M. pneumoniae** on solid or biphasic medium is like **Fried egg appearance and colonies can be examined by Diene's method of staining.Q**
- **Serological test – CAT – Cold agglutination test and streptococcus MG agglutination test.Q**
- **Most sensitive test – PCR.**
- **NGU mainly caused by Ureaplasma urealyticum and M. genitalium are MCC of non-chlamydial cases of NGU.Q**
- **Ureaplasma urealyticum causes NGU, Epididymitis, Bacterial vaginosis.**

MCQs

1. **Positive cold agglutination test is seen in infections with:** *(Recent MCQ)*
   (a) Mycoplasma (b) Chlamydia
   (c) Infectious (d) Varicella
2. **Cell wall deficient organisms are:** *(PGI 01, Recent MCQ)*
   (a) Chlamydia (b) Mycoplasma
   (c) Streptococcus (d) Anaerobes
3. **The following statements are true with references to Mycoplasma *except*:** *(AIIMS 05)*
   (a) They are the smallest prokaryotic organisms that can grow in cell free culture media
   (b) They are obligate intracellular organisms
   (c) They lack a cell wall
   (d) They are resistant to Beta-lactam drugs
4. **In reference to Mycoplasma, the following are true *except*:** *(APPG 13)*
   (a) They are inhibited by penicillins
   (b) They can reproduce in cell free media
   (c) They have an affinity for mammlian cell membranes
   (d) They can pass through fiters of 450 nm pore size
5. **The following is true about Mycoplasma *except*:** *(AIIMS 02, 96, UPPG 10)*
   (a) Multiply by binary fission
   (b) Are sensitive to beta-lactam group of drugs
   (c) Can grow in cell free media
   (d) Requires sterols for their growth
6. **Mycoplasma pneumonia is characterized by all *except*:** *(AIIMS 01)*
   (a) Diagnosed by serum cold antibody (b) Treatment is erythromycin
   (c) Cannot be cultured from sputum (d) Raised ESR

7. **Atypical pneumonia can be caused by the following microbial agents *except*:** (*AI 05*)
   (a) Mycoplasma
   (b) Legionella pneumophilia
   (c) Human corona virus
   (d) Klebsiella pneumonia
8. **All are features of ureplasma urealyticum *except*:** (*AI 01*)
   (a) Non-gongococcal urethritis
   (b) Salpingitis
   (c) Epididymitis
   (d) Bacterial vaginosis
9. **True about Mycoplasma:** (*UP 97*)
   (a) CO_2 is important for growth
   (b) Does not cause hemolysis
   (c) May be commensal in throat
   (d) Acid fast bacillus
10. **True about Mcyoplasma is:** (*Recent MCQ*)
   (a) Not sensitive to antibiotics
   (b) L. form is most common
   (c) Culture in sarbaroudz media
   (d) Most common cause of nongonococcal urethritis
11. **True about Mycoplasma is:** (*AIIMS 09, AI 10*)
   (a) Causes lung infection
   (b) Penicillin is drug of choice
   (c) Thick cell wall
   (d) Thallium acetate inhibits the growth
12. **Diene's method is used for:** (*PGI 99, AIIMS 01*)
   (a) Mycoplasma
   (b) Chlamydiae
   (c) Plague
   (d) Diphtheria

ANSWERS AND EXPLANATIONS

(Harrison, 19th/e, p. 1163; Ananthanarayan, 9th/e, p. 386)

1. **Ans. is 'a'** i.e., Mycoplasma

   Serological test for mycoplasma (Nonspecific Ab detection tests) – **Mycoplasma possess certain heterophile antigens that cross react with I Ag of the RBCs and carbohydrate Ag of group F Streptococci cell wall.** This property is used to detect Abs against Mycoplasma in patient's serum by CAT (cold agglutination test) and streptococcus MG agglutination test.

2. **Ans. is 'b'** i.e., Mycoplasma (***Ref:*** *Ananthanarayan, 8th/e, p. 17-18, 38*)

   Lack cell wall so Pleomorphic and resistant to cell wall active antimicrobials (Beta-lactams).

3. **Ans. is 'b'** i.e., They are obligate intracellular organisms.

   Obligate intracellular bacteria are: M leprae, Chlamydia, Rickettsiae, Coxiella burnetti, Pathogenic treponemes so cannot grow on artificial cell free culture media. Mycoplasma grows on artificial cell free culture media.

4. **Ans. is 'a'** i.e., They are inhibited by penicillins.

   Cell wall is absent so they are not inhibited by β-lactum antibiotics.

5. **Ans. is 'b'** i.e., Are sensitive to beta-lactam group of drugs.

   Already explained in book text.

6. **Ans. is 'c'** i.e., Cannot be cultured from sputum

   Mycoplasma can be cultured from throat swab, respiratory secretions or sputum. Sputum is not very useful as it contains too many contaminants. Colonies of M. pneumoniae on solid or biphasic medium is like Fried egg appearance and colonies can be examined by Diene's method of staining.

7. **Ans. is 'd'** i.e., Klebsiella pneumoniae

   The most common cause of atypical pneumonia is Mycoplasma. The disease is characterized by paucity of respiratory sign on physical examination but radiological evidence of consolidation.

   Organisms causing atypical pneumonia are – Mycoplasma (Most Common), Legionella pneumonia, Francisella tularensis, Chlamydia Psittacosis, Chlamydia pneumoniae, Coxiella burnetti, Pneumocystis carinii, Histoplasma capsulatum, Coccidiodes.

8. **Ans. is 'b'** i.e., Salpingitis

   Some strains of mycoplasma frequently isolated from the urogenital tract of human beings and animals form **very tiny colonies** (15-50 µm). So called T strain or T form of Mycoplasmas (T for Tiny). They are peculiar in their ability to hydrolyse urea. **Human T strain mycoplasma are classified as Ureaplasma urealyticum.**

   Infections caused by Mycoplasma hominis and ureaplasma urealyticum are:

   (a) **Genital infection in men:** Urethritis, proctitis, balanoposthitis, Reiter's syndrome.

   (b) **Genital infection in men:** Acute salpingitis, PID, cervicitis, Vaginitis.

   (c) Infertility, abortion, chorioamnionitis, postpartum fever.

9. **Ans. is 'c'** i.e., May be commensal in throat (***Ref:*** *Ananthanarayan, 8th/e, p. 589, 7th/e, p. 600*)

   Already explained in book text.

10. **Ans. is 'b'** i.e., L. form is most common (***Ref:*** *Ananthanarayan, 8th/e, p. 390; 7th/e, p. 399*)

    Shows gliding motility, Requires sterol for growth reproduces by binary fission and Budding, also known as PPLO (Stable L forms).

11. **Ans. is 'a'** i.e., Causes lung infection (***Ref:*** *Ananthanarayan, 8th/e, p. 590*)

    Already explained.

12. **Ans. is 'a'** i.e., Mycoplasma

    Colonies of M. pneumoniae on solid or biphasic medium is like Fried egg appearance and colonies can be examined by Diene's method of staining.

CHLAMYDIAE

- **Obligate Intracellular bacteria** (can't multiply outside cell) so unable to grow in cell free media.Q
- They can't synthesis ATP, so a/k/a ATP parasites/Energy parasites.
- Their cell wall lacks a peptidoglycan layer and contains tetrapeptide linked matrix with high lipid content.Q

Growth Cycle of C. TrachomatisQ

- Multiply by binary fission and has biphasic life.
- They exist in 2 forms:
  1. **Elementary body (EB)** – Extracellular and infectious.Q
  2. **Reticulate body (RB)** – Intracellular and Replicating.Q

EB	RB
• Mainly found extracellularly	• Only intracellular
• Metabolically inactive	• Metabolically active
• Can't multiply	• Replicates
• Don't replicate	• **Binary fission**
• **Infectious form**	• Can't initiate infection of cell
• **DNA = RNA**	• **RNA > DNA**

Chlamydia TrachomatisQ

- Forms compact inclusion mixed with glycogen matrix and sensitive to sulfonamide.
- Human pathogen and leaves the host cell with a scar.

Biovars

1. **TRIC – Causing trachoma, inclusion conjunctivitis.**Q
2. LGV – Causing Lymphogranuloma venereum.

Serotype

1. **A, B, Ba, C** – Trachoma.
2. **D-K** – Genital chlamydiasis, inclusion conjunctivitis and infant pneumonia, Urethritis.
3. **L1, L2, L3** – Lymphogranuloma venereum (Genital elephantiasis).Q

Contd.

Contd.

Chlamydia PsittaciQ

- Natural pathogen of birds.
- Resistant to sulfonamide.
- Causing Psittacosis (Atypical pnemonia).
- Transmission – inhalation – Pet birds and poultry.
- No man to man transmission.

Chlamydia Pneumoniae – TWAR agentQ

- **Exclusive human pathogen – Community Acquired Atypical pneumonia, Associated with Asthma and Athero-sclerosis.**
- **Resistant to sulfonamide.**

Lab Diagnosis

- **Specimens – Scraping or swabs from infected site, Urethral swab for NGU, Endocervical swab for cervicitis, conjunctival swab, urethral secretions, Nasopharyngeal aspirate, bubo aspirate for LGV.**
- **MicroscopyQ**
  - **Gram staining of samples shows presence of abundant pus cells** but **no bacteria** (Intracellular bacteria).
  - **Castaneda, Machiavello or Gimenez stains are better for demonstrations of Chlamydia.**
  - Lugol's iodine is used for inclusion bodies.
  - **Inclusion bodies – Halberstaedter-Prowazek (HP) in trachoma, LCL body in Psittacosis, Miyagawa corpuscle in LGV.**
  - Direct Immunofluorescence test (DIF) – by monoclonal Abs, More sensitive and specific.
- **Ag detection – ELISA – Preferred for screening.**
- **CultureQ**
  - Embryonated egg (Yolk sac), Mice.
  - Cell lines – **McCoy,** HeLa, Buffalo, green monkey, BHK.
- **NAAT** (Nucleic acid amplification test) – **PCR, LCR (Ligase Chain Reaction).** Most sensitive test in cervical C. trachomatis.Q
- **Ab Detection**
  - Complement fixation test – Genus or group specific LPS Ag is responsible.
  - **Micro IF – Most useful for TRIC (Inclusion conjunctivitis) – Serovar specific major membrane protein is responsible.**
    - **DOC – Azithromycin, Doxycyline, Tetracycline, Erythromycin.Q**

EXTRA EDGE POINTS****Q

- **C. trachomatis** MCC of NGU (Nongonococcal urethritis), postgonococcal urethritis, epididymitis.
- **Reiter's syndrome** (Reactive arthritis) consist of conjunctivitis, Urethritis (or, in female cervicitis) polyarthritis and mucocutaneous lesion.

  Ritter's disease – Severe form of SSSS.
- Isolation of Chlamydia from tissue specimens can be done by **Yolk sac inoculation.**
- **C. trachomatis does not causes** – Parotitis, Rhinitis, Q-fever, Vulvitis.

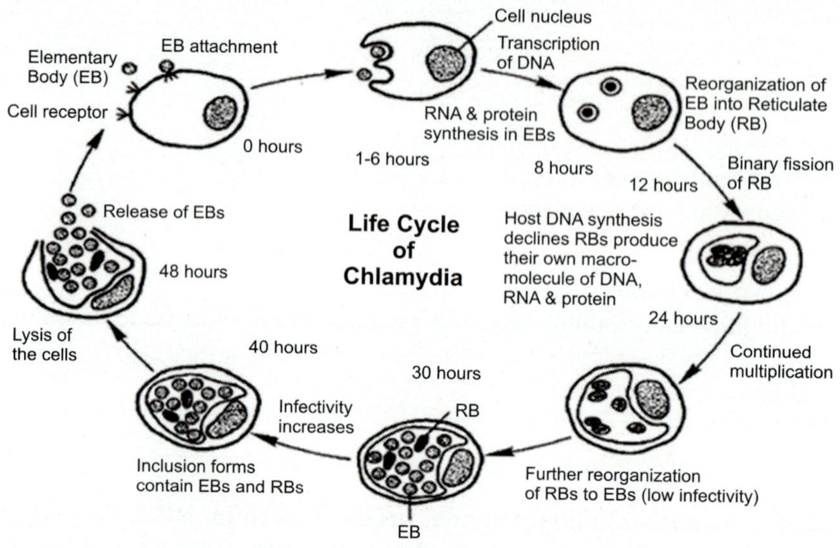

MCQs

1. **Chlamydia causes:** (*PGI 00, Recent MCQ*)
   (a) Infertility
   (b) Pneumothorax
   (c) Pelvic inflammatory disease
   (d) Congenital malformation in fetus
2. **Which of the following is not true regarding chlamydia?** (*AI 07; AIIMS 06*)
   (a) Has biphasic life
   (b) Elementary body is metabolically active
   (c) Reticulate body undergoes binary fission
   (d) Once it invades into cell it abates phagolysosomal fusion
3. **Chlamydia trachomatis is associated with the following *except*:** (*Recent MCQ*)
   (a) Endemic trachoma
   (b) Inclusion conjuncitivitis
   (c) LGV
   (d) Community acquired pneumonia
4. **Which one of the following statements is true regarding Chlamydia pneumonia?** (*AI 05*)
   (a) Fifteen serovars have been identified as human pathogen
   (b) Mode of transmission is by the air-borne bird excreta
   (c) The cytoplasmic inclusions presents in the sputum specimen are rich in glycogen
   (d) The group specific antigen is responsible for the production of complement fixing antibodies
5. **The most sensitive method for detecting cervical Chlamydia trachomatis infection is:** (*Recent MCQ*)
   (a) Direct fluorescent antibody test
   (b) Enzyme immunoassay
   (c) Polymerase chain reaction
   (d) Culture on irradiated McConkey cells
6. **Chlamydia does not cause:** (*Recent MCQ*)
   (a) Q. fever
   (b) Non-gonococcal urethritis
   (c) Trachoma
   (d) Salpingitis
7. **All are true regarding Chlamydia psittaci *except*:** (*APPG 10*)
   (a) Endemic in birds
   (b) Cause non-gonococcal urethritis
   (c) Grow in a specified laboratory
   (d) Tetracycline is treatment of choice
8. **A 45 years female complains of lower abdominal pain and vaginal discharge. On examination there is cervicitis along with a mucopurulent cervical discharge. The gram smear of the discharge shows presence of abundant pus cells but no bacteria. The best approach to isolates the possible causative agent would be:** (*AIIMS 05*)

(a) Culture on chocolate agar supplemented with Haemin
(b) Culture on McCoy cells
(c) Culture on a bilayer human blood agar
(d) Culture on vero cell lines

9. The following is not a method of isolation of Chlamydia from clinical specimens: *(APPG 14)*
(a) Yolk inoculation
(b) Enzyme immunoassay
(c) Tissue culture using irradiated McCoy
(d) Tissue culture using irradiated BHK cells

10. The following statements are true regarding Chlamydia *except*: *(AIIMS 05)*
(a) Erythromycin is effective for therapy of Chlamydial infections
(b) Their cell wall lacks a peptidoglycan layer
(c) They can grow in cell free culture media
(d) They are obligate intracellular bacteria

11. A man presents to STD clinic with urethritis and urethetral discharge. Gram stain shows numerous pus cells but no microorganism. Culture is negative on routine laboratory media. The most likely agent is: *(Recent MCQ)*
(a) Chlamydia trachomatis
(b) H. ducreyi
(c) T. pallidum
(d) N. Gonorrhoeae

12. Chlamydia trachomatis serovars D-K cause: *(Recent MCQ)*
(a) Arteriosclerosis
(b) Trachoma
(c) Lymphogranuloma venereum
(d) Urethritis

13. Triad of Reiter's syndrome: *(PGI 07)*
(a) Conjunctivitis
(b) Uveitis
(c) Polyarthritis
(d) Mucosal lesions
(e) Glaucoma

14. Chlamydia grows in which of the following cell lines? *(PGI 01)*
(a) HeLa
(b) HeP2
(c) McCoy
(d) Human diploid fibroblast series
(e) Vero cells

15. Most sensitive test for diagnosing asymptomatic chlamydia infection is: *(AIIMS 09, Recent MCQ)*
(a) Tissue culture
(b) Nucleic acid amplification
(c) Serology
(d) Serum electrophoresis

16. Isolation of Chlamydia from tissue specimen can be done by: *(AI PGMEE 10)*
(a) ELISA (Enzyme Linked Immune Assay)
(b) Yolk sac inoculation
(c) Direct Immunofluotescence Antibody test (DFA)
(d) Polymerase Chain Reaction (PCR)

17. A male patient with symptoms of urethritis. Examination reveals only pus cells without any organism. Most likely cause is: *(AI 08; UPPG 10)*
(a) Chlamydia trachomatis
(b) H. ducreyi
(c) Treponema pallidum
(d) M. tuberculi

18. Regarding Chlamydia infection of the eyes, true statement includes the following *except*: *(AI 09)*
(a) Mostly asymptomatic
(b) Can be cultured

(c) Inclusion conjunctivitis is an acute ocular infection caused by sexually transmitted C. trachomatis strains (usually serovars D through K)

(d) Penicillin is the treatment

19. In a patient with UTI; on smear, no bacteria are found on gram stain with abundant pus cells, to demonstrate organism, which of the following is useful? (*AI 07; AIIMS May 2012,11, 06*)

(a) McCoy cell line
(b) Thayer Martin medium
(c) L. J. medium
(d) Acid fast staining

ANSWERS AND EXPLANATIONS

(Harrison, 19th/e, p. 1165 and Ananthanarayan, 9th/e, p. 415)

1. **Ans. are 'a, c'** (***Ref:*** *Harrison, 18th/e, p. 1422-1425*)

   Chlamydia causes:

   In women – Cervicitis, salpingitis, urethritis, PID, infertility.

   In men – NGU, epididymitis.

   Neonates – Conjunctivitis, pneumonia.

   Either sex – Proctitis, LGV, Reiter syndrome.

2. **Ans. is 'b'** i.e., Elementary body is metabolically active (***Ref:*** *Jawetz, 25th/e, p. 327*)

   Chlamydia occurs in two forms: Elementary body and Reticulate body. The elementary body is extracellular infective form. The reticulate body is intracellular growing and replicative form.

3. **Ans. is 'd'** i.e., Community acquired Pneumonia (***Ref:*** *Harrison, 18th/e, p. 1422-1425*)

   Most common bacteria causing CAP – Pneumococcus, H. influenzae, Chlamydia pneumoniae, Legionella.

Diseases Caused by Chlamydiae

Species	Character	Serotype	Disease
C. trachomatis	• Form compact inclusions with glycogen matrix • Sensitive to sulfonamide • Natural parasite of human • Leave the host cell with a scar	**Biovar TRIC – A, B, Ba, C**	• Trachoma
		Biovar TRIC – D-K	• Inclusion conjunctivitis • Infant pneumonia • Genital chlamydiasis
		Biovar LGV – L1,L2,L3	• LGV
C. psittaci	• Diffuse vacuolated inclusions without glycogen matrix • R/ to sulfonamide • Natural parasite of birds	Many	• Psittacosis (Pneumonia) • Inhalational route • Poultry ingestion – no role • Occupational spread to human

C.pneumoniae **TWAR agent**	• Exclusively human pathogen
	• Inclusions without glycogen matrix
	• R/ to sulfonamide
		Only 1	• Atypical pneumonia
			• Associated with
			  – **Atherosclerosis**
			  – **Asthma**
			• **Hep2 cell most affective**

4. **Ans. is 'd'** i.e., The group specific antigen is responsible for the production of complement fixing antibodies.

   The group specific LPS antigen is responsible for CFT and serovar specific major membrane protein is responsible for microimmunofluorescence.

5. **Ans. is 'c'** i.e., Polymerase chain reaction (***Ref:*** *Harrison, 17th/e, p. 1074*)

Amplification assays such as ligase chain reaction and polymerase chain reaction are the most sensitive chlamydial diagnostic method.

Other methods are:

(a) **Cell culture:** Sensitivity (60-80%).

(b) **Direct immunofluorescent antibody test:** Sensitivity 70-80% and quite specific.

(c) **ELISA:** 60-80%.

6. **Ans. is 'a'** i.e., Q. fever

   Q fever is caused by Coxiella burnetti.

7. **Ans. is 'b'** i.e., Cause non-gonococcal urethritis

   Already explained.

8. **Ans. is 'b'** i.e., Culture on McCoy cells

   Chlamydiae are usually grown on McCoy cell line and HeLa cell line.

   Genital chlamydiasis is suspected if gram stained smear of urogenital exudates shows significant number of neutrophils. > 4/oil immersion field in urethritis, > 30 in cervicitis in the absence of gonococcal bacteria.

9. **Ans. is 'b'** i.e., Enzyme immunoassay

   Enzyme immunoassay is used for chlamydia antigen detection not for isolation.

   The cell lines on which chlamydia are most commonly isolated are HeLa and McCoy. Other cell lines are HeP2, HL and BHK cell line. It can also be isolated on yolk sac.

10. **Ans. is 'c'** i.e., They can grow in cell free culture media.

    Obligate Intracellular bacteria (can't multiply outside cell) so unable to grow in cell free media.

11. **Ans. is 'a'** i.e., Chlamydia trachomatis

    Gram staining of samples shows presence of abundant pus cells but no bacteria (Intracellular bacteria) and Chlamydia cannot be grown on laboratory media like blood agar, chocolate agar, MacConkey agar etc.

12. **Ans. is 'd'** i.e., Urethritis

    Already explained.

13. **Ans. are 'a, c, d'**

    Reiter's syndrome (Reactive arthritis) consist of conjunctivitis, Urethritis (or, in female cervicitis) polyarthritis and mucocutaneous lesion.

    Ritter's disease – Severe form of SSSS.

14. **Ans. are 'a, b, c'**

    Apart from these it can be grown on HL cell line, BHK cell line and yolk sac.

15. **Ans. is 'b'** i.e., Nucleic acid amplification

    NAAT (Nucleic acid amplification test) – PCR, LCR (Ligase Chain Reaction).

    Most sensitive test in cervical C. trachomatis.

16. **Ans. is 'b'** i.e., Yolk sac inoculation

    Isolation of chlamydia can be done by **using yolk sac or cell lines. NAAT detect DNA of bacteria so it is an identification test so bacteria cannot isolate by using this method.**

17. **Ans. is 'a'** i.e., Chlamydia trachomatis

    Already explained.

18. **Ans. is 'd'** i.e., Penicillin is the treatment

    DOC – Azithromycin, Doxycycline, Tetracycline, Erythromycin.

    Penicillin is not effective against chlamydia.

19. **Ans. is 'a'** i.e., McCoy cell line

    Already explained.

RICKETTSIAE

- They are obligate intracellular organism and cannot grow in cell free media **except Rochalimaea quintana.Q**
- Gram negative coccobacilli, nonmotile and transmitted by an arthropods vectors (tick, flea or mouse).
- Family Rickettsiaceae consists of two genera – **Rickettsia and Orientia.**
- They do not take stain well in gram stating so can be stained by **Giemsa, Gimenez, Castaneda and Machiavello stain.**
- The primary site of multiplication of rickettsia is **vascular and reticuloendothelial cells.**Q
- **Transovarian or Transovarial transmission** (occurs in certain arthropods as they transmit disease causing bacteria from parent to offspring arthropod) is seen in R. rickettsiae.Q

Group	Species	Disease	Vector
Typhus group	**R. prowazekii**	Epidemic typhus Brill Zinsser	Louse **(LET)**
-do-	**R. typhi (R. mooseri)**	Endemic/Murine-typhus	Flea **(FEN)**
Spotted fever group	**R. rickettsii**	Rocky mountain spotted fever (RMSF)	Tick **(TRI)**
-do-	**R. conorii**	Indian tick typhus or Mediterranean spotted fever	Tick
-do-	**R. akari**	Rickettsial pox	Mite **(PSM)**
Scrub typhus	**R. tsusugamushi or orientia tsutsugamushi**	Scrub typhus (chigger-borne typhus)	Mite (trombiculid)
Q fever	**Coxiella burnetti**	Q fever	Nil (Air borne)
Trench fever	**Rochalimaea Quintana (bartonella quintana)**	Trench fever/five-day fever	Louse
Ehrlichiosis	**Ehrlichiae**	Ehrlichiosis	Tick

- **Except** for louse borne typhus, humans are accidental hosts.
- **RMSF – Most severe** rickettsial disease.
- **Rickettsial infections –** Fever, headache, malaise, prostration, skin, rash and hepatosplenomegaly.

Scrub typhus	Coxiella burnetii (Q fever)
• Causing agent is **Orientia tsutsugamushi, transmitted by Mite (trombiculid) Chigger (larva).Q** • It **lacks lipopolysaccharide.** • Affect rats in deserts, rain forest. • Eschar at site, rash, LN↑.Q • ↑**OXK titre** in Weil Felix.Q • Zoonotic disease.	• Causing agent is **Coxiella burnetii** • Zoonotic disease. • Disease – **Interstitial pneumonia** • It survives pasteurization. • **Transmitted without arthropod (respiratory mode)** • **No skin rash in Q fever.Q**

Lab Diagnosis

- **Culture (cannot grow in cell free media)** – Isolation can be done by cell lines (HeLa, primary chick embryo, vero) and egg yolk inoculation or guinea pig inoculation.Q
- **Neil-Mooser/Tunica reaction – Intraperitonially inoculation into male guinea pigs and changes observed in animal – +ve for R. typhi, R. conorii, R. akari** and -ve for R. prowazekii.

- **Weil-Felix Test** (Heterophile agglutination test)Q
  - Based on sharing of alkali stable LPS between typhus rickettsia and some strain of Proteus bacilli (OX-19, OX-2, OX-K).
- **DOC – Doxycycline.**

MCQs

1. **A man presents with fever, chills 2 weeks after a louse bite. There was maculopapular rash on the trunk which spread peripherally. The cause of this infection can be:**
   (a) Scrub typhus
   (b) Endemic typhus
   (c) Rickettsiae pox
   (d) Epidemic typhus
2. **All of the following statements are true regarding Q fever *except*:**
   (a) It is a zoonotic disease
   (b) Human disease is characterized by an interstitial pneumonia
   (c) No rash is seen
   (d) Weil-Felix reactions is very useful for diagnosis
3. **Which of the following statements is true about endemic typhus?** *(MCQ)*
   (a) Is caused by R. rickettsii
   (b) Is transmitted by bites of fleas
   (c) Has no mammalian reservoir
   (d) Can be cultured in chemical defined culture medium
4. **True about scrub typhus:** *(PGI Nov 11)*
   (a) Zoonotic disease
   (b) Positive Weil-Felix reaction
   (c) Spread by adult mite
   (d) Eschar indicates the location of mite bite
   (e) Spread by infected chigger
5. **Lice are not the vectors of:** *(AI 07; AIIMS 06)*
   (a) Relapsing fever
   (b) Q fever
   (c) Trench fever
   (d) Epidemic typhus
6. **All are true about scrub typhus, *except*:** *(AI 2010)*
   (a) Causative organism is R.Tsutsugamushi
   (b) Vector is trombiculid mite
   (c) Adult female feeds on vertebrate hosts
   (d) Tetracycline is the drug of choice
7. **A patient complained of chills and fever following a louse bite 2 weeks before. He had rashes all over the body and was delirious at the time of presentation to the hospital and subsequently went into coma. A provisional diagnosis of vasculitis due to rickettsial infection was made. Which one of the following can be the causative agent?** *(AI 05)*
   (a) Rickettsia typhi
   (b) Rickettsia rickettsiae
   (c) Rickettsia prowazekii
   (d) Rickettsia akari
8. **Scrub typhus is transmitted by:** *(AIIMS Nov. 07, APPG 12)*
   (a) Reduvid bug
   (b) Trombiculid mite
   (c) Enteric pathogens
   (d) Cyclops
9. **It is true regarding endemic typhus that:** *(AIIMS 06)*
   (a) Man is the only reservoir of infection
   (b) Flea is a vector of the disease
   (c) The rash developing into eschar is a characteristic presentation
   (d) Culture of the etiological agent in tissue culture is a diagnostic

10. Following is the etiological agent of Rocky Mountain spotted fever: *(AIIMS 05, UPPG 10)*
(a) R. rickettsii
(b) Rochalimae quintana
(c) R. tsutsugamushi
(d) Coxiella burnetti

11. Mode of transmission of Q-fever is: *(Recent MCQ)*
(a) Bite of infected louse
(b) Bite of infected tick
(c) Inhalation of aerosol
(d) Bite of infected mice

12. Disease caused by both Rickettsia and Orientia is transmitted by: *(PGI 2011)*
(a) Rat flea
(b) Tick
(c) Louse
(d) Trombiculid mite
(e) Gamaxid mite

13. Which is caused by Rickettsia? *(PGI 07, Recent MCQ)*
(a) Weil's disease
(b) Rocky mountain spotted fever
(c) Scrub typhus
(d) Lyme disease

ANSWERS AND EXPLANATIONS

(Harrison, 19th/e, p. 1154; Ananthanarayan, 9th/e, p. 405)

1. **Ans. is 'd'** i.e., Epidemic typhus

Louse borne diseases – Epidemic typhus, Brill Zinsser disease, Trench fever.

Humans are the natural reservoir for R. prowazekii, which is prevalent worldwide and transmitted by body lice when louse feces are scratched or rubbed into bite or other wounds (or sometimes the mucous membranes of the eyes or mouth). **Headache is generalized and intense. Small, pink macules, which appear on the 4th to 6th day, rapidly cover the body, usually in the axillae and on the upper trunk and not on the palms, soles and face.** Later, the **rash becomes dark and maculopapular.**

2. **Ans. is 'd'** i.e., Weil Felix reactions is very useful for diagnosis

Weil-Felix Test (Heterophile agglutination test) **has** no value in – Q fever, Trench fever, R. pox.

Coxiella Burnetii (Q fever)

- Causing agent is Coxiella burnetii. It is a Zoonotic disease.
- Disease – Interstitial pneumonia.
- It survives pasteurization.
- **Transmitted without arthropod (respiratory mode).**
- **No skin rash in Q fever.**

3. **Ans. is 'b'** i.e., is transmitted by bites of fleas

Let's consider other choices.

(a) It is caused by R typhi and R felis.
(b) Rat and Opossum are the reservoir.
(d) Rickettsiae are **unable to in cell free media.**

4. **Ans. are 'a, b, d, e'**

Scrub typhus – Causing agent is Orientia tsutsugamushi, transmitted by Mite (trombiculid) Chigger (larva) not adult mite.

- It lacks lipopolysaccharide.
- Affect rats in deserts, rain forest.
- Eschar at site, rash, LN↑.
- **↑OXK titre in Weil Felix.**
- Zoonotic disease.

5. **Ans. is 'b'** i.e., Q fever

   Q fever is a disease caused by the bacteria Coxiella burnetii which is found worldwide. The bacteria naturally infects some animals, such as goats, sheep and cattle. C. burnetii bacteria are found in the birth products (i.e., placenta, amniotic fluid), urine, feces, and milk of infected animals.

6. **Ans. is 'c'** i.e., Adult female feeds on vertebrate hosts

   Mite feeds on serum of warm blood animals during their larval stage (chiggers) and adult mite feed only on plants.

7. **Ans. is 'c'** i.e., Rickettsia prowazekii

   Louse bite (take a note from this).

8. **Ans. is 'b'** i.e., Trombiculid mite

   Already explained in book text.

9. **Ans. is 'b'** i.e., Flea is a vector of the disease

   Already explained in book text.

10. **Ans. is 'a'** i.e., R. rickettsii

    Rocky Mountain spotted fever is a bacterial infection transmitted by a tick. Serious damage to organs such as your kidneys and heart. Severe headache, high fever are important findings. A few days later, a rash usually appears on the wrists and ankles.

11. **Ans. is 'c'** i.e., Inhalation of aerosol

    Transmitted without arthropod (respiratory mode).

12. **Ans. is 'd'** i.e., Trombiculid mite

    Already explained in book text.

13. **Ans. is 'b'** i.e., Rocky mountain spotted fever

    Other choices:

    (a) Weil's disease is caused by Leptospira interrogans.

    (b) Scrub typhus is caused by Orientia tsutsugamushi.

    (c) Lyme disease is caused by Borrelia burgdorferi.

SPIROCHETES (TREPONEMA PALLIDUM)

TREPONEMA PALLIDUM

- **T. pallidum – Causative agent of syphilis.**
- Syphilis was discovered by **Schaudinn and Hoffman.**Q
- Treponemes cannot be seen by light microscope so dark ground or phase contrast microscope is used.Q
- **IP – 10-90 days.**
- Transmission – Venereal syphilis by sexual contacts, direct contact to lesions, blood transfusion or congenital.

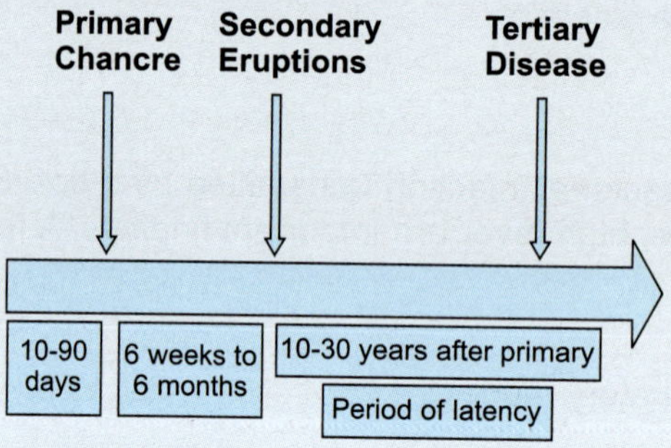

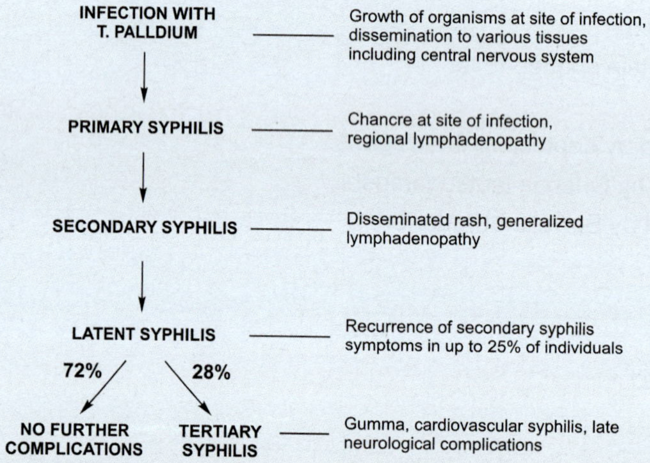

Lab Diagnosis

- Specimens – Lesion exudates.
- **Direct Microscopy**
  - Dark field microscopy.
  - Direct IF staining from sample (DFA-TP).
  - **Silver impregnation method (Levaditi stain for tissue section and Fontana stain for smear).**
- Culture – Pathogenic Treponemes cannot be isolated on artificial media or in tissue culture but Nichole's strain can be maintained in rabbit testes.Q

  Nonpathogenic Reiter's strain can grow in artificial media.
- **Serological tests**Q
  - **Non treponemal or Nonspecific or Standard tests for syphilis** – Ag (cardiolipin) is not specific for T. pallidum which detects nonspecific regain Abs – Wassermann test (CFT), VDRL (slide flocculation test), RPR, TRUST (Toluidine red unheated serum test), USR (unheated serum) test.

- **Advantages** – VDRL or RPR can be used for treatment monitoring as specific tests remains positive (reactive) after the treatment.
- **Biological False Positive (BFP)** – Infectious mononucleosis, viral hepatitis, relapsing fever, Kala azar, Leprosy, Malaria, IV drug user, HIV people.
  - **Treponemal or specific tests for syphilis** – Detects specific Abs against T. pallidum Ag – FTA-ABS, Agglutination assays (MHA-TP, TPHA, TPPA), TPI (dark ground microscope is required for observing Immobilization).
- All reactive/positive Non treponemal tests must be confirmed by specific tests to rule out the BFP. Q

> - **Most sensitive test** – FTA-ABS
> - **Most specific test** – TPI (Now not used)
> - **Test of choice for rapid diagnosis and mass screening in medical camps** – RPR
> - Test of choice for therapy evaluation – VDRL
> - **Test of choice for diagnosis of congenital syphilis – IgM FTA-ABS**
> - **DOC** – Penicillin

EXTRA EDGE POINTS****Q

- **Chancre redux** is a clinical feature of **early relapsing syphilis.**
- T. pallidum is very difficult to demonstrate in Gumma (Tertiary syphilis).
- Nichole strain is used in TPI test.

Non Venereal Treponemes

- Mode of transmission – Direct contact not sexual.
- **Endemic syphilis (Bejel)** – Caused by T. pallidum subsp. **endemicum.**
- **Yaws –** Caused by T. pallidum subsp. **pertenue.**
- **Pinta** – Caused by T. pallidum subsp**. carateum.**
- In Non Venereal Treponematosis, **Yaws and Pinta gives +ve for serological tests for syphilis.Q**

LEPTOSPIRA

- Leptospira interrogans → Hooked end.
- Leptospirosis – **Sewer worker disease, Weil's disease or Icterohemorrhagic fever (jaundice + fever).**
- **'3R' – Rats, Rain, Rice field.**
- Zoonotic infection – Mainly rats.
- In rats organism multiplies in Renal tubules → Rat urine, Rats infests rice field.
- Humans get infected, when bacteria rat urine

  ↓

  H_2O

  ↓

  Mucous membrane/cuts in skin

  Cl/f: – animal – human

  (No person to person transmission) – Man is the dead end host.
- Direct microscopy – Dark field examination of centrifuged urine.
- Culture media – **EMJH, Fletcher and Korthokoff.**
- IOC – serological – **Microscopic agglutination test (MAT) –** Gold standard and Macroscopic agglutination test.Q
- PCR **for Leptospira sps done.**
- DOC – Penicillin (severe form) or oral doxycycline (mild form).

BORRELIA

- Large, retractile spirochetes which can be stained by ordinary methods and gram –ve.
- **Pathogenic species are B. burgdorferi (Lyme's disease), B. recurrentis (Relapsing fever), B. vincenti (Vincent angina).**

Lyme's Disease (Lyme borreliosis)

- Causative agent – **B. burgodoferi.**
- Transmitted by bite of **Ixodid ticks/Hard tick.**
- Replicates locally and invades locally.
- Centre → periphery **Erythema Chronicum migrans (ECM).**
- **Annular rash/bull's eye.**
- Associated with chronic Arthritis (joint movement).
- **BSK media is used to culture Borrelia burgdorferi.**
- **Intrathecal IgA confirms meningitis.**

Relapsing Fever

- Causative agent – **B. recurrentis.**
- **Antigenic variation seen.Q**
- It is of 2 types – Louse borne and tick borne.
- Borellia causing them are indistinguishable.
- **Louse borne relapsing fever occurs as epidemic. Tick (Ornithodorus) borne occurs as sporadic/endemic.**

Vincent Angina

- Causative agent – **B. vincenti.**
- Normal mouth commensal but when associated with fusiform bacilli causes ulcerative gingivostomatitis or oropharyngitis called **Vincent angina.**

MCQs

Spirochaetes

1. **Incubation period of syphilis:** *(AIIMS 11)*
   (a) 1 hour - 5 hours
   (b) 24 hours - 48 hours
   (c) 1 day - 10 days
   (d) 10 days - 90 days
2. **Investigation of choice for detection of syphilis in a patient after 2 course of complete therapy:** *(Recent MCQ)*
   (a) FTAABS
   (b) VDRL
   (c) TPI
   (d) Dark ground microscopy
3. **Syphilis was first identified:** *(Manipal 08, Recent MCQ)*
   (a) Fraenkel
   (b) Nicolair
   (c) Schaudinn and Hoffman
   (d) Ogston
4. **Following is true of T. pallidum *except*:** *(PGI 98)*
   (a) Can be maintained in rabbit testis
   (b) Motile by peritrichate flagella
   (c) To visualise, dark ground microscopy is used
   (d) TPI test is very useful

5. Stain for treponema: *(APPG 09)*

(a) Fontana's
(b) Acid-facid
(c) Methenamine-silver
(d) PAS

6. In a syphilis patient, site which does not help in isolation of organism: *(AIIMS 06)*

(a) Gumma
(b) Primary chancre
(c) Mucosal patch
(d) Maculopapular rash

7. True about primary chancre: *(PGI May 14)*

(a) Painless ulcer
(b) Painless lymphadenopathy
(c) Covered with exudate
(d) Indurated lesion
(e) Organism can be cultured from exudative fluid

8. The skin lesions of secondary syphilis include all of the following *except*: *(Recent MCQ)*

(a) Macules
(b) Nodule
(c) Vesicles and Bullae
(d) Papulosquamous

9. 23 years old male had unprotected sexual intercourse with a commercial sex worker. Two weeks later, he developed a painless, indurated ulcer on the glans that exuded clear serum on pressure. Inguinal lymph nodes in both groins were enlarged and not tender. The most appropriate diagnostic test is: *(AIIMS May 04)*

(a) Gram's stain of ulcer discharge
(b) Dark field microscopy of ulcer discharge
(c) Giemsa stain of lymph node aspirate
(d) ELISA for HIV infection

10. Tabes dorsalis is seen in: *(APPG 11)*

(a) Primary syphilis
(b) Secondary syphilis
(c) Tertiary syphilis
(d) Latent syphilis

11. Confirmatory test for syphilis: *(APPG 12)*

(a) VDRL
(b) FTAABS
(c) RPR
(d) None

12. After giving treatment for syphilis, the response to treatment can be best assessed by: *(AIIMS Nov 99, Recent MCQ)*

(a) FTA- ABS
(b) VDRL
(c) TPHA
(d) Immobilization test

13. Diagnostic test of choice for neurosyphilis is: *(RJ 07, UPPG 10)*

(a) VDRL
(b) FTA-ABS
(c) TPI
(d) RPR

14. Most sensitive test for Treponema: *(APPG 05, Recent MCQ)*

(a) VDRL
(b) RPR
(c) FTA-ABS
(d) Kahn

15. False + ve VDRL, is seen in all *except*: *(AI 00)*

(a) Lepromatous leprosy
(b) Infectious mononucleosis
(c) HIV
(d) Pregnancy

16. True about VDRL test: *(Recent MCQ)*

(a) Non-specific
(b) Slide flocculation test
(c) Best followed for drug therapy
(d) All

17. Regarding syphilis, all are true, *except*: *(AIIMS Nov 93, UPPG 08)*

(a) VDRL titre decreases or even absent after treatment
(b) VDRL becomes positive after 10-14 days of infection

(c) Earliest serological test to become positive in untreated primary syphilis is TPHA
(d) Yaws and Pinta cannot be differentiated

18. All are true about FTA-ABS in Syphilis, *except*: *(Recent MCQ)*
(a) FTA - ABS becomes negative after treatment
(b) Present in secondary syphilis
(c) It is a specific test
(d) May be positive in Lyme's disease

19. 36-year-old labourer 3 years back presented with penile ulcer not treated. Later he presented with neurological symptoms for which he got treated. Test to monitor response to treatment is: *(AIIMS 13)*
(a) VDRL
(c) TPI
(b) FTA-ABS
(d) RPR

20. Congenital syphilis can be best diagnosed by: *(UPPG 13)*
(a) IgM FTA- ABS
(b) IgG FTA-ABS
(c) VDRL
(d) TPI

21. VDRL reactive mother gave birth to an infant. All of the following would help in determining the risk of transmission to the infant *except*: *(AI 06, APPG 12)*
(a) TPHA test on the serum sample of the mother
(b) TPHA test on the serum sample of the infant
(c) VDRL on the paired serum sample of the infant and mother
(d) Time interval between the treatment of the mother and her delivery

22. Regarding yaws, all are true *except*: *(Recent MCQ)*
(a) Caused by T. pertenue
(b) Sexually transmitted
(c) Cross reactive antibodies with syphilis
(d) Drug of choice is penicillin

23. All of the following statements about, Yaws are true *except*: *(AI 2002)*
(a) Caused by Treponema pertenue
(b) Transmitted non venerally
(c) Secondary yaws can involve bone
(d) Late stages of yaws involve heart and nerves

24. The following are true regarding Lyme's disease, *except*: *(APPG 15)*
(a) It is transmitted by ixodid tick
(b) Erythema chronicum migraines may be a clinical feature
(c) Borrelia recurrentis is the aetiological agent
(d) Rodents act as natural hosts

25. Which of the following species of Borrelia are associated with tick borne relapsing fever, *except*? *(AI 09)*
(a) Borrelia recurrentis
(b) Borrelia hennsii
(c) Borrelia turicatae
(d) Borrelia duttoni

26. True about B. recurrentis: *(APPG 14)*
(a) Causes leptospirosis
(b) Water borne disease
(c) Vector borne disease
(d) Transmitted by tick

27. Bacterial disease that has been associated with the 3 "Rs" i.e., rats, ricefields and rainfall is a: *(UPPG 13)*
(a) Leptospirosis
(b) Plague
(c) Melioidosis
(d) Rodent-bite fever

28. Weils' disease is caused by: *(Manipal 14, Recent MCQ)*
(a) Leptospira
(b) Listeria
(c) Mycoplasma
(d) Legionella

29. A 25-year-old farmer presented with history of high grade fever for 7 days and altered sensorium for 2 days. On examination, he was comatosed and had conjunctival hemorrhage. Urgent investigations showed a hemoglobin of 11 gm/dl, serum bilirubin 9 mg/dl and urea 78 mg/dl peripheral blood smear was negative for malarial parasite. What is the most likely diagnosis? (*AIIMS 12*)

(a) Brucellosis (b) Weil's disease
(c) Acute viral hepatitis (d) Q fever

30. Not used in leptospirosis: (*AIIMS May 10*)

(a) Microscopic agglutination test (b) Dark field illumination
(c) Macroscopic agglutination test (d) Weil-Felix reaction

31. Leptospira canicola infection usually present as: (*APPG 16*)

(a) Aseptic meningitis (b) Jaundice
(c) Diarrhoea and vomiting (d) Lobar pneumonia

32. A sewage worker presents to the emergency department with fever and jaundice. Laboratory findings reveal an elevated BUN and serum creatinine suggestive of renal failure. Which of the following antibiotics is recommended? (*UPPG 14*)

(a) Cotrimoxazole (b) Erythromycin
(c) Penicillin G (d) Ciprofloxacin

33. Culture media of leptospirosis: (*AIIMS 13*)

(a) Korthokoff (b) Perkin
(c) Tinsdale (d) Baker's

34. Labourer involved with repair work of sewers was admitted with fever, jaundice and renal failure. The most appropriate test to diagnose the infection in this patient is: (*Manipal 12, Recent MCQ*)

(a) Weil-Felix test (b) Paul Bunnell test
(c) Microscopic agglutination test (d) Microimmunofluorescence test

ANSWERS AND EXPLANATIONS

(Harrison, 19th/e, p. 1132; Ananthanarayan, 9th/e, p. 370)

1. **Ans. is 'd'** i.e., 10 days-90 days (***Ref:*** *Ananthanarayan, 9th/e, p. 372; Harrison, 18th/e, p. 381, 382*)
   IP – 9-90 days
2. **Ans. is 'b'** i.e., VDRL (***Ref:*** *Ananthanarayan, 9th/e, p. 375 and 8th/e, p. 374-375*)
   Test of choice for therapy evaluation – VDRL.
3. **Ans. is 'c'** i.e., Schaudinn and Hoffman (***Ref:*** *Ananthanarayan, 9th/e, p. 371 and 8th/e, p. 372*)
4. **Ans. is 'b'** i.e., Motile by peritrichate flagella (***Ref:*** *Ananthanarayan, 9th/e, p. 371 and 8th/e, p. 372*)
   T pallidum is motile by endoflagella, which are polar flagella.
   Direct Microscopy:
   - Dark field microscopy.
   - Direct IF staining from sample (DFA-TP).
   - Silver impregnation method (Levaditi stain for tissue section and Fontana stain for smear).
5. **Ans. is 'a'** i.e., Fontana's stain (***Ref:*** *Ananthanarayan, 9th/e, p. 371 and 8th/e, p. 372*)
   Fontana's method is used for staining films and Levaditi's method for tissue sections.
6. **Ans. is 'a'** i.e., Gumma (***Ref:*** *Ananthanarayan, 9th/e, p. 372, 373 and 8th/e, p. 374*)
   - T. pallidum is very difficult to demonstrate in **Gumma (Tertiary syphilis).** Infectivity of a patient to the sexual partner is maximum during primary, secondary and early latent stage. During these stages spirochetes are abundant in the lesions.

7. **Ans. are 'a, b, c, d'** (***Ref:*** *Ananthanarayan, 9th/e, p. 372*)

For option 'e' – **Pathogenic Treponemes cannot be isolated on artificial media or in tissue culture but Nichole's strain can be maintained in rabbit testes. Nonpathogenic Reiter's strain can grow in artificial media.**

Hard chancre: Ulcer of primary syphilis – Spirochetes multiply locally at the site of entry, and some spread to nearby lymph nodes and then reach the bloodstream. Within 2–10 weeks after infection, a papule develops at the site of infection and breaks down to form an ulcer with a clean, hard base ("hard chancre").

Soft chancre (chancroid): Ulcer caused by **H. ducreyi.**

8. **Ans. is 'c'** i.e., Vesicles and Bullae

(***Ref:*** *Harrison, 18th/e, p. 1382, 1383; 17th/e, p. 1040-1041; Ananthanarayan, 9th/e, p. 373*)

Vesicles and bullae are seen in congenital syphilis (not in secondary syphilis).

Note: Venereal syphilis is acquired by sexual contact, T. pallidum rapidly penetrates intact mucous membranes or microscopic abrasions in skin.

Tabes dorsalis and general paresis of insane are known us late tertiary or quaternary syphilis.

When syphilis is transmitted by blood transfusion, the primary chancre does not occur.

9. **Ans. is 'b'** i.e., Dark field microscopy of ulcer discharge (***Ref:*** *Harrison, 17th/e, p. 1384 and 18th/e, p. 1043*)

History is indicating towards syphilis and T. pallidum can be seen from ulcer discharge by using Dark field microscopy.

10. **Ans. is 'c'** i.e., Tertiary syphilis

Tabes dorsalis, also known as syphilitic myelopathy, is a slow degeneration (specifically, demyelination) of the nerves primarily in the dorsal columns (posterior columns) of the spinal cord (the portion closest to the back of the body). These nerves normally help maintain a person's sense of position (proprioception), vibration and discriminative touch.

Tabes dorsalis is caused by demyelination caused by advanced syphilis infection (tertiary syphilis), when the primary infection by the causative spirochete bacterium Treponema pallidum is left untreated for an extended period of time (past the point of blood infection by the organism).

11. **Ans. is 'b'** i.e., FTAABS (***Ref:*** *Ananthanarayan, 9th/e, p. 375 and 8th/e, p. 375-377*)

- **Treponemal or specific tests for syphilis – detects specific Abs against T. pallidum Ag – FTA-ABS, Agglutination assays (MHA-TP, TPHA, TPPA), TPI (dark ground microscope is required for observing immobilization).**

12. **Ans. is 'b'** i.e., VDRL (***Ref:*** *Ananthanarayan, 9th/e, p. 375 and 8th/e, p. 375, 377*)

Already explained.

13. **Ans. is 'a'** i.e., VDRL (***Ref:*** *Ananthanarayan, 9th/e, p. 375 and 8th/e, p. 375, 377*)

Among the serological tests, the VDRL CSF test is the standard serological test for CSF and it is considered diagnostic of neurosyphilis.

Specific treponemal tests (TPPA, FTA-ABS, TPHA) have proved to be quite inaccurate in the diagnosis of neurosyphilis because the antibodies against the specific treponemal antigen have the tendency to cross CSF; so enough antibodies may be present in CSF even before neurosyphilis develops. Therefore, specific treponemal tests have no specificity for neurosyphilis. The CSF becomes positive for these tests even when neurosyphilis is not present.

14. **Ans. is 'c'** i.e., FTA-ABS

Most sensitive test – FTA-ABS

- Most specific test – TPI (Now not used).
- Test of choice for rapid diagnosis and mass screening in medical camps – RPR.
- Test of choice for therapy evaluation – VDRL.
- Test of choice for diagnosis of congenital syphilis – IgM FTA-ABS.

15. **Ans. is 'd'** i.e., Pregnancy (***Ref:*** *Harrison, 18th/e, p. 1385*)

Since the test employs a non-treponemal antigen, there are many chances of false positive results. False positivity (other than technical) may be due to physiological of pathological conditions. These are called biological false positives (BFP).

If they remain positive for less than 6 months it is considered acute and they remain positive for longer than 6 months it is called chronic BFP.

The physiological reasons for BFP include pregnancy (Rarely), menstruation, repeated blood loss, vaccination, severe trauma etc., while the reasons for pathological BFP include malaria, infectious mononucleosis, hepatitis, relapsing fever, tropical eosinophilia, lepromatous leprosy, SLE, rheumatoid arthritis, who have recently been immunized etc.

A reactive VDRL test does not necessarily imply that the person is syphilitic. The diagnosis must be made in conjunction with clinical findings. Any reactive VDRL test must be confirmed with a specific or treponemal test such as TPHA, FTA-ABS test.

16. Ans. is 'd' i.e., All

(***Ref:*** *Ananthanarayan, 9th/e, p. 374 and 8th/e, p. 375; Harrison, 19th/e, p. 1385 and 17th/e, p. 1043*)

Type of VDRL test is Slide flocculation test.

17. Ans. are 'b, c'

(***Ref:*** *Ananthanarayan, 9th/e, p. 374, 375 and 8th/e, p. 375; Harrison, 18th/e, p. 1385 and 17th/e, p. 1043*)

The FTA-ABS test is the first to become positive. – *Jawetz, 23rd/e, p. 333*

Reagin antibody tests (VDRL and RPR) become positive 3-5 weeks after acquiring the infection (7-10 days after the appearance of primary chancre).

18. Ans. is 'a' i.e., FTA – ABS becomes negative after treatment

(***Ref:*** *Ananthanarayan, 9th/e, p. 375 and 8th/e, p. 376-377; Harrison, 18th/e, p. 1385 and 17th/e, p. 1043*)

Specific treponemal tests (FTA-ABS, TPHA, TPI) are of little value as indicators of clinical cure, as they tend to remain positive in spite of treatment because of it. Specific tests are not used in monitoring of the treatment. **VDRL or RPR can be used for treatment monitoring as specific tests remain positive (reactive) after the treatment.**

19. Ans. is 'a' i.e., VDRL (***Ref:*** *Ananthanarayan, 8th/e, p. 375*)

For CSF sample (neurosyphilis) VDRL is preferred over RPR.

20. Ans. is 'a' i.e., IgM FTA- ABS (***Ref:*** *Harrison, 16th/e, p. 982*)

Already explained.

* Test of choice for diagnosis of congenital syphilis – IgM FTA-ABS.

IgM can be detected in Acute or recent infection.

21. Ans. is 'b' i.e., TPHA test on the serum sample of the infant

Tests for antibodies in the newborn's blood are not always positive at first, even when infection is present in the infant, possibly because if the infection is acquired late in pregnancy, specific antibody have not had time to form.

ABOUT OTHER OPTIONS

Option 'a' – A positive TPHA on maternal serum confirms the diagnosis of maternal syphilis and depending on the age of gestation indicate the risk of transmission.

Option 'c' – Infant should be evaluated for congenital syphilis if the newborn has a titre four-fold greater than mother (Examination of paired serum example of the infant and mother).

Option 'd' – Early and adequate treatment of mother decreases the risk of transmission.

22. Ans. is 'b' i.e., Sexually transmitted

(***Ref:*** *Anathnarayan, 9th/e, p. 377 and 8th/e, p. 377*)

Penicillin is the drug of choice for all treponematosis.

Non Venereal Treponemes

- Mode of transmission – Direct contact not sexual.
- Endemic syphilis (Bejel) – Caused by T. pallidum subsp. endemicum.
- Yaws – Caused by T. pallidum subsp. pertenue.
- Pinta – Caused by T. pallidum subsp. carateum.
- In Non-Venereal Treponematosis, Yaws and Pinta gives +ve for serological tests for syphilis.

23. Ans. is 'd' i.e., Late stages of yaws involve heart and nerves

(***Ref:*** *Park, 21st/e, p. 314, 315; Ananthanarayan, 9th/e, p. 377 and 8th/e, p. 378*)

Yaw is a chronic contagious non-veneral disease caused by Treponema pertunae. It resembles syphilis in its clinical course and is characterised by a primary skin lesion (mother yaw) followed by a generalised eruption and a later stage of destructive lesions of the skin and bone. However, unlike syphilis, cardiovascular and neurological manifestations are rare. As in syphilis, secondary and tertiary manifestations follow in yaws, but cardiovascular and neurological involvement is rare.

24. Ans. is 'c' i.e., Borrelia recurrentis is the etiological agent

25. Ans. is 'a' i.e., Borrelia recurrentis (***Ref:*** *Ananthanarayan, 9th/e, p. 380*)

Louse borne Epidemic R.F. or LBRF Q	**Tick borne (TBRF) Endemic R.E. Q**
Caused by B. recurrentis	Caused by: B. duttoni, B. parken
	B. hermesii
	B. turicatae
RF – Relapsing fever	B. hispanica

26. Ans. is 'c' i.e., Vector borne disease (***Ref:*** *Ananthanarayan, 9th/e, p. 378 and 8th/e, p. 275*)

Already explained.

27. Ans. is 'a' i.e., Leptospirosis

28. Ans. is 'a' i.e., Leptospira (***Ref:*** *Harrison, 18th/e, p. 1394 and 17th/e, p. 1050*)

- Leptospirosis – Sewer worker disease, Weil's disease or Icterohemorrhagic fever (jaundice + fever).

29. Ans. is 'b' i.e., Weil's disease (***Ref:*** *Harrison, 18th/e, p. 1394 and 17th/e, p. 1050*)

High grade fever, altered sensorium, sign of hemorrhagic diathesis (conjunctival hemorrhage) along with raised BUN and serum bilirubin are suggestive of Weil's disease. The time between a person's exposure to a contaminated source and becoming sick is 2 days to 4 weeks. Illness usually begins abruptly with fever and other symptoms. Leptospirosis may occur in two phases:

- **After the first phase (with fever, chills, headache, muscle aches, vomiting, or diarrhea) the patient may recover for a time but become ill again.**
- **If a second phase occurs, it is more severe; the person may have kidney or liver failure or meningitis. This phase is also called Weil's disease.**

30. Ans. is 'd' i.e., Weil-Felix reaction

(***Ref:*** *Ananthanarayan, 9th/e, p. 382-383 and 8th/e, p. 383; Greenwood Microbiology*)

Weil-Felix reaction (Heterophile agglutination test) is used for diagnosis of Rickettsial infection.

31. Ans. is 'a' i.e., Aseptic meningitis (***Ref:*** *Ananthanarayan, p. 382*)

L. canicola causes Canicola fever which presents either influenza like illness or aseptic meningitis.

32. Ans. is 'c' i.e., Penicillin G (***Ref:*** *Harrison, 18th/e, p. 1396; Greenwood, 16th/e, p. 3551*)

- DOC – Penicillin (severe form) or oral doxycycline (mild form).

33. Ans. is 'a' i.e., Korthokoff (***Ref:*** *Ananthanarayan, 9th/e, p. 381*)

- Culture media – EMJH, Fletcher and Korthokoff.

34. Ans. is 'c' i.e., Microscopic agglutination test (***Ref:*** *Harrison, 18th/e, p. 1395 and 17th/e, p. 1050*)

- IOC – serological – Microscopic agglutination test (MAT) – Gold standard and Macroscopic agglutination test.

MISCELLANEOUS BACTERIOLOGY

MISCELLANEOUS BACTERIOLOGY

1. Anaerobic gram positive bacilli are Eubacterium, propionibacterium, lactobacillus, mobiluncus, bifidobacterium and Actinomyces.
2. Peptostreptococcus is anaerobic gram positive coccus and can cause puerperal sepsis.
3. Regarding the biological activity of lipopolysaccharides of Bacteroides fragilis.
   (a) **"They possess lipopolysaccharides (endotoxins) that are less biologically potent than endotoxins Q associated with aerobic gram negative bacteria. This relative biologic inactivity may account for lower frequency of disseminated intravascular coagulation and purpura in Bacteroides bacteremia than in facultative and aerobic gram negative bacillary bacteremia.**
4. Bacteroides are anaerobes and are commonly, implicated in causing brain abscess. **Prevotella melaninogenica** Q is a species of Bacteroides which gives **characteristic red fluorescence** when exposed to ultraviolet light. **It is also a common cause for brain abscess.Q**
5. **Corynebacterium pseudotuberculosis** is also called **Preisz-Nocard bacillus.**
6. **Fournier's gangrene** is a necrotising fascitis of genitalia, usually affecting the scrotum and penis.
   (a) Majority of cases are due to mixed infection caused both aerobic and anaerobic bacteria.
   (b) Following are common causative organisms: Staphylococcus aureus, streptococcus pyogenes (beta-hemolytic streptococci), Enterobacteriaceae (E. coli, klebsiella, proteus), enterococci, pseudomonas, and anaerobes like bacteroides and peptostreptococcus.
7. **Pyomyositis:** It is common in tropics, therefore also called Tropical pyomyositis. It is a localized infection of skeletal muscles. It is caused most commonly by Staphylococcus aureus.
8. **Necrotizing fasciitis:** Necrotizing fasciitis is an infection of the deeper layers of skin and subcutaneous tissues, easily spreading across the fascial plane within the subcutaneous tissues. There are two types of necrotizing fasciitis:
   (a) **Type 1:** It is a polymicrobial infection, i.e., mixed aerobic and anaerobic infection. It occurs most commonly after surgical procedures in diabetic patients or in those who have peripheral vascular disease.
   (b) **Type 2:** It is caused most commonly by Streptococcus pyogenes (Group A beta hemolytic streptococci).
9. **Clostridial myonecrosis (Gas gangrene):** It is characterized by rapid and extensive necrosis of muscle.
   (a) Accompanied by gas formation and systemic toxicity. It is caused by C. perfringens (most common), C. novyii.
   (b) C. septicum und C. histolyticum. It is also called type III necrotizing fasciitis.
10. **Vancomycin resistance** may be due to:
   (a) Synthesis of low affinity precursors, in which the C terminal D-Ala residue is replaced by D-Lactate (D-Lac) or D-serine (D-Ser thus modifying the Vancomycin-binding target.Q
   (b) Elimination of the high affinity precursors that are normally produced by the host.
   (c) Vancomycin-binding target.
11. Polysaccharide capsule is the primarly virulence factor for Pneumococcus, meningococcus and Haemophilus Influenza (type b).
12. **HACEK** bacteria normally inside in the oral cavity and have been associated with local infections in the mouth and also cause **culture negative endocarditis.**
13. Causes of Rat bite fever – Streptobaciillus moniliformis, spirillum minus.Q
14. Septicemia is defined as Circulation and multiplication of bacteria in blood. Bacteremia is defined as Circulation (not multiplication) of bacteria in blood. Toxemia is defined as Circulation of toxin in blood. Pyaemia is defined presence of pus in blood.

15. Most common cause of Pyomyositis (tropical pyomyositis) – Staphylococcus aureus.
16. Most common cause of upper respiratory tract infection is viral infection. **Rhinovirus is the most common cause.**
17. Among the bacteria group A beta-hemolytic streptococci (Streptococcus pyogenes) is the most common cause and most common type of infection is pharyngitis.
18. **Chancre redux** is the appearance of relapsing lesion at the site of the healed lesion, it is due to relapse of original infection not due to reinfection.
19. Bacterial vaginosis is caused by Gardenella vaginalis, Prevotella and Mobiluncus, Amsler criteria is followed: (1) Clue cells present (2) Whiff test positive – in Discharge when KOH is put, fishy smell comes (3) PH>4.5 of vagina.

RED ALERT POINTS

1. The diagnostic test for Rickettsial infection is: **Weil-Felix reaction (cross reactivity between Nonmotile Proteus strains and Rickettsial family members is a heterophile agglutination test) it is OX-K positive for Scrub typhus.**
2. The causative agent of **Lyme's** disease: **Borrelia burgdorferi, BSK media is used, Erythema Chronicum migrans is seen.**
3. Clostridium tetani is: **Gram positive bacilli Drum stick shape, spore forming, causes tetanus (8th day disease), tetanospasmin acts presynaptically on inhibitory neurotransmitter Glycine and GABA.**
4. The sulphur granules in the wound are diagnostic of: **Actinomyces, oral actinomycosis most common site is cervicofacial and triad of Sulphur granules, Sinus and Swelling.**
5. Legionella pneumonia is: **Can be isolated from lung biopsy and water ingestion from aquatic source (Main mode of transmission).**
6. Botulinum toxin acts by: **Inhibits Ach release** at neuromuscular junction mainly, autonomic ganglia, postganglionic parasympathetic nerve endings and postganglionic sympathetic nerve endings that release acetylcholine. Most potent toxin on earth.
7. Fermentation of mannitol is basis of classification of Shigella sps. Shigella dysentriae is mannitol non-fermenter and Shigella dysentriae type I is Catalase negative.
8. **Elek test** is used for toxin demonstration in: **Diphtheria, Shick test determines suspectibility of an individual to diphtheria, it is a neutralization test.**
9. **Johne's** Bacillus is: **M. Paratuberculosis, Kleb lofflers bacilli is C. diphtheriae, Pffefiers bacilli is Haemophilus influenza, Nicolaire bacilli is Treponema pallidum, Preisz nocard bacilli is Corynebacterium pseudo TB, Friedlanders bacilli is Klebsiella pneumoniae.**
10. **Pikes** medium is used for transport of: **Streptococci pyogenes and Crystal violet blood agar is used as a selective medium, classification is based upon hemolysis.**
11. **Draughtsman** concentric rings on culture are produced by: **Pneumococci, it is Bile soluble, Inulin fermenter, Optochin sensitive (BIO positive).**
12. In **Legionnaire's** disease, the culture medium used is: **BCYE medium, pontaic fever is also caused by legionella pneumophila which is self limiting, common cause of atypical pneumonia, a species legionella micadedi is acid fast in nature.**
13. **Bread crumb** colony appearance is of: **Actinomyces Israeli, it is non acid fast, actinomyces species causes cervicofacial variety of oral actinomycosis with Sulphur granules.**
14. **Weil-Felix** raection is: Heterophile **agglutination reaction, cross reaction of proteus sps with rickettsial family members, other heterophile agglutination reaction are Paul Bunnel test, Streptococcus MG agglutination test.**
15. Shortest incubation period is for which food poisoning: **Bacillus cereus emetic strain (Chinese fried rice) of 1-6 hours which resembles Staphylococcus aureus food poisoning contaminated meat and milk (1-6 hours).**
16. **O 157:H7 strain** of E.coli can be grown in: **Sorbitol macconkey agar and Rainbow agar.**
17. **Buruli ulcer** is caused by: **Mycobacterium ulcerans. Mycobacterium marinum leads to swimming pool granuloma, Mycobacterium avium intracellulare and Mycobacterium kansasii infection mimics tuberculosis in its presentation.**
18. Klebsiella pneumoniae cause typical lobar pneumonia, atypical pneumonia is caused by legionella and mycoplasma sps.
19. Most common species of Pseudomonas causing **intravenous catheter** related infection is: **P. cepacia and pseudomonas aeruginosa is having green colour pigment, plays a role in causing burn wound infection, Shanghai fever, Malignant otitis externa. Best selective media is Cetrimide agar and best for pigment production is Kings media.**

20. Stalactite growth is a feature of Yersinia pestis in ghee broth, Bisected pearl appearance seen on Bordet gengou media of Bordetella pertussis.
21. The most common organism isolated in emphysematous pyelonepharitis is: **E. coli, it causes mainly UTI, Diarrhoea and Neonatal meningitis. IM Vi C is (+ + - -).**
22. Lancefield classification based on: **Carbohydrate antigen and Grp A further typed with help of M protein, called as Griffith typing. Transport media is Pikes media, streptococcus pyogenes is known as Flesh eating bacteria (Necrotizing fasciitis), Streptococcus pyogenes is bacitracin sensitive but Streptococcus agalactiae is Bacitracin resistant.**
23. Selective media for vibrio: **TCBS (Thiosulphate citrate bile salt sucrose), transport media is VR media, Cary Blair media. It shows Fish in stream appearance, Darting motility is seen in Hanging drop preparation.**
24. **Malta fever**, meditteranean fever is caused by: **Brucellamelitensis, Erythritol is added to blood culture bottle to stimulate growth of Brucella species, Tblisi phage typing is done for Brucella typing. Milk ring test, rose Bengal card test and whey agglutination are test performed for milk contamination.**
25. Burkholderia pseudomallei (Whitmore bacilli) causes Melioidosis and is nonmotile, Burkholderia mallei causes Glanders disease and is motile, both are bipolar stained and are non-fermenters. Acinetobacter baumanii is also a nonfermenter and is a common MDR isolate found in ICU settings.
26. Culture media for leptospirosis: **Korthof, EMJH, Fletcher, leptospirainterrogans causes Weil's disease. Rat, Rice and Rain are commonly associated with leptospirosis and National referral centre for leptospira is in Port Blair.**
27. **Campylobacter** is microaerophilic, Gull wing shape bacteria, Fecal leucocytes are visible, charcoal based media like Butzler, skirrow are used for culture.
28. **Clostridium perfringens:** The major enzyme secreted is hyaluronidase, causes gas gangrene, food poisoning, pigbel.
29. BCG (Bacillus calmette guerin) vaccine if constituted has to be used in: **(1 day) reconstituted with normal saline, given by intradermal route and have an efficacy of 0-80% efficacy.**
30. The most common bacterial cause of diarrhea in Travellers is: **Enterotoxigenic Escherichia coli, Enteroaggregative E.coli also leads to travelers' diarrhea. Heat stable and heat labile toxin of E.coli are responsible for diarrhea.**
31. The most common cause of antibiotic induced colitis is due to: **Clostridium difficile (Demonstration of Enterotoxin and cytotoxin is done on Hep2 cell lines. Oral vancomycin is indicated. CDAD (clostridium difficile associated diarrhea), Pseudomembranous colitis are associated with clostridium difficile infection.**
32. Actinomycosis is caused by: **Bacteria (Gram positive bacteria, causing oral actinomycosis (Cervicofacial is most common variety) having sulphur granules and sunray appearance is a feature).**
33. **Tumbling motility** is shown by: **Listeria, Darting – Vibrio cholera, Swarming – Proteus, Falling leaf like – Giardia lamblia, corkscrew motility – Treponema pallidum).**
34. **Eaton** agent is: **Mycoplasma (Dienes method of staining is seen), Sterol in cell membrane and no cell wall).**
35. **Pea-soup stool** is characteristically seen in: **Typhoid and from longitudinal ulcers are seen. Step ladder pattern fever is present, rose spots are also seen.**
36. Reinfection TB is almost exclusively a disease of the: **Lungs (Cavity formation is seen).**
37. **Ito's test** is useful in the diagnosis of: **Chancroid (soft sore), school of fish appearance is a feature.**
38. Dark ground illumination helps to detect: **Leptospira, Treponema, Borrelia using reflected light.**
39. **Satellitism** is seen in culture of: **Hemophilus influenza (Type b PRP is used for Hib vaccine production.**
40. Endemic typhus is transmitted by: **Rat flea and caused by Rickettsia typhi.**
41. Organism detected in ischorectal fossa: **E. coli.**
42. Vi antigen is used for epidemiologic typing, Ab to Vi if absent indicates poor prognosis.
43. Strain of streptococci is implicated in Neonatal meningitis is: **Group B streptococci, infact it is the second most common cause of neonatal meningitis, it is present in normal vaginal flora, it is CAMP test positive, Hippurate hydrolysis test positive.**

44. Weil's disease is caused by: **Leptospira interrogans and concerned with RRR – rat, rice and rain. Infection spread by Contaminated rat urine in paddy field worker and mostly in rainy season.**
45. Causative agent of Yaws: **Treponema pertenue, Pinta – T. carateum, Bejel – Treponema endemicum.**
46. Chlamydia escapes killing by: **Molecular mimicry, Elementary and reticulate bodies are seen. Investigation of choice – NAAT – nucleic acid amplification test.**
47. Generation time of Mycobacterium leprae: **12-14 days.**
48. **Scrub typhus is positive for OX-K, Rocky mountain spotted fever is strongly positive for OX-19 and OX-2, basis of Weil-Felix reaction.**
49. Gonorrhoea is identified by: **Fermentation of glucose from Meningococci which ferments Glucose and maltose both.**
50. Melioidosis is caused by: **Burkholderia pseudomallei (whitmore bacilli), Burkholderia mallei causes Glanders disease and is nonmotile.**
51. Pseudomembrane formation happens in diphtheria. Most common site is Faucial and narrowest site is laryngeal. Bull neck is seen because of Edema and lymphadenopathy.
52. Features of El Tor vibrio: Hardier and survives longer; milder disease with more subclinical cases and less mortality; Low SAR (secondary attack rate).
53. True about V cholerae: Gram (-)ve, curved (comma shaped) rod, obligate aerobe, indole production and nitrate reduction positive, resistant to alkaline pH, best grow at 37°C, produces neuraminidase.
54. Bacillary angiomatosis is caused by: **Bartonella henselae, common in HIV individuals, B. henselae leads to Cat scratch disease.**
55. Drug resistance in TB is due to: **Mutation. Anti-tubercular drug susceptibility** tests are Absolute concentration, resistance ratio, proportion method, molecular method, radiometric broth. **Not a susceptibility test for antitubercular drugs**: **Disc diffusion method.**
56. **Photochromogens** are: M. asiaticum, M. kansasii, M. marinum, M.simiae.

    Scotochromogenes are: M. flovescens. M. gordonae, M. scrofulaceum, M. szulgi.

    Non-chromogens are: MAC (M. intracellulare and M. avium), M. haemophilum, M. gastri, M. ulcerans, M. xenopi. **Rapid growers** are: M. abscessus, M. fortuitum, M. chelonae, M. phlei, M. smegmatis, M. vaccae.
57. M. tuberculosis is differentiated from other mycobacteria by: Niacin test, nitrate reduction test, arylsulfatase test, neutral red test, amidase test, catalase-peroxidase test.
58. Symptoms of pneumonia with demonstration of acid-fast, aerobic gram-positive filament: Nocardia asteroides.
59. Technique used to isolate Nocardia: Paraffin baiting.

    Stains used for Nocardia: Z-Nstain, Kinyoun stain, Fite-faraco stains (Mucicarmine, Alcian blue).
60. **Predominantly saccharolytic** clostridia: Cl perfringens, Cl novyi, Cl septicum, Cl difficile. **Only saccharolytic** (not proteolytic) clostridia: Cl botulinum C, D, E.

    Predominantly proteolytic clostridia: Cl sporogenes, Cl bifermentans, Cl botulinum A, B/F, Cl histolyticum. **Only proteolytic** (not saccharolytic) clostridia: Cl tetani.

    Neither proteolytic nor saccharolytic clostridia: Cl cochlearum.
61. **Levinthal Coles Lillie bodies** are seen in: C. psittacosis, HP bodies, Miyagawa corpuscles.
62. Reiter's syndrome is caused by: C. trachomatis, ureaplasma urealyticum, salmonella spp, shigella, campylobacter spp.
63. Appendicitis like feature can be caused by: Y enterocolitica, Y pseudotuberculosis, Pasteurella septic (Pasteurella multocida).
64. Important virulence factors of H pylori: Cag A, Vac A (vacuolating cytotoxin), Bab A, urease.
65. Selective media for V cholerae: BSA, GTTA, TCBS.

    Transport media for V cholerae: VR medium, Cary-Blair medium, autoclaved sea water. Enrichment media for V cholerae: Alkaline peptone water, Monsur's taurocholate peptone water.

66. Screening test for carrier of typhoid: Vi antibody test.

    Confirmatory test for carrier of typhoid: Culture, either from feces/duodenal aspirate (in fecal carrier) or urine (in urinary carrier).
67. Charbonis: Another name of malignant pustule, Hideporter's disease, Wool sorter's disease.
68. B. anthracis differs from anthracoid bacilli by being: Non-motile, capsulated, non-hemolytic.
69. Tetanus is caused by presynaptic inhibition of GABA and GLYCINE (inhibitory neurotransmitter) which results in constant stimulation with lockjaw and opisthotonus.
70. Mycobacterium leprae is not cultivated on normal media, difficult to grow, grown mostly in foot pad of armadillo, Ridley jopling classification is used to classify.
71. Fecal leucocytes are present in: **Campylobacter infection, with gull wing shape, predispose to GBS (Guillain-Barré syndrome).**
72. HACEK group of organisms does **not** include: **Acinetobacter-baumannii, it is Actinobacillus myceticomitans. Name others.**
73. **N.gonorrhoea** is becoming increasingly resistant to penicillin because of plasmid, Auxotyping and pili based typing is seen.
74. **In Diphtheria:** Maculopapular rash is not present but pseudomembrane formation seen in Faucial and laryngeal lesions mostly.
75. Primary atypical penumonia is **mostly caused by Mycoplasma pneumoniae, Legionella pneumophila.**
76. Plasmid borne – Tetanospasmin of C. tetani, Pertussis toxin, Heat labile toxin of ETEC, Anthrax toxin (TPHA).
77. Chromosomal – Pyrogenic toxin B of S. pyogenes, Pertussis toxin, Cholera toxin, Shiga Toxin and Exotoxin A of P. aeruginosa **(PCS Examination).**
78. Phage encoded – Botulinum toxin, pyrogenic toxin A, C of Streptococcus pyogenes, Verotoxin (shiga like toxin) EHEC, Diphtheria toxin **(Buerger PVD).**
79. Clostridium tetani – Nicolaire's bacillus, klebsiella ozaenae – Abel bacillus.
80. Chromatid body – Entamoeba histolytica precyst, citron bodies – Cl. Septicum, Councilman bodies – Yellow fever, LCL – Levinthal Cole Lillie bodies, Halberstaedter Prowazek body – Chlamydia trachomatis.
81. Rota virus inhibits Na K ATPase is present in BMC CESS – Bacillus cereus (diarrhoeal), Medullary carcinoma thyroid, Cholera, Carcinoid, ETEC labile toxin Salmonella, Staphylococcus.
82. Food poisoning onset >16 hours – Vibrio parahemolyticus, Campylobacter jejuni, clostridium botulinum, E.coli, Salmonella and Shigellasps, CC.
83. Culture media for Clostridium difficile is CCFA – cefoxitin cycloserine fructose Agar CCEY – Cefoxitin cycloserine Egg yolk agar.
84. **CIN** – Cefsulodin Irgasan Novobiocin medium for Yersinia, **Thioglycollate medium, Brain heart infusion agar** used for Actinomyces, **Todd Hewitt broth** – Streptococcus agalactiae, **Ashdown media** for Burkholderia.
85. **Levinthal and Filde agar** for Hemophilus, **Smith Noguchi media** – Reiter treponema.
86. **Middlebrook's medium, Dorset egg medium** used for MTB, **Regan Lowe medium, Lacey DFP** used for Bordetella pertussis.
87. **GTTA** (Gelatin taurocholate tellurite agar), **Alkaline bile salt agar** (BSA), **TCBS** used for V. cholerae.
88. **Pea soup stool** seen in Typhoid fever, **Vi abs used for carriers and for epidemiological typing.**
89. **Important virulence factor** of H. pylori – Cag A, Vac A (Vacoulating cytotoxin), Urease. **Most sensitive and specific test** for H. pylori – Urea breath test.
90. Spirochaetes are motile by endoflagella; Differential motility based on temperature is found in yersinia enterocolitica; listeria sps.
91. **Thumb print appearance** in culture film smear seen in Bordetella pertussis. Ehrlichia chaffensis causes HME – Human Monocytic Ehrlichiosis.

PRACTICE QUESTIONS

Staphylococcus

1. **A 57-year-old man arrives at the emergency room complaining of weakness, fatigue, and intermittent fever that has recurred for several weeks. The patient had a cardiac valvular prosthesis implanted five years earlier. Physical examination reveals petechiae (pinpoint, nonraised, purplish-red spots caused by intra-dermal hemorrhage) on the chest and stomach. Blood cultures grew catalase-positive, coagulase-negative, cocci. The gram-positive organisms failed to ferment mannitol, and their growth was inhibited by novobiocin. What is the most likely infectious agent?**
   (a) Staphylococcus aureus
   (b) Staphylococcus epidermidis
   (c) Staphylococcus saprophyticus
   (d) Streptococcus pneumoniae
2. **A 32-year-old woman became ill four days after the onset of her menstrual period. She presented in the emergency room with fever (104°F; normal = 98.6°F), elevated white blood cell count (16,000/mm^3; normal = 4,000 to 10,000/mm^3), and a rash on her trunk and extremities. She complained of fatigue, vomiting, and diarrhea. She had recently eaten at a fast-food restaurant, but otherwise had prepared all her meals at home. The patient described most likely has:**
   (a) Staphylococcal food poisoning
   (b) Scalded skin syndrome
   (c) Infection with a staphylococcus saprophyticus
   (d) Chickenpox
3. **Staphylococcus does not cause:**
   (a) Osteomyelitis
   (b) Abscess
   (c) Scarlet fever
   (d) Pneumonia
4. **Staphylococcal food poisoning is caused by:**
   (a) Bacterial spores
   (b) Preformed exotoxin
   (c) Multiplication of bacteria
   (d) Preferred endotoxin
5. **The following are characteristic features of staphylococcus food poisoning *except*:**
   (a) Optimum temperature for toxin production is 37°C
   (b) Intradietic toxin is responsible for intestinal symptoms
   (c) Toxin can be destroyed by boiling for 30 minutes
   (d) Incubation period is 1-6 hours
6. **Staphylococcus aureus is differentiated from Staph epidermidis by:**
   (a) Colour of colony
   (b) Shape of bacteria
   (c) Coagulase test
   (d) Catalase test
7. **Incubation period of Staphylococcal food poisoning is:**
   (a) 2-6 hours
   (b) 8-24 hours
   (c) 1-2 days
   (d) 3-6 days
8. **Person consuming contaminated chicken fat develops diarrhoea, pain in abdomen and vomiting within 3-5 hours after ingestion. Most common organism:**
   (a) S. aureus
   (b) Salmonella
   (c) Cl. Botulinum
   (d) B. cereus
9. **Most strains of *Staphylococcus aureus* show:**
   (a) Golden yellow pigment
   (b) β haemolysis on sheep blood agar
   (c) Phosphatase production
   (d) All of the above

10. Which of the following bacteria are inhibited on crystal violet (1:50000) blood agar?

(a) *Staphylococci*
(b) *Streptococci*
(c) Both of the above
(d) None of the above

11. Which of the following bacteria is catalase positive and oxidase negative?

(a) *Staphylococcus*
(b) *Streptococcus*
(c) *Neisseria*
(d) *Pseudomonas*

12. Protein A is present in cell wall of:

(a) *Staphylococcus aureus*
(b) Coagulase negative *staphylococci*
(c) *Micrococci*
(d) None of the above

13. True about Toxic Shock Syndrome all *except*:

(a) Some strains of *Streptococcus pyogenes* may be the causative agent
(b) Enterotoxin I is now known as TSS Toxin
(c) Most of the strains producing TSST belong to phage group I
(d) TSST is non-antigenic

14. A 28-year-old woman seeks medical attention at the emergency room because she is having a very difficult menstrual period. In addition to bleeding profusely, she had a fever that has been as high as 1030F and has felt extremely lethargic. She has had progressively severe diarrhea, which in the last day a tachycardiac, tachypenic female, with cold, damp skin and a blood pressure of 80/40 mm Hg. Faint, diffuse erythema is noted on her neck and the upper half of her thorax. The supportive therapy and administration of antibiotics are initiated. The organism of antibiotics are initiated. The organism most likely responsible for this woman's symptoms release a toxin that:

(a) Dissolves lipid bilayer membranes
(b) Causes epidermolysis
(c) Causes hemolysis
(d) Induces the massive release of proinflammatory cytokines
(e) Causes persistent activation of adenylate cyclase in mucosal cells

15. Clumping factor can be detected by the:

(a) Slide coagulase test
(b) Tube coagulase test
(c) Precipitation test
(d) None of the above

16. CRF (Coagulase reacting factor) is necessary for:

(a) Slide coagulase test
(b) Tube coagulase test
(c) Both of the above
(d) None of the above

17. Which of the following bacteria are novobiocin resistant?

(a) *Staphylococcus aureus*
(b) *Staphylococcus epidermidis*
(c) *Staphylococcus saprophyticus*
(d) None of the above

18. Staphylococcal enterotoxin is detected by:

(a) VDRL
(b) Kahn's test
(c) ELISA
(d) Reversed passive latex agglutination
(e) C + D

19. Which of the following bacteria ferment mannitol?

(a) *Staph epidermidis*
(b) *Staph aureus*
(c) *Streptococcus pyogenes*
(d) *Streptococcus agalactiae*

20. A patient in an ICU, undergone CSF shunt surgery. His blood culture shows growth of grain positive cocci which are catalase positive and coagulase negative. The most likely etiological agent is:

(a) *Staph aureus*
(b) *S. epidermidis*
(c) *Strep. pyogenes*
(d) None of the above

21. Community acquired MRSA differs from hospital acquired MRSA in all the features *except*:
(a) Community isolates have remained susceptible to many non β-lactam antibiotics
(b) CA-MRSA seen in individuals with no prior medical exposure
(c) CA-MRSA strains have been associated with type 4 SCCmec (Staphylococcal cassette chromosomes)
(d) CA-MRSA are resistant pattern is similar to hospital acquired MRSA

Streptococcus

22. A 52-year-old man, generally in good health, is diagnosed with carcinoma and is scheduled for surgery. While waiting for his HMO to arrange for a bed, he develops persistent low-grade fever and constitutional symptoms. Physical examination is unremarkable other than a heart murmur not previously present. Out-patient blood cultures yield gram-positive, cocci. The most likely cause for the clinical picture is:
(a) Spread of carcinoma
(b) Anxiety, with skin flora contamination of the blood cultures
(c) Subacute endocarditis caused by streptococcus bovis
(d) Subacute endocarditis caused by Group B streptococci
(e) AIDS

23. Pikes medium is used for transport of:
(a) Staphylococci
(b) Streptococci
(c) Shigella
(d) Vibrio

24. Strep. pyogenes elaborates the following toxin *except*:
(a) Streptolysin O
(b) Deoxyribonuclease
(c) Enterotoxin
(d) Erytherogenic toxin
(e) Hyalorunidase

25. Bacteria that cause meningitis are all *except*:
(a) Group B streptococcus
(b) Streptococcus gp A
(c) Pneumococcus
(d) Listeria

26. Streptococcus is classified on the basis of:
(a) M protein
(b) Polysaccharide C antigen
(c) Culture Characteristic
(d) Bile solubility

27. Streptococcus pyogenes classifying in subtype on the basis of:
(a) M protein
(b) Polysacchride C
(c) Viridans group
(d) Frikiococcus group

28. Schultz Charlton test is seen in:
(a) Streptococcus
(b) Bacillus anthrax
(c) Pneumococcus
(d) Mycoplasma

29. Infection by group B streptococci:
(a) Can be followed by rheumatic fever
(b) Frequently occurs in persons debilitated by underlying systemic disease
(c) Can be prevented by the vaccine directed against the capsule
(d) Occurs in neonates

30. Streptococcus pyogenes with type 12 m protein:
(a) Fails to adhere to host pharyngeal epithelium

(b) Induces immune response but not protective immunity
(c) Adheres to epithelium but fails to induce an inflammatory response
(d) Induces immune responses that may lead to AGN in 10 to 15% infections

31. Which one of the following bacteria is most likely to be recovered from the cerebrospinal fluid (CSF) of a newborn with meningitis?
(a) *Escherichia coli*
(b) *Streptococcus agalactiae*
(c) *Haemophilus influenzae type b*
(d) *Listeria monocytogenes*
(e) *Streptococcus pneumoniae*

32. Cell wall protein of *Streptococcus pyogenes* cross reacts with human:
(a) Synovial fluid
(b) Myocardium
(c) Cardiac valves
(d) Vascular intima

33. A non-specific protein associated with the M protein is:
(a) T protein
(b) R protein
(c) M AP
(d) SOF
(e) None of the above

34. Which of the following enzymes are used for liquefaction of thick exudates as in empyema?
(a) Streptokinase and NADase
(b) Streptokinase and Streptodornase
(c) NADase and Hyaluronidase
(d) Streptokinase and N acetyl glucosaminidase

35. The antibody that increases in streptococcal skin infection and glomerulonephritis:
(a) ASO
(b) Anti DNAse-B
(c) Anti M
(d) Anti-streptokinase

36. Rapid identification of *Streptococcus pyogenes* is demonstrated by:
(a) Sensitivity to bacitracin
(b) Resistance to crystal violet
(c) Susceptibility to sulfonamide
(d) All of the above
(e) None of the above

37. Antibodies to following protein of Streptococci are protective:
(a) M protein antigen
(b) R protein antigen
(c) T protein antigen
(d) None of the above
(e) All of the above

38. Which of the following conditions is/are nonsuppurative sequelae of *Streptococcus pyogenes* infections?
(a) Acute rheumatic fever
(b) Acute glomerulonephritis
(c) Erythema nodosum
(d) All of the above

39. Which of the following bacteria is/are involved in the production of dental caries?
(a) *Streptococcus mutans*
(b) *Streptococcus sanguis*
(c) Both of the above
(d) None of the above

40. Individuals suffering from primary atypical pneumonia have agglutinins to:
(a) *Streptococcus MG*
(b) *Streptococcus faecalis*
(c) *Streptococcus avium*
(d) *Streptococcus mutans*

41. Serological test useful to diagnose *Streptococcus pyogenes* infection include:
(a) ASO
(b) Anti DNAase B
(c) Antihyaluronidase
(d) Anti M type specific antibodies
(e) All of the above

42. Which of the following is not bacteriophage mediated?
(a) Cholera toxin
(b) Botulinum toxin
(c) Diphtheria toxin
(d) Streptococcus pyrogenic exotoxin B

43. Causes of Pseudomembrane are all *except*:
(a) Corynebacterium diphtheriae
(b) Strept viridans
(c) Strept pyogenes
(d) Infectious mononucleosis

44. A patient admitted to an ICU is on central venous line for the last one week. He is on ceftazidime and amikacin. After 7 days of antibiotics he develops a spike of fever and his blood culture is positive for gram positive cocci in chains, which are catalase negative. Following this, vancomycin was started but the culture remained positive for the same organism even after 2 weeks of therapy. The most likely organism causing infection is:
(a) Staphylococcus aureus
(b) Viridans streptococci
(c) Enterococcus faecalis
(d) Coagulase negative Staphylococcus

45. A 55-year-old man was admitted to a local hospital with fever and chills. The patient was HIV positive and had received multiple courses of antibiotics. Blood cultures grew gram-positive cocci, which tested positive with Group D streptococcal antisera. The isolate was resistant to penicillin and vancomycin. Which one of the following is the most likely pathogen?
(a) Streptococcus pneumoniae
(b) Enterococcus faecium
(c) Streptococcus pyogenes
(d) Streptococcus agalactiae
(e) Enterococcus faecalis

46. Which among the following statements about *Enterococcus species* are not true?
(a) *Enterococcus faecium* is usually much more antibiotic resistant than *E.faecalis*
(b) *Enterococcus faecalis* causes 85-90% of the clinical infections
(c) *Van*A phenotype is manifested by inducible high level resistance to both vancomycin and teicoplanin
(d) VanC phenotype is plasmid mediated

Pneumococcus

47. Culture of Streptococccus viridans resemble:
(a) Staphylococcus
(b) Strept pyogenes
(c) Pneumococcus
(d) Strept fecalis

48. Draughtsman concentric rings on culture are produced by:
(a) Yersinia pestis
(b) H ducreyi
(c) B. pertussis
(d) Pneumococci
(e) B anthracis

49. Pneumococcus can be differentiated from streptococcus by:
(a) Type of Hemolysis
(b) Gram staining
(c) Growth characteristics
(d) Bile solubility

50. Specific soluble substance of Pneumococci which protect organism from phagocytosis:
(a) Haemolysin
(b) Capsular polysachharide acid
(c) Leucocidin
(d) Receptors destroying enzyme

51. Bile solubility by pneumococci is based on:
(a) Presence in pneumococci of an autolytic amidase
(b) Amidase cleaves the bond between alanine and muramic acid in peptidoglycan
(c) Amidase is activated by bile or bile salts resulting in lysis of organisms
(d) All of the above
(e) None of the above

52. The bacterial agent most likely to be associated with meningitis in a 2-year-old child who has been properly immunized is:

(a) *Escherichia coli*
(b) *Haemophilus influenzae type b*
(c) *Listeria monocytogenes*
(d) *Streptococcus agalactiae*
(e) *Streptococcus pneumonia*

53. True about CRP is all *except*:

(a) It is known as C Reactive Protein because it precipitates with C antigen of pneumococci
(b) It is an antibody
(c) Its production is stimulated by bacterial infection, inflammation and malignancy
(d) Can be detected by capillary precipitation or latex agglutination

Neisseria

54. A 14-month-old presented to his family physician with fever, vomiting, and lethargy of 24 hours duration. There was no neck stiffness or photophobia, but a nonblanching rash was found on the boy's chest. The boy's tonsils were inflamed. The child was diagnosed with upper respiratory viral infection and transported to the hospital. That evening, the child became increasingly irritable and drowsy. He was started on parenteral fluids and ceftriaxone. Several hours later, the patient developed seizures. The boy was transferred to the pediatric intensive care unit, where he developed unreactive pupils and central nonresponsive hypothermia. Later that next day, he showed no recordable brainstem activity. The child died two days after admission. Group B meningococcal infection was diagnosed by rapid antigen screen and confirmed on blood culture. The most likely source of the meningococcal infection was:

(a) Activation of endogenous Neisseria meningitidis
(b) Close contact with a carrier
(c) Contaminated fomites
(d) Close contact with an infected pet
(e) Contaminated food

55. Thayer Martin medium is used for:

(a) Gonococci
(b) Borellia
(c) Clostridia
(d) Shigella

56. A gram-negative diplococcus was isolated from a chocolate agar culture of a cerebrospinal fluid sample. Which one of the following tests or observations would be most informative in identifying the organism as N. meningitidis?

(a) Appearance of colonies
(b) Growth on Thayer-Martin medium
(c) Direct oxidase test on spinal fluid
(d) Growth in air
(e) Positive oxidase test and ability of culture isolate to ferment glucose and maltose

57. Incubation period for gonorrhea is:

(a) Less than 24 hours
(b) 1-3 days
(c) 2-15 days
(d) 15-18 days

58. Which one of the following is characteristic of N. meningitidis but not N. gonorrhoeae?

(a) Ferments glucose
(b) Contains a polysaccharide capsule
(c) Is oxidase-positive
(d) Most isolates show resistance to penicillin
(e) No effective vaccines are available

59. Gonococcus ferments:

(a) Glucose
(b) Maltose
(c) Sucrose
(d) Fructose

60. Best site to obtain swab in asymptomatic gonorrhoea is:

(a) Endocervix
(b) Lateral vaginal wall
(c) Urethra
(d) Posterior fornix

61. *Neisseria gonorrhoea* possesses which of the following antigens?

(a) Pilins
(b) LPS
(c) Outer membrane protein I
(d) All of the above

62. Prophylaxis against meningococcal meningitis is done with:

(a) Rifampicin
(b) Penicillin
(c) Ciprofloxacin
(d) Chloramphenicol

63. The causative agent of NGU is/are:

(a) C trachomatis
(b) Ureaplasma urealyticum
(c) Trichomonas vaginalis
(d) All of the above

64. Which among the following is not true?

(a) *Neisseria meningitidis* capsulated and utilizes both glucose and maltose
(b) Group C is responsible for both epidemics and outbreaks
(c) Associated with C5 to C9 deficiency
(d) Strict human pathogens inhabiting the nasopharynx

65. Characteristics of outer membrane of meningococci are all *except*:

(a) Contains lipo oligosaccharide
(b) Induces tumor necrosis factor
(c) Induces interlukein III
(d) May cause complications like shock and hemorrhage
(e) Lipopolysaccharide endoxin is analogous to lipo oligosaccharide

66. Neisseria bacteriemia is favoured by complementdeficiency of:

(a) C1 to C2
(b) C1 to C3
(c) C1 to C4
(d) C5 to C8
(e) C1 to C6

67. *N. gonorrhoeae* is a fastidious pathogen and found in sites often contaminated with normal flora. The best medium for isolation is:

(a) Sheep blood agar
(b) Löffler's medium
(c) Modified Newyork medium
(d) Thiosulfate citrate bile salts sucrose medium

68. Which of the following is not true about *Neisseriagonorrhoeae*?

(a) It is an exclusive human pathogen
(b) Some stains may cause disseminated disease
(c) Acute urethritis is the most common manifestation in males
(d) All stains are highly sensitive to penicillin

Corynebacterium

69. A diagnosis of diphtheria is confirmed by:

(a) Microscopic appearance of organisms stained with methylene blue
(b) Isolation of a typical colony on tinsdale's agar
(c) Isolation of typical organisms from materials such as blood, showing invasiveness
(d) Detection of β phage plaques in cultures of suspicious isolates
(e) Demonstration of toxin production by a suspicious isolate

70. Diphtheria toxin acts by:

(a) Increasing levels of cAMP
(b) Inhibiting protein synthesis
(c) Inhibiting Acetylcholine release
(d) Inhibiting glucose transport

71. Which of the following organisms produces toxins that act in organs and tissues distant from the site of colonization?

(a) V cholera
(b) S typhi
(c) E coli
(d) C diphtheria

72. Which of the following bacterium is used to stimulate immune system?

(a) *Corynebacterium diphtheriae*
(b) *Mycobacterium bovis*
(c) *Corynebacterium parvum*
(d) *Corynebacterium jakeium*

73. A child was having respiratory infection with membrane in peritonsillar area swab was taken from site which will be medium of choice?

(a) Tellurite
(b) Cary Blair
(c) LJ
(d) LSS

74. Septicaemic spread of the bacteria is the cause of the following diseases *except*:

(a) Enteric fever
(b) Diphtheria
(c) Bacterial endocarditis
(d) Miliary tuberculosis
(e) Brucellosis

75. Which of the following statements about diphtheria are untrue?

(a) Immunity to diphtheria depends circulating antitoxin
(b) Humans are the only hosts for the organisms
(c) Toxin is produced by only strains lysogenic for bacteriophages carrying the tox gene
(d) Fragment A of the toxin is responsible for attachment to host cells

76. True statement regarding diphtheria toxin is:

(a) Toxin produced by all corynebacteria
(b) Positive Schick test suggest immunity
(c) Toxin production is influenced by critcal conc of iron
(d) It is an Endotoxin

77. Virulence of corynebacterium diphtheria is associated in Lab by:

(a) Metachromatic granules
(b) Elecks gel precipitation
(c) Glycogen production
(d) Daisy head colony as growth

78. Which of true about infectivity of diphtheria?

(a) Some patients are infectious for life long
(b) Patients are infectious during 2-4 weeks of the illness
(c) Nasal carriers are most important
(d) Has a long incubation period

79. Which biotypes of *Corynebacterium diphtheriae* is/are predominant in endemic areas?

(a) Gravis
(b) Intermedius
(c) Mitis
(d) Mitis and gravis

80. Earliest growth of diphtheria bacilli can be detected of:

(a) Blood agar
(b) Blood tellurite agar
(c) Loeffler serum slope
(d) Nutrient agar

81. Daisy head appearance of colonies of Corynebacterium diphtheria on blood tellurite agar is shown by:
(a) Gravis biotype
(b) Intermedius biotype
(c) Mitis biotype
(d) None of the above

Bacillus

82. Medusa head colonies are produced by:
(a) Bordetella
(b) Corynebacterium
(c) Anthrax bacilli
(d) Anthracoid bacilli

83. Which of the following is a tripartite toxin?
(a) *Diphtheria toxin*
(b) *Anthrax toxin*
(c) *Botulinum toxin*
(d) *Cholera toxin*

84. Which of the following is not bacteriophage mediated?
(a) Cholera toxin
(b) Botulinum toxin
(c) Diphtheria toxin
(d) Streptococcus pyrogenic exotoxin B

Anaerobes

85. The best method of obtaining sputum for anaerobic culture is:
(a) Endobronchial aspiration
(b) Expectoration
(c) Gastric lavage
(d) Transbronchial aspiration

86. Which of the following bacilli swarms on blood agar and produces hemolytic colonies under suitable conditions?
(a) Cl. welchii
(b) Cl. tetani
(c) Proteus vulgaris
(d) Bacillus spp

87. The most common form of infection caused by Clostridium botulinum in this country is:
(a) Infant botulism
(b) Wound infection
(c) Food poisoning
(d) Primary septicemia
(e) Anaerobic cellulitis

88. Clostridium perfringens infections are commonly associated with:
(a) Contamination of wounds
(b) Antibiotic treatment
(c) Consumption of water contaminated with sewage
(d) Immunosuppression
(e) Preexisting lung disease

89. Specific antitoxin is an important part of treatment in:
(a) Gas gangrene
(b) Tetanus
(c) Enteritis necroticans
(d) Pseudomembranous colitis
(e) Bacteroides and prevotella infections

90. Which of the following about *Clostridium* are true?
(a) *Cl. histolyticum* do not grow aerobically
(b) Proteolytic species turn the meat pink
(c) Spores are highly sensitive to Phenolic disinfectant
(d) *Cl. perfringens* are toxigenic and also invasive

91. Lecithinase produced by which of the following bacteria is neutralized by *Clostridium perfringens* anti-toxin?

(a) *Clostridium novyi*
(b) *Clostridium bifermentans*
(c) *Bacillus cereus*
(d) *Vibrio species*

92. **The entire following are true of Botulism, *except*:**
(a) It causes a symmetric descending paralysis
(b) Botulinum toxin acts on GABA neurotransmitter
(c) All produce neurotoxin except C2 which shows enterotoxic activity
(d) *Cl. botulinum* can be isolated from food or the patient's feces

93. **A 25 years old male on chronic antibiotic therapy presented with fever, abdominal pain and diarrhoea associated with occasional blood in stools. Which among the following are true?**
(a) Easily isolated in culture
(b) Presence of large central spores
(c) Toxin is neutralized by Clostridium sordelii antitoxin
(d) Vancomycin is the drug of choice

94. **The bowel contains many microorganisms but the most prevalent bacterium is:**
(a) *B. fragilis*
(b) *Lactobacillus*
(c) *S. epidermidis*
(d) *E. coli*

95. **With reference to bacteroides fragilis the following statements are true, *except*:**
(a) B. fragilis is the same frequent anaerobe isolated from clinical samples
(b) B. fragilis is not uniformaly sensitive to metronidazole
(c) The lipopolysaccharide formed by B. fragilis is structurally and functionally different from the conventional endotoxin
(d) Shock and disseminated intravascular coagulation are common in bacteroides bacteriemia

ENTEROBACTERIACEAE

Salmonella

96. **All are correct regarding Widal test, *except*:**
(a) Baseline titres differ depending on the endemicity of the disease
(b) Even one high titre is not enough for conclusive diagnosis
(c) O antibody lasts longer and hence is not indicative of recent infection
(d) H antibody cannot differentiate between types

97. **Identify non motile salmonella:**
(a) Salm typhi
(b) Salm gallinarum
(c) Salm pullorum
(d) A+B
(e) B+C

98. **Phase variation of Antigens is typically seen in bacteria:**
(a) Shigella
(b) Salmonella
(c) Clostridium
(d) Vibrio

99. **Which of the following Salmonella is most common in India?**
(a) A
(b) B
(c) C
(d) None of the above

100. **Most common typhoid vaccine used in India:**
(a) Polyvalent TAB
(b) Divalent typhoid paratyphoid
(c) Oral (typhi 21a)
(d) Typhium V

101. Salmonella typhi is the causative agent of typhoid fever. The infective dose of S. typhi is:

(a) One bacillus
(b) $10^8 - 10^{10}$ bacilli
(c) $10^2 - 10^5$ bacilli
(d) 1 – 10 bacilli

102. All the following statements of typhoid carrier state are true *except*:

(a) Carrier presents even after the treatment of disease
(b) In carriers the organism rest in gallbladder
(c) In Japan, urinary carrier state is common
(d) Detection of carrier state is by antibodies to "O" and "H" antigens

103. In typhoid, Widal test detects:

(a) Antigens
(b) H antigens
(c) Vi antigen
(d) Antibody

104. Which of the following about *Salmonella Typhi Vi* antigen are correct *except*?

(a) Total absence of Vi antibody in a proven case of typhoid carries good prognosis
(b) Vi antigen provides a method of epidemiological typing of *S.Typhi* by phage typing
(c) Vi antigen is strongly immunogenic
(d) Vi antibody is usually present in carriers

105. Salmonella septicemia in particular associated with:

(a) *Salm gallinarum*
(b) *Salm paratyphi B*
(c) *Salm cholerae*
(d) *Salm anatum*

106. Which of the following bacteria is known as Ebert Gaffky bacillus?

(a) Klebsiella
(b) H. aegipticus
(c) Salmonella
(d) Corynebacterium

107. The following diseases caused by bacteria are due to the exotoxins produced by them *except*:

(a) Diphtheria
(b) Cholera
(c) Salmonellosis
(d) Tetanus
(e) Botulism

108. True about blood culture is following *except*:

(a) Salmonella 1st week
(b) Equal vol of both culture and specimen
(c) First put on liquid and then on solid media
(d) Repeat culture often useful

109. Which of the following are not gas producing salmonella?

(a) S typhi
(b) S enteritidis
(c) S cholera
(d) S typhimurium

110. Stool culture can be used in the diagnosis of typhoid fever during:

(a) 1st week
(b) 2nd week
(c) 3rd week
(d) 4th week

111. A patient with a fever of 103F, bradycardia and leukopenia probably has:

(a) Brucellosis
(b) Typhoid
(c) Malaria
(d) Meliodesis

112. Which of the following statement is incorrect?

(a) S typhi causes gastroenteritis
(b) S paratyphi produces acid and gas on glucose
(c) Vi antigen is related to virulence
(d) Persistence of Vi antibody indicates development of carrier state

113. Agglutination with O antigen of S typhi is inhibited by:

(a) Vi antigen
(b) Pili antigen
(c) Flagellar antigen
(d) All of the above

ENTEROBACTERIACEAE – PART-II

114. Lac$^+$, glucose-fermenting, gram-negative rod isolated from a previously healthy child with bloody diarrhea is most likely to be:

(a) Shigella sonnei
(b) Pseudomonas aeruginosa
(c) Escherichia coli
(d) Salmonella enterica
(e) Helicobacter pylori

115. An elderly, alcoholic male develops severe, necrotizing lobar pneumonia. The organism is Lac$^+$ and produces a luxuriant capsule. The most likely agent is:

(a) Klebsiella pneumoniae
(b) Serratia species
(c) Yersinia pseudotuberculosis
(d) Pseudomonas aeruginosa
(e) Campylobacter fetus

116. A 20-year-old male had pain abdomen and mild fever followed by gastroenteritis. The stool examination showed presence of pus cells and RBCs on microscopy. The etiological agent responsible is most likely to be:

(a) *Enteroinvasive E. coli.*
(b) *Enterotoxigenic E. coli.*
(c) *Enteropathiogenic E. coli.*
(d) *Enteroaggregative E. coli.*

117. Travellers diarrhoea is caused by:

(a) EPEC
(b) EHEC
(c) ETEC
(d) EIEC

118. The mechanism of action of EPEC is:

(a) Adherence to enterocytes
(b) Stimulates adenylcyclase
(c) Produce secretary diarrhoea
(d) None of the above

119. It has been hypothesized that their exists a strong association between haemolytic uraemic syndrome:

(a) Salmonellae
(b) Bacteriophages and corynebacteria
(c) Verocytotoxin producing E coli
(d) Clostridium difficile

120. Which of the following is usual complication of shigellosis?

(a) Arthritis
(b) Pneumonitis
(c) Panophthalmitis
(d) Meningitis

121. An infant is brought to the emergency room with hemolytic uremic syndrome and thrombocytopenia. Stool sample was cultured and non-lactose fermenting colonies grown on Sorbitol MacConkey agar, which also fermented glucose with gas. Which one of the following bacteria would most likely be isolated from a stool specimen?

(a) *Shigella*
(b) *Salmonella*
(c) *Aeromonas*
(d) *E. coli* 0157/H7

122. Invasive property of Shigella dysentry type I can be demonstrated by:

(a) Sereny test
(b) Ability to penetrate Hela or Hep 2 cells
(c) Congo red binding
(d) A+B+C
(e) Skin test

123. Atypical pneumonia can be caused by the following microbial agents *except*:

(a) *Mycoplasma pneumonia*
(b) *Legionella pneumophila*
(c) *Human Corona virus*
(d) *Klebsiella pneumoniae*

124. Generation time of coliform bacilli:

(a) 20 minutes (b) 2 hours

(c) 20 hours (d) 20 days

125. Verocytotoxin has been in individual suffering from hemolytic uraemic syndrome in their:

(a) Blood (b) Tissues

(c) Faeces (d) Saliva

126. Eiken test is which type of reaction used for E. coli.?

(a) Precipitation (b) Agglutination

(c) Toxin antitoxin assay (d) CFT

127. The direct method of study of bacteriophages is:

(a) Electron microscopy (b) Plaque study

(c) Serological testing (d) Lysogenic conversion

128. Classification of shigella is on the basis of fermentation of:

(a) Lactose (b) Sucrose

(c) Mannitol (d) Glucose

129. Shigella dysentriae type I may have complications:

(a) Arthritis (b) Toxic neuritis

(c) Conjunctivitis (d) Myocarditis

(e) All of the above

130. Surface antigen of *E coli* acting as virulence factors are:

(a) LPS O antigen (b) Enveloper K antigen

(c) Fimbriae (d) All of the above

(e) None of the above

131. True about EPEC is:

(a) Diarrhoea in infants (b) Least infectious

(c) Affects immunocompromised (d) Affects adults most

132. One of the following bacteria does not show swarming:

(a) *Vibrio alginolyticus* (b) *Clostridium tetani*

(c) *Proteus mirabilis* (d) *Morganella morganii*

133. True about Enterobacteriacea:

(a) Oxidase positive (b) Polar flagella

(c) Resistant to antibiotics (d) Urease positive

134. Identify late lactose fermenters:

(a) *E coli* (b) *Salmonella typhi*

(c) *Shigella sonnei* (d) *Klebsiella*

(e) *Proteus*

135. Strain of *E coli* carrying K antigen are:

(a) Responsible for pyelonephritis (b) Liable to cause cystitis

(c) Known to cause diarrhea (d) Capable of causing all of the above

136. True about binding of *E coli* to epithelial cells receptors by means of adhesion causing UTI:

(a) Six antigenic types F_1 to F_{12} of fimbriae have been identified from UNO pathogenic *E coli* strains

(b) Detection of fimbriae using EM

(c) Uropithelial adhesion assay can be demonstrated
(d) Demonstration of aerobactin production, *i.e.,* siderophase
(e) All of the above

137. Characteristic biochemical test of proteins:

(a) PPA
(b) Urease
(c) A+B
(d) Catalase
(e) Phosphatase

138. E.coli is an important causative agent of pyelonephritis in man. The property that helps the bacteria in this is most likely to be:

(a) Adhesive property
(b) Toxigenecity
(c) Haemolytic property
(d) Presence of capsule

Vibrio

139. Cholera toxin:

(a) Increases the levels of intracellular cyclic GMP
(b) Acts through the receptor for opiates
(c) Cause continued activations of adenylate cyclase
(d) Inhibition of EF2

140. All about *Vibrio O139* are wrong *except*:

(a) Noncapsulated
(b) 1st reported from Calcutta in 1992
(c) Now it's the only pathogenic serovar prevalent
(d) Invasive and might cause extra intestinal manifestation

141. *Vibrio vulnificus,* which is a marine Vibrio of medical importance, mostly found in the temperate and tropical climates is best characterized as:

(a) Three serotypes—Ogawa (AB), Inaba (AC), Hikojima (ABC)
(b) Rare human pathogen, halophilic, lactose-positive
(c) Produce yellow colony on TCBS
(d) Shows positive kanagawa phenomena

142. All are true about *Vibrio mimicus except*:

(a) Failure to ferment sucrose
(b) Oxidase positive
(c) Acquired from eating sea food
(d) Grows in presence of 8% NaCl conc

143. String test is used for:

(a) B. anthracis
(b) Vibrio cholerae
(c) Brucella abortus
(d) Ps mallei

144. Person having open wound is in leg comes in contact with sea water and develop wound injection organism implicated is:

(a) V. Parahaemolyticus
(b) V. vulfinicus
(c) Cl. botulinum
(d) S. paratyphi

145. The endotoxin of the following gram-negative bacteria does not play any part in the pathogenesis of the natural disease:

(a) Escherichia coli
(b) Klebsiella sp.
(c) Vibrio cholerae
(d) Pseudomonas aeruginosa

Pseudomonas

146. An elderly man, hospitalized and recovering from cardiac bypass surgery, develops pneumonia. Sputum culture reveals a gram-negative rod that produces a green pigment but does not ferment carbohydrates. The most likely organism is:

(a) Klebsiella pneumoniae
(b) Serratia species
(c) Proteus species
(d) Enterobacter species
(e) Pseudomonas aeruginosa

147. Toxin which interfere with protein synthesis is:

(a) E coli toxin
(b) Pseudomonas toxin
(c) Staphylococcal toxin
(d) Cholera toxin

148. An alginate-producing, aerobic, oxidase-positive, Gram-negative bacillus is isolated from the sputum of a patient with cystic fibrosis. The organism is likely to be:

(a) *Bacteroides fragilis*
(b) *Escherichia coli*
(c) *Klebsiella pneumonia*
(d) *Pseudomonas aeruginosa*
(e) *Streptococcus faecalis*

Yersinia, Pasteurella, Francisella

149. Stalactite growth in ghee broth is due to:

(a) H influenzae
(b) C. diphtheria
(c) Y. pestis
(d) T. pallidum

150. *Yersinia pestis* produces plague by virtue of:

(a) F1 antigen
(b) V antigens
(c) W antigen
(d) Exotoxin and endotoxin
(e) All of the above

151. Predominant vector in north India for transmission of *Yersinia pestis* are:

(a) Xenopsylla astia
(b) Xenopsylla cheopis
(c) Ceratosphyllus fasciatus
(d) Louse

152. Biotypes of *Yersinia pestis* are:

(a) Yersinia pestis orienttalis
(b) Yersinia pestis antigua
(c) Yersinia pestis mediavelis
(d) All of the above
(e) None of the above

153. A young boy had a flea bite while working in a wheat grain godown. After 5 days he developed fever and had axillary lymphadenopathy. A smear was sent to the laboratory to perform a specific staining. Which one of the following staining method would help in the identification of the suspected pathogen?

(a) Albert staining
(b) Zeihl-Neelsen staining
(c) Mc Fadyean staining
(d) Wayson staining

Haemophilus

154. Satellitism is seen in culture of:

(a) Haemophilus
(b) Streptococcus
(c) Klebsiella
(d) Proteus
(e) Salmonella

155. Epiglottitis is caused by:

(a) Strept pneumoniae
(b) Strept haemolyticus
(c) H. influenzae
(d) Staph albus

156. Haemophilus ducreyi is causative agent of:

(a) Hard chancre
(b) Soft chancre
(c) LGV
(d) Granuloma inguinale

157. A 2 years old child is brought to the emergency with history of fever and vomiting. On examination he has neck rigidity. The CSF examination shows polymorphs more than 2000/ul, protein 100 mg/dl and glucose 10 mg/dl. The Gram stain shows the presence of Gram-negative coccobacilli. The culture shows growth of bacteria only on chocolate agar and not on blood agar. The causative agent is:

(a) *Neisseria meningitides*
(b) *Haemophilus influenzae*
(c) *Branhamella catarrhalis*
(d) *Legionella pneumophila*

158. Biotypes of *H influenza* are grouped into 8 (I-VIII) on the basis of production of:

(a) Indole
(b) Urease
(c) Ornithine decarboxylase
(d) All of the above

159. Biotypes of H influenza most frequently responsible for meningitis:

(a) 8 (b) 2 (c) 7 (d) 6 (e) 1

Bordetella

160. What is true about Bordetella pertussis?

(a) Adheres to normal mucosa
(b) Destroys cilia
(c) Local tissue destruction
(d) All of the above

161. Which of the following media is used for transporting Bordetella pertussis?

(a) VR medium
(b) Peptone water
(c) Stuarts' transport medium
(d) Any of the above

162. True about Bordetella pertussis is:

(a) Strict aerobes
(b) Facultative anaerobe
(c) Ferment sugars
(d) Needs X and V factors for growth

163. Culture media for pertussis is:

(a) L J media
(b) Chocolate agar
(c) Wilson and Blair medium
(d) Bordet Gengou medium

164. Virulence factors of Bordetella pertussis are:

(a) Tracheal cytotoxin
(b) Adenylate cyclase
(c) Pertussis toxin
(d) Filamentous hemagglutinin
(e) All of the above

Brucella

165. A veterinary doctor had pyrexia of unknown origin. His blood culture in special laboratory media was positive for gram negative short bacilli which was oxidase positive. Which one of the following is the likely organism grown in culture?

(a) *Pasturella spp.*
(b) *Francisella spp.*
(c) *Bartonella spp.*
(d) *Brucella spp.*

166. A farmer rearing sheep presented with complaints of fever and weakness for lasting one month. There is generalized LNP. There was also associated hepatomegaly. Biopsy of liver showed non casting granuloma due to:

(a) Br. Mellitensie
(b) Br. Casis
(c) Francisella tularensis
(d) Yersinia pestis

167. Which of the following test would you recommend for a farmer suffering from fever of unknown origin who raises goats and had a history of drinking raw milk?

(a) Standard agglutination test
(b) Weil-Felix test
(c) Widal test
(d) Microscopic agglutination test

Mycobacterium

168. Which one of the following is characteristic of mycobacteria?
(a) They contain mycolic acids
(b) They are resistant to inactivation by heat
(c) They grow extracellularly
(d) They are anaerobic
(e) They are spore-forming

169. An acid-fast smear on a patient's sputum is positive. The tuberculin test, however, is negative. A more definitive diagnosis could be obtained by:
(a) Paying attention to the patient's history
(b) A more extensive physical examination
(c) A chest radiograph
(d) Repeat of the sputum smear
(e) Laboratory culture and speciation

170. The treatment of tuberculosis:
(a) Is initiated with a single first-line drug
(b) Is initiated after the results of sensitivity testing are available
(c) Is most effective in patients with chronic or arrested tubercles
(d) May last two to three weeks
(e) Should be directly observed in individuals who have a history of noncompliance

171. Virulence in mycobacteria is most strongly correlated with:
(a) Mycotoxin production
(b) Slow growth
(c) Composition of the cell envelope
(d) Small size of cells
(e) Dependence on oxygen for growth

172. Dorset egg medium is used for cultivation of:
(a) Staphylococcus
(b) Streptococcus
(c) Gonococcus
(d) M TB

173. True about M. tuberculosis is:
(a) Strict aerobes
(b) Gram negative
(c) Thin cell wall
(d) Curved rod

174. Acid fastness of tubercle bacilli is attributed to:
(a) Presence of mycolic acid
(b) Integrity of cell wall
(c) Both of the above
(d) None of the above

175. The medium used for Mycobacterium tuberculosis is:
(a) Sabouraud's medium
(b) L J medium
(c) Pick's medium
(d) NIH medium

176. The factor which promotes virulence of M. tuberculosis:
(a) Wax D
(b) Cord factor
(c) Muramyl dipeptide
(d) Mycolic acid

177. Reactivation of TB is almost exclusively a disease of:
(a) Bone
(b) Lymph nodes
(c) Lung
(d) Brain

178. The most common focus of Scrofuloderma is:
(a) Lung
(b) Lymph node
(c) Larynx
(d) Skin

179. Collection of urine sample of a patient of TB/kidney:

(a) 24 hours urine
(b) 12 hours urine
(c) In early morning
(d) Any time

180. Rapid examination of Tubercle bacilli is possible with:

(a) Ziehl-Neelsen stain
(b) Kin young stain
(c) Auramine–Rhodamine stain
(d) Giemsa stain

181. Anti-tubercular drug susceptibility can be done by all of the following methods, *except*:

(a) Resistance ratio method
(b) Disc diffusion method
(c) Molecular method
(d) Radiometric broth method

182. Drug resistance in Tuberculosis is due to:

(a) Transformation
(b) Transduction
(c) Conjugation
(d) Mutation

183. Tuberculin test positive is depended on:

(a) Erythema
(b) Nodule formation
(c) Induration
(d) Ulcerative change

184. True about Mantoux is:

(a) False negative in fulminant diseases
(b) If once done, next time it is always positive
(c) Results are given in terms of positive and negative
(d) Indurations given in terms of length and breadth
(e) Always indicate active TB infection

185. True about Mantoux test:

(a) < 5 cm always +ve
(b) Positive reaction in children < 2 years is not important than adult
(c) Usually read after 48-72 hours
(d) False +ve in post measles state

186. True regarding mycobacterium tuberculosis is:

(a) Produces visible colonies in 1 weeks' time on Lowenstein-Jensen media
(b) Decolorized by 5% sulfuric acid
(c) Facultative aerobe
(d) Niacin positive

187. Mycobacterium tuberculosis is diffentiated from other atypical mycobacteria:

(a) Niacin test
(b) AFB staining
(c) PAS staining
(d) None

188. Test for differentiating tubercle bacilli from atypical mycobacteria:

(a) Aryl sulphate test
(b) Niacin test
(c) Tellurite reduction
(d) Growth on Mac Conkey Agar

189. Most common mycobacterial infection is patient is tropical contries:

(a) M.Leprae
(b) M.avium intracellulare
(c) M.tuberculosis
(d) M.kansasii

190. All the following are true of Tuberculosis *except*:

(a) For sputum to be positive, bacilli should be > 10^4/ml
(b) Niacin test differentiates M.tuberculosis and M.bovis

(c) Pathogenicity to rabbits differentiates M.tuberculosis and M.bovis
(d) Culture techniques have low sensitivity

191. Basanti, 29 years aged female from Bihar present with active TB. She delivers baby. All of the following are indicated *except*:
(a) Administer INH to baby
(b) Withhold breastfeeding
(c) Give ATT to mother for 2 years
(d) Ask mother to ensure proper disposal of sputum

192. Which one of the following statement is true regarding pathogenicity of Mycobacteria species?
(a) M.tuberculosis is more pathogenic than M.bovis to the humans
(b) M.kansasii can cause a disease indistinguishable from tuberculosis
(c) M.africanum infection is acquired from the environmental source
(d) M.marinum is responsible for tubercular lymphadenopathy

193. Which of the following is photochromogenic?
(a) M.kansasii
(b) M.scrofulorum
(c) M.intracellulare
(d) M.avium
(e) M.xenopi

194. Battey bacillus or mycobacterium intracellulare is:
(a) Photochromogen
(b) Scotochromogen
(c) Non-photochromogen
(d) Rapid grower

195. Which of the following is not a pathogenic mycobacteria?
(a) M.Kansasii
(b) M.scrofulaceum
(c) M.cheolonei
(d) M.smegmatis

196. Cutaneous lesions may be produced by the following mycobacteria *except*:
(a) M.intracellulare
(b) M.Leprae
(c) M.marinum
(d) M.tuberculosis
(e) M.ulcerans

M.Leprae

197. Which of the following is true regarding globi in a patient with lepromatous leprosy?
(a) Consists of lipid laden macrophages
(b) Consists of macrophages filled with AFB
(c) Consists of neutrophils filled with bacteria
(d) Consists of activated lymphocytes

198. For experimental work, Lepra bacilli are best cultured in:
(a) Armadillos
(b) Mouse foot pad
(c) Guinea pigs
(d) Rabbit testes

199. Leprosy spreads by:
(a) Skin to skin contact
(b) Blood transfusion
(c) Droplet spread
(d) Ingestion

200. Neurological involvement is pronounced in which type of leprosy?
(a) Tuberculoid
(b) Lepromatous
(c) Borderline
(d) Lucio leprosy

201. The characteristic finding in a case of leprosy is:
(a) Culture test is positive in 2-3 months in LJ media
(b) Long contact with tuberculoid leprosy can transmit the disease

(c) CMI is seen in Lepromatous leprosy
(d) Macule lesion heals spontaneously

202. The following test is not used for diagnosis of leprosy:
(a) Lepromin test
(b) Slit skin smear
(c) Fine needle aspiration cytology
(d) Skin biopsy

203. Mitsuda reaction is read after:
(a) 3 days
(b) 3 hours
(c) 3 weeks
(d) 3 months

204. In the management of leprosy, lepromin test is most useful for:
(a) Herd immunity
(b) Prognosis
(c) Treatment
(d) Epidemiological investigations

205. The main cytokine, involved in erythma nodosum leprosum (ENL) reaction is:
(a) Interleukin – 2
(b) Interferon – gamma
(c) Tumor necrosis factor – alpha
(d) Macrophage colony stimulating factor

206. The following drug is used for the treatment of type II lepra reaction, *except*:
(a) Chloroquine
(b) Thaliodomide
(c) Cyclosporine
(d) Corticosteroid

207. Under leprosy eradication programme the management of single lesion is:
(a) Single dose of Rifampicin and Dapsone
(b) Rifampicin and Dapsone for 6 months
(c) Rifampicin, ofloxacin and minocycline single dose
(d) Rifampicin and minocycline for 6 months

208. True about lepra bacilli is:
(a) INH inhibits their growth
(b) Antileprosy vaccine can give lifelong protection
(c) Mycobacterium leprae can be grown in foot pad of mice
(d) Incubation period is 3-4 months

Spirochetes

209. Which is not a test for syphilis?
(a) TPHA
(b) Freis test
(c) Dark ground microscopy
(d) RPR

210. In a syphilitic patient, which one of the following test combinations is most appropriate?
(a) FTA-Abs (IgG)/FTA-Abs (IgM)
(b) RPR/FTA-Abs
(c) RPR/culture of the lesion
(d) VDRL/RPR

211. Which of the following statement about serological tests for syphilis is/are untrue?
(a) FTA-ABS test is positive in almost all patients with secondary, latent or tertiary syphilis
(b) The VDRL test detects antibodies that react with the nontreponemal antigen cardiolipin
(c) TPI test is an indirect fluorescent antibody test for antitreponemal antigen in serum

212. Most sensitive investigation for syphilis is:
(a) FTA-ABS
(b) VDRL
(c) Wasserman's reaction
(d) Kahn test

213. All are true about syphilis *except*:
(a) VDRL becomes positive after 10-14 days of chancre

(b) The earliest serological test to appear in untreated primary syphilis in TPHA

(c) Yaws and pinta cannot be differentiated

(d) VDRL titres ↓ or even negative after Rx

214. A 38-year-old businessman presents with a penile lesion that is crateriform, moist and peripherally indurated. Upon questioning, the patient reveals that the lesion has been present for approximately 10 days, and is not noticeably painful. Which one of the following tests should be performed to further narrow?

(a) Blood cultures

(b) Culture of the exudates

(c) Gram stain of the exudates

(d) Microhemagglutination *Teponema pallidum* (MHA-TP) test

(e) Veneral Disease Research Laboratory (VDRL) test

215. The minimum no of treponemes that must be present to be detected by dark ground microscopy:

(a) 10^2/ml (b) 10^3/ml

(c) 10^4/ml (d) 10^5/ml

216. The following are true regarding Lyme's disease, *except*:

(a) It is transmitted by Ixodes tick

(b) Erythema chronicum migrans may be a clinical feature

(c) *Borrelia recurrentis* is the aetiological agent

(d) Rodents act as natural hosts

217. A 32-year old swimmer presented with history of high grade fever for 7 days and altered sensorium for 2 days. On examination, he was comatosed and had sub conjunctival hemorrhage. Urgent investigations showed a haemoglobin of 9 gm/dl, serum bilirubin 10 mg/dl and urea 88 mg/dl. Peripheral blood smear was negative for malarial parasite. What is the most likely diagnosis?

(a) Brucellosis (b) Leptospirosis

(c) Acute viral hepatitis (d) Rickettsiosis

218. Noguchi medium is used for:

(a) Bordetella (b) Brucella

(c) Borrelia (d) Corynebacterium

Mycoplasma

219. True about Mycoplasma:

(a) Also called PPLO

(b) Requires cholesterol as growth factor

(c) *Mycoplasma pneumonia* and *Ureaplasma urealyticum* are pathogenic

(d) Free living Pleomorphic

(e) All of the above

220. Wrong about *Ureaplasma urealyticum*:

(a) T strain (b) Colonies are 5 to 25u

(c) Does not require cholesterol for growth (d) Hydrolyse urea

221. Fried egg colony is seen in culture of:

(a) Mycoplasma (b) Legionella

(c) Trachoma (d) Haemophilus

222. *Mycoplasma pneumoniae* pneumonia (causing atypical pneumonia) may be rapidly identified by which of the following procedures?

(a) Detection of specific antigen in urine
(b) Cold agglutinin test
(c) Electron microscopy of sputum
(d) Culture of respiratory secretions in HeLa cells

Actinomycetes

223. Which of the following statements regarding Actinomyces and Nocardia is true?

(a) Both organisms have branching growth but are prokaryotes
(b) Neither stains with Gram stain
(c) Nocardia infections are endogenous, and often initiated by trauma
(d) Actinomyces usually causes infections in systemically compromised patients
(e) Neither is sensitive to anti-bacterial drugs

Miscellaneous Bacteria

224. Listeria monocytogenes shows which of the following characteristics?

(a) It can grow at refrigerator temperatures (4°C)
(b) It is an extracellular pathogen
(c) It is catalase-negative
(d) It is a gram-negative coccus
(e) It is strictly a human pathogen

225. A 26-year-old woman, eight months pregnant, visits her obstetrician complaining of fever, myalagia and backache of recent onset. Three weeks earlier, the patient had been a weekend guest at a rural farmhouse. A culture of the patient's blood shows gram-positive rods that are catalase-positive and display a distinctive tumbling motility in liquid medium. What is the most likely source of the woman's infection?

(a) Well-done roast beef
(b) Fresh, raw cow's milk
(c) Home-baked bread
(d) Homemade apple sauce
(e) Baked apple pie

226. Donovanosis is best diagnosed by:

(a) Microscopy
(b) Culture
(c) Skin testing
(d) Serology

227. All are true about Bacterial vaginosis *except*:

(a) Vaginal pH < 4.5
(b) Nugent scoring is used for diagnosis
(c) Foul smelling discharge accentuated by KOH
(d) Presence of clue cells is pathognomic

228. All are true about *Moraxella catarrhalis except*:

(a) Causes angular conjunctivitis
(b) Gram negative cocci in pair
(c) It is part of normal pharyngeal flora
(d) Produces β lactamase

229. A 70-year-old patient presented with high-grade fever, cough and pain abdomen. Sample collected from patient, culture shows gram-negative organisms grow only charcoal yeast extract agar the causative organism is:

(a) listeria monocytogens
(b) B. Psudomalaei
(c) M. Catarrhalis
(d) Legionella

230. Which of the following about *Legionella pneumophilla* is true?

(a) Causes Weil's disease
(b) Culture is done in MYPA medium

(c) Widely distributed in natural and artificial aquatic environment
(d) Transmits mainly by ingestion

231. Which of the following bacteria is/are blamed to cause bacterial vaginitis?
(a) Gardnelle vaginalis
(b) Bacteroides sp
(c) Mobiluncus
(d) All of the above

Rickettsiaceae

232. An army jawan posted in a remote forest area with history of louse bite, had fever and headache. His fever was 104°F and pulse was 70 per min. He had an erythematous lesion of about 1 cm on the leg surrounded by small vesicles, along with generalized lymphadenopathy at the time of presentation to the referral hospital. His blood sample was collected to perform serology for the diagnosis of Rickettsial disease. Which one of the following results in Weil-Felix reaction will be diagnostic in this clinical setting?
(a) High OX-2
(b) High OX-19
(c) High OX-K
(d) High OX-19 and OX-2

233. A patient complained of chills and fever following a louse bite 2 weeks before. He had rashes all over the body and was delirious at the time of presentation to the hospital and subsequently went into coma. A provisional diagnosis of vasculitis due to Rickettsial infection was made. Which one of the following can be the causative agent:
(a) *Rickettsia typhi*
(b) *Rickettsia rickettiae*
(c) *Rickettsia prowazekii*
(d) *Ricketssia* akari

234. Blood clot of a patient with suspected Rickettsiosis was inoculated intraperitoneally into male guinea pig. After 2 weeks animal developed fever, scrotal necrosis and later died. Most probable pathogen here is:
(a) *Rickettsia prowazekii*
(b) *Rickettsia typhi*
(c) *Rickettsia rickettsii*
(d) *Rickettsia conori*

235. A patient complained of chills and fever following a louse bite 2 weeks before. He had rashes all over the body and was delirious at the time of presentation to the hospital and subsequently went into coma. A provisional diagnosis of vasculitis due to Rickettsial infection was made. Which one of the following can be causative agent?
(a) *Rickettsia typhi*
(b) *Rickettsia rickettsiae*
(c) *Rickettsia prowazekii*
(d) *Rickettsia akari*

236. An ill patient presented with interstitial pneumonia, denied being bitten by insects. Of the following rickettsial diseases, which one has he most likely contracted?
(a) Scrub typhus
(b) Rickettsial pox
(c) Brill-Zinsser disease
(d) Q fever

237. Which one of the following statements best describes human monocytic ehrlichiosis (HME)?
(a) The HME agent is both intracellular and extracellular pathogen
(b) Transmitted by the bite of a dog and cats
(c) Clinical diagnosis is based on the presence of erythema migrans (EM)
(d) Morulae may be seen in the cytoplasm of monocytes

Chlamydia

238. *C. trachomatis* can be distinguished from *C. psittaci* by which of the following criteria?
(a) *C. trachomatis* is sensitive to sulfonamides
(b) *C. trachomatis* has a different lipopolysaccharide antigen
(c) *C. trachomatis* is more infective to mice
(d) *C. psittaci* forms inclusions that contain glycogen

239. Skin test done to diagnose LGV is called:

(a) Freis test
(b) Schick test
(c) Dick test
(d) Bunn test

240. Which of the following techniques can be used for isolation chlamydia?

(a) Inoculation into mice
(b) Inoculation in yolk sac of chick embryo
(c) Inoculation cell culture
(d) All of the above

241. Which of the following character is shown by chlamydiae?

(a) Seck of peptidoglycen
(b) Seck of ability to produce their own ATP
(c) Production of inclusion bodies
(d) All of the above

242. Which of the serovars of chlamydia trachomatis cause trachoma?

(a) A,B,Ba, C
(b) D-K
(c) L_1-L_3
(d) All of the above

243. Which of the serovars of C trachomatis cause genital tract infections?

(a) A, B, B a c
(b) D-K
(c) Both of the above
(d) None of the above

244. Which of the serovars of chlamydia are responsible for inclusion conjunctivitis?

(a) A, B, Ba,c
(b) D-K
(c) L_1-L_3
(d) None of the above

245. The following is true of C. trachomatis:

(a) It is a gram -ve organism
(b) It can be cultivated on the Theyer Martin medium
(c) It causes trachoma
(d) It is susceptible to penicillin

246. LCL bodies are seen in:

(a) LGV
(b) Psittacosis
(c) Kala azar
(d) Chicken pox

247. Which is an obligatory intracellular organisms?

(a) Chlamydia
(b) Borrelia
(c) Actinomycetes
(d) Campylobacter

248. A man with chills, fever, and headache is thought to have "atypical" pneumonia. History reveals that he raises chickens and that approximately 2 weeks ago he lost a large number of them to an undiagnosed disease. The most likely diagnosis of this man's condition is:

(a) Ornithosis (psittacosis)
(b) Q fever
(c) Relapsing fever
(d) Leptospirosis

249. Which one of the following statements best characterizes lymphogranuloma venereum (LGV)?

(a) The causative agent is *C. trachomatis A,B,C*
(b) In India, it is more common among men
(c) It is most common in temperate regions
(d) Penicillin is effective in early treatment

ANSWERS

1.	(b)	2.	(e)	3.	(c)	4.	(b)	5.	(c)	6.	(c)	7.	(a)	8.	(a)
9.	(d)	10.	(a)	11.	(a)	12.	(a)	13.	(d)	14.	(d)	15.	(a)	16.	(b)
17.	(c)	18.	(e)	19.	(b)	20.	(b)	21.	(d)	22.	(c)	23.	(b)	24.	(c)
25.	(b)	26.	(b)	27.	(a)	28.	(a)	29.	(d)	30.	(d)	31.	(a)	32.	(c)
33.	(c)	34.	(b)	35.	(b)	36.	(a)	37.	(a)	38.	(a)	39.	(c)	40.	(a)
41.	(e)	42.	(d)	43.	(b)	44.	(c)	45.	(b)	46.	(d)	47.	(c)	48.	(d)
49.	(d)	50.	(b)	51.	(d)	52.	(e)	53.	(b)	54.	(b)	55.	(a)	56.	(e)
57.	(c)	58.	(b)	59.	(a)	60.	(a)	61.	(d)	62.	(a)	63.	(d)	64.	(b)
65.	(c)	66.	(d)	67.	(c)	68.	(d)	69.	(e)	70.	(b)	71.	(d)	72.	(c)
73.	(a)	74.	(b)	75.	(d)	76.	(c)	77.	(b)	78.	(c)	79.	(c)	80.	(c)
81.	(a)	82.	(c)	83.	(b)	84.	(d)	85.	(d)	86.	(b)	87.	(a)	88.	(a)
89.	(b)	90.	(d)	91.	(b)	92.	(b)	93.	(c)	94.	(a)	95.	(d)	96.	(c)
97.	(e)	98.	(b)	99.	(a)	100.	(c)	101.	(c)	102.	(d)	103.	(d)	104.	(c,a)
105.	(c)	106.	(c)	107.	(c)	108.	(b)	109.	(a)	110.	(d)	111.	(b)	112.	(a)
113.	(a)	114.	(c)	115.	(a)	116.	(a)	117.	(c)	118.	(a)	119.	(c)	120.	(a)
121.	(d)	122.	(d)	123.	(d)	124.	(a)	125.	(c)	126.	(a)	127.	(b)	128.	(c)
129.	(e)	130.	(d)	131.	(a)	132.	(d)	133.	(c)	134.	(c)	135.	(a)	136.	(e)
137.	(a)	138.	(a,d)	139.	(c)	140.	(d)	141.	(b)	142.	(d)	143.	(b)	144.	(b,a)
145.	(c)	146.	(e)	147.	(b)	148.	(d)	149.	(c)	150.	(e)	151.	(b)	152.	(d)
153.	(d)	154.	(a,b)	155.	(c)	156.	(b)	157.	(b)	158.	(d)	159.	(e)	160.	(d)
161.	(c)	162.	(a)	163.	(d)	164.	(e)	165.	(d)	166.	(a)	167.	(a)	168.	(a)
169.	(e)	170.	(e)	171.	(c)	172.	(d)	173.	(a)	174.	(c)	175.	(b)	176.	(b)
177.	(c)	178.	(b)	179.	(c)	180.	(c)	181.	(b)	182.	(d)	183.	(c)	184.	(a)
185.	(c)	186.	(d)	187.	(a)	188.	(a,b,c,d)	189.	(c)	190.	(d)	191.	(b)	192.	(b)
193.	(a)	194.	(c)	195.	(d)	196.	(a)	197.	(b)	198.	(a)	199.	(c)	200.	(a)
201.	(b)	202.	(a)	203.	(c)	204.	(d,b)	205.	(c)	206.	(c)	207.	(c)	208.	(c)
209.	(b)	210.	(b)	211.	(c)	212.	(a)	213.	(b)	214.	(e)	215.	(c)	216.	(c)
217.	(b)	218.	(c)	219.	(e)	220.	(c)	221.	(a)	222.	(b)	223.	(a)	224.	(a)
225.	(b)	226.	(a)	227.	(a)	228.	(a)	229.	(d)	230.	(c)	231.	(d)	232.	(b)
233.	(c)	234.	(c)	235.	(d)	236.	(d)	237.	(d)	238.	(b)	239.	(a)	240.	(d)
241.	(d)	242.	(a)	243.	(b)	244.	(b)	245.	(c)	246.	(b)	247.	(a)	248.	(a)
249.	(b)														

Chapter 6

MYCOLOGY

Group of **non-motile eukaryotic organisms** which exist as saprophytes, parasites or commensals.

- The cells possess rigid cell wall **composed of chitin (polymer of N-acetylglucosamine).**
- Cell membrane which surrounds the cytoplasm contains **sterols (ergosterol).**
- The cytoplasm contains **true nuclei with nuclear membrane, mitochondria, 80 S ribosomes, food reserves (fat, oil or glycogen).**
- Fungi may be **unicellular or multicellular.**
- They divide asexually, sexually or by both processes.

SYSTEMATIC CLASSIFICATION

Four classes (type of sexual spore formed):

- **Zygomycetes** (zygospores) – Rhizopus.
- **Ascomycetes** (ascospores) – Aspergillus.
- **Basidiomycetes** (basidiospores) – Cryptococcus neoformans.
- **Deuteromycetes:**
  - Lack known sexual state.
  - Also called as **Fungi Imperfecti.**
  - Most medically important fungi belong to this group.

MORPHOLOGICAL CLASSIFICATION

Yeasts

- Reproduce **asexually by budding or fission.**
- Round or oval unicellular fungi.
- Form moist or mucoid colonies.

  E.g.: Saccharomyces cerevisae, Cryptococcus neoformans.

Yeast-like

- Formation of **pseudohyphae** (chains of elongated cells having constriction at the septa).

  E.g.: Candida spp.

Molds

- **Produce branching filaments called hyphae.**
- Hyphae may be septate or nonseptate (coenocytic).
- **Tangled mass of hyphae is called as mycelium.**
- In culture medium part of the mycelium projecting above the surface is called as aerial mycelium and part growing in the medium is called as vegetative mycelium.

  E.g.: Aspergillus spp., Penicillium spp., dermatophytes, Mucor spp. etc.

Dimorphic Fungi

- **Yeast** form in the host tissue and in-vitro at 37°C on enriched media.
- **Mould** form in-vitro at 25°C.
  E.g.: **Sporothrix schenkii,** Histoplasma capsulatum, Blastomyces dermatitidis, Coccidiodes immitis, Paracoccidiodes brasilienses, Penicillium marneffei.Q

CLASSIFICATION OF FUNGAL SPORES

Sexual Spores (Z A B)Q

- Zygospore.
- Ascospore.
- Basidiospore.

Asexual Spores (A B C)

- **Blastospore** (budding yeast cell, Candida spp.).
- **Arthrospore** (mold form of C. immitis).
- **Chlamydospore** (Candida albicans).
- **Microconidia** (single-celled conidia).
- **Macroconidia** (multicelled conidia, Microsporum spp.).
- **Sporangiospore** (Rhizopus spp., Mucor spp.).

Perfect state (sexual stage) of a fungus is known as **Teleomorph** whereas imperfect state (asexual stage) is known as **Anamorph.** Both are separately classified and named for a genus and the species. A single organism may produce both anamorphs and teleomorphs therefore; many fungi have more than one name.

CLINICAL CLASSIFICATION

Superficial Mycoses

- Infection of skin, hair, nails.
  E.g.: Dermatophytosis, Pityriasis versicolor, Tinea nigra, Black piedra, White piedra.

Subcutaneous Mycoses

- Infection of skin, subcutaneous tissue and bones.
- Inoculation of saprophytic fungi.
  E.g.: Mycetoma, Chromoblastomycosis, Sporotrichosis, Rhinosporidiosis.

Systemic Mycoses

- Inhalation of airborne spores.
  E.g.: Blastomycosis, Histoplasmosis, Coccidioidomycosis and Paracoccidioidomycosis.

Opportunistic Mycoses

- Produced by opportunistic pathogens.
  E.g.: Aspergillosis, Penicilliosis, Zygomycosis, Candidiasis, Cryptococcosis.

Miscellaneous Mycoses

- Otomycosis, keratomycosis.

SUPERFICIAL MYCOSES

Pityriasis Versicolor

- Chronic superficial infection of stratum corneum.

- White to brown colored lesions covered with scales.
- Caused by **lipophilic** fungus **Malassezia furfur.**
- **Common sites:** Chest, back, abdomen, neck.

Laboratory Diagnosis

Direct Examination: 10% KOH mount of scrapings from the lesion shows yeast cells (2-7 μm) along with short curved hyphae (**banana and grapes; spaghetti and meat ball** appearance).Q

Culture: On SDA overlaid with olive oil (lipophilic fungus); creamy colonies develop in 5-7 days.

In wood lamp examination – Golden yellow fluorescence is seen.

PIEDRA

Fungal infection of hair, characterized by appearance of firm, irregular nodules along the hair shaft.

Black Piedra

Caused by **Piedrae hortae.**Q

Discrete black, gritty, hard nodules on the hair of the scalp.

10% KOH mount of the crushed nodule reveals **dark septate hyphae** with club shaped asci, each containing 2-8 ascospores.

White Piedra

Caused by Trichosporon beigelii.Q

Soft, mucilaginous, greyish nodules on the hair of genital area, beard, moustache.

10% KOH mount reveals mycelia which fragment into arthrospores.

Tinea Nigra

Caused by **dematiaceous fungus Exophiala werneckii.Q**

Brown to black discoloration of the thickly keratinised sites such as palms and soles.

10% KOH mount shows **brown septate branching hyphae** and budding yeast cells (1-5 μm). On SDA it forms moist, dark colored colonies.

DERMATOPHYTOSIS

Dermatophytosis, tinea or ringworm is the most common superficial mycosis.

It infects keratinised tissues of the skin, hair and nails.

Caused by 42 species of dermatopytes belonging to three genera:

- **Trichophyton:** 24 species (infect skin, hair and nails).
- **Microsporum:** 16 species (infect skin and hair).
- **Memory aid: M does not affect contain N.**
- **Epidermophyton:** 2 species (infect skin and nails).

On the basis of natural habitat they are classified into three groups:

- **Geophilic:** Found in soil.
- **Zoophilic:** Found in domestic or wild animals.
- **Anthropophilic:** Found exclusively in humans.

Geophilic	Zoophilic	Anthropophilic
T. ajelloi **M. gypseumQ**	T. equinum **T. mentagrophytes var. mentagrophytesQ** **T. verrucosumQ**	T. mentagrophytes var. intedigitale **T. rubrumQ** **T. schoenleniiQ**

Contd.

Contd.

	M. canisQ	**T. tonsuransQ** T. violaceum M. audounii **E. floccosumQ**

Secondary eruptions may occur in sensitized patients due to circulation of antigen from the primary site. It is called as **dermatophytid or id reaction.**

Clinically it is classified depending upon the site involved:

Clinical Classification	Etiological Agent
Tinea corporis (non hairy region) Tinea imbricata **(Indian ringworm, hanuman ringworm)**	T. rubrum T. concentricum
Tinea pedis **(athlete's foot)**	T. rubrum, T. mentagropytes
Tinea capitis **(Favus, Kerion)**	Trichopyton spp., Microsporum spp.
KerionQ	T. verrucosum, T. mentagrophytes
FavusQ	T. schoenlenii, T. violaceum, M. gypseum
Tinea cruris (jock itch)Q	E. floccosum, T. rubrum, T. mentagrophytes
Tinea barbae (barbers itch)Q	T. rubrum, T. mentagrophytes
Tinea unguium (nail)	T. rubrum, T. mentagrophytes
Tinea manuum (hands)	T. rubrum, E. floccosum

Two types of hair invasion are seen with dermatophytes:

- **Ectothrix:** Arthroconidia appear as sheath on the surface of the hair shaft.
- **Endothrix:** Arthrospores formation occurs entirely within the hair completely filling the hair shaft.

Ectothrix	Endothrix (TVS)
T. mentagrophytes T. rubrum T. verrucosum M. canis M. gypseum M. audouinii	T. **t**onsurans T. **v**iolaceum T. **s**choenlenii

Laboratory Diagnosis:

KOH wet mount: Branching hyaline mycelium, arthrospores formation.

Culture: Grow on SDA. Septate hyaline hyphae, microconidia and macroconidia. The differentiation of three genera based on the nature of macroconidia.

Dermatophytes	Macroconidia	Microconidia
Trichophyton	Rare, thin walled, smooth, **pencil shapedQ**	**AbundantQ**
Microsporum	Numerous, thick walled, rough, **spindle shaped**	Rare
Epidermophyton	Numerous, smooth walled, **club shaped**	**AbsentQ**

Hair Perforation Test:

- Filter paper soaked in distilled water.
- Sterilized prepubertal/infant hair is taken.
- Inoculate the hair, incubate for four weeks at 25°C.

- **Wet mount:** Conical perforation of the hair shaft.
- **T. mentagrophytes and M. canis** (+); T. rubrum and M. equinum (-).

Urease Test:

- Christensen's urea agar inoculated.
- Incubated at room temperature for 5 days.
- **T. mentagrophytes (+)** and T. rubrum (-).Q

SUBCUTANEOUS MYCOSES

MYCETOMA

- **Chronic granulomatous infection** of the exposed part of the body.
- First observed in **Madurai district of South India** (1842).
- Infection follows traumatic inoculation of the organism into the subcutaneous tissue.

Triad of symptoms: Tumefaction of involved tissue + draining sinus tracts + grains or granules.

Three Types:

- **Eu**mycetoma (more prevalent in north India).
- **Actino**mycetoma (more prevalent in south India).
- **Botryo**mycosis (Mycetoma like lesion caused by staphylococcus aureus).Q

Genus	Colour of Grains
Eumycetoma	
• **Ma**durella mycetomatis	Black
• **Ma**durella grisea	Black
• **Exo**phiala jeanselmei	Black
• **Acremonium** kilienseQ	White
• **Pseudoallescheria boydiiQ**	White
Actinomycetoma	
• Actinomadura madurae	White, Yellow
• **Actinomadura pellitieriQ**	Red
• Nocardia asteroides	White
• Nocardia brasiliensis	White
Streptomyces somaliensisQ	Yellow

	Actinomycotic	**Eumycotic**
Tumor	Multiple tumour masses with ill defined margins	Single, well defined margins
Sinuses	Appear early, numerous, raised inflamed opening	Appear late, few in no.
Discharge	Purulent	Serous
Granule	White/red	Black/white
Bone	Osteolytic lesions	Osteosclerotic lesions
Filament	< 2 μm (bacilli)	>2 um (hyphae)

CHROMOBLASTOMYCOSIS

Chronic localized infection of the skin and subcutaneous tissue.

Irregular, rough, cauliflower-like lesions involving mostly lower legs and feet.

Caused by following **dematiaceous fungi:**

- **Phialo**phora verrucosa.
- **Fonas**ecaea pedrosoi, F. compacta.
- **Clados**porium bantiana.
- **Rhino**cladiella aquaspersa.

Infection follows traumatic inoculation of the organism into the subcutaneous tissue.

Microscopy of biopsy shows: Thick walled **Fonas**ecaea pedrosoi, brown cells divided by transverse septa called **SCLEROTIC BODIES/COPPER PENNY/MURIFORM CELLS/MEDLAR BODIES.Q**

PHAEOHYPHOMYCOSIS

The fungus in the tissue is present in the **form of darkly pigmented septate hyphae** and not as thick walled cluster of cells.

- Caused by exogenous dematiaceous fungi which normally occur in the nature.
- **Commonly implicated fungi: Wangiella dermatitidis, Exophiala jeanselmei.**

CHROMOMYCOSIS

Term chromomycosis includes chromoblastomycosis and a variety of diseases by other dematiaceous fungi, like phaeohyphomycosis of subcutaneous tissue, CNS, paranasal sinuses.

RHINOSPORIDIOSIS

Caused by **Rhinosporidium seeberi.**

- **Chronic granulomatous disease** characterised by friable sessile or pedunculated polyps or wart like lesions.
- **Nasal (Most common),** ocular, cutaneous, other mucocutaneous sites.
- 90% cases have been reported from Srilanka, India, South America.
- **India:** Tamilnadu, Kerala, Orissa, Andhra Pradesh.
- Very little known about its mode of transmission.
- **Persons bathing in stagnant pools of water.Q**

Laboratory Diagnosis: Non-cultivable.

Biopsy stained with H&E, GMS, PAS, Carminophilic **(Mayer's muciarmine stains inner layer of sporangium and outer layer of endospore).**

Sporangia (350 µm in diameter) filled with endospores (6-9 µm in diameter).Q

Treatment – Dapsone or surgical polypectomy.

SPOROTRICHOSIS

Chronic pyogenic granulomatous infection of the skin and subcutaneous tissue.

- Caused by dimorphic fungus **Sporothrix schenkii.**
- Fungus is found in soil, decaying wood, thorns.
- Infection seen in rural workers, **gardeners,** florists, carpenters.
- **India:** Prevalent in sub-Himalayan areas from Himachal Pradesh to Assam.
- **Infection is due to implantation of spores through injured skin.**

Clinical Forms:

- **Lymphocutaneous (Most common type).Q**
- Fixed cutaneous.

- Mucocutaneous.
- Disseminated.
- Pulmonary.

The initial lesion is a **small ulcerated nodule** on the arm or forehand. Nodules and abscesses occur along the draining lymphatics and the regional lymph nodes enlarge and ulcerate. The primary lesion may remain localized or disseminate.

LABORATORY DIAGNOSIS

Direct microscopic examination:

- PAS, methenamine silver or fluorescent staining shows oval, **cigar shaped** yeast cells.Q
- **Splendore-Hoeppli** or **Asteroid phenomenon Q:** Central basophilic yeast cell with eosinophilic (immune complex deposition) material radiating from it.

Culture:

Growth on SDA at 25°C shows delicate hyphae bearing pyriform conidia arising directly from hypha or developing in a **rosette pattern** at the ends of conidiophore **(Flower like sporulation).Q**

SYSTEMIC MYCOSES

HISTOPLASMOSIS

Classical Histoplasmosis/Darlings Disease.Q

Caused by dimorphic fungus Histoplasma capsulatum.

Infection of reticuloendothelial system

- Occurs predominantly in America and Africa.
- 25 cases have been reported from India but no definite endemic focus is known.
- Grows in the soil with high nitrogen content enriched with excreta of bats and chickens.

Infection is due to inhalation of spores.

Clinical Features:

Asymptomatic in 90-95% cases.

Clinical Types:

- Acute pulmonary.
- Chronic pulmonary.
- Cutaneous/subcutaneous/mucocutaneous.
- Disseminated.

Laboratory Diagnosis:

Specimens: Sputum, biopsy of bone marrow, cutaneous, mucosal lesions.

Direct Microscopic Examination:

Giemsa, Wright, calcofluor white staining.

Round/oval yeast cells (2-4 μm diameter) found intracellular within macrophages **(Narrow based budding yeast cells).**Q

Culture:

Growth on SDA at 25°C shows septate branching hyphae with two types of unicellular asexual spores. **Large round tuberculate macroconidia Q** (8-14 μm) and smooth walled, pyriform microconidia (2-4 μm).

BLASTOMYCOSIS

Gilchrist's disease, Chicago disease, North American Blastomycosis

- Caused by dimorphic fungus **Blastomyces dermatitidis.**
- Occurs predominantly in central and mid western USA and eastern Canada.
- Few reports from India.
- Infection is due to inhalation of spores, natural habitat unknown.

Clinical Features

Laboratory Diagnosis:

Specimens: Pus from abscess, sputum, tissue.

Direct microscopic examination:

- Methenamine silver, H&E, PAS staining.
- **Thick walled spherical yeast cells** (8-15 μm), single bud with broad base of attachment **(figure of eight appearance).**
- **On PAS staining** shows **Splendore-Hoeppli phenomenon.**

Culture:

Growth on SDA at 25°C shows **septate branching hyphae** with smooth walled, spherical or pyriform microconidia (2-10 μm) that are located on short terminal or lateral branches.

PARACOCCIDIODOMYCOSIS

South American Blastomycosis, Lutz's Mycosis

- Caused by dimorphic fungus **Paracoccidiodes brasilienses.**
- Occurs predominantly in humid mountain forests of South and Central America.
- No reports from India.
- Infection is due to inhalation of spores, fungus has been isolated from soil.

Clinical Features

Clinical Types:

Acute or subcutaneous form (Juvenile type).

Chronic form (Adult type)

- Unifocal.
- Multifocal.

There is a primary pulmonary infection that spreads by haematogenous routes to mucosa of the nose, mouth, gastrointestinal tract, skin, lymphatics, internal organs producing chronic granulomatous reaction.

Laboratory Diagnosis:

Specimens: Pus from abscess, sputum, biopsy from lesions.

Direct Microscopic Examination:

Methenamine silver, H and E staining.

Yeast cell (2-30 μm) with multiple buds **(Mariner's wheel, pilot wheel, mickey mouse appearance).**

COCCIDIODOMYCOSIS

San Joaquin Valley Fever, Desert Rheumatism

- Caused by dimorphic fungus **Coccidiodes immitis.**

- Occurs predominantly in semi-arid areas of South-West USA and North Mexico.
- No reports from India.
- Infection is due to **inhalation of arthroconidia.**

Clinical Features

Clinical Types:

Primary pulmonary type (influenza like illness), some people [mainly white females develop hypersensitivity reaction after 1-2 weeks which is called as **(San Joaquin Valley fever or Desert rheumatism)**].

- **Primary cutaneous type.**
- **Scrofuloderma type (enlargement of cervical lymph nodes).**
- **Disseminated type** (osteoarticular lesions, CNS involvement).

Laboratory Diagnosis:

Specimens: Pus from abscess, sputum, CSF.

Direct Microscopic Examination:

Methenamine silver, H and E and PAS staining.

Doubly refractile thick walled spherule (30-60 μm diameter) containing endospores.Q

Culture:

Growth on SDA at 25°C shows septate hyphae. **Aerial mycelia form alternate barrel shaped arthroconidia.Q**

OPPORTUNISTIC MYCOSES

CANDIDIASIS

Most common mycosis involving skin and its appendages, mucosa and internal organs.

- Caused by **yeast like fungus.**
- **Candida albicans** (most common species 80-90% of cases, **germ tube positive**).
- **C. stellatoidea** (germ tube positive).Q
- **C. dubliniensis** (germ tube positive).Q
- C. tropicalis.
- C. guilliermondi.
- C. krusei.
- C. glabrata.
- C. lusitaniae.

They occur as normal flora of skin, mucous membranes, gastrointestinal tract. Therefore, it is an **endogenous infection.**

Predisposing Factors:

AIDS, Diabetes, IV catheters, neutropenia, malignancy etc.

Clinical Types:

Mucocutaneous: Oral (thrush), oesophageal, vulvovaginitis, balanitis, conjunctivitis, keratitis.

Skin and nail infections: Intertrigenous areas (axilla, groin, perineum, submammary folds).

Systemic: UTI, pulmonary, endocarditis, meningitis, arthritis, osteomyelitis.

Laboratory Diagnosis:

Specimens: Exudates from lesions, skin and nail scrapings, blood culture.

Direct Microscopic Examination:

Gram staining, KOH mount.

Oval or spherical gram positive yeast cells with pseudohyphae (buds continues to grow but fails to detach, elongated cells are constricted at septations).Q

Culture:

Growth on SDA at 37°C **shows cream colored smooth pasty colonies.**Q

Identification:

Germ tube test: Culture inoculated in sheep or human serum and incubated at 37°C for 2-4 hours. A drop of suspension examined under microscope. **Long tube like projections extending from yeast cell (true hypha).** There is no constriction at the point of attachment. Called as **Reynolds-Braude phenomenon.**Q

Growth on corn-meal agar (C. albicans produces chlamydospores).

- Sugar fermentation tests.
- Sugar assimilation tests.

CRYPTOCOCCOSIS

Caused by **encapsulated true yeast, Cryptococcus neoformans.**

Five serotypes based on **polysaccharide capsular antigen (A,B,C,D,AD).**

C. neoformans var. neoformans	C. neoformans var. gattii
Serotype A,D,AD	Serotype B,C
Prevalent throughout the world	Parts of California, Australia
Isolated form **pigeon excretaQ**	Associated with **eucalyptus trees (river reed gum)**
More common	Less common
Spherical yeast cell	Oval yeast cell
Susceptible to canavanine	**Resistant to canavanineQ**
Cannot utilize glycine and d-proline as sole source of nitrogen	**Can utilize glycine and d-proline** as sole source of nitrogenQ
Urease not sensitive to EDTA	**Urease sensitive to EDTA**

- Infection occurs after **inhalation of yeast cells.**
- From lungs yeast can metastasize to any organ of the body.

Clinical Forms:

- **Pulmonary (Most common type).**
- CNS (meningitis).
- Cutaneous.
- Osseous.
- Visceral.

Laboratory Diagnosis:

Specimens: CSF, tissue sections.

Direct Microscopic Examination:

Negative staining (nigrosin/India ink) to demonstrate capsule, PAS, methenamine silver, H&E, Mayer's mucicarmine staining.

Spherical budding yeast (5-20 μm in diameter) cells surrounded by wide capsule that may be twice as thick as diameter of the cell.

Culture:

- Growth on SDA at 37°C shows **cream colored smooth pasty colonies.**
- Identification.
- **Produces enzyme phenoloxidase (brown colored colonies on bird seed agar, niger seed agar).**
- **Produces enzyme urease.**
- Inositol and nitrate assimilation test positive.
- Mice pathogenicity test positive.

Serology

Antigen detection: In serum and CSF by Latex agglutination; diagnostic and prognostic importance.

ASPERGILLOSIS

Important species: A. fumigatus, A. niger, A. flavus, A. terreus, A. nidulans.

Inhalation of **conidia or mycelial fragments.**

Predisposing factors: AIDS, immunosuppressive therapy, neutropenia, malignancy.

Clinical Forms:

- **Allergic bronchopulmonary aspergillosis.Q**
- **Aspergilloma (fungus ball).Q**
- **Invasive aspergillosis.**
- **Endocarditis.**
- **Paranasal granuloma.**

Laboratory Diagnosis:

Specimens: Sputum, BAL, transbronchial biopsy.

Direct Microscopic Examination:

10% KOH preparation, H&E, methenamine silver staining; special fungal stains better than H&E staining.

Hyaline, septate hyphae, 3-5 μm in diameter, dichotomus branching at acute angle mostly 45 degree.Q

Culture:

SDA at 25°C, isolate identified by growth characteristics and microscopic morphology.

ZYGOMYCOSIS/MUCORMYCOSIS

Caused by fungi of the class Zygomycetes.

Rhizopus spp., Mucor spp., Absidia spp.

Most common species: Rhizopus arrhizus.

Predisposing factors: Diabetes mellitus, metabolic acidosis, leukaemia, lymphoma etc.

Clinical Forms:

Rhinocerebral: Serious fulminating infection, **angioinvasive,** thrombosis and ischaemic necrosis of the tissue.

- **Pulmonary.**
- **Gastrointestinal.**
- **Disseminated.**
- **Dermal.**
- **Subcutaneous.**

Laboratory Diagnosis:

Specimens: Tissue biopsy.

Direct Microscopic Examination:

- H and E staining best, special fungal stains not useful.
- Hyaline, aseptate hyphae, ribbon like, 7-15 µm in diameter, irregular branching at the obtuse angle.Q

Culture:

SDA at 37°C, isolate identified by growth characteristics **(dense, hairy colony)** and microscopic morphology **(aseptate hyphae, sporangiophore, sporangiospores).**

Rhizoids Arrangement:

- **No rhizoids** – Mucor.Q
- **Internodal arrangement** – Absidia.Q
- **Directly opposite to sporangia** – Rhizopus.

MISCELLANEOUS FUNGAL INFECTIONS

PENICILLIOSIS

- More than 150 known species.
- Occur as saprophytes in soil and decomposing organic matter.
- Only dimorphic species is **P. marnefii.**
- Caused infection in **AIDS patients.Q**
- Mainly in southeast Asian countries.
- **India:** Cases have been reported from northeastern states.
- **Animal reservoir:** Chinese bamboo rats.
- Infection acquired by respiratory route.
- **Infects reticuloendothelial system.Q**

Clinical features: Tuberculosis like illness characterized by fever, weight loss, anaemia, involvement of liver, spleen, lungs.Q

Histologic sections: Ellipsoidal yeast cell (2-6 µm in length), divided by transverse septations (fission). **Stained well by PAS, methenamine silver.**

Mold form: SDA at 25°C, **brush like arrangement of conidia, produces brick red colored diffusible pigment.Q**

PNEUMOCYSTOSIS

Pneumocystis Carinii

Features in favor of fungi: 16s RNA, attacked by chitinase, lack of intracellular or sexual stages not typical of sporozoa, **stained with fungal stains.**

Features in favor of protozoa: 5s-rRNA similar to sporozoa, lacks ergosterol, responds better to anti-protozoal treatment.

- Greater similarity to fungi than to protozoa therefore classified as fungus.
- One of the most common opportunistic infection in AIDS.

Morphological forms: Trophozoite, sporozoites and cyst.

Trophozoites: Fill the alveoli of the lungs, pleomorphic, 2-12 µm.

Cysts: Most commonly observed, 5-8 µm, oval, thick walled, containing upto 8 sporozoites.

Cysts: Stained by **Methanamine silver** (black), Toluidine blue O (red purple).

Infection acquired by respiratory route; reactivation of latent infection.

Attaches and damages type I pneumocytes.

Clinical Features:

Fever; non-productive cough, hypoxia, cyanosis, gradual and progressive dyspnoea, alveolar or interstitial infiltrates (usually involves whole lung after beginning in the hilus), **CXR – perihilar haziness with diffuse mottling.Q**

Nosocomial spread – premature infants, debilitated, malnourished, congenital immunodeficiency.

Diagnosis: Bronchoalveolar lavage fluid, Lung Bx, Sputum, Direct microscopic examination, Direct Fluorescent antibody staining, not been successfully cultured.

Treatment: TMP – SMX, drug of choice (Cotrimoxazole).Q

OTOMYCOSIS

Subacute/chronic infection of external auditory canal.

Common Agents:

- **A. Niger (Blackish crust seen).**
- A. Fumigatus.
- Penicillium spp.
- C. Albicans.

Diagnosis by microscopic examination and culture.

KERATOMYCOSIS

Invasive Fungal Infection of the Cornea

Common Agents:

- **A. fumigatus.**
- A. flavus.
- A. glaucus.
- A. niger.
- **Fusarium** spp.
- **Curvularia** spp.
- **Penicillium spp.**
- **Alterneria** spp.

It usually follows trauma.

Diagnosis by microscopic examination and culture.

MYCOTOXICOSIS AND MYCETISMUS

Mycotoxicosis:

Illness or death of man or domesticated animals **following consumption of food contaminated with mycotoxins** (secondary metabolites and their affects are not dependent on fungal infection or viability), e.g., Aflatoxins produced by Aspergillus flavus (Turkey X disease) leads to Hepatocellular carcinoma.

Mycetismus:

Due to the **consumption of fleshy fungi,** e.g., Ergot poisoning caused by eating bread made of rye flour which is contaminated with **Claviceps** purpurea **(St. Anthony's fire, St. Vitus Dance), mushroom poisoning.Q**

RESPIRATORY ALLERGIC DISEASES CAUSED BY FUNGI AND ACTINOMYCETES

Allergic Disease	Source	Etiology
Farmer's lung	Stored hay	Thermoactinomyces vulgaris, **Micromonospora faeniiQ**
Bagassosis	Sugar cane	**T sacchariiQ**
Maple bark strippers lung	Maple tree bark	Cryptostroma corticale
Cheese washers lung	Cheese	**Penicillium caseicolum**
Maltster's lung	Barley malt	**Aspergillus clavatusQ**
Sequoiosis	Red wood saw dust	**Aureobasidium pullulans**
Suberosis	Cork	**Penicillium frequentans**
Wood pulp workers lung	Wood pulp	**Alterneria spp.**
Humidifier lung	Humidifier	**T. vulgaris**, T. candidus

MCQs

GENERAL PROPERTIES OF FUNGUS

Classification of Fungi

1. **Aseptate hyphae are seen in:** *(Recent MCQ)*
   (a) Phycomycetes
   (b) Ascomycetes
   (c) Basidiomycetes
   (d) Deutromycetes
2. **Which of the following is produced sexually?** *(AIIMS 81)*
   (a) Ascospore
   (b) Conidium
   (c) Blastoconidia
   (d) Yeast buds
3. **Fungal spores may be produced:** *(AIIMS 02)*
   (a) Singly
   (b) In chains
   (c) In sporangium
   (d) All of the above
4. **Budding reproduction in tissue is seen in:** *(Recent MCQ)*
   (a) Cryptococcus, Candida
   (b) Candida, Rhizopus
   (c) Rhizopus, Mucor
   (d) Histoplasma, Candida

Morphology

5. **Which of the following is only yeast?** *(Recent MCQ)*
   (a) Candida
   (b) Mucor
   (c) Rhizopus
   (d) Cryptococcus
6. **In HIV infected individual Gram stain of lung aspirate shows yeast like morphology. All of the following are the most likely diagnosis *except*:** *(AIIMS Nov 05)*
   (a) Candida tropicalis
   (b) Cryptococcus neoformans
   (c) Penicillium marneffi
   (d) Aspergillus fumigatus
7. **A 25 years old female complains of recurrent rhinitis, nasal discharge and bilateral nasal blockage since one year. She has history of asthma and allergy. On examination multiple ethmoidal polyps are noted with mucosal thickening and impacted secretions in both the nasal cavities. Biopsy is taken and the material is cultured which shown the growth of many hyphae and pseudohyphae with dichotomous branching typically at 45°. Which of the following is the most likely responsible organism?** *(AI 10)*
   (a) Aspergillus fumigatus
   (b) Rhizopus
   (c) Mucor
   (d) Candida

8. Gram stained periorbital exudates in severe panophthalmitis with cellulitis in an elderly diabetic shows irregular branching aseptate and broad hyphae. Which of the following is the most likely diagnosis? *(AI 12)*

(a) Candida (b) Aspergillus
(c) Pencillium (d) Apophysomyces species

9. Acute angled septate hyphae are seen in: *(Recent MCQ)*

(a) Aspergillus (b) Mucor
(c) Penicillium (d) Candida

Laboratory Diagnosis

10. KOH wet mount can be prepared for:

(a) Bacteria (b) Virus
(c) Fungus (d) Parasite

11. Stain used for staining fungal elements:

(a) Acid fast stain (b) Mucicarmine
(c) Methanamine silver (d) Gram stain

12. Which dye is most suitable for fungus demonstration in biopsy?

(a) Alizarin red (b) Veirhoff dye
(c) Masson's trichome (d) PAS

13. Which of the following fungi difficult to isolate culture?

(a) Candida (b) Dermatophytes
(c) Cryptococcus (d) Malassezia furfur

14. Which organism cannot be cultured? *(PGI Nov 14)*

(a) Klebsiella rhinoscleromatis (b) Klebsiella ozaenae
(c) Klebsiella granulomatis (d) Pneumocystis jiroveci
(e) Rhinosporidium seeberi

Dimorphic Fungi

15. Which of the following is false regarding dimorphic fungi? *(Recent MCQ)*

(a) Occurs in two growth forms
(b) Can cause systemic infection
(c) Cryptococcus is an example
(d) Coccidioides is an example

16. All are dimorphic fungi *except*: *(AIIMS May 09)*

(a) Blastomyces dermatitidis (b) Histoplasma
(c) Pencillium marneffi (d) Phialopora

17. Dimorphic fungus: *(Recent MCQ)*

(a) Candida (b) Histoplasma
(c) Rhizopus (d) Mucor

Fungal Infections

18. White piedra is caused by: *(MH 11)*

(a) Piedra hortae (b) Pityrosporum orbicularea
(c) Hortae wernickii (d) Trichosporum beigelli

DERMATOPHYTES

Classifications

19. Which of the following infects hair, skin and nails? *(Recent MCQ)*

(a) Trichosporum
(b) Trichophyton
(c) Microsporum
(d) Epidermophyton

20. A patient made a self-diagnosis of athlete's foot (Tinea pedis) and began using a product advertised on television. The condition improved but did not clear and then the patient showed himself to a Dermatologist. A skin scraping was sent to the laboratory for culture, including culture for fungi. The fungal culture yielded a slow growing colony, which produced a few small microconidia. This is consistent with isolation of a dermatophyte of the genera: *(AIIMS Nov 03)*

(a) Trichophyton
(b) Microsporum
(c) Epidermophyton
(d) Trichosporon

TINEA CAPITIS AND TINEA VERSICOLOR

21. Most common cause of Tinea capitis: *(Recent MCQ)*

(a) M. canis
(b) Epidermophyton floccosum
(c) T. Tonsurans
(d) M. distortum

22. Kerion is caused by: *(PGI 98)*

(a) Candida
(b) Streptococcus
(c) Dermatophytes
(d) Herpes

23. Black dot ring worm is caused by: *(Recent MCQ)*

(a) Microsporum
(b) Trichophyton
(c) Epidermophyton
(d) Candida

24. T. capitis (endothrix) is caused by: *(PGI Dec 2000)*

(a) Epidermophyton
(b) T. tonsurans
(c) T. violaceum
(d) Microsporum
(e) T. rubrum

25. Pityriasis versicolor is caused by: *(Recent MCQ)*

(a) E. floccosum
(b) M. gypseum
(c) M. furfur
(d) T. tonsurans

26. Selenium sulfide is indicated for treating: *(Recent MCQ)*

(a) Tinea versicolor
(b) Tinea corporis
(c) Mixed mycotic infections
(d) Candidiasis only

27. Trichophyton species which is zoophilic?

(a) T. tonsurans
(b) T. violaceum
(c) T. schoenleinii
(d) T. mentagrophytes

28. Which of the following is spread from animals to man? *(AI 92)*

(a) T. rubrum
(b) T. tonsurans
(c) T. floccosum
(d) T. verrucosum

29. Tinea cruris is caused by: *(PGI 97)*

(a) Epidermophyton
(b) Trichophyton
(c) Microsporum
(d) Candida

30. Hair perforation test is positive in infection with:

(a) Trichophyton
(b) Microsporum
(c) Epidermophyton
(d) All of the above

SUBCUTANEOUS MYCOSIS AND SYSTEMIC MYCOSIS

Mycetoma

1. A farmer has an ulcer on leg with indurated margin and multiple sinuses with discharging granules. The likely diagnosis is: (*AIIMS Dec 94*)

(a) Nocardia (b) Dimorphic fungus
(c) Aspergillus (d) Dermatophytes

2. The causative organism in Madura Mycosis Mycetomatis: (*AI 96*)

(a) Madurella mycetomatis (b) Nocardia
(c) Aspergillus (d) Dermatophytes

3. Color of granules in mycetoma caused by:

Actinomadura pelleteri

(a) Black (b) Red
(c) Yellow (d) Brown

4. The granules discharged in mycetoma contains:

(a) Pus cells (b) Inflammatory cells
(c) Bone spicules (d) Fungal colonies

5. Which of the following is false about mycetoma? (*AI 95*)

(a) Can affect lower and upper extremities (b) Caused by actinomycetes and filamentous fungi
(c) Diagnosis is by examination of pus (d) Uncommon in India

CANDIDA

Morphology

6. Reynold Braude phenomenon is seen in:

(a) Candida albicans (b) Candida parapsilosis
(c) Histoplasma (d) Cryptococcus

7. The following is not true of candida albicans:

(a) Yeast like fungus (b) Forms chlamydospores
(c) Blastomeres seen in isolates (d) Causes meningitis in immunocompromise

8. Candida albicans causes all of the following *except*: (*AI 95*)

(a) Endocarditis (b) Mycetoma
(c) Meningitis (d) Oral thrush

9. Which fungal infection is the most common in neutropenia? (*AIIMS 99*)

(a) Candida (b) Histoplasma
(c) Aspergillus niger (d) Aspergillus fumigates

10. Most common fungal infection in febrile neutropenia is:

(a) Aspergillus niger (b) Candida
(c) Mucormycosis (d) Aspergillus fumigates

CRYPTOCOCCUS

Morophology, Diagnosis and Transmission

11. Primary site of infection in cryptococcosis is:

(a) Adrenal gland (b) Bone
(c) Central nervous system (d) Lung

12. The capsule of cryptococcus neoformans in a CSF sample is best seen by:

(a) Gram stain
(b) India ink preparation
(c) Giemsa stain
(d) Methanamine-silver stain

Virulence Factors and Clinical Features

13. Phagocytosis of C. neoformans is inhibited by: (*PGI 83*)

(a) Cryptococcal capsular material
(b) The size of the yeast cells
(c) The cell walls
(d) Toxins produced by the organism

14. Cryptococcus is least likely to cause infection of: (*GI 951*)

(a) Skin
(b) Bone
(c) Brain
(d) Kidney

15. Eucalyptus camaldulensis is associated with the transmission of: (*PGI 99*)

(a) Blastomyces dermatitidis
(b) Histoplasma
(c) Cryptococcus
(d) Coccidioides immitis

16. Fungi that possess a capsule is:

(a) Candida
(b) Aspergillus
(c) Cryptococcus
(d) Mucor

ASPERGILLUS

Morphology and Clinical Features

17. What is the most probable portal of entry of an Aspergillus?

(a) Puncture wound
(b) Blood
(c) Lungs
(d) Gastrointestinal tract

18. Aspergillus causes all *except*:

(a) Bronchopulmonary allergy
(b) Otomycosis
(c) Dermatophytosis
(d) Keratitis

Differential Diagnosis

19. An elderly diabetic has left sided orbital cellulites, CT scan of paranasal sinuses shows evidence of left maxillary sinusitis. Gram stained smear of the orbital exudates shows irregularly branching septate hyphae. The following is the most likely aetiological: (*AIIMS Nov 03*)

(a) Aspergillus
(b) Mucor
(c) Candida
(d) Rhizopus

20. In a patient, corneal scraping reveals narrow angled septate hyphae, which of the following is likely etiologic agent?

(a) Mucor
(b) Histoplasma
(c) Aspergillus
(d) Candida

21. Which of the following is the most common etiological agent in paranasal sinus mycoses?

(a) Aspergillus spp
(b) Histoplasma
(c) Conidiobolus coronatus
(d) Candida albicans

22. Aflatoxins are produced by:

(a) Aspergillus flavus
(b) Aspergillus niger
(c) Aspergillus fumigatus
(d) Candida

P. CARINII

Developmental Stages and Clinical Features

23. Pneumocystis carnii is a:
(a) Fungi
(b) Gram negative
(c) Protozoa
(d) Virus

24. P. carnii causes infection of primarily:
(a) Rats
(b) Mice
(c) Rabbits
(d) Humans

Diagnosis and Treatment

25. A patient of acute leukemia is admitted with febrile neutropenia. On day four of being treated with broad-spectrum antibiotics, his fever increases. X-ray chest shows trilateral fluffy infiltrates. Which of the following should be the most appropriate next step in the management?
(a) Add antiviral therapy
(b) Add antifungal therapy
(c) Add cotrimoxazole
(d) Continue chemotherapy

ENDEMIC MYCOSIS

26. Which of the following is endemic mycosis?
(a) Candidiasis
(b) Blastomycosis
(c) Cryptococcosis
(d) None of the above

Histoplasmosis

27. True about Histoplasma capsulatum: *(Recent MCQ)*
(a) Dimorphic fungus
(b) Causative organism of moniliasis
(c) Causative organism of valley fever
(d) Capsulated

28. What is true about Histoplasmosis? *(AIIMS May 08)*
(a) In early stage it is indistinguishable from TB
(b) Culture is not diagnostic
(c) Hyphal forms are infectious form
(d) Person to person spread occurs by droplet infection

29. Tuberculate spores are features of:
(a) Candidia
(b) Histoplasma
(c) Coccidiodomyces
(d) Cryptococcus

Coccidiodes

30. In tissue, Coccidioides immitis produces:
(a) Spherules and endospores
(b) Encapsulated yeast cells
(c) Fine, delicate hyphae
(d) Coarse, septate hyphae

31. Valley fever desert rheumatism is caused by:
(a) Sporothrix
(b) Coccidioides
(c) Phialophora
(d) Histoplasma

32. Coccidioides immitis is identified in tissues on the basis of which of the following? *(AIIMS, Orissa 90)*
(a) Budding yeast cells with pseudohyphae
(b) Yeast like forms with very large capsules
(c) Arthrospores
(d) Endosporulating spherules

CHROMOBLASTOMYCOSIS

33. Causative microorganism of chromoblastomycosis:

(a) Cladosporium
(b) Blastomyces
(c) Sporothrix
(d) Histoplasma capsulatum

34. Sclerotic bodies is seen: *(AIIMS, May 93)*

(a) Sporotrichosis
(b) Blastomycosis
(c) Chromoblastomycosis
(d) Coccidiodes

SPOROTRICHOSIS

35. A plant prick can produce sporotrichosis. All are true statements about sporotrichosis *except*:

(a) Is a chronic mycotic disease that typically involves skin, subcutaneous tissue and regional lymphatics
(b) Most cases are acquired via cutaneous inoculation
(c) Enlarged lymph nodes extending centripetally as a beaded chain are a characteristic findings
(d) It is an occupational disease of butchers-doctors

36. A gardener has multiple vesicles on hand and multiple eruptions along the lymphatics. Most common fungus responsible is: *(AIIMS Nov 08)*

(a) Sporothrix schenckii
(b) Cladosporium
(c) Histoplasma
(d) Candida

37. A patient, resident of Himachal Pradesh presented with a series of ulcers in a row, on his right leg. The biopsy from the affected area was taken and cultured on Sabouraud's Dextrose agar. What would be the most likely causative organism? *(AIIMS Nov 03)*

(a) Sporothrixschenckii
(b) Cladosporium spp.
(c) Pseudoallescheria boydii
(d) Nocardia brasiliensis

38. Asteroid bodies and cigar shaped globi may be produced by: *(AIIMS 87)*

(a) Sporothrix
(b) Sporotrichosis
(c) Phialophora
(d) Aspergillus

39. A diabetic patient presents with pus from eye. Colonies of isolated organisms are black with microscopic feature of non-septate hyphae and obtuse branching. Diagnosis is:

(a) Aspergillosis
(b) Candidiasis
(c) Mucormycosis
(d) Histoplasmosis

MISCELLANEOUS

40. Which is false about penicillium marneffi?

(a) Black colonies
(b) Dimorphic fungi
(c) Amphotericin B used for treatment
(d) Causes fulminant infections in immunocompromised patients

41. Which of the following is the most common fungal infection in immunocompetent patient?

(a) Candida
(b) Aspergillus
(c) Cryptococcus
(d) Penicillium

42. Which is not a fungus?

(a) Rhinosporidiosis
(b) Sporotrichosis
(c) Torulosis
(d) Candidiasis

43. A diabetic patient present with bloody nasal discharge, orbital swelling and pain. Culture of periorbital pus showing branching septate hyphae. Which of the following is the most probable organism involved? *(AI 10)*

(a) Mucor
(b) Candida
(c) Aspergillus
(d) Rhizopus

44. The culture media for fungus is: *(Recent MCQ)*

(a) Tellurite medium
(b) NNN medium
(c) Chocolate agar
(d) SDA

45. Correctly matched stain: *(PGI 01)*

(a) Mucicarmine: Cryptococcus
(b) Giemsa: Candida
(c) Methamine sliver: Histoplasma
(d) Gram's: Pneumocystis carinii

46. Wood's light can be used for evaluation of: *(PGI 02)*

(a) Tinea capitis
(b) Freckles
(c) Vitiligo
(d) Tuberous sclerosis
(e) All

47. The medium of choice culturing yeast form of dimorphic fungi is: *(Recent MCQ)*

(a) BHI
(b) SDA
(c) SDA with antibiotics
(d) Any medium incubated at 35-37° C

48. Tinea pedis is caused by which of the following? *(Recent MCQ)*

(a) E. floccosum
(b) M. furfur
(c) M. canis
(d) E. werneckii

49. Which of the following does not produce Dermatophytosis in India? *(PGI 04)*

(a) Trichophyton rubrum
(b) Trichophyton mentagrophytes
(c) Microsporidium distortum
(d) Epidermophyton floccosum

50. Mycetoma is caused by the following agents *except*: *(Recent MCQ)*

(a) Allescheria boydii
(b) Madurella mycetomii
(c) Trichosporum beigelli
(d) Nocardia asteroids

51. All of the following cause sulfur granules *except*: *(AMU 05)*

(a) Chromoblastomycosis
(b) Botryomycosis
(c) Mycetoma
(d) Actinomycosis

52. Sulphur granules are composed of: *(Recent MCQ)*

(a) Organism
(b) Leukocytes
(c) Erythrocytes
(d) Keratinocytes

53. Mycetoma foot can be caused by following: *(PGI 10)*

(a) Cladosporium
(b) Phialophora jeanselmei
(c) Madurella mycetomi
(d) Allescheria boydii

54. Actinomycetoma is caused by: *(PGI 05)*

(a) Actinomycetes
(b) Nocardia
(c) Streptomyces
(d) Madura mycosis

55. The most common cause of Mycetoma in India: *(Recent MCQ)*

(a) Nocardia braziliensis
(b) Acetinomadura madurae
(c) Piedra
(d) Tinea cruris

56. Which of the following organism is implicated in the causation of botryomycosis? *(PGI 01)*

(a) Staphylococcus aureus
(b) Staphylococcus albus
(c) Pseudomonas aeruginosa
(d) Streptococcus pneumoniae
(e) Streptococcus pyogenes

57. A farmer presents with multiple discharging sinuses in the leg not responding to antibiotics. Most likely diagnosis is: *(AIIMS 02)*

(a) Madurella
(b) Actinomycetoma
(c) Nocardiosis
(d) Sporothrix

58. True about madura mycetoma: *(PGI 05)*

(a) Fungal infection
(b) Presented as non-painful nodular lesion for many months
(c) Discharging sinus
(d) Bone involvement seen
(e) All

59. True about Candida albicans is: *(AIIMS)*

(a) Candida is pathogenic to mice
(b) Its growth is inhibited by Griseofulvin
(c) Candida shows mycelia and Chlamydospore on corn meal agar
(d) Candida is present in normal feces

60. Candida is most often implicated in causation: *(Recent MCQ)*

(a) Conjunctivitis
(b) Tinea capitis
(c) Desert rheumatism
(d) Thrush

61. Candidiasis is associated with all *except*: *(Recent MCQ)*

(a) OCP user
(b) IUCD user
(c) Diabetes
(d) Pregnancy

62. All are true regarding cryptococcal infection *except*: *(AIIMS)*

(a) Occurs in immune-deficient states
(b) Capsular Ag in CSF is a rapid method of detection
(c) Anticapsular Abs is protective
(d) Urease test +ve

63. Which is false regarding cryptococcus neoformans? *(AI 05)*

(a) Grows at 5°C and 37°C
(b) It has 4 serotypes
(c) Urease negative
(d) Causes superficial skin infections

64. Most fulminant fungal meningitis is caused by: *(AP 01)*

(a) Coccidioides
(b) Histoplasma
(c) Cryptococcus
(d) Mucormycosis

65. Cryptococcal meningitis is common in: *(PGI 2000)*

(a) Renal transplant recipient
(b) A gamma globulinemia
(c) Neutropenia
(d) IgA deficiency

66. Aspergilloma has: *(JIPMER 99)*

(a) Septate hyphae
(b) Pseudohyphae
(c) Metachromatic hyphae
(d) Nn hyphae

67. Common fungus causing corneal ulcer: *(PGI)*

(a) Aspergillus
(b) Mucor
(c) Fusarium
(d) Sprothrix

68. Pneumocystis carinii is a fungus because: *(PGI 00)*

(a) rRNA, mitochondrial protein gene sequence and presence of thymidine synthase
(b) Cell wall contain glucans
(c) Antifungals are effective
(d) Most common infection in AIDS

69. Select the false statement about P. jiroveci: *(AI 08)*

(a) It is seen only in immunocompromised individuals
(b) Frequently associated with CMV
(c) May be associated with pneumatocele
(d) Diagnosed with sputum microscopy

70. Darling disease is caused by: *(Recent MCQ)*

(a) Histoplasma
(b) Candida
(c) Cryptococcus
(d) Rhizopus

71. Cigar body is seen in: *(Recent MCQ)*

(a) Cryptococcus
(b) Histoplasmosis
(c) Sporotrichosis
(d) Aspergillosis

72. Mucormycosis: *(PGI 02)*

(a) Angio-invasion
(b) Lymph: invasion
(c) Long term deferoxamine therapy is predisposing factor
(d) It may lead to blindness
(e) Septate hyphae

73. Vascular involvement and thrombosis is seen in: *(Recent MCQ)*

(a) Coccidiodomycosis
(b) Aspergillosis
(c) Mucormycosis
(d) Histoplasmosis

ANSWERS AND EXPLANATIONS

Classification of Fungi

1. **Ans. is 'a'** i.e., Phycomycetes (***Ref:*** *Ananthanarayan, 8th/e, p. 601*)
   - Lower fungi (Phycomycetes or Zygomycetes) → Aseptate hyphae.
   - Higher fungi (Ascomycetes, Basidiomycetes, Deutromycetes) → Septate hyphae (Memory Aid – **BAD**).
2. **Ans. is 'a'** i.e., Ascospore (***Ref:*** *Ananthanarayan, 8th/e, p. 601*)
   - **Sexual spores:** Oospore, Zygospore, Ascospore, Basidiospore (Memory Aid – **BOZA**).
   - **Asexual spores (Conidia):** Sporangiospore, Arthrospore, Blastospore, Chlamydospore **(CABS).**
3. **Ans. is 'd'** i.e., All of the above (***Ref:*** *Jawetz, 23rd/e, p. 626*)
   - Fungal spores have different morphology. They may be unicellular, multicellular or in chains.
   - Sporangium contains asexual spores of phycomycetes, called sporangiospores.
4. **Ans. is 'a'** i.e., Cryptococcus, candida (***Ref:*** *Ananthanarayan, 8th/e, p. 600*)
   - Budding is a method of asexual reproduction.
   - **Unicellular yeasts** (e.g., cryptococcus) reproduce by **simple budding.**
   - Candida grows partly as yeast and partly as elongated cells resembling hyphae. Therefore, it is classified as **yeast like fungi.**

Morphology

5. **Ans. is 'd'** i.e., Cryptococcus (***Ref:*** *Harrison, 19th/e, p. 1339*)
   - Cryptococcus is a yeast.
6. **Ans. is 'd'** i.e., Aspergillus fumigatus
   (***Ref:*** *Greenwood Micro, 16th/e, p. 588; Ananthanarayan, 8th/e, p. 607, 610, 613*)
   - Cryptococcus is a yeast and candida is yeast like fugus. Penicillium is a dimorphic fungi which can produce yeast like form (all dimorphic fungi have yeast form in host tissue or cultures).
   - Aspergillus is neither a yeast nor yeast like. It is a mould (hyphae).
7. **Ans. is 'a'** i.e., Aspergillus fumigatus (***Ref:*** *Harrison, 18th/e, p. 1655, 1656 and 17th/e, p. 1257*)
   - Information provided in this question are:
     (i) Recurrent rhinitis, nasal discharge, bilateral nasal blockade.
     (ii) History of asthma and allergy.
     (iii) **Hyphae with dichotomous branching at 45°C.**
   - All suggest the diagnosis of Aspergillus fumigatus.
     (i) **Most common type of fungal infection of nose and paranasal sinuses** are due to **Aspergillus.**
     (ii) Most common **fungus causing allergy** is aspergillus.
     (iii) Aspergillus has septate hyphae that branch typically at 45°C (V shaped).
8. **Ans. is 'd'** i.e., Apophysomyces species (***Ref:*** *Read below*)
   - This question is slightly different from previous one.
   - Here, organism is having aseptate hyphae (not septate).
   - Branching aseptate hyphae suggests the diagnosis of mucormycosis (mucor infection).
   - Apophysomyces is a novel pathogen belonging to the family Mucoraceae.
9. **Ans. is 'a'** i.e., Aspergillus (***Ref:*** *Previous explanations*)
   - Septate hyphae with acute branching is characteristic of Aspergillus.

Laboratory Diagnosis

10. **Ans. is 'c'** i.e., Fungus
    (***Ref:*** *Harrison's 17th/e, Chapter 14; Greenwood, 16th/e, p. 570; Ananthanarayan, 9th/e, p. 601*)
    - Tissue specimens such as skin scarpings, are generally examined as wet mounts after treatment with 10% KOH.
    - KOH (alkali) digests cells and other tissue materials, enabling the fungus elements to be seen clearly.
11. **Ans. is 'c'** i.e., Methanamine silver (***Ref:*** *Ananthanarayan, 8th/e, p. 601*)
    - Routinely used stains for the **demonstration of fungal elements in tissue sections** are:
      (i) **Methenamine silver.**
      (ii) **Periodic acid schiff (PAS).**
12. **Ans. is 'd'** i.e., PAS (***Ref:*** *Ananthanarayan, 8th/e, p. 601*)
    "The Periodic acid schiff (PAS) and methenamine silver stains are valuable methods for the demonstration of fungal elements in tissue sections."
13. **Ans. is 'd'** i.e., Malassezia furfur (***Ref:*** *Harrison, 19th/e, p. 1353*)
    - Malassezia furfur does not grow on regular Sabouraud's medium.
    - It requires complex media to grow.
    - M. furfur is a lipid dependent fungus and 1% emulsified olive oil is added to sabouraud medium for its cultivation **(Dixon media).**

14. Ans. is 'd' i.e., Pneumocystis jiroveci 'e' i.e., Rhinosporidium seeberi

(***Ref:*** *Ananthanarayan, 8th/e, p. 609-610; Harrison, 18th/e, p. 1671 and 17th/e, p. 1267*)

"The life cycle of Pneumocystis probably involves sexual and asexual reproduction, although definitive proof awaits the development of a reliable culture system." *– Harrison*

"Rhinosporidium seeberi **has not been cultivated in media".** *– Ananthanarayan*

Dimorphic Fungi

15. Ans. is 'c' i.e., Cryptococcus is an example (***Ref:*** *Ananthanarayan, 9th/e, p. 601, 609; Jawetz, 23rd/e, p. 645*)

Dimorphic Fungi

- Fungi that have two growth forms, such as mold (filaments) and a yeast, which develop under different growth conditions.
- In host tissues or cultures at 37°C they occur as yeasts, while in the soil and in cultures at 22°C they appear as moulds.
- Most fungi causing systemic infections are dimorphic fungi.

Examples:

- **Coccidioides.**
- **Histoplasma.**
- **Blastomyces.**
- **Paracoccidioides.**
- **Sporothrix (Sporotrichum).**
- **Penicillium marneffi.**

16. Ans. is 'd' i.e., Phialophora

17. Ans. are 'b > a' i.e., Histoplasma > Candida (***Ref:*** *Ananthanarayan, 8th/e, p. 601, 609; Jawetz, 23rd/e, p. 645*)

- Histoplasma is a dimorphic fungi.

Fungal Infections

18. Ans. is 'd' i.e., Trichosporum beigelii (***Ref:*** *Ananthanarayan, 8th/e, p. 603*)

- Two varieties of piedra are there:
  (i) **Black piedra** caused by Piedra hortae.
  (ii) **White** piedra caused by Trichosporon beigelii.

DERMATOPHYTES

Classification

19. Ans. is 'b' i.e., Trichophyton (***Ref:*** *Ananthanarayan, 8th/e, p. 604*)

Dermatophytes

Trichophyton	**Microsporum**	**Epidermophyton**
Skin	Skin	Skin
Hair	Hair	Nail
Nail		

20. Ans. is 'b' i.e., Microporum (***Ref:*** *Ananthanarayan, 8th/e, p. 603*)

- Dermatophytes can be identified by their colonial appearance and microscopic morphology after growth for 2 weeks at 25°C on Sabouraud's dextrose agar.

Tinea Capitis and Tinea Versicolor

21. Ans. is 'c' i.e., T. Tonsurans (***Ref:*** *Read below*)

- Harrison has mentioned that T tonsurans is the most common cause of T capitis.
- But most textbooks of dermatology have mentioned that Ectothrix is the most common type of T capitis and is caused mostly by M canis.
- Thus, the answer of this question is M canis.
- **Most common cause of 'Endothrix' – Tinea capitis by T. tonsurans.**
- **Most common cause of 'Ectothrix' – Tinea capitis by M. canis.**

22. Ans. is 'c' i.e., Dermatophytes (***Ref:*** *Harrison, 18th/e, p. 401 and 17th/e, p. 318; Jawetz, 23rd/e, p. 631*)

- Kerion is a **hypersensitivity and inflammation reaction in Tinea capitis caused by zoophilic species of dermatophytes (T. verrucosum and T. mentagrophytes).**

23. Ans. is 'b' i.e., Trichophyton (***Ref:*** *Jawetz, 23rd/e, p. 631*)

- T. tonsurans is the chief cause of "black dot" tinea capitis.

24. Ans. is 'b' i.e., T. tonsurans; 'c' i.e., T. violaceum (***Ref:*** *Greenwood, 16th/e, p. 574; Ananthanarayan, 9th/e, p. 606*)

Ectothrix → M. canis, M. audouinii, T. mentagrophytes.

Endothrix → T. tonsurans, T. voilaceum, T. schoenleinii **(TVS – Memory aid).**

25. Ans. is 'c' i.e., M. furfur (***Ref:*** *Harrison, 18th/e, p. 402 and 17th/e, p. 318; Ananthanarayan, 8th/e, p. 603*)

- Tinea versicolor is caused by a non-dermatophyte dimorphic fungus – Malassezia furfur.

26. Ans. is 'a' i.e., Tinea versicolor (***Ref:*** *Harrison, 18th/e, p. 402 and 17th/e, p. 318*)

Drugs for T. Versicolor

Topical → **Selenium sulfide, salicylic acid,** solution containing sulfur.

Oral → Ketoconazole.

27. Ans. is 'd' i.e., T. mentagrophytes (***Ref:*** *Harrison, 18th/e, p. 401; Jawetz, 23rd/e, p. 631*)

- Zoophilic dermatophytes are the species which primarily infect animals and occasionally transmitted to humans.
- **Zoophilic species** of trichophyton are **T. mentagrophytes and T. verrucosum.**
- Other zoophilic species of dermatophytes is M. canis.

28. Ans. is 'd' i.e., T. verrucosum (***Ref:*** *Ananthanarayan, 9th/e, p. 607; Greenwood, 16th/e, p. 572*)

29. Ans. is 'a' i.e., Epidermophyton; **'b'** i.e., Trichophyton (***Ref:*** *Jawetz, 23rd/e, p. 631*)

30. Ans. is 'a' i.e., Trichophyton (Mycology online)

- **Hair perforation test is done to distinguish between isolates of dermatophytes, particularly trichophyton mentagrophytes and its variants.**

SUBCUTANEOUS MYCOSIS AND SYSTEMIC MYCOSIS

Mycetoma

1. Ans. is 'a' i.e., Nocardia (***Ref:*** *Ananthanarayan, 9th/e, p. 608*)

2. Ans. is 'a' i.e., Madurella mycetomatis

Actinomycetoma caused by Actinomadura madurae, Actinomadura pelletri, Nocardia brasilensis, Nocardia caviae.Q

Eumycetoma – Madurella mycetomatis, Pseudoallescheria boydii, Acremonium.Q

3. Ans. is 'b' i.e., Red

Colour of Grains in Mycetomas of Various Etiologies:

White to Yellow

(1) Nocardia asteroides.

(2) Nocardia brasiliensis.

(3) Actinomadura madurac.

(4) Streptomyces somaliensis.

(5) Pseudoallescheria boydii.

Brown to Black

(1) Madurella mycetomatis.

(2) Madurella grisea.

(3) Phialophora jeanselmei.

Red

Actinomadura pelletierri.

4. **Ans. is 'd'** i.e., Fungal colonies (***Ref:*** *Ananthanarayan, 9th/e, p. 60*)

   Granules are microcolonies of the etiological agents.

5. **Ans. is 'd'** i.e., Uncommon in India (***Ref:*** *Ananthanarayan, 8th/e, p. 60g*)

   Mycetoma was originally reported from 'Madura', South India, and is, therefore, commonly known as Madura mycosis or **Madurafoot.** It is **quite common in Tamil Nadu in India.**

CANDIDA

Morphology

6. **Ans. is 'a'** i.e., Candida albicans

   Germ tube test: Culture inoculated in sheep or human serum and incubated at 37°C for 2-4 hours. A drop of suspension examined under microscope. Long tube like projections extending from yeast cell (true hypha). **There is no constriction at the point of attachment.** Called as **Reynolds-Braude phenomenon.**

7. **Ans. is 'c'**

   Growth on corn-meal agar **(C. albicans produces terminal chlamydospores).**

8. **Ans. is 'c'** i.e., Meningitis

   Clinical Types:

   - **Mucocutaneous:** Oral (thrush), oesophageal, vulvovaginitis, balanitis, conjunctivitis, keratitis.
   - **Skin and nail infections:** Intertrigenous areas (axilla, groin, perineum, submammary folds).
   - **Systemic:** UTI, pulmonary, endocarditis, meningitis, arthritis, osteomyelitis.

9. **Ans. is 'a',** i.e., Candida

10. **Ans. is 'b'**

    - Gram staining, KOH mount.
    - Oval or spherical gram positive yeast cells with pseudohyphae (buds continues to grow but fails to detach, **elongated cells are constricted at septations**).

CRYPTOCOCCUS

Morphology

11. **Ans. is 'd'** i.e., Lung

12. **Ans. is 'b'** i.e, Indian ink staining is **Negative staining** (Background is stained not the organism).

Virulence Factors and Clinical Features

13. **Ans. is 'a'** i.e., Cryptococcal Capsular material (*Jagdish Chander Book of Mycology*)

Virulence factor of cryptococcus neoformans

1. Polysaccharide capsule.
2. Melanin production.

Inhibits phagocytosis by WBC.

Due to **enzyme phenolic oxidase.**

14. Ans. is 'd' i.e., Kidney (***Ref:*** *Harrison, 18th/e, p. 1649, 1650 and 17th/e, p. 1252; Greenwood, 16th/e, p. 5831*)

15. Ans. is 'c' i.e.' Cryptococcus (***Ref:*** *Harrison, 16th/e, p. 1183*)

- C. neoformans has been isolated from the litter around trees of the species Eucalyptus camaldulensis.
- Eucalyptus isolates belong to serotype B.

16. Ans is 'c' i.e., Cryptococcus

Polysaccharide capsule – not immunogenic. No anti capsular ab formed.

ASPERGILLUS

Morphology and Clinical Features

17. Ans. is 'c' i.e., Lungs (***Ref:*** *Harrison, 18th/e, p. 1655 and 19th/e, p. 1257; Ananthanarayan, 9th/e, p. 613*)

Mode of transmission – Inhalation of Aspergillus spores (Conidia).

18. Ans. is 'c' i.e., Dermatophytosis (***Ref:*** *Harrison, 18th/e, p. 1655, 16561*)

- Dermatophytosis is caused by dermatophytes and Aspergillus is not a dermatophyte. Other options are correct.

Differential Diagnosis

19. Ans. is 'a' i.e., Aspergillus (***Ref:*** *Harrison, 18th/e, p. 1655, 1656 and 17th/e, p. 1251*)

- Septate hyphae and involvement of sinuses suggests the diagnosis of Aspergillus infection.
- **Aspergillus can cause sinusitis and the hyphae of Aspergillus are septate and branched.**

20. Ans. is 'c' i.e., Aspergillus (***Ref:*** *Harrison, 18th/e, p. 1655, 1656 and 19th/e, p. 1257*)

21. Ans. is 'a' i.e., Aspergillus spp.

- Many different species of fungi are found to involve the paranasal sinuses, the more common being the **Aspergillus, Alternaria, Mucor or Rhizopus.**

"Most common type of fungal infection of nose and paranasal sinuses are due to Aspergillus, **Aspergillus fumigatus, Aspergillus niger and Aspergillus flavus** are most frequent offenders."

Remember Fungi which do not have Septate Hyphae belong to the family Zygomycetes. They are:

- **Mucor.**
- **Rhizopus.**
- **Absidia.**
- **Pilobolus.**
- **Cunninghamella.**

22. Ans. is 'a' i.e., Aspergillus flavus (***Ref:*** *Ananthanarayan, 9th/e, p. 625*)

Aflatoxins are produced primarily by filamentous fungi Aspergillus flavus and Aspergillus parasiticus.

P. CARINII

23. Ans. is 'a' i.e., Fungi

24. Ans. is 'a' i.e., Rats (***Ref:*** *Harrison, 18th/e, p. 167 and 19th/e, p. 1267*)

- Although the organisms within the pneumocystis genus are morphologically very similar, they are genetically diverse and host specific **P. jirovecii infects humans, whereas P. carinii infects rats.**

Diagnosis and Treatment

25. Ans. is 'c' i.e., Add cotrimoxazole (***Ref:*** *Harrison, 18th/e, p. 717, 1672*)

- First see the infectious causes of chest infiltrate in an immunocompromised patient.

Infiltrate Infectious Cause of Pneumonia

1. **Localized:** Bacteria, Legionella, Mycobacteria.
2. **Nodular:** Fungi (Aspergillus, Mucor), Nocardia.
3. **Diffuse:** CMV, Chlamydia, Toxoplasma mycobacteria.

So, a febrile neutropenic (immunocompromised) patient is predisposed to chest infections with variety of organisms.

The clue to the diagnosis here is **fluffy chest infiltrate** which are seen in Pneumocystis carinii pneumonia.

"The typical radiographic appearance of Pneumocystis carinii pneumonia is **bilateral symmetric interstitial infiltration that often progress to fluffy alveolar infiltrates as the disease progresses.**"Q

The treatment of choice for Pneumocystis carinii pneumonia is cotrimoxazole.

Endemic Mycosis

26. Ans. is 'b' i.e., Blastomycosis (***Ref:*** *Jawetz, 22th/e, p. 636*)

Endemic mycosis are Coccidioidomycosis, Paracoccidioidomycosis, Histoplasmosis and Blastomycosis.

Histoplasmosis

27. Ans. is 'a' i.e., Dimorphic fungus (***Ref:*** *Ananthanarayan, 8th/e, p. 612; Harrison, 18th/e, p. 1640 and 17th/e, p. 1244*)

Histoplasma is a non-capsulated dimorphic fungus.

About Other Options

Moniliasis is caused by Candida.

- **Valley fever is caused by coccidioides immitis.**

28. Ans. is 'a' i.e., In early stages indistinguishable from T.B.

29. Ans. is 'b' i.e., Histoplasma (***Ref:*** *Ananthanarayan, 8th/e, p. 612*)

- On Sabourauds agar, at room temperature, white cottony mycelia growth appears, with large (8-20 micrometer) thick walled, spherical spores with **tubercles or finger-like projections.** This appearance of "tuberculate spores" is diagnostic of Histoplasma capsulatum.

Coccidiodes

30. Ans. is 'a' i.e., Spherules and endospores

(***Ref:*** *Ananthanarayan, 8th/e, p. 611, 612; Harrison, 18th/e, p. 1643, 17th/e, p. 1244*)

C. imitis reproduces in host tissue by forming small endospores within mature spherules.

31. Ans. is 'b' i.e., Coccidiodes (***Ref:*** *Ananthanarayan, 9th/e, p. 612*)

Valley fever or desert rheumatism is a self-limited influenza like fever caused by Coccidioides immitis.

32. Ans. is 'c' i.e., Arthrospores; **'d'** i.e., Endosporulating spherules (***Ref:*** *Harrison, 18th/e, p. 1643 and 17th/e, p. 1247*)

C. immitis is identified by its appearance **(endosporulating spherules)** and by the formation of thick walled, barrel shaped spores, called **arthrospores.**

Chromoblastomycosis

33. Ans. is 'a' i.e., Cladosporium (***Ref:*** *Ananthanarayan, 9th/e, p. 608, 609*)

Chromoblastomycosis is caused by **Cladosporium, Phialophora and Fonsecae** (all are members of family Dematiacea.

34. Ans. is 'c' i.e., Chromoblastomycosis (***Ref:*** *Ananthanarayan, 9th/e, p. 609*)

Histologically, the lesions of chromoblastomycosis show the presence of the fungus as round or irregular, dark brown, yeast-like bodies with septae, called **sclerotic bodies.**

SPOROTRICHOSIS

35. Ans. is 'd' i.e., It is an occupational disease of butchers-doctors

36. Ans. is 'a' i.e., Sporotrichosis schenckii

Sporotrichosis is caused by the thermally **dimorphic fungus sporothrix schenckii.**

Because S. schenckii naturally found in soil, hay, sphagnum moss, and plants, it usually affects farmers, gardeners, and agricultural workers (not butchers, doctors). Also known as Rose gardeners disease.

37. Ans. is 'a' i.e., Sporothrix schenckii (***Ref:*** *Harrison, 18th/e, p. 1665; Jawetz, 23rd/e, p. 633-634*)

Series of ulcers in a row suggests the diagnosis of sporotrichosis.

38. Ans. is 'b' i.e., Sporotrichosis (***Ref:*** *Ananthanarayan, 9th/e, p. 609*)

- Sometimes **'asteroid bodies'** are seen in the lesion of sporotrichosis, composed of a central fungus cell with eosinophilic material radiating from it.

39. Ans. is 'c' i.e., Mucormycosis (***Ref:*** *Harrison, 19th/e, p. 661; Ananthanarayan, 8th/e, p. 613-614*)

- Information in this question are:
  - (i) Patient is diabetic.
  - (ii) Orbital mycosis.
  - (iii) **Non-septate hyphae with obtuse branching (seen in Rhizopus and Mucor).**

These suggest the diagnosis of mucormycosis, most common organism being Rhizopus.

MISCELLANEOUS

40. Ans. is 'a' i.e., Black colonies

- The most distinguishing characteristic of mould phase (at 25°C) of Penicillium is the **early presence of red pigment that diffuses into agar.** The colonies start as pinkish-yellow and evolve into a bluish-green color in the center with a white periphery.

41. Ans. is 'a' i.e., Candida

- Candida is the most common fungal infection both in immunocompetent person and as well as opportunistic infection in immunocompromised persons.

42. Ans. is 'a' i.e., Rhinosporidiosis

Rhinosporidium Seeberi is not a fungus.

"Molecular studies have shown that the organism is not a fungus, but a primitive aquatic bacterium."

Torulosis: Fungal infection by Cryptococcus neoformans affecting CNS and lungs.

43. Ans. is 'c' i.e., Aspergillus

- Hint is branching septate hyphae.
- Mucor and Rhizopus have broad aseptate hyaline hyphae with wide angle branching.
- Candida is a yeast like fungi.

44. Ans. is 'd' i.e., SDA

- Sabouraud's dextrose agar media is comprised enzymatic digest of casein and animal tissues which provide a nutritious source of amino acids and nitrogenous compounds for the growth of fungi and yeasts. Dextrose is the fermentable carbohydrate incorporated in high concentration as a carbon and energy source. Low pH (5.6) makes it more selective. Agar is the solidifying agent. Addition of antibiotics like Chloramphenicol and/or tetracycline acts as broad spectrum antimicrobials to inhibit the growth of a wide range of gram-positive and gram-negative bacteria. Gentamicin is added to further inhibit the growth of gram-negative bacteria.
- SDA with chloramphenicol (to prevent bacterial contamination) is used in isolation of all fungus.
- SDA with chloramphenicol and cycloheximide (to prevent fungal contamination like Aspergillus species and Zygomycetes) is used in isolation of dermatophytes.

45. Ans. are 'a,c'

The yeast forms of cryptococcosis are usually widely separated by their thick mucoid capsules. PAS stain decorates the yeasts and mucicarmine stain decorates the highly characteristic gelatinous capsule a bright pink.

Histoplasmosis is diagnosed by visualizing intracellular microorganisms in biopsy and/or culture. Periodic-acid Schiff (PAS) and Gomori methenamine silver (GMS) staining methods are routinely used for identification.

46. Ans. is 'e' i.e., All

Wood lamp examination is a diagnostic test in which the skin or hair is examined while exposed to the black light emitted by Wood lamp. Black light is invisible to the naked eye because it is in the ultraviolet spectrum, with wavelength just shorter than the colour violet. The lamp glows violet in a dark environment, because it also emits some light in the violet part of the electromagnetic spectrum.

A Wood Lamp for Skin Examination may reveal:

1. Increase in pigmentation (e.g., melasma, postinflammatory pigmentation) to determine whether the pigmentation is epidermal (pigmentation enhanced by Wood lamp examination) or dermal (pigmentation unchanged by Wood lamp examination). Pigmented lesions have a clear border under Wood light because the light is absorbed by increased melanin.
2. Loss of pigmentation (e.g., vitiligo, ash-leaf macules in tuberous sclerosis, and hypomelanosis of Ito) to identify affected areas in light skinned people. Hypopigmented skin has sharper borders under black light and fluoresces bright blue-white (or sometimes, yellowish green) due to accumulated biopterins. In contrast, areas of reduced blood flow are unchanged.
3. Pityriasis versicolor—a slightly scaly persistent rash on anterior chest and back caused by malassezia yeasts. When active, the scale emits a yellowish or orange glow.
4. Malassezia folliculitis—hair follicles fluoresce bluish-white.
5. Tinea capitis—areas of scale and baldness due to fungal infection. Microsporum species fluoresce blue-green (M canis, M audouinii, M ferrugineum, M distortum); Trichophyton schoenleinii fluoresces dull blue. Fungal infection due to other organisms does not fluoresce.
6. Head lice and scabies.
7. Erythrasma—corynebacteria bacteria cause a pigmented rash in skin folds that fluoresces a coral-pink colour.
8. Pseudomonas in spa pool folliculitis and wound infection fluoresces green.
9. Acne fluoresces orange-red due to cutibacteria in hair follicles.
10. Porphyria causes red-pink fluorescence of the skin (porphyria cutanea tarda), or teeth (erythropoetic porphyria).
11. Porphyrins used as the photosensitiser in photodynamic therapy.
12. Drugs on the skin surface—tetracyclines and mepacrine fluoresce after oral ingestion.
13. The evenness of application of a salicylic acid-containing chemical peel (this fluoresces green).

47. Ans. is 'c' i.e., SDA with antibiotics

SDA with antibiotics (Chloramphenicol) is always preferred over plain SDA to avoid bacterial contamination and make it more selective.

48. Ans. is 'a' i.e., E. floccosum

Tinea pedis is a foot infection due to a dermatophyte fungus. Tinea pedis thrives in warm humid conditions and is most common in young adult men.

Tinea pedis is most frequently due to:

1. Trichophyton (T.) rubrum.
2. T. interdigitale, previously called T. mentagrophytes var. interdigitale.
3. Epidermophyton floccosum

49. Ans. is 'c' i.e., Microsporidium distortum

50. Ans. is 'c' i.e., Trichosporum beigelli

51. Ans. is 'a' i.e., Chromoblastomycosis

52. Ans. is 'a' i.e., Organism

Ultrastructurally, the center of the sulfur granule was composed of a cluster of hyphae, and the periphery was surrounded by clubs arranged radially. The clubs were made of electron-dense fine granules and had a degenerated hypha at the center. These granules varied in amount from small to large.

53. Ans. are 'b,c,d'

54. Ans. are 'a,b,c'

55. Ans. is 'a' i.e., Nocardia braziliensis

Over 75% of persons with mycetoma have a lesion of a lower extremity, most commonly in the foot (70%). Next in frequency is disease of the hand (15%), followed by the upper extremities and other areas of the body that may be exposed by carrying firewood or thorny brush, including the upper back and adjacent neck, top of the head and, rarely, the face The causative agents of mycetoma vary from region to region and with climate. Worldwide, M. mycetomatis is the most common cause of this affliction, but A. madurae, M. mycetomatis, and S. somaliensis are more commonly reported from drier regions, whereas P. boydii, Nocardia species, and A. pelletieri are more common in those areas with higher annual rainfall. In India, Nocardia species and M. grisea are the most common causes of Mycetoma.

56. Ans. is 'a' i.e., Staphylococcus aureus

Botryomycosis (bacterial pseudomycosis) is a rare chronic bacterial granulomatous disease that usually involves skin and rarely viscera. Main etiological agent is Staphylococcus aureus and less commonly Pseudomonas spp., Escherichia coli, Proteus spp., Streptococcus spp.

57. Ans. is 'a' i.e., Madurella

It is the case of eumycetoma and antifungal therapy of eumycetoma most commonly includes the use of azole antifungals, because amphotericin B has not been effective in producing long-term cures. Itraconazole (400 mg/day) or ketoconazole (200 to 400 mg/day) are considered first-line azole agents in the treatment of this disease.

58. Ans. is 'e' i.e., All

59. Ans. are 'c, d'

60. Ans. is 'd' i.e., Thrush

61. Ans. is 'b' i.e., IUCD user

62. Ans. is 'c' i.e., Anticapsular Abs is protective

63. Ans. is 'c' i.e., Urease negative

64. Ans. is 'c' i.e., Cryptococcus

65. Ans. is 'a' i.e., Renal transplant recipient

Predisposing factors of cryptococcal meningitis are AIDS, hematologic malignancies, transplant recipients and patients on immunosuppressive or steroid therapy.

66. Ans. is 'a' i.e., Septate hyphae

Aspergilloma is caused by Apergillus.

67. Ans. are 'a, c'

68. Ans. are 'a, b, c'

69. Ans. is 'b' i.e., Frequently associated with CMV

70. Ans. is 'a' i.e., Histoplasma

It usually causes lung disease called Histoplasmosis or Darling's disease. It is called Darling's disease because it was found by Samuel Darling in histopathologic specimens about a century ago.

71. Ans. is 'c' i.e., Sporotrichosis

S. schenckii is yeast-like, appearing as spherical or cigar-shaped bodies measuring 4 to 6 μm in length that reproduce by budding at 37°C. Nonpathogenic Sporothrix species do not convert to yeast phase at 37°C on media.

72. Ans. are 'a, c'

73. Ans. is 'c' i.e., Mucormycosis

PRACTICE QUESTIONS

1. **All are yeast or yeast like fungi *except*:**
   (a) Candida
   (b) Geotrichum
   (c) Cryptococcus
   (d) Trichophyton
2. **Fungi which do not have sexual stage:**
   (a) Phycomycetes
   (b) Ascomycetes
   (c) Basidiomycetes
   (d) Fungi imperfecti
3. **All are asexual spores of fungi *except*:**
   (a) Arthrospores
   (b) Chlamydospores
   (c) Blastospores
   (d) Ascospores
4. **Fungi which grow by budding:**
   (a) Cryptococci and Candida
   (b) Pityriasis versicolor and Sporothrix
   (c) Rhinosporidium and Cryptococcus
   (d) Tinea and Candida
5. **Which stain is most suitable for fungus demonstration in biopsy?**
   (a) Alizarian red
   (b) Verihoof dye
   (c) Mason's Trichrome
   (d) PAS
6. **Which antimicrobial is added in SDA to prevent growth of contaminant moulds?**
   (a) Griseofulvin
   (b) Cycloheximide
   (c) Ketoconazole
   (d) Clotrimazole
7. **Example for fungus having Branching, Aseptate hyphae are all *except*:**
   (a) Rhizopus
   (b) Penicillium
   (c) Mucor
   (d) Absidia

Superficial and Subcutaneous Mycosis

8. **About Dermatophytes all true *except*:**
   (a) Superficial skin layer involvement
   (b) Epidermophyton does not involve hair
   (c) Microsporum does not involve nail
   (d) Systemic involvement
9. **Hair perforation test is positive in:**
   (a) Trichophyton
   (b) Microsporum
   (c) Epidermophyton
   (d) Trichosporon
10. **Pityriasis Versicolor is caused by:**
    (a) E. floccosum
    (b) M. furfur
    (c) M. gypseum
    (d) T.Tonsurans
11. **Organism that does not affect hair:**
    (a) Trichophyton rubrum
    (b) Epidermophyton floccosum
    (c) Microsporum
    (d) Hortaea werneckii
12. **The causative agent of Favus is:**
    (a) Microsporum audonii
    (b) Microsporum canis
    (c) Trichophyton mentagrophytes
    (d) Trichophyton schoenleinii
13. **Microconidia are absent in:**
    (a) Trichophyton rubrum
    (b) Trichophyton mentagrophytes
    (c) Microsporum audonii
    (d) Epidermophyton floccosum

14. All are dermatophyte infections of hair *except*:

(a) Favus
(b) Kerion
(c) Piedra
(d) Tinea capitis

15. Patient presents with vesicular, itchy lesions on plams. Examination of vesicle fluid or scraping from vesicles do not yield any fungus. Probable diagnosis is:

(a) Dermatophyte infection
(b) Candidiasis
(c) 'id' reaction
(d) Cryptococcosis

16. How the skin scrapings collected for Dermatophyte infection transported to lab?

(a) In Sabouraud's broth
(b) Peptone water
(c) In transport medium
(d) Dark coloured paper packets

17. Examination of skin scraping from a patient having hypopigmented, non-itchy lesions on chest show yeast like cells and branched filaments (Sphagetti – meat ball appearance) Probable fungus is:

(a) Malassezia furfur
(b) Dimorphic fungus
(c) Candida albicans
(d) Dermatophyte

18. Dark, hard nodules along the hair short caused by:

(a) Piedraia hortae
(b) Microsporum gypseum
(c) Hortae werneckii
(d) Trichophyton violaceum

19. Which is not a fungal infection of hair?

(a) Endothrix
(b) Ectothrix
(c) Piedra
(d) Dermatophytid

20. Which of the following is not useful in diagnosing dermatophyte infection?

(a) Lott
(b) Lactophenol cotton blue stain
(c) Wood's lamp
(d) India ink

21. A patient coming from Himachal Pradesh, presents with multiple skin lesions. Microscopy reveals cigar shaped yeast cells and Asteroid bodies microscopy of culture shows 'Flower like' pattern most likely fungus is:

(a) Trichophyton rubrum
(b) Epidermophyton floccosum
(c) Sporothrix schencki
(d) Aspergillus flavus

22. Red coloured grains are seen in mycetoma caused by:

(a) Madurella mycetoniatis
(b) Actino Madura Pelletieri
(c) Madurella grisea
(d) Actino Madura madurae

23. Superficial mycosis is caused by all *except*:

(a) Madurella mycetomatis
(b) Malassezia furfur
(c) Hortae werneckii
(d) Piedraria hortae

24. Drug of choice for extensive Tinea corporis is:

(a) Topical clotrimazole
(b) Amphotericin – B
(c) Oral Griseofulvin
(d) Topical miconazole

25. Tinea imbricata is caused by:

(a) Trichophyton verruconsum
(b) Trichophyton rubrum
(c) Trichophyton concentricum
(d) Trichophyton tonsurans

Candidiasis

26. Most common fungal infection in febrile neutropenia:

(a) Aspergillus Niger
(b) Candida albicans
(c) Aspergillus fumigatus
(d) Mucormycosis

27. Candida infection is predisposed by all *except*:

(a) Menstruation
(b) Diabetes
(c) Minipill users
(d) Combined pill users

28. An HIV infected female has an ulcer over the tongue. Lab findings show growth in corn meal agar at 20°C. Microscopy shows Pseudo hyphae and growth in human serum at 37°C show budding yeast cells. The probable cause is:

(a) Candida albicans
(b) Histoplasmosis
(c) Blastomyces
(d) Cryptococcus neoformans

29. Germ tube test is diagnostic for:

(a) Candida kefyr
(b) Cryptococcus neoformans
(c) Coccidiodes immitis
(d) Candida albicans

Cryptococcosis

30. The most common type of deep mycosis in India is:

(a) Blastomycosis
(b) Histoplasmosis
(c) Coccidioidomycosis
(d) Cryptococcosis

31. Capsulated fungus is:

(a) Histoplasma capsulatum
(b) Candida albicans
(c) Cryptococcus neoformans
(d) Rhinosporidium seeberi

32. True about Cryptococcus neoformans is all *except*:

(a) Capsular antigen detected in CSF
(b) Common in immunocompromised
(c) Anticapsular antibody prevents recurrence
(d) Strongly positive mucicarmine stain of the organism intissue is diagnostic

33. The capsule of Cryptococcus neoformans in CSF sample is best seen by:

(a) Gram stain
(b) Giemsa stain
(c) Indian ink preparation
(d) Methanamine silver stain

Dimorphic Fungi

34. Blastomycosis is characterized by all *except*:

(a) Yeast like fungus
(b) Commonly involves lung and skin
(c) Common in North America
(d) Broad based budding yeast cells in tissues

35. What is true about Histoplasmosis?

(a) In early stages it is indistinguishable from TB
(b) Blood culture is not diagnostic
(c) Hyphal forms NOT infectious
(d) Person to person spread occurs by droplet infection

36. A gardener has multiple vesicles on hand and multiple eruptions along the lymphatic channels. Most common fungus responsible is:

(a) Cladosporium
(b) Sporothrix
(c) Histoplasma
(d) Candida

37. All of the following are true about Histoplasmosis *except*:

(a) Very rare in patients with AIDS
(b) Bone marrow is involved
(c) Gomori methanamine silver stain is used
(d) Dimorphic fungus

38. All of the following are dimorphic fungi *except*:

(a) Sporothrix schenckii
(b) Histoplasma capsulatum
(c) Blastomyces dermatitidis
(d) Penicillium griseofulvin

39. All of the following are thermally dimorphic *except*:

(a) Coccidioides immitis
(b) Paracoccidioides brasiliensis
(c) Sporothrix schenckii
(d) Cryptococcus neoformans

40. Which of the following is NOT an opportunistic fungus?

(a) Cryptococcus
(b) Mucor mycosis
(c) Mycetoma
(d) Penicillium marneffi

41. Which rays are used in Wood's lamp?

(a) X-rays
(b) Gamma rays
(c) Infra red rays
(d) UV rays

42. A patient presents with chronic congh, resistant to routine antibiotics; whose X-ray chest shows cavity filled with mass. Sputum microscopy shows acutely branching septate hyphae. Probable organism:

(a) Histoplasma capsulatum
(b) Aspergillus fumigatus
(c) Mycobacterium tuberculosis
(d) Actinomyces

43. Not true about Rhinosporidiosis is:

(a) Can be cultured on Sabouraud's dextrose Agar
(b) Fungal Spherules in biopsy
(c) Bleeds to touch
(d) Most common site is nose

44. Aflatoxin is produced by:

(a) A. flavus
(b) A. fumigatus
(c) A. nidulans
(d) A. niger

45. Sclerotic bodies are seen in:

(a) Chromoblastomycosis
(b) Sporotrichosis
(c) Histoplasmosis
(d) Rhinosporidiosis

46. All are true about Botryomycosis *except*:

(a) Clinical features similar to mycetoma
(b) Caused by staphylococcus aureus
(c) Microscopy shows branching filaments
(d) Multiple discharging sinus

47. Most common fungus causing orbital cellulitis in a patient with diabetic ketoacidosis is:

(a) Mucor
(b) Aspergillus
(c) Candida
(d) Cryptococcus

48. In a patient, corneal scraping reveals narrow angled septate hyphae. Which of the following is the likely etiologic agent?

(a) Mucor
(b) Aspergillus
(c) Histoplasma
(d) Candida

49. Which of the following is the most common etiologic agent in paranasal sinus mycoses?

(a) Aspergillus species
(b) Histoplasma
(c) Coccidioides coronatus
(d) Candida albicans

50. Most common fungus implicated in otomycosis is:

(a) Aspergillus
(b) Candida
(c) Cryptococcus
(d) Trichophyton

51. Pneumocystis carinii is diagnosed by:

(a) Silver nitrate staining
(b) Leishman stain
(c) Fontana stain
(d) Acid fast stain

52. Neurotrophic fungus is all *except*:

(a) Cryptococcus neoformans
(b) Piedraria hortae
(c) Cladosporium castellani
(d) Histoplasma capsulatum

ANSWERS

1.	(d)	2.	(d)	3.	(d)	4.	(a)	5.	(d)	6.	(b)	7.	(b)	8.	(d)
9.	(a)	10.	(b)	11.	(b)	12.	(d)	13.	(d)	14.	(c)	15.	(c)	16.	(d)
17.	(a)	18.	(a)	19.	(d)	20.	(d)	21.	(c)	22.	(b)	23.	(a)	24.	(c)
25.	(c)	26.	(b)	27.	(a)	28.	(a)	29.	(d)	30.	(d)	31.	(c)	32.	(c)
33.	(c)	34.	(a)	35.	(a)	36.	(b)	37.	(a)	38.	(d)	39.	(d)	40.	(c)
41.	(d)	42.	(b)	43.	(a)	44.	(a)	45.	(a)	46.	(c)	47.	(a)	48.	(b)
49.	(a)	50.	(a)	51.	(a)	52.	(b)								

Chapter 7

PARASITOLOGY

INTRODUCTION

- **Medical Parasitology** is the science dealing with parasites that infect man, causing disease and misery in most countries of the tropics.
- The most acceptable taxonomic classification of human parasites includes Endoparasites and Ectoparasites.
- **Endoparasites** are sub-classified into Helminthic parasites (multicellular organisms) and Protozoan parasites (unicellular organisms).
- **Helminthic parasites** are either flat worms (Trematodes), segmented ribbon like worms (Cestodes) or cylindrical worms (Nematodes).

Different Kinds of Parasites	Different Kinds of Hosts
• **Ectoparasite** – A parasitic organism that lives on the outer surface of its host, e.g., lice, ticks, mites etc. • **Endoparasites** – Parasites that live inside the body of their host, e.g., Entamoeba histolytica. • **Obligate Parasite** – This parasite is completely dependent on the host during a segment or all of its life cycle, e.g., Plasmodium spp. • **Facultative parasite** – An organism that exhibits both parasitic and non-parasitic modes of living and hence does not absolutely depend on the parasitic way of life, but is capable of adapting to it if placed on a host, e.g., Naegleria fowleri.	• **Definitive host** – A host that harbors a parasite in the adult stage or where the parasite undergoes a **sexual method** of reproduction. • **Intermediate host** – Harbors the larval stages of the parasite or an **asexual cycle** of development takes place. In some cases, larval development is completed in two different intermediate hosts, referred to as first and second intermediate hosts. • **Paratenic host** – **A host that serves as a temporary refuge** and vehicle for reaching an obligatory host, usually the definitive host, i.e., it is not necessary for the completion of the parasites life cycle. • **Reservoir host** – A host that makes the parasite available for the transmission to another host and is usually not affected by the infection. • **Natural host** – A host that is naturally infected with certain species of parasite. • **Accidental host** – A host that is under normal circumstances not infected with the parasite.

CLASSIFICATION OF MEDICALLY IMPORTANT PARASITES

PROTOZOA	METAZOA (HELIMINTHS)
Sarcodina (Amoebae) (a) Genus, Entamoeba: E.g., Entameba histolytica (b) Genus Endolimax: E.g., Endolimax nana (c) Genus Iodamoeba: E.g., Iodameba butschlii	**Platyhelminthes** **Trematodea** (a) Genus Schistosoma: E.g., S. mansoni (b) Genus Fasciola: E.g., F. hepatica

Contd.

Contd.

(d) Genus Dientamoeba: E.g., Dientameba fragilis — E^2 ID **Mastigophora (Flagellates)** (a) Genus Giardia: E.g., G. lamblia (b) Genus Trichomonas: E.g., T. vaginalis (c) Genus Trypanosoma: E.g., T. brucei (d) Genus Leishmania: E.g., L. donovani (a)–(d): GL T^2 **Sporozoa** 1. Genus Plasmodium: E.g., P. falciparum 2. Genus Toxoplasma: E.g., T. gondi 3. Genus Cryptosporidum: E.g., C. parvum 4. Genus Isospora, E.g., I. belli **Ciliates** E.g., Balantidium coli	**Cestoda** (a) Genus Diphyllobotrium: E.g., D. latum (b) Genus Taenia: E.g., T. saginata (c) Genus Echinococcus: E.g., E. granulosus (d) Genus Hymenolepsis: E.g., H. nana **Nemathelminthes** (a) Intestinal Nematodes: E.g., A. lumbricoides (b) Somatic Nematodes: E.g., W. bancrofti

PROTOZOOLOGY

- Prokaryotes – Monera (e.g., Bacteria, Blue green algae, archaebacteria.
- Eukaryotes – Protista (Protozoal parasite), Fungi (e.g., fungus), Plantae (e.g., plants), Animalia (e.g., Helminths, Arthropods and higher animals).
- KINGDOM – PHYLUM – CLASS – ORDER – FAMILY – GENUS – SPECIES.

PROTOZOA

Amoebae:

(a) Intestinal species – Entamoeba histolytica, E.coli.

(b) Free living – Acanthamoeba, Naegleria.

Ciliates: Balantidium coli.

Flagellates:

(a) Intestinal – Giardia lamblia, Trichomonas hominis.

(b) Oral and vaginal – Trichomonas vaginalis.

(c) Blood and tissue (Haemoflagellates).

Sporozoa:

(a) Blood species – Plasmodium sps, Babesia.

(b) Tissue sps. – Toxoplasma.

(c) Intestinal – Isospora, Cryptosporidium.

ENTAMOEBA HISTOLYTICA

- **Source of infection:** Cyst passing patient/asymptomatic carrier. Acutely ill patients do not act as reservoirs as they excrete non-infective trophozoites.
- **Transmission:** Contaminated food and water.
- **Life Cycle:** Completed in single host (Man).
- **Infective stage (Quadrinucleate cyst)Q** ingested in contaminated food/water → excysts in caecum → trophozoite with four nuclei liberated → divides by binary fission giving rise to 8 daughter trophozoites → migrate to ileocaecal region

Contd.

Contd.

→ penetrate the muscular mucosa and localize in the submucosal layer of the large intestine → lesion by necrosis and destruction of the tissue → penetrate portal circulation → reach different organs of the body.

- **Zymodeme analysis:** Isoenzyme electrophoretic mobility have identified seven potentially and 11 non-pathogenic zymodemes.
- Isolates of E. histolytica from patients with invasive amoebiasis have unique isoenzymes, surface antigens, DNA markers, and virulence properties and are now recognized as distinct species from the non-invasive E. dispar.

- **Extraintestinal amoebiasis:**
  Amoebic liver abscess is the most common extra intestinal manifestation of amoebiasis. Most common in **postero-superior surface** of the **right lobe.** Usually there is one large solitary abscess. The necrotic contents of liver abscess are classically described as **anchovy-sauce pus.** Pleuropulmonary involvement is the most frequent complication of amoebic liver abscess.
- Other sites of involvement are lung, brain and genitourinary system.

Diagnosis of Amoebiasis

Stool examination – For amoebic colitis definitive diagnosis is made by the **demonstration of hematophagous trophozoites.Q**

Fecal findings are:

(i) Positive test for heme.
(ii) Paucity (lack) of neutrophils (pus cells).
(iii) Presence of amoebic cysts or trophozoites.
(iv) **Charcot-leyden crystals.**

DOC – Metronidazole and Tinidazole

Clinical Features:

- Asymptomatic (85-95%), Symptomatic (5-15%).
- **Intestinal** – Most common infection is asymptomatic cyst passage.
- Symptomatic invasive infection causes amoebic colitis and dysentry.
- Invasive infection causes amoebic ulcer, a classical flask shaped ulcer, water bottle, undermined ulcer.
- Most frequent site of involvement is caecum and ascending colon, followed in order by sigmoid, rectum and appendix.
- Intestinal amoebiasis (95% of symptomatic cases) – Amoebic dysentery, Non-dysenteric colitis, Amoebic appendicitis, Amoeboma.
- **Complications:** Perforation, Peritonitis, Haemorrhage, Obstruction.
- **Extraintestinal amoebiasis** (5% of symptomatic cases) – Diet in excess of cholesterol and carbohydrate predisposes to invasive amoebiasis. Invasive amoebiasis is three times more common in men than in women.

Laboratory Diagnosis:

Faecal examination: Saline mount **(trophozoites with ingested RBCs, erythrophagocytosis, pathognomic feature) Iodine mount (morphological details of the cyst), permanent mount (iron-haematoxylin, trichrome stain), after concentration (only cysts seen).**

- **Trophozoite:** 15-30 µm, **pseudopodia, eccentrically placed nucleus with central karyosome,** inner surface of nuclear membrane lined with chromatin granules.
- **Cyst:** 15 µm, smooth wall, **early cyst shows chromatoid bars, glycogen mass, disappear as cyst matures.** Initially uninuclear, mature quadrinuclear.

Proctosigmoidoscopy Scrapings/Biopsy

Pus aspirate (only seen trophozoites, no cysts seen).

- **Culture: Philip's mediumQ, Craig's medium, Balamuth's medium, Robinson's medium, Diamond's medium (BD– PCR).**
- **Serological Diagnosis:** Extremely useful for diagnosis of extra-intestinal amoebiasis:
  – IHA: 1:256
  – ELISA

Molecular methods: DNA probes.

PATHOGENIC FREE LIVING AMOEBAE

Naeglaria fowleri (Brain eating amoeba)	Acanthamoeba spp.
Primary Amoebic Meningoencephalitis (PAM) • **Trophozoite:** Amoeboid form: 10-35 μm, motile by lobopodia; flagellate form: pear shaped, motile by 2 flagella, non-replicating (Baveja, 5th edition). • **Cyst:** 7-10 μm, smooth double cyst wall, not found in tissues. • **Infective form:** Trophozoites. • **Source of infection: Swimming in lakes and ponds; amoebae invade nasal mucosa → pass through olfactory plate → reach meninges and cause acute purulent meningitis.** **Laboratory Diagnosis:** • **CSF: Neutrophilic leukocytosis**, detection of trophozoites (no cysts seen), can be cultivated.	It causes **Contact lens keratitis but sometimes causes Granulomatous amoebic encephalitis (GAE).** • **Trophozoite:** 15-45 μm, Acanthopodia, no flagellate form. • **Cyst:** 10-25 μm, double walled, also found in tissues. • **Source of infection:** Inhalation, ingestion, traumatized skin/eyes (contact lenses). Chronic disease with prolonged course. **Laboratory Diagnosis:** • **CSF: Lymphocytes:** Detection of cysts and trophozoites is done. • **Serological tests:** Immunofluorescence is done to diagnose.

GIARDIA LAMBLIA/GIARDIA INTESTINALIS

- **Giardia is a flagellate protozoa.**
- It is the only common protozoa that inhibit the duodenum and jejunum (upper small intestines of human.
- **Mode of transmission** – Ingestion of cysts.
- **Habitat:** Duodenum and upper jejunum.
- **Trophozoite:** Vegetative stage, pear shaped (monkey faced appearance), 10-20 × 6-15 μm, convex dorsal surface, 2 axostyles, 2 nuclei, four pairs of flagella. Multiply by binary fission, motile **(falling leaf motility).Q**
- **Cyst:** Oval, 8-14 × 6-10 μm, four nuclei, axostyle.
- **Infective dose** is low ingestion of **as few as 10 cysts** are sufficient to cause infection in humans.
- **Infective form** – **Quadrinucleate Cyst.**
- **Life cycle:** Excystation in duodenum, trophozoites attach to the intestinal villi and multiply by binary fission.

Clinical Features:

- Asymptomatic, diarrhoea, **Malabsorption syndrome (due to loss of brush border enzyme activities).**
- Giardia may also cause **traveller's diarrhea.**

Predisposing conditions to giardiasis are:

Agammaglobulinemia, common variable immunodeficiency and **selective IgA-deficiency.**

Laboratory Diagnosis:

- **Faecal examination:** Cysts and trophozoites.
- **Duodenal aspirate:** Trophozoites (Enterotest).
- **Antigen detection in stool:** ELISA, CIEP, immunofluorescence.
- **Antibody detection:** ELISA, IFAT.

DOC – Metronidazole and Tinidazole.

TRICHOMONAS VAGINALIS

- **Only one form:** Trophozoite (no cystic stage).Q
- **Trophozoite: Pear shaped,** 10-30 μm × 5-10 μm, 4 anterior flagellae, wobbling or rotatory motility, multiplies by binary fission.
- **Habitat:** Vagina, cervix in females; anterior urethra in males.
- **Mode of transmission:** Venereal disease.

Contd.

Contd.

Clinical Features:
20% asymptomatic.
Females: Vaginal discharge, foul smelling frothy, itching **(strawberry appearance). Males:** Urethritis, balanoposthitis.

DOC – Metronidazole and Tinidazole.

Laboratory Diagnosis:
Wet mount preparation.
Stained smear: Giemsa, Leishman, Papanicolaou.
Culture: Bushley's, Feinberg-Whittington's, Johnson-Trussel.

Hemoflagellates

The family Trypanosomatidae (includes hemoflagellates) contain only two genera that parasitize humans.

(a) **Genus Leishmania** are always intracellular, **principally in cells of the reticuloendothelial system.**
(b) **Genus Trypanosoma** contains members that may be found both in the circulating blood and intracellularly in cardiac muscle.

TRYPANOSOMA

Trypanosoma brucei gambiense	Trypanosoma cruzi
• West African sleeping sickness (western, central parts of Africa) • Trypomastigote: Actively motile, spindle shaped • Antigenic variation: Shed outer **variant surface glycoprotein** (VSG) and replace with another. **Life cycle:** • **Definitive host**: Man, Domestic animals • **Intermediate host**: Tsetse fly (**Glossina palpalis**, Glossina species) Stumpy trypomastigote in human blood → ingested by fly → multiply in mid gut → migrate to salivary glands → transform into epimastigotes → **transform into metacyclic trypomastigotes (EIP: 25-50 days) (infective stage for man)** → fly bites → transform into slender trypomastigotes → in peripheral circulation → some transform into stumpy trypomastigotes **Note –** Infective form for humans is **Metacyclic trypomastigotes.Q** • Reservior: Man only **Clinical features:** **Trypanosomal chancre** → febrile attacks **(Winterbottom's sign: Enlargement of posterior cervical lymph nodes Q)** → CNS involvement (**Kerandel's sign:** Pressure on palms of the hand or over ulnar nerve is followed by severe pain after pressure is removed).Q **Laboratory diagnosis:** **Trypomastigote** is demonstrated in chancre, peripheral blood, bone marrow, lymph node aspirate, CSF.	• **American trypanosomiasis/Chaga's disease (Central/South America)** • **Trypomastigote form: C shaped,** 20 μm long • **Amastigote form:** Oval, 2-4 μm, nucleus, kinetoplast **Life cycle:** • **Definitive host:** Humans, wild, domestic animals • **Intermediate host: Reduvid bug (kissing bug)** Trypomastigote form → taken up by reduvid bug after biting human → transformed into amastigote in mid gut and multiply by binary fission → migrate to hind gut → transformed into metacyclic trypomastigotes → excreted in faeces → defecate soon after biting → invade human tissue cells → converted into amastigote forms → mutiply by binary fission and after passing through promastigote and epimastigote forms are transformed into trypomastigotes → liberated in the blood. **Clinical features:** **Romana's sign** (facial swelling, oedema of one eyelid), **chagoma,** systemic complications (fever, LAP, hepatosplenomegaly), chronic phase (destruction of muscle, nerve cells: **Cardiac myopathy, megaesophagus, megacolon**) **Laboratory diagnosis:** Peripheral blood smear examination Xenodiagnosis Culture: **NNN medium, Warren medium** **In lymph node** biopsy, muscle biopsy: Amastigote form demonstrated. **Serological tests: CFT (Machado guerreiro testQ),** IFAT, ELISA

Trypanosoma Brucei Rhodesiense

- **East African sleeping sickness (eastern, central Africa).**
- **Life cycle:** Morphology, antigenic variation, life cycle similar, **(Glossina morsitans).**
- **Clinical features:** More rapid and fatal course.

LEISHMANIA

Leishmania donovani

Kala-Azar

- **Habitat:** Amastigote form is found in cells of RE system (liver, spleen, bone marrow).
- Promastigote form is found in the gut of sand flies (phlebotomus argentipes).
- **Amastigote:** 2-4 μm, round, oval, kinetoplast (**LD body** – Leishman Donovan bodies).
- **Promastigote:** 15-20 μm × 1-2 μm, flagellum.
- **Mode of transmission:** Sandfly (Phlebotomus), Vertical transmission, Blood transfusion.

Life Cycle:

Blood meal → transform into promastigotes in the gut of the insect → migrate to mouth parts (partial or complete blockage) (EIP: 8-20 days) → parasites dislodged when blocked sandfly tries to ingest blood → in human convert into amastigote forms → multiply in the RE system.

Clinical Features:

IP: 3-6 months, fever, hepatosplenomegaly, pigmentation of skin, weight loss.

Laboratory Diagnosis:

- **Nonspecific tests:** Progressive neutropenia with relative lymphocytosis.
- **Reversed albumin: Globulin ratio Hypergammaglobulinaemia** demonstrated by **Napier aldehyde test, Chopra's antimony test.**
- **Demonstration of LD bodies: Spleen (most sensitive)** > bone marrow > liver > liver > lymph nodes; D/D Toxoplasma gondii, H. capsulatum.

Culture:

Monophasic media: Grace's, Schneider's.

Biphasic media: NNN, Tobie's, BHI agar 24°C for 7 days.

- Leishmanin (Montenegro skin test).
- **Detection of the antigen:** ELISA, immunofluorescence.
- **Detection of the antibodies:** CFT, CIEP, IFAT ≥ 1:32, ELISA, Direct agglutination, IHA.
- **ELISA using rk39 antigenQ** has been found to have 100% sensitive and 96% specific. It has both diagnostic as well as prognostic importance (antibody titer falls with the successful treatment).

Post Kala-Azar Dermal Leishmaniasis:

2-10% cases of visceral leishmaniasis treated with antimony/spontaneously cured presents after 2 years of successful treatment with depigmented macules, erythematous patches, nodular lesions.

Diagnosis: Biopsy, culture, no role of serology.

Treatment: Prolonged course of antimonials.

Leishmania Tropica

Oriental sore, Delhi boil, Baghdad boil, Aleppo button.Q

Leishmania Brasiliensis

Mucocutaneous leishmaniasis (Espundia).Q

Sandfly: Lutzomyia spp.

Reservoir: Small rodents.

BALANTIDIUM COLI

- **Ciliate** causes dysentery like feature.
- Largest protozoal parasite and only ciliate infecting humans.
- **Habitat:** Large intestine, caecum, terminal ileum.
- **Reservoir:** Pig.
- **Trophozoite:** 80-120 μm, Peristome, Cytostome, Cytopharynx, Cytopyge, two nuclei **(macronucleus, micronucleus).**
- **Cyst:** Spherical, ellipsoid, 50-75 μm, double layered cyst wall.
- **Life Cycle:**
  Natural host: Pig, man incidental host.
  Infective stage: Cyst.
  Transmission: Pig to pig, pig to man, man to man, man to pig.

Laboratory Diagnosis:

Faecal examination: Trophozoite, cyst.

DOC – Tetracycline.

PLASMODIUM SPECIES

- **Species are:**
  P. vivax, P. malariae
  P. ovale
  P. falciparum
  Plasmodium vivax, Plasmodium falciparum account for 80% of infections.
- **Habitat:** Hepatic parenchymal cells, RBCs.

Life Cycle:

Intermediate host: Man.

Definitive host: Female anopheles mosquito.

Human cycle (Schizogony/asexual cycle): Female anopheline mosquito bites → Sporozoites injected Q → general circulation → invade hepatocytes → preerythrocytic schizogony → merozoites → invade RBCs → erythrocytic schizogony → some merozoites develop into gametocytes.

P. vivax (Schuffner's dots).

P. malariae (Zeimann's dots).

P. ovale (James dots).

P. falciparum (Maurer's dots).

Mosquito cycle (Sporogony/sexual cycle): Female anopheline mosquito bites → picks macrogametocyte and microgametocyte → exflagellation of microgametocyte → penetrates one macrogamete → zygote → ookinete → penetrates the epithelial lining and muscular wall and lies below the outer limiting membrane of the stomach → oocyst → sporocyst containing sporozoites → rupture, sporozoites liberated in the body cavity → reach salivary gland.

In Plasmodium vivax and Plasmodium ovale hepatic forms **(hypnozoites)Q** persist and remain dormant and are responsible for **relapses.**

In P. falciparum and P. malariae there is persistence of erythrocytic stages leading to **recrudescence.Q**

Extrinsic incubation period: 8-21 days.

Intrinsic incubation period:

- P. falciparum: 12 days.
- P. vivax: 14 days.
- P. malariae: 28 days.
- P. ovale: 17 days.

Contd.

Contd.

Clinical Features:

Fever, anaemia, massive splenomegaly.

Complications: Blackwater fever, pernicious malaria, cerebral malaria.

In-vivo Anti-malarial Susceptibility Testing:

Sensitive: If asexual parasites have cleared by **day 6** from the beginning of treatment without subsequent recrudescence until **day 28.**

RI: If asexual parasites have **cleared for atleast 2 consecutive days, latest on day 6** from the beginning of the treatment, followed by recrudescence (early, before day 14; late, between days 15 and 28).

RII: Showing **marked reduction of asexual parasitaemia to less than 25% of the pretreatment count within 48 hours of the initiation of treatment,** but no subsequent disappearance of parasitaemia **(positive on day 6).**

RIII: Showing only **modest reduction, no change,** or an increase in asexual parasitaemia, during the first 48 hours following the implementation of treatment and no subsequent clearance of parasitaemia.

Laboratory Diagnosis:

- **Peripheral blood film examination:** Thick, thin film.
- Thick film is used for prevalence of parasite and thin film is used for speciation.Q
- Quantitative buffy coat examination using Kawamoto technique with acridine orange.
- **Antigen detection:** P. falciparum uses HRP2 **(Parasight F test),** pLDH **(Optimal test).**
- **Molecular methods:** DNA/RNA hybridization, **PCR.**
- **Antibody detection:** IFAT, IHA.

TOXOPLASMA GONDII

- It causes Toxoplasmosis.
- **Trophozoite (tachyzoites): Crescent shaped,** 3 × 7 μm, multiply by **endodyogeny,** found in tissues during acute stage. Appear rounded enclosed within the host cell **(Pseudo cyst).**
- **Tissue cyst:** Formed during **chronic infection.** Skeletal, heart muscle, brain, 200 μm Bradyzoites.
- **Oocyst:** Found in the definitive host (cat). 10-12 μm round. Shed in faeces. **Freshly passed contain a single sporoblast. Sporoblast divides into 2 sporocysts and 4 sporozoites develop in each sporocyst (infective form for humans).**

Life Cycle:

Enteric cycle: Cat.

Exoenteric cycle: Human, mouse.

Enteric cycle: Sporozoites released from ingested mature oocyst → penetrate epithelial cells of the intestine → merozoites → some merozoites form tissue cysts in various extraintestinal tissues; some develop into gametocytes → fertilization → oocyst → shed in faeces.

Exenteric cycle: Ingestion of oocyst, tissue cyst. Only asexual development occurs in man, oocysts are not formed. Merozoites enter lymphatics → blood → tissue cysts in various organ.

- **Mode of Transmission:**

  Contaminated food (oocysts).
- **Vertical transmission (congenital infection).**

  Blood transfusion.

Clinical Features:

- **Congenital toxoplasmosis:** Chorioretinitis, blindness, epilepsy, mental retardation.

Disseminated infection: Immunocompromised (AIDS) – MCC of Neurological deficits.

Laboratory Diagnosis:

- **Direct examination:** Giemsa, immunofluoresence.
- **Animal inoculation:** I/P inoculation in mice.
- **Serology:** LA, Direct agglutination test, IHA, ELISA, CFT, IFAT.
- **Sabin and Feldman dye test** (specific inhibition by antibody of the staining of trophozoites by **alkaline methylene blue**).Q

CRYPTOSPORIDIUM PARVUM

- It causes **Cryptosporidiosis.**
- **Oocyst:** 4-5 µm, mature contains 2-4 sporozoites, thin walled reinfect the host, thick walled is excreted out.

Life Cycle:

Completed in one host, infective stage: Oocyst → excystation in the small intestine → invade epithelial cells → trophozoites → merozoites → micro and macrogametocytes → zygote → oocyst.

Clinical Features:

Protracted diarrhoea in immunocompromised patients (AIDS).Q

Laboratory Diagnosis:

Faecal examination: Wet mount (oocysts), modified ZN staining (0.5% sulphuric acid, acid fast), IFAT, ELISA, PCR.

Cyclospora cantonensis – Oocyst size 8-10 Micron, acid fast in nature.Q

Isospora belli is having largest size oocyst (23-36 micron), acid fast in nature.Q

BABESIA SPECIES

- Human infection **(Babesiosis)** caused by B. bovis, B. divergens, B. microti.
- Organisms show Antigenic variation.
- **Mode of transmission:** Ticks.
- **Reservoir of infection:** Ticks (transovarial transmission).

Clinical features: Fever, myalgia, hepatosplenomegaly.

Life Cycle:

Sexual cycle in insect host, asexual cycle in mammals. In mammals invades RBCs **(Maltese cross).**

Laboratory Diagnosis:

- Peripheral blood smear examination. Parasite arrange in form of **(Maltese cross).Q**
- **Serological diagnosis:** IFAT, IHA, ELISA.

HELMINTHES

INTRODUCTION

- The sources of the parasites are different. Exposure of humans to the parasites may occur in one of the following ways: The helminthes are classified into three major groups. These are:
  1. **Trematodes** (Flukes).
  2. **Nematodes** (Round worms).
  3. **Cestodes** (Tape worms) – The Trematodes and Cestodes are groups of flat worms.

CLASSIFICATION OF HELMINTHES

Helminthes	Cestodes	Trematodes	Nematodes
Shape	Tape like	Leaf like (Flukes)	Cylindrical
Sex	Monoecious	Mainly monoecious but Schistosomes are dioecious	Dioecious
Head end	Suckers with hooks	Sucker without hooks	Buccal capsule
Alimentary canal	Present	Incomplete, anus absent	Complete
Body cavity	Absent	Absent	Present

METAZOA (Sub-kingdom) – Platyhelminthes (Phylum)

Class: Cestoda (Tape worms)

- **Intestinal species** – Taenia saginata, Taenia solium, Hymenolepis nana, Diphyllobothrium latum.
- **Intestinal tissue species** – Echinococcus granulosus.

Class: Trematode (Flukes)

- **Intestinal species** – Fasciolopsis buski.
- **Blood species** – Schistosoma species.
- **Tissue species** – Fasciola hepatica (liver fluke), Paragonimus westermanii (lung fluke).

METAZOA – Nemathelminthes (Phylum)

Class: Nematoda (Round worms)

- **Intestinal species** – Enterobius vermicularis, Trichuris trichura, Ascaris lumbricoides, Necator americanus, Ancylostoma duodenale, Strongyloides stercolaris.
- **Intestinal tissue species** – Trichinella sps, Dracunculus medinensis.
  Blood borne species – Wucheria bancrofti, Brugia malayi, Loa loa, Onchocerca volvulus

INFECTIVE FORMS

Eggs	Cysticercus	Plerocercoid	Metacercaria	Cercaria	Larva
T. solium	T. solium	Diphyllobothrium Latum	Fasciola sp	Schistoma sps.	Strongyloides Stercoralis (Filariform larva)
E. granulosus	T. saginata		Clonorchis sinensis		Ancylostoma duodenale (Filariform larva)
Ascaris			Paragonimus westermanii		Necator americanus (Filariform larva)
Enterobius					Trichinella spiralis (Encysted larva)

Contd.

Contd.

Trichuris trichiura					Wucheria bancrofti (3rd stage larva)
					Loa-Loa (3rd stage larva)
					Onchocerca volvulus (3rd stage larva)
					Dracunculus Medinensis (3rd stage larva)

IMPORTANT CESTODES

Name	Definitive host	Intermediate host
Taenia solium	Man	Pig and manQ
Taenia saginata	Man	Cattle
Echinococcus granulosus	Dog	Man, sheep
H. nana	Man	Man
Diphylobothrium latum (Fish Tape worm)	Man	Cyclops and Fresh water fish

***Taenia* species**	**Definitive host**	**Intermediate host**	**Organ affected**	**Disease**
T. saginata	Man	Cattle	Intestine	Intestinal taeniasis
T. solium	Man	Pig	Intestine	Intestinal taeniasis
T. solium	Man	Man	Muscle, CNS, eye	Cysticercosis
T. asiatica	Man	Pig (Liver)	Intestine	Intestinal taeniasis
T. multiceps	Dog	Sheep, rarely man	CNS	Coenurosis

TAENIA

TAENIA SAGINATA

- **Beef tape worm, unarmed tape worm.**
- **Habitat:** Scolex of the adult worm is embedded in the mucosa of the ileum.

Life Cycle:

- **Definitive host: Man.**
- **Intermediate host:** Cow, buffalo.
- **Eggs/gravid segments** → passed in feces → cow/buffalo swallow → penetrate the gut wall → portal circulation → systemic circulation → muscle → **cysticercus bovis** → humans infected by eating uncooked beef → develop into adult worm → mating → eggs/gravid segments.

Clinical Features:

Abdominal pain, diarrhea, constipation, intestinal obstruction.

Laboratory Diagnosis:

Faecal examination – Proglottids/eggs (spherical, bile stained, **oncosphere**).

TAENIA SOLIUM

- **Pork tape worm, armed tape worm.Q**
- **Habitat:** Adult worm found in small intestine of man.

Life Cycle:

- **Definitive and intermediate host:** Man.
- **Intermediate host:** Pig.
- Eggs/gravid segments → passed in feces → pig swallow → penetrate the gut wall → portal circulation → systemic circulation → muscle → **cysticercus cellulosae in pig** → humans infected by eating uncooked pork → develop into adult worm → mating → eggs/gravid segments.

Contd.

Contd.

- Man also acquires infection by ingesting eggs in contaminated food/water, auto infection → larval form **(cysticercus cellulosae)** develops in humans (brain, eyes, subcutaneous tissue) and this forms the route to cause **Neurocysticercosis.Q**
- **Most common site** – Subarachnoid > Parenchymal.Q
- **IOC – Radiological – MRI and CT scan.**

Clinical Features:

- **Adult worm:** Abdominal pain, diarrhea, loss of appetite.
- **Cysticercus cellulosae (larva): Neurocysticercosis:** Epilepsy, hydrocephalus, increased intracranial tension, blurred vision.

Laboratory Diagnosis:

- **Fecal examination:** Proglottids/eggs (spherical, bile stained, oncosphere).
- **Cysticercus cellulosae:**
  IOC-Radiology (CT scan, MRI).
  FNAC, serology (CFT, IHA, ELISA, IFAT).

DOC – Albendazole.

Difference between Taenia Solium and Taenia Saginata

	T. saginata	T. solium
Length	**5-10 metres**	**2-3 metres**
Head	**Large, quadrate without rostellum and hooks** Suckers may be pigmented	**Small, globular, with rostellum and hooks,** suckers not pigmented
Number	1000-2000	Below 1000
Expulsion	Expelled singly	Expelled passively in chains of 5-6
Uterus	Lateral branches (15-30) on each side	Lateral branches 5-10 on each side
Vagina	Vaginal sphincter present	Vaginal sphincter absent
Testes	300-400 follicles	150-200 follicles
Ovary	2 without any accessory lobe	2 with accessory lobe

ECHINOCOCCOSIS

(Echinococcus Granulosus/Dog Tapeworm)

- Four species causing disease in humans:
  - **E. granulosus** (most common).Q
  - E. multilocularis (second most common).Q
    (Multilocular alveolar hydatid disease)
  - E. oligarthus (America).
  - E. vogeli (Latin America)–Causes polycystic hydatid disease.Q

Habitat:

Humans harbor the larval form (hydatid cyst); adult worm in small intestine of dog and other canines.

Life Cycle:

- **Definitive host:** Dog, jackal, fox; adult worm resides in the small intestine and discharges eggs in the feces.
- **Intermediate host:** Sheep, pig, goat, cattle, man (dead end host).

Dog discharges eggs in feces → man acquires infection by ingestion of food/water → **Hexacanth embryo hatches in duodenum** → **penetrates gut wall** → portal circulation → systemic circulation → hydatid cyst (**liver** > **lung** > brain > kidneys > spleen).

Clinical Features:

Pressure effects due to cyst, cerebral (epilepsy), renal (hematuria), rupture of cyst (allergic manifestation).

Contd.

Contd.

Laboratory Diagnosis:
- **Radiology:** X-ray, CT scan, MRI.
- **Casoni's test:** Immediate hypersensitivity, I/D, wheal in 30 minutes.
- **Serology:** IHA, CIEP, ELISA, IFAT, **Immunoelectrophoresis Arc 5 test is done.Q**

HYMENOLEPIS NANA

- **Dwarf tapeworm.**
- **Habitat:** Adult worm found in ileum.
- **Mode of infection:** Food/water contaminated with eggs, **Auto infection** happens.

Life Cycle:

Only tape worm for which humans act as both definitive and intermediate host:

Eggs ingested → Oncosphere penetrates the intestinal villi → develop into **cysticercoid stage** → released in the lumen → reattaches to another villus → develops into adult worm → mating → eggs.

Clinical Features: Abdominal pain, diarrhea, weight loss.

Laboratory diagnosis: Fecal examination – Eggs **(Polar filaments emanating from little knobs at either end of embryophore).Q**

Adult worm/proglottids: Rarely seen in feces.

DOC – Praziquantel.Q

DIPHYLLOBOTHRIUM LATUM

- **Fish tape worm.**
- **Habitat:** Adult worm found in small intestine.

Life Cycle:

- **Definitive host:** Man, dog, cat, pig.
- **First intermediate host:** Cyclops.
- **Second intermediate host:** Fresh water fish.

Eggs liberated through feces of definitive host in water → develops into ciliated embryo **(coracidium)** → ingested by cyclops → develops into second stage larva **(procercoid)** → Cyclops containing procercoid larvae eaten by fish → penetrates the gut wall → liver/muscle/fat → develops into third stage larva (sparganum/**plerocercoid larva** Q) → man ingests infected fish → in gut develops into adult worm → mating → eggs.

Clinical Features: Abdominal pain, diarrhea, **megaloblastic anaemia.Q**

Laboratory Diagnosis:

Segments of worm: Fecal examination.

Egg: Fecal examination.

Serology: ELISA, LA.

TREMATODES

IMPORTANT FEATURES

(a) **Flat leaf like.**
(b) Trematodes are monoecious except schistosomes.
(c) Always have two intermediate hosts and definitive host.
(d) Trematodes are oviparous and lay operculated eggs except for schistosomes which lay nonoperculated eggs.
(e) Fasciola buski – largest fluke and cause GI symptoms.

SCHISTOSOMIASIS

Bilharziasis

Five main species infect humans:

S. mansoni	eggs with lateral spine
S. haematobium	eggs with terminal spine
S. intercalatum	eggs with terminal spine
S. japonicum	round eggs with minute spine (Lateral knob)
S. mekongi	round eggs with minute spine

Only S. haematobium found in India.

Life Cycle:

All schistosomes share basic life cycle:

Eggs passed in urine (S. haematobium), feces (S. japonicum, S. mansoni, S. intercalatum) → eggs contain **miracidium** → hatch in water → miracidium penetrate fresh water snail → develops into **mother sporocyst** → **daughter sporocyst** → **cercariae** → released in water → penetrate the skin of humans → **schistosomula** → lymphatics/venous vessels → portal vessels (all species migrate mesenteric veins except S. haematobium which migrates to **vesical plexus**) → develop into adults → mate → eggs.

Clinical Features:

- **Acute schistosomiasis (katayama fever):** S. mansoni **(Inferior mesenteric vein),** S. japonicum **(superior mesenteric vein).Q**
- **Chronic intestinal schistosomiasis:** S. mansoni, S. japonicum, S. intercalatum, S. mekongi (abdominal pain, dysentery, obstruction, Hepatosplenomegaly, portal hypertension).
- **S. hematobium:** Resides in veins of vesical and pelvic plexuses hematuria, dysuria, urgency, frequency and causes **(painless terminal haematuriaQ)** and have strong association with **Squamous cell carcinoma.Q**
- **Fairley's test (Intradermal test)** is done for Schistosomiasis.Q

Laboratory Diagnosis:

- **Fecal specimen:** Eggs.
- **Urine specimen:** Eggs.
- **Biopsy (liver, rectal, bladder):** Eggs.
- **Serology:** IFAT, ELISA.

FASCIOLA HEPATICA

(Sheep Liver Fluke)

- **Mode of infection:** Ingestion of aquatic vegetation contaminated with **encysted metacercaria.**

Life Cycle:

- **Definitive host:** Sheep, goat, cattle.
- **Intermediate host:** Snail.

In sheep eggs laid in the biliary tract → faeces → **miracidium hatches from egg → penetrates snail → sporocyst → rediae → cercariae → cercariae emerge from snail → encyst on aquatic vegetation (metacercariae)** → ingested by definitive host → excyst in duodenum → penetrate intestinal wall → penetrate liver → reach bile duct → develop into adult → mating → eggs.

Clinical Features: Epigastric pain, fever, diarrhea, jaundice, urticaria, arthralgia, eosinophilia.

- **Acute fascoliasis:** Tender hepatomegaly, fever, eosinophilia.
- **Chronic:** Obstruction/inflammation of bile duct.

Laboratory Diagnosis:

- **Eggs:** Feces.
- **Serology:** ELISA, CFT, LA, IHA, IFAT.

Halzoun syndrome (Laryngeal edema due to eating sheep liver), Bile duct obstruction and sometimes Cholangiocarcinoma.

PARAGONIMUS WESTERMANI

- **Mode of infection: Ingestion of raw/undercooked crab/cray fish.**

Life Cycle:

- **Definitive host:** Man, tiger, leopards.
- **First intermediate host:** Fresh water snail.
- **Second intermediate host:** Fresh water crab, cray fish.

Eggs reach bronchioles → coughed up → swallowed → passed in feces → **miracidium hatch in water → penetrate snail → sporocyst → rediae → cercariae → emerge from snail → penetrate crab/cray fish → encyst (metacercariae) in gills/ muscles** → ingestion of raw/undercooked intermediate host → excyst in duodenum → young worms penetrate through gut wall → penetrate diaphragm → **penetrate lung capsule** → develop into adult worm → mating → eggs.

Clinical Features:

- Chronic cough, hemoptysis **(Endemic hemoptysis),** pleural pain, dyspnoea, secondary bacterial infection.

Laboratory Diagnosis:

- **Sputum, stool:** Eggs.
- **Serology:** ELISA, CFT.

CLONORCHIS SINENSIS

- **Mode of infection:** Ingestion of raw/undercooked fresh water fish.

Life Cycle:

- **Definitive host:** Man, dog, pig, cat.
- **First intermediate host:** Snail.
- **Second intermediate host:** Fish.

  Eggs containing **miracidium from bile duct to intestine → excreted in feces → miracidium hatch in water → penetrate snail → sporocyst → rediae → cercariae → emerge from snail → penetrate beneath the scales of fish → encyst (metacercariae)** in subcutaneous tissue → ingestion of raw/undercooked fish → excyst in duodenum → young worms migrate up the bile duct → develop into adult worm → mating → eggs.

Clinical Features:

Cholangitis, portal hypertension, biliary obstruction, implicated in **cholangiocarcinoma.Q**

Laboratory Diagnosis:

Eggs: Stool examination.

HELMINTHOLOGY

NEMATODES

CLASSIFICATION BASED ON LOCATION OF ADULT WORM

Intestinal	Somatic
Small intestine	***Lymphatic system***
Ascaris lumbricoides	W. bancrofti
Ancylostoma duodenale	B. malayi
Necator americanus	***Subcutaneous tissue***
Trichinella spiralis	Loa loa
Strongyloides stercoralis	Onchocerca volvulus
Large intestine	***Mesentery***
Trichuris trichiura	D. perstans
Enterobius vermicularis	Mansonella ozzardi
	Dracunculus medinensis
	Conjunctiva
	Loa loa

CLASSIFICATION BASED ON MODE OF INFECTION

Ingestion (EAT mnemonic)	Cutaneous penetration (ANS mnemonic)	Insect
A. lumbricoides	Ancylostoma duodenale	W. bancrofti
T. trichiura	Necator americanus	Loa loa
E. vermicularis	S. stercoralis	O. volvulus
T. spiralis		

NEMATODES LAYING EGGS/LARVAE

Oviparous	Viviparous
Unsegmented ovum	T. spiralis
A. lumbricoides	W. bancrofti
T. trichiura	B. malayi
Segmented ovum	D. medinensis
A. doudenale	**Ovo-viviparous**
N. americanus	S. stercoralis.Q
Egg containing larvae	
Enterobius vermicularis	

TRICHURIS TRICHIURA (Whip worm)

- **Habitat:** Large intestine, caecum, appendix.
- **Egg: Barrel shaped, bile stained, Mucus plugs at each pole,** unsegmented ovum.

Life Cycle:

Egg → develop in moist soil (2 weeks) → embryonated egg → ingested → larvae released → migrate to caecum → develop into adult worm → fertilization → egg.

Clinical Features:

Abdominal pain, weight loss, anaemia, acute appendicitis.

Contd.

Contd.

Laboratory Diagnosis:

Stool examination

Sigmoidoscopy: "Coconut cake rectum".Q

TRICHINELLA SPIRALIS

- **Habitat:** Adult worm found in small intestine of pig, rat, man.

Morphology

Adult worm: Smallest nematode infecting humans, 1-3 mm in length.

Larva: 100 × 6 μm.

Life Cycle:

Man is a **dead end host,** pig is a reservoir host. Ingestion of infected meat (pig) → larvae released in duodenum → adult worm → mating → larvae → penetrate intestinal wall → lymphatic vessel → blood stream → skeletal muscles (diaphragm, intercostals muscles, pectoral muscles).

Clinical Features:

Intestinal invasion phase: First week, nausea, vomiting and diarrhea.

Muscle invasion phase: Second week, orbital edema, chemosis, photophobia; death due to myocarditis, neurological complications.

Laboratory Diagnosis:

X-ray: Calcified cysts.

Increased muscle enzymes.

Muscle biopsy.

Skin test: Brachman's antigen.Q

Serological test: Main stay, CFT, IFAT.

STRONGYLOIDES STERCORALIS

Morphology: Adults worm, egg, larvae.

Egg: Embryonated, hatch in mucosal epithelium.

Larvae: Rhabditiform larvae → filariform larvae.

Internal reinfection.

External reinfection.

Life Cycle:

Direct phase: Filariform larvae → penetrate skin → venous circulation → right heart → lungs → leave pulmonary capillaries → alveoli → bronchi → trachea → larynx → swallowed → intestinal tract → develop into adults in duodenum/jejunum → mating → eggs → immediately hatched into rhabditiform larvae → filariform larvae.

Free living phase (heterogenetic development): Rhabditiform larvae → soil → free living males and females → mating in soil → rhabditiform larvae → filariform larvae.

Hyperinfection syndrome: Immunocompromised (HIV/AIDS), massive larval invasion of the lungs, other organs.Q

Clinical Features:

- **Larva currens** (intra dermal migration of the filariform larvae at a faster speed).Q
- Diarrhea, nausea, vomiting, **Loeffler's syndrome,** infection of brain, meninges.

Laboratory Diagnosis:

Stool examination: Only larvae are seen.

- **Concentration methods: Bearmann's method, Charcoal based methods.**
- **Stool culture** for **Rhabditiform larvae: Harada mori technique.**
- **Disseminated infection:** Sputum, urine, CSF culture can be tried etc.
- **Serological test:** ELISA, IFAT.

ASCARIS LUMBRICOIDES

Roundworm

- **Habitat:** Adult worm in jejunum/upper ileum.

Life Cycle:

Fertilized egg containing unsegmented ovum → develop in soil (3 weeks) → Egg containing **second stage rhabditiform larva (first moulting)** → Ingestion → larva released → penetrate the wall of small intestine → portal circulation → liver → venous circulation → right heart → pulmonary circulation **(moult twice 2nd, 3rd Q)** → penetrate capillary wall → alveoli → bronchi → trachea → larynx → pharynx → swallowed → **localize in upper part of small intestine (fourth moulting)** → develop into adult worms → mating → egg.

Clinical Features:

Asymptomatic, malnutrition, **intussusception, intestinal obstruction,** perforation, appendicitis, obstructive jaundice, pancreatitis**, Loffler's syndrome.**

Laboratory Diagnosis:

Adult worm: Stool, vomitus.

Egg: Bile stained, unsegmented ovum; stool (Pic in Image based section).

Sputum: Larvae are demonstrated.

HOOKWORM (ANCYLOSTOMA DUODENALE/NECATOR AMERICANUS)

Life Cycle:

Egg containing segmented ovum → develop in soil → first stage rhabditiform larva → (1st moult) → (2nd moult) filariform larvae → penetrate skin → venous circulation → right heart → lungs → leave pulmonary capillaries → alveoli → bronchi → trachea → larynx → swallowed → intestinal tract (3rd moult, third stage larva) → **(4th moult) develop into adults in jejunum** → mating → eggs.

Clinical Features:

Nausea, vomiting, diarrhea, epigastric pain, **microcytic hypochromic anaemia**, **wakana disease (seen in Japan),** rash.

Laboratory Diagnosis:

Demonstration of eggs in stool, duodenal aspirate; **non-bile stained, segmented ovum.**

ENTEROBIUS VERMICULARIS

- **Thread worm, pin worm, seat worm, oxyuriasis.Q**

Life Cycle:

Adult female emerges from anus at night → lay eggs → **perianal pruritis** → scratch → contaminated nails and finger tips → mouth → eggs hatch → develop into adult worms in small intestine → mating → female migrates to caecum and colon.

Mode of Infection:

Direct transfer of eggs from anus to mouth through contaminated fingers.

Retroinfection: Eggs hatch in the perianal area and larvae migrate back in the bowels through contaminated night clothes, bed linen.

Clinical Manifestation:

Pruritis ani, nocturnal enuresis, anorexia, weight loss, salpingitis, omentitis, cervicitis, peritonitis.

Laboratory Diagnosis:

- **Demonstration of adult worms:** Stool.
- **Demonstration of eggs:** Stool examination not recommended, NIH swab, cellulose tape.

LARVA MIGRANS

Infection with helminth larvae not adapted to humans.

Cutaneous larva migrans (creeping eruption)	**Visceral larva migrans**
Ancylostoma brasilienses (most common)Q A. caninum Gnathostoma spinigerum	Toxocara canis (most common)Q T. catis Angiostrongylus cantonensis – it also leads to Eosinophilic meningitis.Q Anisakine spp.

	CLM	VLM
Tissue involved	Skin	Viscera (liver, lungs)
Infecting organism	Zoophilic hook worm	Zoophilic roundworm
Route of infection	Larvae penetrate the skin	Ingestion of infected eggs
Eosinophilia	Rare	Present
Anti-A, anti-B agglutinins	Not present	Present
Serodiagnosis (ELISA)	No role	Well established

FILARIASIS

Lymphatic filariasis caused by **W. bancrofti** (90%), B. malayi (10%), B. timori.

W. Bancrofti

- **Habitat:** Adult worm in lymphatics, sheathed microfilaria in blood.

Life Cycle:

- **Definitive host:** Humans.
- **Intermediate host:** Mosquito **(culex, aedes, anopheles),** India: **Culex pipens fatigans.**

  Adult worm in lymphatics → sheathed microfilaria in blood → mosquito bite → exsheathing in stomach → penetrate stomach wall → migrate to thoracic muscles → first stage larva → second stage larva → **third stage filariform larva (infective stage)Q** → mosquito bites humans → larvae reach lymphatics → adult worm.

  Extrinsic incubation period: 10-20 days.

  Pre-patent period (biological incubation period): Time taken for the third stage infective larvae to develop into adult worms → sexually mature → liberate microfilariae in the peripheral blood (patent period).

  Clinical incubation period: 8-16 months.

Clinical Features:

Fever, lymphangitis, lymphadenitis, chylocele, chyluria, chylous ascites, chylothorax, lymphedema, elephantiasis, occult filariasis.

	CLASSICAL FILARIASIS	OCCULT FILARIASIS
Cause	Adult, developing worms	Microfilariae
Organs involved	Lymphatic vessels, lymph nodes	Lymphatic vessels, lung, liver, spleen
Microfilariae	Present in peripheral blood	Absent
Lesion	Lymphangitis, lymphadenitis	**Eosinophilic granuloma**
Response to DEC	No response	Good response

Laboratory Diagnosis:

Demonstration of Microfilaria

Direct film – Microfilariae is having nocturnal periodicity and is characterized by **Tail tip free of nuclei.Q**

Concentration (Knott's)

DEC provocation test: 2 mg/kg, blood sample after one hour.

Demonstration of Adult Worm

Biopsy of lymph node.

Immunodiagnosis

Detection of antibody: ELISA, IHA, IFAT.

Detection of antigen: ELISA, immunochromatography.

Various radiological investigations are done like Ultrasound, CT scan and Chest X-ray to demonstrate Microfilariae.

In USG Scrotum – Dancing worm sign is seen.Q

Nowadays best test to distinguish is PCR for Wucheria Bancrofti.

B. MALAYI

Vector: Mosquito, mansonia annulifera (in India), Important feature to be remembered that **Microfilariae tail have terminal two nuclei.**

B. Timori

Timor in Indonesia; vector: Anopheles barbirostris (not found in India).

ONCHOCERCA VOLVULUS

- Onchocerciases, **River blindness.**
- Tropical Africa.
- **Habitat:** Adult worm in subcutaneous tissue (onchocercomas); microfilariae found in skin.

Life Cycle:

Definitive host: Man.

Intermediate host: Female black flies (**simulium spp.**/buffalo gnats) breed in fast flowing rivers.

Bite of mosquito → ingests microfilaria → **develop into third stage larva (infective stage)** → bite → in humans develop into adults → microfilaria.

Clinical Features:

- Adult worm relatively non-pathogenic (onchocercomas).
- Microfilariae main cause of disease: Dermatitis, keratitis, iridocyclitis.

Laboratory Diagnosis:

- **Adult worm:** Biopsy of subcutaneous nodules.
- **Microfilaria:** Skin snip technique is employed (iliac crest); **Mazzotti reaction:** 50 mg DEC → pruritis, erythema.

LOA LOA

- **Loiasis, calabar swellings, fugitive swelling.Q**
- **West and Central Africa.**
- **Habitat:** Adult worm in subcutaneous tissue; microfilariae found in blood.

Life Cycle:

Definitive host: Man.

Intermediate host: Female chrysops (mango fly/deer fly/soft fly).Q

Bite of mosquito → ingests microfilaria → develop into infective larva (infective stage) → bite → in humans develop into adults → microfilaria.

Clinical Manifestations:

- **Adult worm: Migratory swellings (Calabar/fugitive swellings),** glomerulonephritis, retinopathy, peripheral neuropathy, meningitis, Jacksonian epilepsy.
- **Microfilariae:** Relatively non pathogenic.

Laboratory Diagnosis:

- **Adult worm:** Biopsy.
- **Microfilariae:** Blood.

DRACUNCULUS MEDINENSIS

- **Guinea worm, medina worm.Q**
- **Habitat:** Adult female found in subcutaneous tissue.

Life Cycle:

Definitive host: Humans.

Intermediate host: Cyclops.

Patient enters water → adult female worm emerges from blister/ulcer → **anterior end of worm ruptures** → thousands of larvae released in water → ingested by cyclops → **develops in coelomic cavity to third stage larva** → **human drink water (contaminated with Cyclops)** → penetrate the gut wall → **migrate to retroperitoneal connective tissue** → mature into adult worms → mating → male dies → fertilized female migrates to subcutaneous tissue of the body → blister → blister/ulcer on the skin.

Clinical Features: Blister, ulcer, secondary bacterial infection, urticaria, nausea, calcified worm (arthritis, spinal cord compression).

Laboratory Diagnosis:

- Emerging adult worm.
- **Embryo:** Contact with water, larvae released in water, examined under microscope.
- **X-ray:** Calcified worm.
- **Serology:** ELISA, IHA.
- **India achieved eradication of Guinea worm disease in 1999 and declared in year 2000.Q**

CLASSIFICATION OF MICROFILARIA

Unsheathed and non-periodic microfilaria	Sheathed periodic microfilaria found in blood
Found in blood • Pointed tail tip with nuclei: M. perstans. • Pointed tail tip without nuclei: M. ozzardi. **Found in skin** • Tail tip hooked, nuclei upto tip: M. streptocerca. • Tail tip free of nuclei: O. vovulus.	**Tail tip free of nuclei** • W. bancrofti.Q **Nuclei upto tail tip** • **Blunt tail with two terminal nuclei: B. malayi.Q** • Pointed tail tip with nuclei upto tail tip: Loa loa.

Contd.

Contd.

List of non-bile stained eggs (Memory aid (NEHA))	Eggs that float in saturated salt solution (FATEH)
Necator americanus	**F** – Fertilised egg of ascaris
Enterobius vermicularis	**A** – Ancylostoma duodenale
Hymenolepis nana	**T** – Trichuris trichiura
Ancylostoma duodenale	**E** – Enterobius vermicularis
	H – H. nana

MCQs

PROTOZOA 'A': AMOEBA and CILIATES

Entamoeba

1. **True about amoebic colitis is:** *(AI 10)*
   (a) Caused by E histolytica
   (b) Cyst contains eight nuclei
   (c) Flask-shaped ulcers are present
   (d) Cecum is most commonly affected
2. **Culture medium used for Entamoeba histolytica:** *(Recent MCQ)*
   (a) Blood agar
   (b) Philip's medium
   (c) CLED medium
   (d) Trypticase serum
3. **All the following amoebae are non-pathogenic *except*:**
   (a) E.coli
   (b) E.histolytica
   (c) E.gingivalis
   (d) I. butschii

Morphology

4. **Glycogen mass and chromidial bars are absent in the cyst of Entamoeba histolytica in:**
   (a) Uninucleate
   (b) Binucleate
   (c) Quadrinucleate
   (d) Octanucleate
5. **Which one of the following statements is false:** *(AIIMS Nov 03)*
   (a) The presence of ingested erythrocytes is seen only in Entamoeba histolytica
   (b) Young adult male of low socioeconomic status are most commonly affected by invasive amoebiasis
   (c) A low iron content in the diet predisposes to invasive amoebiasis
   (d) The pathogenic and non-pathogenic strains of E.histolytica can be differentiated by the electrophoretic study of zymodemes
6. **Which of the following is true about mature cysts of E. histolytica?** *(AI 96)*
   (a) Endoplasm and ectoplasm are clearly defined
   (b) Eight chromatid bodies
   (c) Shows chromatid bodies and glycogen mass
   (d) Nuclear structure retains characteristics of trophozoite
7. **Which is true of trophozoites of E.histolytica?** *(AI 93)*
   (a) Has eccentric karyosome
   (b) Nuclear membrane with chromatin
   (c) Shows erythrophagocytosis
   (d) Presence of bacteria inside cell

Clinical Features, Diagnosis and Treatment

8. **Charcot leyden crystals in stool are seen in:** *(Recent MCQ)*
   (a) Bacillary dysentery
   (b) Amoebic dysentery
   (c) Giardiasis
   (d) Cholera

9. **Amoebic liver abscess can be diagnosed by demonstrating:** *(AI 91)*
   (a) Cysts in the sterile pus
   (b) Trophozoites in the pus
   (c) Cysts in the intestine
   (d) Trophozoites in the feces

10. **A patient presents with lower gastrointestinal bleed. Sigmoidoscopy shows ulcer in the sigmoid. Biopsy from this area shows flask-shaped ulcers. Which of the following is the most appropriate treatment?** *(AIIMS 98)*
   (a) Intravenous ceftriaxone
   (b) Intravenous metronidazole
   (c) Intravenous steroids and sulphasalazine
   (d) Hydrocortisone enemas

11. **Most common extrahepatic complication of amoebic hepatitis is:** *(Recent MCQ)*
   (a) Meningitis
   (b) Lung abscess
   (c) Nephritis
   (d) Encephalitis

12. **Stain with parasite having Charcot-Layden crystals but no pus cells:** *(Recent MCQ)*
   (a) Giardia
   (b) Taenia
   (c) E.histolytica
   (d) Trichomonas

Amoebic Meningoencephalitis

13. **Acute Primary Amoebic meningoencephalitis true is:** *(AIIMS May 08)*
   (a) Meningitis caused by acanthamoeba species is acute in nature
   (b) Diagnosis is by demonstration of trophozoite in CSF
   (c) Caused by feco-oral transmission
   (d) More common in tropical climate

Amoeba

14. **The pathogenicity of E. histolytica is indicated by:** *(APPGE 05)*
   (a) Zymodeme pattern
   (b) Size
   (c) Nuclear pattern
   (d) ELISA test

15. **The main reservoir for Entamoeba histolytica is:** *(AI 91)*
   (a) Man
   (b) Dirty water
   (c) Soil
   (d) Ponds

16. **Amoebiasis is transmitted by all *except*:** *(AIIMS 10)*
   (a) Cockroach
   (b) Faeco-oral
   (c) Vertical transmission
   (d) Oro-rectal

17. **All are seen in cyst of E. histolytica *except*:** *(Kerala 02)*
   (a) Glycogen mass
   (b) Chromatid bars
   (c) Eccentric nucleus
   (d) Refractile nucleus

18. **Primary amoebic meningitis caused by:** *(SGPGI 05)*
   (a) Naegleri fowleri
   (b) E. histolytica
   (c) E. coli
   (d) B. coli

19. **The most distinctive feature of pathogenic E. histolytica on fresh stool examination is:** *(UP 08)*
   (a) Presence of active pseudopodia
   (b) Erythrophagocytosis
   (c) Presence of intracytoplasmic vacuole
   (d) Presence of two nucleoli

20. **Regarding cutaneous amoebiasis, which is not true?** *(Manipal 06)*
   (a) It is a spreading necrotizing inflammation of the skin and cutaneous tissue
   (b) Rapid improvement with anti-amoebic treatment occurs
   (c) Can occur in the perianal region
   (d) The infection reaches the skin through the blood stream

21. Invasive amoebiasis can be best diagnosed by: *(AIIMS 01)*

(a) ELISA
(b) Countercurrent immunoelectrophoresis
(c) Indirect Hemagglutination test
(d) Complement fixation test

22. Significant titers of IHA is seen in all types of amoebiasis *except*: *(AIIMS 08)*

(a) Acute amoebic dysentery
(b) Brain abscess
(c) Liver abscess
(d) Cyst passers

23. Which one of the following statements is false? *(AIIMS 12)*

(a) The presence of ingested RBC is seen only in E. histolytica
(b) Young adult male of low socioeconomic status are most commonly affected by invasive amoebiasis
(c) A low iron content in the diet predispose to invasive amoebiasis
(d) The pathogenic and non-pathogenic strains of E. histolytica can be differentiated by the electrophoretic study of zymodemes

24. Neuropathogenic amoeba are: *(JIPMER)*

(a) Acanthamoeba
(b) Ent. coli
(c) Nageleria
(d) Ent. Histolytica

25. A 30 years old patient presented with features of acute meningoencephalitis in the casualty. His CSF on wet mount microscopy revealed motile unicellular microorganism. The most likely organism is: *(AIIMS 05)*

(a) Naegleria fowleri
(b) Acanthamoeba castellani
(c) E. histolytica
(d) Ent. coli

26. Acute primary meningoencephalitis true is: *(AIIMS 08)*

(a) Meningitis caused by acanthamoeba species is acute in nature
(b) Diagnosis is done by demonstration of trophozoites in CSF
(c) Caused by feco-oral transmission
(d) More common in tropical climate

27. Eosinophilic meningoencephalitis is caused by: *(PGI 2000)*

(a) Gnathostoma spinigerum
(b) Naegleria
(c) Toxocara canis
(d) Angiostrongylus

28. Most fatal amoebic encephalitis is caused by: *(Bihar 09)*

(a) E. histolytica
(b) Naegleria
(c) E. dispar
(d) Acanthamoeba

29. Fulminant Amoebic meningoencephalitis is caused by: *(AP 06)*

(a) Acanthamoeba
(b) Naegleria
(c) E. histolytica
(d) Entamoeba coli

30. Selective medium for Naegleria fowleri: *(AI 12)*

(a) Nutrient agar rich with E. coli
(b) NNN media
(c) Non-nutrient agar with E. coli
(d) Diamond media

ANSWERS AND EXPLANATIONS

PROTOZOA 'A': AMOEBA and CILIATES

Entamoeba

1. **Ans are 'a, c, d'** (***Ref:*** *D.R. Arora, 3rd/e, p. 26, 27, 28*)
   - Cysts range in size from 10-20 μm. The immature cyst has inclusions namely; glycogen mass and chromatoidal bars. As the cyst matures, the glycogen and chromatoidal bars completely disappears.
2. **Ans. is 'b'** i.e., Philip's medium (***Ref:*** *Chatterjee, 13th/e, p. 274; D.R. Arora, 3rd/e, p. 23*)
   - Cultures media used for cultivation of E. histolytica are:
     I. Boeck and Drbohlav's medium.
     II. Balamuth's medium.
     III. Diamond's medium.
     IV. Nelson's medium.

     All these solid and liquid media are **polyaxenic media** which consist of Enteric bacteria, T.cruzi, as well as starch or rice for the amoebae to grow.

     * **Note that Diamond first reported cultivation in absence of bacteria axenic cultivation – useful to study pathogenicity, immunological and biochemical properties, in vitro drug suspectibility, preparation of axenic amoebic antigen.**
3. **Ans. is 'b'** i.e., E. histolytica (***Ref:*** *D.R. Arora, 3rd/e, p. 26-32; Chatterjee, 13th/e, p. 43*)
   - **E. Gingivalis** is a parasite of human mouth.
   - Other three are intestinal amoebae.
   - **Non-pathogenic amoebae** are **E. hartmanni, E.coli, E.polecki, Endolimax nana, Iodamoeba botschlii, and Dientamoeba fragilis.**

Morphology

4. **Ans is 'c'** i.e., Quadrinucleate (***Ref:*** *D.R. Arora, 3rd/e, p. 22*)
   - Glycogen mass, chromatoid bars are seen in uninucleate and binucleate stage but absent in quadrinucleate stage and infective stage for Entamoeba histolytica is Quadrinucleate stage.
5. **Ans. is 'c'** i.e., A low iron content in the predisposes to invasive amoebiasis (***Ref:*** *Panikar, 6th/e, p. 28*)
   - Invasive amoebiasis and iron content don't have any relation.
   - **Pathognomic sign of infection** is Erythrophagocytosis.
   - Infection is more common in adult males with low socioeconomic status and more association seen in HIV +ve, **it is severe in pregnant and lactating mothers and in neonates.**
   - There are distinct invasive and non-invasive strain of E. histolytica. These strains vary according to their isoenzyme patterns (zymodemes). **E. Histolytica strains have 22 zymodemes (isoenzyme patterns) of these 10 zymodemes are invasive and 12 are non-invasive.Q**
6. **Ans. is 'd'** i.e., Nuclear structure retains characteristics of trophozites

   (***Ref:*** *Parasitology by Chatterjee, 12th/e, p.15; 13th/e, p.19; D.R. Arora, 3rd/e, p. 23*)

   "A mature cyst is quadrinucleate spherical body. Its cytoplasm is clear and hyaline, and the nuclear structure retains the characteristics of the trophozoite."

   About Other Options:
   - **Trophozoites have clear ectoplasm and endoplasm,** not in mature cyst.
7. **Ans. is 'b'** i.e., Nuclear membrane with chromatin; **'c'** i.e., Shows erythrophagocytosis

   (***Ref:*** *Chatterjee, 12th/e, p. 15; 13th/e, p. 19s*)
   - Nuclear membrane is lined with a single layer of uniformly distributed fine chromatin granules.
   - Karyosome is central in position (not eccentric).Q

Clinical Features, Diagnosis and Treatment

8. **Ans. is 'b'** i.e., Amoebic dysentery (***Ref:*** *Harrison, 18th/e, p. 1685*)

   Charcot-Leyden crystals are slender and pointed at both ends, consisting of a pair of hexagonal pyramids joined at their bases. They consist of lysophospholipase (galectin 10), an **enzyme** synthesized by **eosinophils,** and are produced from the breakdown of these cells.

9. **Ans. is 'b'** i.e., Trophozoites in the pus (***Ref:*** *Chatterjee, 12th/e, p. 31*)
   - Exploration by puncture is one of the most practical methods for confirming the diagnosis of amoebic liver abscess.The aspirated pus may be examined for the demonstration of trophic forms (trophozoites) of E. histolytica.
   - **Aspiration from the center of amoebic liver abscess** do not show trophozoites, while **aspirates from the margins show trophozoites.**

   About Other Options:

   Option 'a'

   "Cysts are never seen in extraintestinal lesions."Q

   Option 'c and d'

   In extraintestinal amoebiasis, often stool examination is negative.Q

10. **Ans. is 'b'** i.e., Intravenous metronidazole (***Ref:*** *Harrison, 18th/e, p. 1686; 17th/e, p. 1278*)
    - **Flask-shaped ulcer** in a patient of GI bleed suggests **amoebiasis (amoebic dysentery).**
    - **Metronidazole or Tinidazole** are the DOCs.

11. **Ans. is 'b'** i.e., Lung abscess (***Ref:*** *Harrison, 18th/e, p. 1684*)
    - **Pleuropulmonary involvement** is the **most frequent complication of amoebic liver abscess (amoebic hepatitis).**

12. **Ans. is 'c'** i.e., E. histolytica

    (***Ref:*** *Harrison, 19th/e, p. 1685; D.R. Arora, 2nd/e, p. 26, 27*)
    - **Fecal finding in amoebiasis are:**
      - I. Charcot-Leyden crystals.
      - II. Positive test for heme.
      - III. Paucity (lack) of neutrophils (pus cells).

Amoebic Meningoencephalitis

13. **Ans. is 'b'** i.e., Diagnosis is by demonstration of trophozoite in CSF

    (***Ref:*** *Jawetz, 23rd/e, p. 676; Harrison, 18th/e, p. 1687; 17th/e, p. 1279, 2632*)
    - **Diagnosis of acute primary amoebic meningoencephalitis** is established by microscopic examination of the cerebrospinal fluid which contains trophozoite and red cell but no bacteria.

    About Other Options:
    - **Acanthamoeba causes chronic meningoencephalitis, while Naegleria fowleri is responsible for acute cases of meningoencephalitis.**
    - The Amoebae trophozoites enter via the nose and the cribriform plate of the ethmoid passing directly into the brain tissue **where they forms nests of amoebas that causes hemorrhage and damage,** chiefly in the basilar portion of the cerebrum and cerebellum.
    - **Naegleria fowleri causes primary amoebic meningoencephalitis.Q**
    - **Acanthamoeba causes granulomatous amoebic encephalitis.Q**
    - **Balamuthia mandrillaris causes amoebic meningoencephalitis.Q**

Amoeba

14. Ans. is 'a' i.e., Zymodeme pattern

Zymodeme (isoenzyme) analysis: E. histolytica possesses several isoenzymes like malic enzyme, hexokinase, isomerase and phosphoglucomutase and these isoenzymes contribute in pathogenesis. When these isoenzymes are subjected to electrophoresis based on electrophoretic pattern (Zymodeme pattern) and mobility of these isoenzymes, Entamoeba can be diagnosed and speciated.

15. Ans. is 'a' i.e., Man

There are no animal reservoirs; however, asymptomatic human carries serve as reservoirs for the spread of E. histolytica.

16. Ans. is 'c' i.e., Vertical transmission

Mode of Transmission:

1. Feco-oral transmission (MC).
2. Sexual transmission (homosexual).
3. Vector (Rare)–Flies and cockroaches (mechanical transmission).

17. Ans. is 'd' i.e., Refractile nucleus

Cystic stage of E. histolytica

1. Size and shape – 12-15 μm, spherical.
2. Cyst wall – Highly refractive membrane.
3. Nucleus – Eccentric nucleus, mature cyst contain 4 nucleuses.
4. Cytoplasm – 1-4 chromatid bodies, glycogen mass (stain brown with iodine), both gradually disappear as the cyst matures from uninucleate to quadrinucleate.

18. Ans. is 'a' i.e., Naegleri fowleri

Pathogenic free living Amoeba (BAN)

1. **N**aegleria fowleri – Acute and fulminating primary amoebic meningoencephalitis (PAM).
2. **A**canthamoeba – Ulcerative keratitis and granulomatous amoebic encephalitis (GAE).
3. **B**alamuthia (Rare) – Chronic granulomatous amoebic encephalitis.

19. Ans. is 'b' i.e., Erythrophagocytosis

In acute dysenteric stools, trophozoites often contains phagocytosed RBC which are not found in E. hartmanni and in other commensal amoebae.

20. Ans. is 'd' i.e., The infection reaches the skin through the blood stream

Cutaneous amoebiasis–It is usually seen over the region adjoining a visceral lesion, e.g., area of drainage of liver abscess or colostomy wound or from the rectum perianally.

21. Ans. is 'a' i.e., ELISA

Detection of 170 kDa lectin Ag in stool by ELISA.

22. Ans. is 'd' i.e., Cyst passers

Serological tests (IHA, ELISA etc.) become positive only in Invasive amoebiasis.

23. Ans. is 'c' i.e., A low iron content in the diet predispose to invasive amoebiasis

There is no relation between iron content in diet and amoebiasis.

24. Ans. are 'a, c'

Already explained in Ans No. 18.

25. Ans. is 'a' i.e., Naegleria fowleri

Already explained in Ans No. 18.

26. Ans. is 'b' i.e., Diagnosis is done by demonstration of trophozoites in CSF

Lab diagnosis of Naegleria: Diagnosis is done by demonstration of trophozoites in CSF or by histopathology of brain at autopsy. Cysts are not found in tissues.

27. Ans. are 'a, d'

Eosinophilic meningitis can be the result of noninfectious causes and infectious agents. Among the infectious agents, Angiostrongylus cantonensis (rat lungworm) and Gnathostoma spinigerum are the most common.

28. Ans. is 'b' i.e., Naegleria

Already explained .

29. Ans. is 'b' i.e., Naegleria

Already explained.

30. Ans. is 'c' i.e.,Non-nutrient agar with E. coli

Culture – CSF sample can be cultivated on non-nutrient agar (Page's saline and 1.5% agar), lawn cultured with E. coli.

MCQs

PROTOZOA 'B': FLAGELLATES

Morphology

1. A mother takes her 4-year-old to day care, she has noticed the child's frequent stools are non-bloody, foul smelling and fatty, what attribute of this parasite imparts its pathogenicity? *(AI 09)*

(a) Lytic enzymes
(b) Flagella
(c) Ventral sucking disc
(d) Encystment

2. True about Giardiasis: *(Recent MCQ)*

(a) Only cyst is infective
(b) Reside in caecum
(c) Only man to man transmission
(d) Exist in one phase

Clinical Features and Diagnosis

3. A 4-year-old child presents with acute watery diarrhea and abdominal cramps. Stool microscopy reveals trophozoites with falling leaf motility without RBCs and pus cells. The etiological agent is: *(Recent MCQ)*

(a) Entamoeba histolytica
(b) Giardia lamblia
(c) Trichomonas tenax
(d) Balantidium coli

4. Giardia lamblia: *(Recent MCQ)*

(a) Is the only flagellate parasite without a cystic stage
(b) Infection happens by ingestion of trophozoites in food and water
(c) Is the only protozoan parasite found in the lumen of small intestine
(d) May sometimes invade the blood stream and cause ectopic lesions

Trichomonas

5. Strawberry vagina and PH > 4.5 of vagina is seen in:

(a) E. histolytica
(b) Giardia
(c) Trichomonas
(d) Toxoplasma

6. The cystic form of all are seen in man *except*: *(Recent MCQ)*

(a) E.histolytica
(b) Giardia
(c) Trichomonas
(d) Toxoplasma

Trypanosoma

7. Chagas disease is the parasitic disease affecting intestine, tell the Vector for the same: *(Recent MCQ)*

(a) Reduvid bug
(b) Tse tse fly
(c) Sand fly
(d) Hard tick

8. Protozoa associated with Megaesophagus, Megacolon, Romanas sign, chagoma: *(Recent MCQ)*

(a) Trypanosome
(b) Amoeba
(c) Giardia
(d) Gnathostoma

T. Brucei

9. Winter bottom sign in sleeping sickness caused by T. brucei Gambiense refers to: *(Recent MCQ)*

(a) Unilateral conjunctivitis
(b) Posterior cervical lymphadenopathy
(c) Narcolepsy
(d) Transient erythema

10. Infective form of T. brucei Gambiense transmitted by Tse Tse fly is: *(Recent MCQ)*

(a) Amastigote
(b) Trypomastigote (Metacyclic trypomastigote)
(c) Egg
(d) None

11. In trypanosomal infections all are true *except*: *(AI 05)*

(a) Trypomastigote form is seen in vertebrate host
(b) T. brucei has posterior station development
(c) Intermediate host of African trypanosomiasis is Tse Tse fly
(d) Tse Tse fly bite during day

Leishmania

12. Mucocutaneous leishmaniasis is caused by: *(PGI 97)*

(a) L. braziliensis
(b) L. tropica
(c) L. donovani
(d) L. orientalis

13. Most common cause of disseminated cutaneous leishmaniasis is: *(DCL)*

(a) L.donovani
(b) L.tropica
(c) L.mexicana
(d) L.brasilensis

Clinical Features and Treatment

14. 40-year-old male from Bihar complains of pain abdomen, having hepatosplenomegaly, peripheral smear on stain shows: *(Manipal 08)*

(a) Plasmodium vivax
(b) Leishmania
(c) Microfilaria
(d) None

15. Drug not used in visceral leishmaniasis: *(AIIMS Nov 09)*

(a) Sitamoqine
(b) Paromycin
(c) Miltefosine
(d) Hydroxychloroquine

Laboratory Diagnosis

16. In case of kala azar aldehyde test become positive after: *(Recent MCQ)*

(a) 2 weeks
(b) 4 weeks
(c) 8 weeks
(d) 12 weeks

17. Leishmania is cultured in which media? *(Recent MCQ)*

(a) Chocolate agar
(b) NNN
(c) Tellurite
(d) Sabourauds

18. The following tests helps in laboratory diagnosis of kala azar *except*: *(AI 02)*

(a) Bone marrow examination
(b) Immobilisation test
(c) Blood smear examination
(d) Aldehyde test

Giardia

19. Giardiasis is associated with: *(AIIMS*

(a) Common variable immunodeficiency
(b) C1 esterase deficiency
(c) C8 deficiency
(d) Anemia

20. The normal habitat of giardia is: *(Recent MCQ)*
(a) Duodenum and Jejunum (b) Stomach
(c) Caecum (d) Ileum

21. True about Giardia is: *(AIIMS 04)*
(a) May cause traveler's diarrhea (b) Giardia inhabits ileum
(c) Trophozoites are infective to man (d) None of the above

22. Digestion in intestinal mucosa is inhibited by: *(Manipal 05)*
(a) V. cholerae (b) G. lamblia
(c) Enterokinase (d) S. haematobium

23. A patient presents with diarrhea, analysis of stool on wet mount shows motile protozoa without RBCs and pus cells. The diagnosis is: *(AI 00)*
(a) B. coli (b) Giardiasis
(c) Trichomonas hominis (d) E. histolytica

24. The following is true of Giardiasis: *(AI 07)*
(a) Complement fixation test (CFT) is diagnostic (b) Stool contains only cysts
(c) Habitat is colon (d) Trophozoites and cysts are found in duodenum

25. Which of the following is true about Giardia? *(PGI)*
(a) CFT is diagnostic (b) Trophozoites and cysts are seen in man
(c) Lives in lower intestine (d) Invades normal mucosa

Trypanosoma

26. Vector for T. cruzi: *(JIPMER 09)*
(a) Reduvid bug (b) Tsetse fly
(c) Sand fly (d) Hard tick

27. Parasitic disease affecting intestine is: *(Recent MCQ)*
(a) Chagas disease (b) Malaria
(c) Kala azar (d) Oriental sore

28. Tsetse fly transmits: *(Recent MCQ)*
(a) T. brucei (b) T. cruzi
(c) Kala azar (d) Oriental sore

29. Sleeping sickness is transmitted by: *(PGI)*
(a) Tsetse fly (b) House fly
(c) Sand fly (d) Simulium fly

Leishmania

0. Amastigote forms are seen in: *(PGI 10)*
) Leishmania donovani (b) Toxoplasma gondi
ishmania major (d) Entamoeba

form is seen in: *(Delhi 06)*
s (b) RES
(d) RBC

voir of Leishmaniasis in India is: *(JIPMER 09)*
(b) Rodents
(d) Case of post kala azar dermal leishmaniasis

24 hours is seen in case of: *(JIPMER 02)*
(b) Malaria
(d) Hodgkin's lymphoma

02)

34. Visceral leishmaniasis: *(PGI 01)*

(a) Caused by L. tropica
(b) Post leishmaniasis dermatitis is common
(c) Antimonials are useful drugs
(d) Diagnosed by blood smear
(e) Vector is phlebotomus sergenti

35. Which of the following is most severely affected in kala azar? *(JIPMER 99)*

(a) Spleen
(b) Liver
(c) Adrenal gland
(d) Bone marrow

36. The following are true of kala azar *except*: *(Recent MCQ)*

(a) Persistent hypergammaglobulinemia
(b) Pancytopenia
(c) Cancrum oris can occur
(d) Full treatment prevents PKDL

37. A 20 years female has hepatosplenomegaly, fever, pallor and generalized lymphadenopathy. Lab test useful for diagnosis is/are: *(PGI 09)*

(a) ESR
(b) Electrophoresis
(c) Parasite detection in aspirate
(d) ELISA
(e) Routine haemogram

38. The following tests help in lab diagnosis of kala azar *except*: *(AI 02)*

(a) Bone marrow examination
(b) Immobilization test
(c) Blood smear examination
(d) Aldehyde test

ANSWERS AND EXPLANATIONS

PROTOZOA 'B': FLAGELLA

GIARDIA LAMBLIA

Morphology

1. **Ans. is 'c'** i.e., Ventral sucking disc
   - **Important part of parasite responsible for clinical manifestation is ventral sucking disc by which the parasite attaches to intestinal epithelium, parasite exists in cyst and trophozoite form, infection manifest as diarrhoea, steatorrhoea and malabsorption syndrome. Diagnosis is established by stool examination for the cyst and the trophozoites.** Giardia can cause traveller's diarrhea.
   - Other protozoal causes of traveller's diarrhea:
     - Entamoeba histolytica
     - Cyclospora
     - Cryptosporidium.
2. **Ans. is 'a'** i.e., Only cyst is infective (***Ref:*** *Chatterjee, 12th/e, p. 39; Harrison, 19th/e, p. 915*)
   - Trophozoite and cysts, both are present in the feces, but it is the resistant cysts that survive outside the body and is responsible for transmission.
   - **Infective dose is low ingestion of as few as 10 cysts is sufficient to cause infection in humans (Quadrinucleate cyst).**
   - Giardia **resides in duodenum and jejunum.**
   - Giardia is usually **transmitted from man to man by fecal-oral route. But infection can also be transmitted from animals to man.**

     Giardiasis exists in two forms, i.e., Trophozoite and cyst.

Clinical Features and Diagnosis

3. **Ans. is 'b'** i.e., Giardia lamblia (***Ref:*** *D.R. Arora, p. 43*)
   - **Mature cyst is the infective form of the parasite acquires infection by contaminated water and food.** Infection may be acquired by **anal oral sexual practices among male homosexuals.**

- Within 30 minutes of ingestion excystation occurs in the duodenum, cyst hatches out two trophozoites which multiplies and **colonize in duodenum and upper part of jejunum.**
- In acute Giardiasis trophozoite show the typical **'falling-leaf'** motility in wet mount examination of faeces.

4. **Ans. is 'c'** i.e., is the only protozoan parasite found in the lumen of small intestine

(***Ref:*** *Harrison, 19th/e, p. 1930; 18th/e, p. 1730; D.R. Arora, 3rd/e, p. 44*)

- Only protozoan found in the small intestine, patient complain of dull epigastric pain, flatulence, and chronic diarrhoea, steatorrhoea, stool is voluminous, foul smelling and contain large amount of mucus, **patient loses weight.**
- **Enterotest is employed** and **ELISA test is developed for the detection of Giardia antigen in faeces.**

Trichomonas

5. **Ans. is 'c'** i.e., Trichomonas
   - **Trichomonas vaginalis** is vaginal flagellate causes strawberry vagina and PH>4.5 and grows on **Bushley, Johnson and trussel media.**
6. **Ans. is 'c'** i.e., Trichomonas (***Ref:*** *Chatterjee, 12th/e, p. 39*)
   - **Cystic phase** is not seen in: Trichomonas gingivalis and Dientamoeba fragilis.Q

TRYPANOSOMA

T. Cruzi

7. **Ans. is 'a'** i.e., Reduvid bug (***Ref:*** *Chatterjee, 12th/e, p. 52*)
   - **T. cruzi (C shaped parasite)** causes **Chagas disease** and vector is **reduvid bug.**
8. **Ans. is 'a'** i.e., Trypanosoma (***Ref:*** *Chatterjee, 12th/e, p. 52*)
   - **Megaesophagus and Megacolon** occur as complications of Chronic Chagas disease.
   - T. cruzi causes Chagas disease **(Romana sign, chagoma)** also seen.
   - **ECG changes** like **sinus tachycardia, increased PR interval, T wave changes and low QRS voltage, Myocarditis occurs.**

T. Brucei

9. **Ans. is 'b'** i.e., Posterior cervical lymphadenopathy (***Ref:*** *Harrison, 18th/e, p. 1720; 17th/e, p. 1304*)
   - Lymphadenopathy, **particularly of the posterior triangle of the neck** – **Winter bottom's sign.**
10. **Ans. is 'a'** i.e., Trypanosoma brucei (***Ref:*** *Chatterjee, 12th/e, p. 45*)
    - T. brucei (causative agent of sleeping sickness) is transmitted by Tse Tse fly.
    - T. brucei gambiense – West African sleeping sickness.
    - T. brucei rhodesiense – East African sleeping sickness.
11. **Ans is 'b'** i.e., T. brucei has posterior station development.

T.brucei causes sleeping sickness/African trypanosomiasis.

Vector is tse tse fly which bit during the day.

Infective form is **Metacyclic** trypomastigote.

In African trypanosomiasis: The trypomastigote forms are seen in vertebrate hosts are of two types – **Short stumpy and long thin.**

Clinical Features – **Trypanosomal chancre** – Febrile attacks, lymphadenopathy **(Winterbottom sign: Enlargement of posterior cervical lymphadenopathy).**

CNS involvement (**Kerandel's sign:** Pressure on palms of the hand or over ulnar nerve is followed by severe pain after pressure is removed).

DOC of sleeping sickness – **Suramine** in early stages and **Melarsoprol** in later stages.

Leishmania

12. Ans. is 'a' i.e., L. braziliensis (***Ref:*** *Chatterjee, 12th/e, p. 54*)

- **Visceral leishmaniasis (Kala azar)** – L. donovani.
- **Cutaneous Leishmaniasis**
  - (a) **Oriental sore** – L. tropica.
  - (b) **Mucocutaneous leishmaniasis (Espundia)** – L. brasiliensis

    Leishmania brazilensis causes mucocutaneous or nasopharyngeal leishmaniasis in Amazonian South America.

13. Ans is 'c'

Diffuse cutaneous leishmaniasis: Develops in an anergic host with poor immune response, infection is characterized by a primary lesion, which spreads to involve multiple areas of skin. Plaques, ulcers and nodules may form over the entire body, resembling lepromatous leprosy.

Clinical Features and Treatment

14. Ans. is 'b' i.e., Leishmania (***Ref:*** *Harrison, 18th/e, p. 1712*)

- The information in question are:
  - I. Patient is from Bihar.
  - II. Hepatosplenomegaly with abdominal pain.
- Kala azar typically presents with splenomegaly and hepatomegaly, and is common in Bihar. Thus **the most probable diagnosis is kala azar caused by leishmania donovani.**
- Thus among the given scenario, Leishmania is the best answer.

15. Ans. is 'd' i.e., Hydroxychloroquine (***Ref:*** *Harrison, 19th/e, p. 1712; 18th/e, p. 1299*)

- Drugs used for treatment are:
  - **I. First line:** Pentavalent antimony **(Sodium stibogluconate is the drug of choice), and amphotericin-B (Now drug of choice).**
  - **II. Alternatives:** Paromomycin, pentamidine, miltefosine.

About Option 'a'

- **Sitamaquine (WR-6026)** is an **orally active 8-aminoquinoline analog,** which has been developed as an oral treatment for visceral leishmaniasis.
- Sitamaquine has **low therapeutic range and high nephrotoxicity.**

Laboratory Diagnosis

16. Ans. is 'd' i.e., 12 weeks (***Ref:*** *Chatterjee, 12th/e, p. 61, 62*)

Aldehyde test (formal gel test of Napier)

- The test depends upon an **increase of serum gamma globulin.**
- **Test is positive in:**
  - (a) Kala azar (V.L).
  - (b) S. japonicum infection.
  - (c) T.brucei infection (African trypanosomiasis).
- It is positive after 3 months.
- **Method:**

Serum of patient

Plus

One or two drops of 40% formalin

Jellification of milk-white opacity like the white of a hardboiled egg.

***Chopra antimony test is also employed for Hypergammaglobulinaemia.**

17. Ans. is 'b' i.e., N.N.N. (***Ref:*** *Chatterjee, 12th/e, p. 62, 56*)

- L.donovani can be cultured in **N.N.N. (Novy, Neil and Nicolle)** medium. Hockmeyer and Scheinder liquid media.
- In N.N.N. medium **amastigote form changes into promastigote form.Q**

18. Ans. is 'b' i.e., Immobilization test (***Ref:*** *Chatterjee, 12th/e, p. 61*)

- Immobilization test is not used for kala azar.
- **K39 antigen test** is latest test employed for rapid diagnosis of kala azar.
- **LD bodies (Amastigote forms of L.donovani)** are demonstrated by Splenic and Bone marrow biopsy.

Giardia

19. Ans. is 'a' i.e., Common variable immunodeficiency

Explained in book text.

20. Ans. is 'a' i.e., Duodenum and Jejunum

Explained in book text.

21. Ans. is 'a' i.e., May cause traveler's diarrhea

Explained in book text.

22. Ans. is 'b' i.e., G. lamblia

Giardia causes abnormalities of villous structure that causes a disturbance of intestinal function leading to malabsorption, particularly of lipids and lipids soluble vitamins.

23. Ans. is 'b' i.e., Giardiasis

Giardia causes noninvasive diarrhea so there will be no RBCs.

24. Ans. is 'd' i.e., Trophozoites and cysts are found in duodenum

Explained in book text.

25. Ans. is 'b' i.e., Trophozoites and cysts are seen in man

Explained in book text.

26. Ans. is 'a' i.e., Reduvid bug

Explained in book text.

27. Ans. is 'a' i.e., Chagas disease

In chronic stage infection, damage occurs to Auerbach's plexus leads to dilatation of various parts of alimentary canal, especially the colon and esophagus the mega disease.

28. Ans. is 'a' i.e., T. brucei

Explained in book text.

29. Ans. is 'a' i.e., Tse tse fly

Forms of Human African Trypanosomiasis

Human African trypanosomiasis takes 2 forms, depending on the parasite involved:

Trypanosoma brucei gambiense is found in 24 countries in west and central Africa. This form currently accounts for 97% of reported cases of sleeping sickness and causes a chronic infection.

Trypanosoma brucei rhodesiense is found in 13 countries in eastern and southern Africa. Nowadays, this form represents under 3% of reported cases and causes an acute infection. Only Uganda presents both forms of the disease, but in separate zones.

30. Ans. are 'a,c'

Explained in book text.

31. Ans. is 'b' i.e., RES

Amastigote (Non-flagellate form) occurs in the infected lesion of man in reticuloendothelial cells. Amastigote form also called as LD body.

32. Ans. is 'c' i.e., Acute visceral Leishmaniasis

Visceral Leishmaniasis (Indian kala azar) is caused by L. donovani affects chiefly young adults, Man is reservoir of infection, Disease is not zoonotic, and Vector is P. argentipes. Sequelae is PKDL.

33. Ans. is 'a' i.e., Kala azar

In the early stages of the disease, there is a mild irregular fever becoming intermittent at later stage and in 20% cases pyrexia shows a double rise in 24 hours.

34. Ans. are 'c, d'

Pentavalent antimonial is the drug of choice in most endemic regions of the world, except Bihar due to resistance. Amphotericin B is used when initial antimonial treatment fails.

35. Ans. is 'a' i.e., Spleen

Splenic enlargement is one of the striking features and spleen progressively enlarges.

36. Ans. is 'd' i.e., Full treatment prevents PKDL

PKDL is a cutaneous form of leishmaniasis that occurs in about 2-10% kala azar patients generally one or two years after completion of antimonial treatment. When the visceral infection disappears but the skin infections persists.

37. Ans. are 'a, c, e'

Explained in book text.

38. Ans. is 'b' i.e., Immobilization test

Explained in book text.

MCQs

PROTOZOA 'C': SPOROZOA and MISCELLANEOUS PROTOZOA

Plasmodium

1. The scientists who discovered the malarial parasite and the transmission of malaria by anopheline mosquito: *(Recent MCQ)*

(a) Laveran and Ronald Ross
(b) Paul Muller and Laveran
(c) Ronald Ross and Laveran
(d) Pampania and Ronald Ross

Life Cycle

2. In transmission of malaria, mosquito bite transfers: *(PGI 79, 80)*

(a) Sporozoite
(b) Merozoite
(c) Hypnozoite
(d) Gametocyte

3. Malaria carriers contain: *(Recent MCQ)*

(a) Trophozoite
(b) Gametocytes
(c) Merozoites
(d) Trophozoites

4. The cycle of malaria parasite is in sequence of:

(1) Exoerythrocytic stage
(2) Gametocytic stage
(3) Erythrocytic stage
(4) Sporogony

(a) 1,2,3,4
(b) 1,3,2,4
(c) 1,4,2,3
(d) 1,4,3,2

5. **In which type of malarial parasite is the exoerythrocytic stage absent?** *(PGI 96)*
   (a) P. ovale (b) P. vivax
   (c) P. falciparum (d) P. malariae

Characteristics of Different Species

6. **Plasmodium falciparum infection of man is characterized by:** *(AI 97)*
   (a) The erythrocytes are increased in size
   (b) All stages of erythrocytic schizogony are seen in peripheral blood
   (c) Multiple infection of erythrocytes are seen
   (d) Each erythrocytic cycle lasts 72 hours
7. **Ziemann's stippling of erythrocyte is caused by which species of plasmodium?** *(Recent MCQ)*
   (a) Vivax (b) Falciparum
   (c) Malariae (d) Ovale
8. **Which of the following is true about P. falciparum?** *(AI 96)*
   (a) James dots are seen (b) Accole forms are seen
   (c) Relapses are frequent (d) Longest incubation period
9. **In plasmodium falciparum following are seen in blood *except*:** *(PGI 97)*
   (a) Schizonts (b) Mature trophozoite
   (c) Mature gametocytes (d) None
10. **Thick PBS is made for:** *(PGI 99)*
   (a) Speciation (b) Prevalance of parasite
   (c) Both speciation and prevalence (d) None
11. **Plasmodium falciparum infection of man is characterised by:** *(Recent MCQ)*
   (a) The erythrocytes are increased in size
   (b) All stages of erythrocytic schizogony are seen in peripheral blood
   (c) Multiple infection of erythrocytes are seen
   (d) Each erythrocytic cycle lasts 72 hours
12. **Patient diagnosed to have malaria, smear shows all stages of schizonts 14-20 merozoites, yellowish-brown pigment. The type of malaria is:** *(AIIMS 01)*
   (a) Pl. Falciparum (b) Pl. Malariae
   (c) Pl. Vivax (d) Pl. Ovale
13. **Malarial pigment is formed by:** *(Recent MCQ)*
   (a) Parasite (b) Bilirubin
   (c) Hemoglobin (d) Any of the above
14. **Shortest incubation period in malaria:** *(Recent MCQ)*
   (a) P. Vivax (b) P. Falciparum
   (c) P. Malariae (d) P. Ovale

Complications

15. **Malaria causing nephrotic syndrome:** *(Recent MCQ)*
   (a) P. Vivax (b) P. Falciparum
   (c) P. Malariae (d) P. Ovale

16. Which type of malaria is associated with renal failure? *(NBE Based NEET 2012-13)*

(a) Falciparum
(b) Vivax
(c) Malariae
(d) Ovale

Laboratory Diagnosis

17. JSB stain is used for which parasite? *(Recent MCQ)*

(a) Malaria
(b) Filaria
(c) Kala azar
(d) Sleeping sickness

18. All of the following are true regarding transfusion malaria *except*: *(AI 11)*

(a) Sporozoites transmit it
(b) Incubation period is shorter
(c) Transmitted by merozoites and erythrocytic stages
(d) there is no pre-erythrocytic stage

19. Which one of the following is detected by the antigen detection test used for the diagnosis of P. falciparum malaria? *(AIIMS Nov 04)*

(a) Circumsporozoite protein
(b) Merozoite surface antigen
(c) Histidine – Rich – Protein I (HRP - I)
(d) Histidine – Rich – Protein II (HRP - II)

Treatment

20. What is the treatment of choice for benign tertian malaria? *(UPSC 07)*

(a) Sulfamethaxazole – pyrimethamine
(b) Quinine
(c) Mefloquine
(d) Chloroquine

Babesia

21. Maltese cross is characteristic feature of: *(AI 09)*

(a) Cryptococcus neoformans
(b) Babesia microti
(c) Blastomycosis
(d) Penicillium marfeni

TOXOPLASMA

Life Cycle

22. Tachyzoites are seen in: *(PGI 97)*

(a) Toxoplasma
(b) Toxocara
(c) Pulmonary eosinophilia
(d) Ascaris

23. Intermediate hosts for toxoplasma are all *except*: *(Recent MCQ)*

(a) Human
(b) Sheep
(c) Cat
(d) Pig

24. All of the following statements about toxoplasmosis are true *except*: *(AI 97)*

(a) Oocyst in freshly passed cat's faeces is infective
(b) May spread by organ transplantation
(c) Maternal infection acquired after 6 months has high risk of transmission
(d) Arthalgia, sore throat and abdominal pain are the most common manifestations

25. A 24-year-old primi in her 8th month of pregnancy develops a positive IgM titer to T. Gondii for the first time. She should be advised by her physician that:

(a) This child and all future foetuses will be infected

(b) Newborn with antitoxoplasma IgG response should be treated with antiparasitics

(c) Future infections avoided by proper vaccination and deworming of cats

(d) Chorioretinitis can be treated by drug treatment of an infant with positive IgM response

Cryptosporidium and Isospora

26. 24-year-old AIDS patient develops chronic abdominal pain, low grade fever, diarrhoea, malabsorption. Oocysts demonstrated in stool. Likely cause of his diarrhoea is: *(HP 2006)*

(a) E.histolytica
(b) G.lamblia
(c) Microsporidia
(d) Isospora belli

27. In humans, cryptosporidiosis presents as: *(Recent MCQ)*

(a) Meningitis
(b) Diarrhea
(c) Pneumonia
(d) Hepatitis

ANSWERS AND EXPLANATIONS

PROTOZOA 'C': SPOROZOA AND MISCELLANEOUS PROTOZOA

Plasmodium

1. **Ans. is 'a'** i.e., Laveran and Ronald Ross (***Ref:*** *Paniker, 6th/e, p. 66*)
   - The **mode of transmission** of the disease was established in 1897 by **Ronald Ross.**
   - The specific causative agent of malaria **was discovered** in the red blood cells of a patient in 1880 by **Alophonse Laveran,** a French army surgeon in Algeria.

Life Cycle

2. **Ans. is 'a'** i.e., Sporozoite (***Ref:*** *Chatterjee, 12th/e, p. 73*)
   - Sporozoites are infective to man. Human infection begins when a female anopheline mosquito inoculates plasmodial sporozoites from its salivary gland during a blood meal.
     – **Infective from for human** → Sporozoite.
     – Infective from for mosquito → Gametocyte.
3. **Ans. is 'b'** i.e., Gametocytes (***Ref:*** *Chatterjee, 12th/e, p. 113*)
4. **Ans. is 'b'** i.e., 1,3,2,4 (***Ref:*** *Chatterjee, 12th/e, p. 73-74*)

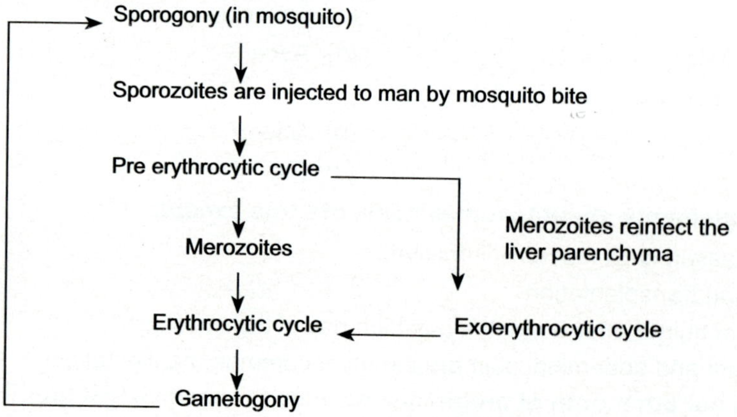

5. **Ans. is 'c'** i.e., P. falciparum (***Ref:*** *Chatterjee, 12th/e, p. 79-80*)

Characteristics of Different Species

6. **Ans. is 'c'** i.e., Multiple infection of erythrocytes are seen
   (***Ref:*** *Chatterjee, 12th/e, p. 79; Panikar, 6th/e, p. 75, 76*)
   - Multiple infection of red blood cell, i.e., more than one parasite (from 2 to 6) invading a single red blood cell is very common with P. falciparum.
   - Infected erythrocytes are normal in size.
   - **Erythrocytic Schizogony** occurs **inside the capillaries of the internal organs (spleen, liver and bone marrow),** hence only the ring forms (not the growing trophozoites and schizonts) and gametocytes are seen in peripheral blood.
   - **Each erythrocytic cycle (schizogony) lasts 48 hours (not 72 hours).**
7. **Ans. is 'c'** i.e., Malariae
   - P. Vivax – Schuffner's dot
   - P. Malariae – Ziemann's stippling
   - P. Falciparum – Maurer's dot
   - P. Ovale – Schuffner's dot
8. **Ans. is 'b'** i.e., Accole forms are seen (***Ref:*** *Chatterjee, 12th/e, p. 79*)
   The parasite often attaches itself to the margin or the edge of the host cell, the nucleus and a small part of the cytoplasm remaining almost outside. This is known as form **appliqué or accole.**
9. **Ans. are 'a' and 'b'** i.e., Schizonts and Mature trophozoite
   (***Ref:*** *Chatterjee, 12th/e, p. 79, 82; D.R. Arora, 3rd/e, p. 75*)
   - Only ring forms (young trophozoites) and gametocytes are seen in peripheral blood not the amoeboid forms (mature trophozoites) or schizonts.
10. **Ans. is 'b'** i.e., Prevalence of parasite (***Ref:*** *D.R. Arora, 3rd/e*)
    - Thin PBF – For Speciation.
    - Thick PBF – For Prevalence and Presence of Malarial parasites.
11. **Ans. is 'c'** i.e., Multiple infections of erythrocytes are seen
    (a) **Multiple infections of the RBC is hallmark of P. falciparum.**
    (b) RBC's are increased in size and vivax malaria.
    (c) Each erythrocytic cycle lasts 48 hours.
12. **Ans. is 'c'** i.e., Plasmodium Vivax (***Ref:*** *Chatterjee, 12th/e, p. 82*)
    - All stages of schizoints in peripheral smear, yellowish brown pigment and 14-20 merozoites suggest the diagnosis of P.vivax malaria.
    - Colour of pigment

      P. vivax – **Yellow brown**
      P. ovale – Dark brown
      P. malariae – Brown black
      P. falciparum – **Black**
    - No. of merozoites per schizonts

      P. vivax – 14-20
      P. ovale – 6-12
      P. malariae – 6-12
      P. falciparum – 8-32 (very rare in peripheral blood)
13. **Ans. is 'c'** i.e., Hemoglobin (***Ref:*** *Parasitology, Panicker, 6th/e, p. 71*)
    - The malarial parasite (plasmodium) feeds on the haemoglobin of the erythrocyte. **Haematin globin pigment – Haemoglobin left behind as a residue after metabolism of parasite.**

- These iron containing pigments formed from haemoglobin accumulate in the body of the parasite as **dark granules, which becomes more prominent, as the parasite grows.**
- The appearance of malaria pigments varies in the different species.
  - **P. vivax – Yellowish brown**
  - **P. falciparum – Dark brown**
  - P. malariae – Dark brown
  - P. ovale – Yellowish brown

Note: The malaria pigment released when the parasitized cells rupture is taken up by reticuloendothelial cells. **Such pigment laden cells in the internal organs provide histological evidence of previous malarial infection.**

14. Ans. is 'b' i.e., P. falciparum (***Ref:*** *Park, 20th/e, p. 237*)

Species	Incubation period		
P. vivax	**14 (8-17) days**		
P. falciparum	**12 (9-14) days**	-	**Minimum**
P. malariae	28 (18-40) days	-	**Maximum**
P. ovale	17 (16-18) days		

- Plasmodium malariae causes quartan malaria.
- P. Falciparum causes malignant tertian malaria (also called **pernicious malaria**).
- P. Vivax causes benign tertian malaria.
- P. Ovale causes ovale tertian malaria.

Complications

15. Ans. is 'c' i.e., P. malariae (***Ref:*** *Harrison, 19th/e; 18th/e, p. 1692-1695*)

- **Nephrotic syndrome is seen in Quartan malarial nephropathy,** caused by repeated or chronic infection with P. malariae.

16. Ans. is 'a' i.e., Falciparum (***Ref:*** *Harrison, 18th/e, p. 1692-1695*)

- Nephrotic syndrome – quartan malaria (P. malariae).
  Malignant tertian malaria.
- **Pernicious malaria (caused by P. falciparum) – Acute tubular necrosis (renal failure).**

Laboratory Diagnosis

17. Ans. is 'a' i.e., Malaria

- **JSB (Jaswant-Singh-Bhattacharya) stain** is a fairly rapid staining method for detection of malarial parasites.
- **This stain is superior to the field's stain** because the parasites stain clearer and both thick and thin smears can be stained.
- However, preparations fade quite rapidly and this stain is, therefore, not recommended when permanent slides are desired.

Stains Used for Staining Malarial Smears

- A number of Romanowsky stains are used for example Field's, Giemsa's, Wright's and Leishman's.
- For **thick smear,** the stains used are: (i) **Field's** or (ii) **Giemsa.**
- For **thin smear,** the stains used are: (i) **Giemsa** or (ii) **Leishman.**
- **JSB stain** is used for both thick and thin smears, and is the standard method used by laboratories under the **National Malaria Eradication Programme in India.**

18. Ans. is 'a' i.e., Sporozoites transmit it

Transfusion malaria is transmitted by **merozoites and RBC stages.**

As the hepatic stage (Preerythrocytic stage) is absent, the incubation period is shorter.

19. Ans. is 'd' i.e., Histidine-Rich-Protein II (HRP-II)

(***Ref:** Harrison, 19th/e, p. 1287 and D.R. Arora, 3rd/e, p. 82*)

- **Detection of histidine rich protein – 2 (HRP-2) antigen is a sensitive and specific diagnostic test for P. falciparum.**

Treatment

20. Ans. is 'd' i.e., Chloroquine

(***Ref:** Harrison, 18th/e, p. 1702; 17th/e, p. 1288*)

- **Benign tertian malaria** is caused by **plasmodium vivax.**
- "Despite recent evidence of chloroquine resistance in P. vivax, **Chloroquine remains the treatment of choice for the benign human malarias (P. vivax, P. ovale, P. malariae).**"

Babesia

21. Ans. is 'b' i.e., Babesia microti (***Ref:** Jawetz, 24th/e, p. 680; Clinical Hematology, 4th/e, p. 108*)

- Intraerythrocytic infection of Babesiosis is characterised by **Maltese cross** and it is transmitted by tick.

TOXOPLASMA

Life Cycle

22. Ans. is 'a' i.e., Toxoplasma (***Ref:** Harrison, 18th/e, p. 1722; 17th/e, p. 1305*)

- **Bradyzoites (released from tissue cyst) and sporozoites (released from oocyst)** enter the small – intestinal epithelium and transform into rapidly dividing tachyzoites.

23. Ans. is 'c' i.e., Cat (***Ref:** Harrison, 18th/e, p. 1722*)

- **Definitive host for toxoplasma: Cat.**
- **Intermediate host for toxoplasma: Human, mouse, sheep or pig.**

24. Ans is 'd' i.e., Arthalgia, sore throat and abdominal pain are the most common manifestations

Definite host in toxoplasmosis is Cat.

The intermediate host is man or any other mammal like sheep or pig.

Stages

Trophozoites (tachyzoites) – Crescent shape multiply by endodyogeny, found in tissue during acute stage, appear rounded enclosed within host cell **(Pseudocyst).**

Tissue cyst – Formed during chronic infection – skeletal, heart, muscle and brain **(Bradyzoites).**

Oocyst – Found in the definitive host cat, shed in faeces. Freshly passed contain a single sporoblast. **Sporoblast divides into two sporocysts and 4 sporozoites** develop in each sporocyst **(infective form for human).**

25. Ans is 'd' i.e., Chorioretinitis can be prevented by drug treatment of an infant with positive IgM response

(a) Presence of IgM in the primi in 8th month of pregnancy indicates primary infection.

(b) Infection acquired in the first trimester by women who are not treated with anti T. Gondii drugs results in congenital infection in 10-25% cases.

(c) Majority of children born of women who acquire their infection during third trimester as in this case born with the subclinical form of the infection.

(d) Signs and symptoms of congenital toxoplasmosis can be prevented by **Pyrimethamine with sulfadiazine.**

26. Ans is 'd' i.e., Isospora belli (***Ref:** Harrison, 18th/e, p. 1731, 1732; 17th/e, p. 1313*)

- Cryptosporidia, microsporidia and Isospora belli are the most common opportunistic protozoa that infect the GI tract and cause diarrhea in HIV-infected patients.

HIV Infected Patient

- Cryptosporidia **(6-8 micron)**
  - Acid fast oocyst in stool
- Microsporidia **(8-10 micron)**
  - Presence of organism in stool
  - No oocyst
- Isospora belli **(23-36 micron)**
  - Acid fast oocyst in stool

27. Ans is 'b' i.e., Diarrhoea (***Ref:*** *Harrison, 18th/e, p. 1731*)

Cryptosporidium parvum – Causes cryptosporidiosis, the main symptom of which is diarrhea. It is most severe in immunocompromised patients, e.g., those with AIDS.

- The jejunum is the site most heavily infested.

MCQs

HELMINTH 'A': PLATYHELMINTHS

1. Operculated eggs are seen in: *(Recent MCQ)*

(a) Nematodes (b) Cestodes
(c) Trematodes (d) Protozoa

2. Which if the following diseases is transmitted by egg ingestion? *(AI 95)*

(a) Taeniasis (b) Trichinosis
(c) Hydatidosis (d) Strongyloidosis

3. Leaf like helminths are also called: *(Recent MCQ)*

(a) Flukes (b) Roundworms
(c) Tapeworms (d) Cestodes

4. Cercariae are infective form of: *(Recent MCQ)*

(a) S. hematobium (b) P. westermanii
(c) F. hepatica (d) T. solium

Taenia

5. Cysticercosis is caused by: *(PGI June 05)*

(a) T. Solium (b) T. Saginata
(c) A. duodenale (d) E. granulosus

6. Which of the following is the most common location of intracranial neurocysticercosis? *(AIIMS Nov 05)*

(a) Brain parenchyma (b) Subarachnoid space
(c) Spinal cord (d) Orbit

7. Neurocysticerosis, following are true *except*: *(PGI 98)*

(a) Not acquired by eating contaminated vegetables
(b) Caused by regurgitation of larva
(c) Acquired by oro-fecal route
(d) Acquired by eating pork

Echinococcus Granulosus

8. Least common site of calcified hydatid cyst is: *(Recent MCQ)*

(a) Lung (b) Mediastinum
(c) Extraperitoneal site (d) Liver

9. ARC-5 in countercurrent electrophoresis of serum is diagnostic of: *(Recent MCQ)*

(a) Cysticercosis
(b) Cryptococcosis
(c) Hydatidosis
(d) Brucellosis

10. Which of the following show regressive metamorphosis?

(a) Hydatid cyst
(b) Cysticercoid
(c) Cysticercus bovis
(d) Cysticercus cellulosae

Hymenolepsis Nana

11. Dwarf tapeworm refers to: *(Recent MCQ)*

(a) Echinococcus
(b) Loa Loa
(c) Hymenolepsis nana
(d) Schistosoma mansoni

Schistosoma

12. Painless terminal hematuria is seen as one of the manifestations in the infection caused by: *(Recent MCQ)*

(a) Schistosoma japonicum
(b) Schistosoma mansoni
(c) Schistosoma haematobium
(d) Plasmodium falciparum

13. A man on return from a country complains of pain in abdomen, jaundice, with increased alkaline phosphatase and conjugated hyperbilirubinemia. USG shows blockage in the biliary tree. What could be the cause? *(AIIMS May 09)*

(a) Fasciola buski
(b) Clonorchis sinensis
(c) Strongyloides
(d) Ancylostoma

14. Which is not a liver fluke? *(PGI Nov 10)*

(a) Paragonimus
(b) Whipworm
(c) Clonorchis sinensis
(d) Gnathostoma spinigerum
(e) Opisthorchis

15. The only ovo-viviparous parasite: *(Recent MCQ)*

(a) Ascaris
(b) Strongyloides
(c) Enterobius
(d) Ancylostoma

16. Natural habitat of Schistosoma (blood flukes): *(PGI 99)*

(a) Veins of the urinary bladder
(b) Portal and pelvic veins
(c) Vesical plexuses
(d) All of the above

17. Terminal spined eggs are seen in: *(PGI 95)*

(a) Schistosoma haematobium
(b) Sch. mansoni
(c) Sch. japonicum
(d) Chlonorchis sinensis

ANSWERS AND EXPLANATIONS

HELMINTH 'A': PLATYHELMINTHS

1. **Ans. are 'b and c'** i.e., Cestodes and Trematodes (***Ref:*** *D.R. Arora, 2nd/e, p. 139*)
   - Operculated eggs (possess lids) has a little cap like structure (operculum) at the end. The operculum pops open when the next stage is ready to emerge.
   - Cestodes lay operculated eggs.
   - The trematodes (flukes) also lay operculated eggs. **An exception is schistosoma egg, which are not operculated.Q**
2. **Ans. are 'a' and 'c'** i.e., Taeniasis, hydatidosis

- Infection of Echinococcus granulosus (hydatidosis) occur by ingestion of eggs.
- Infection of H.nana is also by **egg ingestion.**
- Taenia solium infection usually occurs by ingestion of cysticercus in the pork but also occur by ingestion of egg.
- Transmitted by larva – Strongyloides and Trichenella.

3. **Ans. is 'a'** i.e., Flat leaf like worms
   - Cylindrical helminthes – Nematodes (roundworms)
   - Flat, segmented helminthes – Cestodes (tapeworms)
   - Flat, leaf like helminthes – Trematodes (flukes)
4. **Ans. is 'a'** S. hematobium

   Schistosoma infection to man takes place during bathing or swimming. The cercariae penetrate the skin, are carried into the systemic circulation and pass through to the portal vessels. Within the intrahepatic portion of the portal system, the worms feed and grow to maturity.

Taenia

5. **Ans. is 'a'** i.e., T. Solium (***Ref:*** *D.R. Arora, 3rd/e, p. 131; Chatterjee, 12th/e, p. 118*)

Tapeworms

T. solium	T. saginata
• Larval stage – cysticercus cellulosae • Develops in the muscles of pig • Has also been found in the man causing cysticercosis	• Larval stage – cysticercus bovis • Develops in the muscles of cattle • Not found in man.

6. **Ans. is 'a'** i.e., Brain parenchyma (***Ref:*** *Harrison, 18th/e, p. 3431; 17th/e, p. 2637*)
   - **Most common site of neurocysticercosis is Brain parenchyma.Q**
   - "Parenchymal brain calcification is the most common finding on MRI and CT scan.
   - In India, **neurocysticercosis is regarded as the second most important cause of intracranial space occupying lesions following tuberculosis and the most common cause of epilepsy.**
7. **Ans. are 'a and d'** i.e., Not acquired by eating contaminated vegetables and Acquired by eating pork (***Ref:*** *Chatterjee, 12th/e, p. 120; D.R. Arora, 2nd/e, p. 122*)
   - Cysticercus cellulosae usually develops in pig (intermediate host).
   - Cysticercus cellulosae (cysticercosis) can also develop in man as follows:
     (i) By ingestion of eggs with contaminated water or food (uncooked vegetables).
     (ii) A man harbouring adult worms may auto-**infect oneself either by unhygienic personal habits or by reverse peristaltic movement (regurgitation) of the intestine where by the gravid segments are thrown into the stomach** (Mechanism of Autoinfection in T.solium).
   - Cysticercosis is not acquired by eating pork. Occasionally man gets infected in the same way as pig.
   - **By ingestion of eggs (either by drinking contaminated water or by eating uncooked vegetables infected with eggs). In this cycle man acts both as definitive as well as intermediate host** (More chance of developing neurocysticercosis).

Echinococcus Granulosus

8. **Ans. is 'a'** i.e., Lung (***Ref:*** *D.R. Arora, 3rd/e, p 141*)
   - The pulmonary hydatid cyst almost never calcify, unlike mediastinal cyst.
9. **Ans. is 'c'** i.e., Hydatidosis (***Ref:*** *Harrison, 19th/e, p. 1433*)
   - **Serological test for hydatid cyst:** Precipitin reaction, Complement fixation test, Haemagglutination test, Flocculation test, IFA, **Immuno electrophoresis (Arc 5) test.**

Detection of antibody to specific echinococcal antigens by immunoblotting has the highest degree of specificity.Q

10. **Ans. is 'a'** i.e., Hydatid cyst (***Ref:*** *D.R. Arora, 3rd/e, p. 141*)
    - **Regressive metamorphosis:** Sometimes, hydatid cyst (containing protoscolices) may rupture in intermediate host to release its content in the tissue. If such a patient survives, **the released protoscolices may revert to hydatid cyst instead of developing into an adult worm** (Normally protoscolex give rise to adult worm).

Hymenolepsis Nana

11. **Ans. is 'c'** i.e., Hymenolepsis nana (***Ref:*** *Chatterjee, 12th/e, p. 128*)
    - H. Nana is the smallest intestinal cestode infecting man.
    - It is also known as **dwarf tapeworm.**
    - Egg is peculiar have **onchosphere with six hooklets polar filaments.**
    - Shows autoinfection.
    - **DOC** – Praziquantel. *(AIIMS May 2016)*

Schistosoma

12. **Ans. is 'c'** i.e., Schistosoma haematobium (***Ref:*** *D.R. Arora, 3rd/e, p. 155*)
    - Painless terminal hematuria is characteristic of bilharziasis (urinary schistosomiasis) caused by S haematobium and characteristically have terminal spine.
13. **Ans. is 'b'** i.e., Clonorchis sinesis (***Ref:*** *Harrison, 18th/e, p. 1757, 1758; 19th/e, p. 1498; Chatterjee, 12th/e, p. 136*)
    - Among the given option only **Clonorchis sinensis is a liver fluke which can cause hepatic dysfunction with jaundice and hyperbilirubinemia.**
14. **Ans. are 'a'** i.e., Paragoniomus; **'b'** i.e., Whipworm; **'d'** i.e., Gnathostoma spinigerum
    (***Ref:*** *D.R. Arora, 3rd/e, p. 155-170*)
    - **Liver fluke are:** Clonorchis sinensis, Opisthorchis felineus and Fasciola hepatica.
15. **Ans. is 'b'** i.e., Strongyloides (***Ref:*** *Harrison, 19th/e, p. 1415*)
    - **Strongyloides stercoralis is ovo-viviparous. Trichinella is viviparous.**
16. **Ans. is 'd'** i.e., All of the above (***Ref:*** *Chatterjee, 12th/e, p. 136*)
    - S. Haematobium – Veins of **Vesical and Pelvic plexuses,** less commonly in portal vein and its mesenteric branch.
    - S. Mansoni – Mesenteric veins draining **Sigmoidorectal region (inferior mesenteric veins).**
    - S. Japonicum – Mesenteric veins draining **Ileocaecal region (superior mesenteric vein).**
17. **Ans. is 'a'** i.e., Schistosoma haematobium (***Ref:*** *Chatterjee, 12th/e, p. 138*)

Schistosoma haematobium	–	Egg has terminal spine Q
Schistosoma mansoni	–	Egg has lateral spine Q
Schistosoma japonicum	–	Egg has lateral knob Qs

MCQs

HELMINTH 'B': NEMATHELMINTHES

Strongyloides Stercoralis

1. The cause of larva currens: *(Recent MCQ)*

(a) Strongyloides stercoralis (b) Necator americanus
(c) Ankylostoma duodenale (d) H. nana

2. **Infection with colitis is caused by:** (*PGI 2000*)
   (a) Enterobius vermicularis
   (b) Trichuris trichiura
   (c) Strongyloides
   (d) Clonorchis

Hookworm

3. **The hookworm thrives on:** (*Recent MCQ*)
   (a) Whole blood (b) Plasma (c) Serum (d) RBC
4. **The average blood loss in ankylostomiasis per worm is:** *PGI 79*)
   (a) 0.2 ml/day (b) 2 ml/day (c) 0.33 ml/day (d) 1 ml/day

Enterobius Vermicularis

5. **Child having perianal pruritus with following eggs is due to:** (*Recent MCQ*)
   (a) E. vermicularis
   (b) Ascaris
   (c) Ankylostoma duodenale
   (d) S. stercoralis
6. **Most common presenting symptom of threadworm infection amongst the following is:** (*AI 97*)
   (a) Abdominal pain
   (b) Rectal prolapsed
   (c) Urticaria
   (d) Vaginitis

Ascaris Lumbricoides

7. **Ascariasis causes:** (*Manipal 07*)
   (a) Appendicitis
   (b) Intestinal obstruction
   (c) Bile duct obstruction
   (d) All of the above

FILARIOIDEA

Characterstic Morphological Features

8. **Sheathed microfilaria is/are:** (*PGI Dec 04*)
   (a) W. Bancrofti (b) Loa loa (c) M. Perstans (d) B. Malayi
9. **Wuchereria bancrofti, true is:** (*Recent MCQ*)
   (a) Unsheathed
   (b) Tail tip free from nuclei
   (c) Non-periodic
   (d) All
10. **All of the filarial worms are found in blood *except*:** (*Recent MCQ*)
    (a) W. Bancrofti (b) B. Malayi (c) L. Loa (d) O. Volvulus
11. **Which is false about Wuchereria bancrofti?** (*AI 90*)
    (a) Causes filariasis
    (b) Body is long and slender
    (c) Terminal nuclei absent
    (d) Man and anopheles are host
12. **A child from Bihar comes with fever. Blood examination shows sheathed microfilaria with nuclei upto tail tip. The diagnosis is:** (*AI 2000*)
    (a) B. Malayi
    (b) W. Bancrofti
    (c) Loa loa
    (d) Oncocerca volvulous
13. **Which is non-lymphatic filariasis?** (*Recent MCQ*)
    (a) Loa loa
    (b) Wuchereria bancrofti
    (c) Brugia malayi
    (d) Brugia timori

Lymphatic Filariasis

14. **All are TRUE regarding filariasis *except*:** (*AIIMS Feb 97*)
    (a) Man is an intermediate host
    (b) Caused by Wuchereria bancrofti
    (c) Involves lymphatic system
    (d) DEC is used in treatment

15. Meyers Kouwenaar syndrome is a synonym for: *(PGI 88)*

(a) Tropical pulmonary eosinophilia
(b) Larva migrans
(c) Occult filariasis
(d) Cutaneous allergic reactions to Ascariasis

16. In which stage of filariasis are microfilaria seen in peripheral blood?

(a) Tropical eosinophilia
(b) Early adenolymphangitis stage
(c) Late adenolymphangitis stage
(d) Elephantiasis

Onchocerca and Loa Loa

17. Kallu, a 30-year-old man, presented with subcutaneous itchy nodules over the left iliac crest. On examination they are firm, non tender and mobile. Skin scraping contains microfilaria and adult worms of: *(AIIMS May 01)*

(a) Loa Loa
(b) Onchocerca volvulus
(c) Brugia malayi
(d) Mansonella perstans

18. River blindness is caused by: *(Recent MCQ)*

(a) Onchocerca (b) Loa Loa (c) Ascaris (d) B. malayi

19. Calabar swelling is produce by: *(Recent MCQ)*

(a) Onchocerca volvulus
(b) Loa Loa
(c) Brugia malayi
(d) Wuchereria bancrofti

Trichuris Trichiura

20. Chronic dysentery, abdominal pain and rectal prolapse in children is caused by: *(UP 07)*

(a) Enterobius vermicularis
(b) Ascariasis
(c) Trichuris trichiura
(d) Trichinella spiralis

Dracunculus Medinensis

21. The slender rhabditiform larvae of which of the following helminths move about in water and are ingested by species of cyclops? *(Manipal 05)*

(a) D. Latum (b) D. Medinensis (c) W. Bancrofti (d) S. Mansoni

22. Dragon or serpent worm is: *(AIIMS 01)*

(a) Enterobius (b) Trichuris (c) Dracunculus (d) T. Solium

Larva Migrans

23. Visceral larva migrans is associated with: *(AI 11)*

(a) Strongyloides stercoralis
(b) Ankylostoma brazilensis
(c) Toxocara canis
(d) Visceral leishmaniasis

24. Cutaneous larva migrans is due to: *(Recent MCQ)*

(a) Ankylostoma braziliensis
(b) W. Bancrofti
(c) B. Malayi
(d) D. Medinensis

ANSWERS AND EXPLANATIONS

HELMINTH 'B': NEMATHELMINTHS

Strongyloides

1. **Ans. is 'a'** i.e., Strongyloides stercoralis (***Ref:*** *Harrison, 19th/e, p.1415*)
   - The migrating filariform larva of Strongyloides moves rapidly in a **short line at the rate of 3-4 cm in an hour,** hence it is termed "larva currens".

2. **Ans. is 'c'** i.e., Strongyloides (***Ref:*** *Harrison, 19th/e, p. 1415; D.R. Arora, 3rd/e, p. 180*)
    - Strongyloides causes mild colitis and necrotizing bowel disease.

Hookworm

3. **Ans. is 'b'** i.e., Plasma (***Ref:*** *Chatterjee, 12th/e, p. 175*)
    - Plasma forms the main source of nourishment for hookworm.
4. **Ans. is 'a'** i.e., 0.2 ml/day (***Ref:*** *Harrison, 19th/e, p. 1412*)
    - **Average blood loss:**
        - **Ankylostoma duodenale** – 0.2 ml/day
        - **Nector americanus** – 0.03 ml/day

Enterobius Vermicularis

5. **Ans. is 'a'** i.e., E. Vermicularis (***Ref:*** *Harrison, 19th/e, p. 1416*)
    - Most pinworm infections are asymptomatic, the others name of **Enterobius vermicularis are Pinworm, thread-worm, seatworm.**
    - **Perianal pruritis** is the cardinal symptom. The itching is worse at night and disturbes sleep.
    - Heavy infections can cause abdominal pain and weight loss.
    - **NIH swab** is used for diagnosis.
6. **Ans. is 'a'** i.e., Abdominal pain (***Ref:*** *Harrison, 18th/e, p. 1743; 19th/e, p. 1416*)
    - Amongst the given options, abdominal pain appears to be the best answer.

    Rectal prolapsed (coconut cake rectum) associated with Trichuris trichiura infection.

Ascaris Lumbricoides

7. **Ans. is 'd'** i.e., All of the above (***Ref:*** *Harrison, 18th/e, p. 1739, 1740; 19th/e, p. 1413*)
    - Ascaris causes all the given symptoms (see text of the chapter).

FILARIOIDEA

Characteristic Morphological Features

8. **Ans. is 'a'** i.e., W. Bancrofti; **'b'** i.e., Loa loa; **'d'** i.e., B. Malayi (***Ref:*** *D.R. Arora, 3rd/e, p. 202*)

    Remember Sheathed are LBW-Loa Loa, Brugia malayi, Wuchereria bancrofti.

Sheathed microfilaria	**Non Sheathed microfilaria**
1. Loa Loa	1. M. Perstans
2. B. Malayi	2. M. Ozzardi
3. Wuchereria bancrofti **(LBW)**	3. M. Streptocerca
	4. O. Volvulus

9. **Ans. is 'b'** i.e., Tail tip free from nuclei (***Ref:*** *Chatterjee, 12th/e, p. 189*)
    - **W. Bancrofti is sheathed and periodic with tail tip free from nuclei and same is distinguished from Brugia malayi which have terminal two nuclei in tail tip.Q**
10. **Ans. is 'd'** i.e., O. Volvulus

	W.bancrofti	B.malayi	Loa.Loa	M.perstans	M.ozzardi	M.streptocerca	O.volvulus
Found in	Blood	Blood	Blood	Blood	Blood,Skin	Skin	Skin

11. Ans. is 'd' i.e., Man and anopheles are host (***Ref:*** *Paniker, 6th/e, p. 196*)

- Man is the definitive host and culex (C. fatigons) is the intermediate host (not Anopheles).
- W. Bancrofti has long and slender body.
- Its microfilaria has **tail tip free from nuclei** (terminal nuclei absent).
- It causes lymphatic filariasis.

12. Ans. is 'a' i.e., Br. Malayi (***Ref:*** *Chatterjee, 12th/e, p. 189*)

- 'Sheathed microfilaria with nuclei upto the tip' is a feature of Brugia malayi.

13. Ans. is 'a' i.e., Loa Loa (***Ref:*** *Harrison, 17th/e, p. 1324; Panikar, 6th/e, p. 196*)

I. Lymphatic filariasis	II. Subcutaneous filariasis	III. Serous cavity filariasis
• W. Bancrofti • B. Malayi • B. timori	• Loa Loa • Onchocerca volvulus • Mansonella streptocerca	• M. Ozzardi • M. perstans

Lymphatic Filariasis

14. Ans. is 'a' i.e., Man is an intermediate host (***Ref:*** *Chatterjee, 12th/e, p. 192*)

- For filarial parasite
  - Man – Definitive host
  - Mosquito – Intermediate host
- Lymphatic filariasis is caused by W. bancrofti, B. malayi and B. timori.
- **Drug of choice:** Diethylcarbamazine.

15. Ans. is 'c' i.e., Occult filariasis (***Ref:*** *Chatterjee, 12th/e, p. 195*)

One is Weingarten syndrome – Tropical eosinophilia.

16. Ans. is 'b' i.e., Early Adeno – Lymphangitis stage (***Ref:*** *D.R. Arora, p. 201; Parasitology, 12th/e, p. 197*)

- **The inflammatory phase is characterised by lymphangitis, lymphadenitis and adenolymphangitis.**
  It lasts for a few days, then subsides spontaneously and recurs at irregular intervals for a period of weeks to months. Although this is usually caused by inflammation of lymphatic vessels, due to the adult worm, **blood may reveal the presence of microfilarae in the early phase.** *– Chatterjee, 12th/e, p. 197*

Onchocerca and Loa Loa

17. Ans. is 'b' i.e., Onchocerca Volvulus (***Ref:*** *Harrison, 18th/e, p. 1748; 19th/e, p. 1421*)

- Subcutaneous itchy nodules over the left illiac crest, Skin scrapings containing microfilaria and adult worms confirms the diagnosis of Onchocerca volvulus.

18. Ans. is 'a' i.e., Onchocerca (***Ref:*** *Harrison, 19th/e, p. 1421*)

- Onchocerciasis is also known as **River blindnessQ** and fly involved is Simulium fly.

19. Ans. is 'b' i.e., Loa Loa (***Ref:*** *Chatterjee, 12th/e, p. 202*)

- Calabar (fugitive) swelling is caused by Loa Loa. And fly involved Chrysops fly.

Trichuris Trichiura

20. Ans. is 'c' i.e., Trichuris trichiura (***Ref:*** *Harrison, 18th/e, p. 1743; 17th/e, p. 1322*)

- Clinical manifestations of Trichuris trichiura infection are abdominal pain, anorexia, bloody diarrhea (dysentery) or mucoid diarrhea, rectal prolapse and growth retardation and egg consists of mucus plugs at both ends.

Dracunculus Medinensis

21. Ans. is 'b' i.e., D. Medinensis (***Ref:*** *Harrison, 19th/e, p. 1422-1423; Chatterjee, 12th/e, p. 204*)

- Larva of D. Medinensis is ingested by Cyclops in the water.

22. Ans. is 'c' i.e., Dracunculus (***Ref:** Harrison, 19th/e, p. 1422-1423; Chatterjee, 12th/e, p. 203*)

- **Dracunculus medinensis** is also known as **Guinea worm, Serpent worm, Dragon worm, Medina worm.**

Larva Migrans

23. Ans. is 'c' i.e., Toxocara canis

- Toxocara canis is the most common cause of visceral larva migrans.

24. Ans. is 'a' i.e., Ankylostoma braziliense (***Ref:** Chatterjee, 12th/e, p. 206*)

Larva migrans

Cutaneous

- **Ankylostoma brazilienses (Most Common)**
- **A. Caninum**
- N. Americans and A. Duodenale
- Gnathostoma spinigerum
- Strongyloides
- Loa Loa

Visceral

- **Toxocara Canis (Most common)**
- Toxocara catis
- Gnathostoma
- Anisakis (large ascarid)

MCQs

Helminthology

1. Man is both intermediate and definitive host for: *(Recent MCQ)*
(a) T. solium (b) T. saginata
(c) D. latum (d) Dicroftis fominis

2. Consumption of uncooked pork is likely to cause which of the following helminthic disease? *(AI 01)*
(a) T. saginata (b) T. solium
(c) Hydatid cyst (d) Trichuris trichura

3. The larval form of Taenia is referred as: *(Delhi 08)*
(a) Cysticercus (b) Cysticercoid
(c) Echinococcus (d) Conerus

4. The most commonly affected tissues in cysticercosis is: *(AIIMS 01)*
(a) Brain (b) Eye
(c) Muscles (d) Liver

5. Spinal cord compression may be caused by: *(Kerela 02)*
(a) Cysticercus (b) Ankylostomiasis
(c) E. granulosus (d) Visceral larva migrans

6. Hydatid disease of liver is caused by: *(PGI)*
(a) Strongyloides (b) Echinococcus granulosus
(c) T. solium (d) Trichinella spiralis
(e) Echinococcus multilocularis

7. Intermediate host for hydatid disease: *(AIIMS 09)*
(a) Man (b) Dog
(c) Cat (d) Foxes

8. A company executive, who travels worldwide, present with upper abdominal mass and +ve Casoni's test. The organism is: *(AI 00)*
(a) Echinococcus (b) E. histolytica
(c) Hepatitis (d) Ascariasis

9. The following infection resembles malignancy: *(JIPMER 02)*
(a) Echinococcus granulosus
(b) Echinococcus multilocularis
(c) Echinococcus vogeli
(d) Echinococcus oligarthus

10. What is malignant hydatid disease? *(Recent MCQ)*
(a) Malignant changes into hydatid cyst
(b) Infection with E. multilocularis
(c) Hydatid disease in immunocompromised host
(d) None of the above

11. Natural habitat of schistosoma: *(PGI)*
(a) Veins of the urinary bladder
(b) Portal and pelvic veins
(c) Vesical plexuses
(d) All of the above

12. Terminal spined eggs are seen in: *(AI 05)*
(a) Schistosoma haematobium
(b) Schistosoma mansoni
(c) Schistosoma japonicum
(d) Chlonorchis sinensis

13. Katayama fever is caused by: *(Recent MCQ)*
(a) F. hepatica
(b) C. sinensis
(c) S. haematobium
(d) A. lumbricoides

14. Parasitic intestinal infestation seen in immunocompromised patient is: *(PGI 04)*
(a) Giardiasis
(b) Ascariasis
(c) Liver fluke
(d) Schistosomiasis
(e) Strongyloides

15. Ankylostoma enters the human body by: *(Kerela 05)*
(a) Ingestion
(b) Inhalation
(c) Penetration of skin
(d) Inoculation

16. Habitat of hookworm is: *(Recent MCQ)*
(a) Jejunum
(b) Ileum
(c) Colon
(d) Duodenum

17. Highest incidence of anemia in the tropics is due to: *(Recent MCQ)*
(a) Hookworm
(b) Thread worm
(c) Ascaris
(d) Guinea worm

18. Seat worm is: *(AIIMS 84)*
(a) Enterobius
(b) Dracunculus
(c) Ankylostoma
(d) Necator

19. A child from Bihar comes with fever. Blood examination shows sheathed microfilaria with nuclei upto tail tip. The diagnosis is: *(AI 00)*
(a) B. malayi
(b) W. bancrofti
(c) Loa loa
(d) Oncocerca volvulous

20. All of the following are true about Brugia malayi *except*: *(AI 95)*
(a) The intermediate hosts in India are Mansoni
(b) The tail tip is free from nuclei
(c) Nuclei are blurred, so counting is difficult
(d) Adult worm is found in the lymphatic system

21. Lymphatic filariasis is/are caused by: *(PGI 10)*
(a) W. bancrofti
(b) Brugia malayi
(c) Schistosoma
(d) B. timori
(e) Onchocera volvulus

22. Which is not a feature of tropical eosinophilia? *(Recent MCQ)*

(a) Eosinophilia more than 3000/mm^3
(b) Microfilaria in tissue
(c) Microfilaria in blood
(d) Lymphadenopathy

23. Dracunculosis infection occurs through: *(JIPMER 07)*

(a) Ingestion of water containing cyclops
(b) Ingestion of water containing parasite
(c) Ingestion of fish
(d) Penetration of skin

24. Definitive host for guinea worm is: *(AI 01)*

(a) Man
(b) Cyclops
(c) Snail
(d) Cyclops and man

25. Second intermediate host of Dichyllobothrium latum: *(PGI)*

(a) Cyclops
(b) Man
(c) Snail
(d) Fresh water fish

26. 24 years old AIDS patient develops chronic abdominal pain, low grade fever, diarrhea, and malabsorption. Oocyst demonstrated in stool. Likely cause of his diarrhea is: *(HP 2006)*

(a) E. histolytica
(b) Giardia
(c) Microsporidia
(d) Isospora belli

27. HIV patient with malabsorption, fever, chronic diarrhea with acid fast organism. What is the causative agent? *(AIIMS 10)*

(a) Giardia
(b) Microsporidia
(c) Isospora
(d) E. histolytica

28. Definitive host is one: *(PGI 2000)*

(a) In which sexual multiplication takes place
(b) In which asexual multiplication takes place
(c) Harbors adult form
(d) Harbors larval form

29. Man is secondary host for: *(Recent MCQ)*

(a) Malaria
(b) Tuberculosis
(c) Filariasis
(d) Relapsing fever

30. All float in a saturated salt solution *except*: *(AIIMS 05)*

(a) Clonorchis
(b) Fertilized eggs of ascaris
(c) Larva of strongyloides
(d) Trichuris trichura

ANSWERS AND EXPLANATIONS

Helminthology

1. **Ans. is 'a'** i.e., T. solium
   Explained in book text.
2. **Ans. is 'b'** i.e., T. solium
   Explained in book text.
3. **Ans. is 'a'** i.e.,Cysticercus
   T. solium – Cysticercus cellulosae
   T. saginata – Cysticercus bovis
4. **Ans. is 'c'** i.e., Muscles
   Common sites affected by Cysticercus cellulosae include subcutaneous tissue, skeletal muscle and brain.

5. Ans. is 'a' i.e., Cysticercus

Based on the site of involvement, NCC of two types:

1. **Parenchymal:** Parenchyma.
2. **Extra-parenchymal:** Meningitis, ventricles and spinal cord.

6. Ans. are 'b, e'

Explained in book text.

7. Ans. is 'a' i.e., Man

Explained in book text.

8. Ans. is 'a' i.e., Echinococcus

Casoni's test: This is an immediate hypersensitivity (Type I) skin test used for diagnosis of hydatid disease.

9. Ans. is 'b' i.e., Echinococcus multilocularis

It mimics a carcinoma with enlargement of liver.

10. Ans. is 'b' i.e., Infection with E. multilocularis

Already explained.

11. Ans. is 'd' i.e., All of the above

Explained in book text.

12. Ans. is 'a' i.e., Schistosoma haematobium

Explained in book text.

13. Ans. is 'c' i.e., S. haematobium

Katayama fever is a manifestation of acute schistosomiasis. Typical features include fever, an urticarial rash, enlarged liver, spleen and bronchospasm.

14. Ans. is 'e' i.e., Strongyloides

Explained in book text.

15. Ans. is 'c' i.e., Penetration of skin

Explained in book text.

16. Ans. is 'a > b > d'

Explained in book text.

17. Ans. is 'a' i.e., Hookworm

18. Ans. is 'a' i.e., Enterobius

Pinworm, also called seat worm, or threadworm.

19. Ans. is 'a' i.e., B. malayi

20. Ans. is 'b' i.e., The tail tip is free from nuclei

21. Ans. are 'a, b, d'

22. Ans. is 'c' i.e., Microfilaria in blood

23. Ans. is 'a' i.e., Ingestion of water containing cyclops

24. Ans. is 'a' i.e., Man

25. Ans. is 'd' i.e., Fresh water fish

26. Ans. is 'd' i.e., Isospora belli

27. Ans. is 'c' i.e., Isospora

28. Ans. are 'a, c'

29. Ans. is 'a' i.e., Malaria

30. Ans. are 'a, c'

MISCELLANEOUS IMPORTANT MCQs

1. **In formal ether concentration technique which layer contain parasites?** *(Recent MCQ)*
   (a) Ether (b) Faecal debris
   (c) Formal water (d) Sediment

   Ans. is 'd', Sedimentation techniques use solutions of lower specific gravity than the parasitic organisms, thus concentrating the latter in the sediment. The sedimentation technique used is the formalinethyl acetate technique and floatation technique.

   Floatation techniques (most frequently used: zinc sulfate or Sheather's sugar) use solutions which have higher specific gravity than the organisms to be floated so that the organisms rise to the top and the debris sinks to the bottom.

2. **Which organism can be isolated from sputum?**
   (a) Paragonimus westermanii (b) Fasciola
   (c) Clonorchis (d) Leishmania donovani

   Ans. is 'a', Paragonimus westermanii is also known as lung fluke and is known to be most common cause of Endemic hemoptysis.

3. **Gynaecophoric canal is seen in case of male worm of:**
   (a) Fasciola hepatica (b) Paragonimus westermanii
   (c) Clonorchis sinensis (d) Schistoma mansoni

   Ans. is 'd'

4. **Dog heart worm is:**
   (a) Babesiosis (b) Hookworm infections
   (c) Strongyloidosis (d) Dirofilaria immitis

   Ans. is 'd', Dog is definitive host and mosquito is intermediate host, in humans they obstruct pulmonary arterioles and develop into local granulomatous nodules.

5. **Not transmitted by fish:**
   (a) Paragonimus westermanii (b) Clonorchis sinensis
   (c) Diphyllobothrium latum (d) Schistosoma japonicum

   Ans. is 'd', Schistosoma species have snail and man in the life cycle whereas in all others option 2nd intermediate host is fish.

6. **Which of the following is true with Microsporidia?**
   (a) It is fungus (b) It is a protozoa
   (c) It is a bacteria (d) It is associated with diarrhoea in HIV

   Ans. are 'b and d', Microsporidian species most frequently reported in association with AIDS are Enterocytozoon bieneusi, E.hellem and E. intestinalis and in AIDS patient **ocular involvement** is often the presenting sign of Microsporidiosis and E.hellem is the most common causing it.

7. **Ascariasis causes:**
   (a) Appendicitis (b) Intestinal obstruction
   (c) Bile duct obstruction (d) All of the above

   Ans. is 'd', Ascaris leads to malnutrition and night blindness due to Vitamin A deficiency and retardation of growth is also seen.

8. **Frenkel skin test is positive in:**
   (a) Spinal cord compression (b) Toxoplasmosis
   (c) Pemphigus (d) Pemphigoid

   Ans. is 'b'

9. Plasmodium falciparum causes:

(a) Thrombocytopaenia
(b) DIC
(c) Hemolysis
(d) Haematemesis

Ans. are 'a, b, c, d'

10. Autoinfection is seen in:

(a) Cryptosporidium
(b) Strongyloides
(c) Giardia
(d) Gnathostoma

Ans. is 'b'

11. People with which HLA type are protected from Plasmodium falciparum?

(a) HLA Bw 53
(b) HLA B27
(c) HLA B1
(d) HLA B2

Ans. is 'a', Class 1 antigen HLA Bw53 is found at high frequency in West African population and is related with protection from plasmodium falciparum.

12. Most sensitive index of recent transmission of malaria in community:

(a) Spleen rate
(b) Infant parasite rate
(c) Annual parasite rate
(d) Slide positivity rate

Ans. is 'b', Annual parasite index measures incidence, **spleen rate** measures endemicity, **ABER** – Annual blood examination rate (index of operational efficiency) and **SPR** (slide positivity rate) – forecasting malaria and defining any area to be high risk or low risk.

13. Which of the following is not a coccidian parasite?

(a) Isospora
(b) Cyclospora
(c) Cryptospridium
(d) Enterocytozoon

Ans. is 'd', Enterocytozoon belongs to order Microsporida formerly were grouped with the sporozoa.

14. Which of the following is viviparous?

(a) S.stercoralis
(b) Trichenella spiralis
(c) Enterobius
(d) Ascaris

Ans. is 'b', Muscle cell carrying larva of T.spiralis is known as **Nurse cell.**

15. Protozoa associated with myocarditis:

(a) Trichenella spiralia
(b) Ascaris
(c) Hookworm
(d) Strongyloides

Ans. is 'a'

16. Which of the following doesnot pass through lungs?

(a) Hookworm
(b) Ascaris
(c) Strongyloides
(d) Enterobius vermicularis

Ans. is 'd'

17. Which of the following is toxic to parasite?

(a) Peroxidase
(b) Interferon
(c) IL-2
(d) IL-6

Ans. is 'a'

18. Most common nematode in South India is:

(a) Brugia malayi
(b) Brugia timori
(c) Onchocerca volvulus
(d) Wuchereria bancrofti

Ans. is 'a'

19. All causes malabsorption *except*:

(a) Giardiasis
(b) Ascaris lumbricoides
(c) Strongyloides
(d) Capillaria phillipensis

Ans. is 'b'

20. Simple life cycle means:

(a) One host
(b) Two host
(c) Three host
(d) Four host

Ans. is 'a'

21. Parasitic encephalitis is caused by:

(a) Naegleria
(b) Acanthamoeba
(c) Balamuthia
(d) Gnathostoma

Ans. are 'a, b, c, d', All of the above leads to encephalitis.

22. Most common affected tissue in cysticercosis is:

(a) Brain
(b) Eye
(c) Muscles
(d) Liver

Ans. is 'c', Rarely neurocysticercosis happens and most common site is Parenchymal and associate with Ingestion of infected eggs of Taenia solium with food and water.

23. Parasitic disease affecting intestine is:

(a) Chagas disease
(b) Malaria
(c) Kala azar
(d) Fasciola

Ans. is 'a', Chagas disease is caused by Trypanosoma cruzi and spread by Reduvid bug and leads to Megaesophagus and megacolon.

24. Eosinophilic meningoencephalitis is caused by:

(a) Gnathostoma spinigerum
(b) Naegleria
(c) Toxocara canis
(d) Angiostrongylus cantonensis

Ans. are 'a, d', Gnathostoma spinigerum worm migrate to deeper tissues and produce visceral gnathostomiasis or visceral larvae migrans and can lead to encephalomyelitis in case of **Angiostrongylus cantonensis** L3 larvae enters brain and leads to eosinophilic meningoencephalitis and sometimes may lead to ocular angiostrongyliasis.

25. Selective media for Naegleria fowleri is:

(a) Nutrient agar rich with E.coli
(b) NNN media
(c) Nonnutrient agar with E.coli
(d) Diamond media

Ans. is 'c', It is cultivated on nonnutrient agar with E.coli or Enterobacter aerogenes and incubated at 37 degree, Amoebae will grow on moist agar surface and will use the bacteria as food producing plaques as they clear the bacteria.

RED ALERT POINTS

1. **Napiers aldehyde test, chopra antimony test are used for Hypergammaglobulinaemia. NNN media and Scheinder liquid media are used for culturing promastigotes form.**
2. Duffy blood group antigen negativity confers protection against infection by: **P. vivax and Thalassemic trait, sickle cell anaemic trait, Excess of fetal HB confers protection against P. falciparum.**
3. **Autoinfection** is seen with CHEST – **C**ryptosporidium parvum and **C**apillaria phillipensis, **H.** nana, **E**nterobius vermicularis, **S**trongyloides stercoralis, **T**aenia solium.
4. Infective stage for mosquito in case of P. vivax is: **Gametocyte and for Humans it is sporozoite which is infective, Accole forms, maurer dots are seen, Banana shaped gametocytes are features of Plasmodium falciparum.**
5. R-2 type of drug resistance in malaria is: **Decline by 75% in hours followed by persistence.**
6. Giardiasis is best diagnosed by: **Presence of both cysts and trophozoites in stools, enterotest is done for the same, Malabsorption syndrome is a feature, Common variable immunodeficiency is associated with recurrent Giardiasis.**
7. Metronidazole can be used to treat infections caused by: **Gardenella vaginalis, E. histolytica, Trichomonas vaginalis.**
8. **H. nana** is dwarf tapeworm and H.dimunita is Rat tapeworm belongs to Cestodes.
9. **Cutaneous larve migrans** us due to**: Ancylostoma brasilenses and visceral larvae migrans by Toxocaracanis and catis.**
10. Ova floats in saturated saline are of: **(FATEH) Fertilised egg of ascaris, Ancylostoma duodenale, Trichuris trichiura, Enterobius vermicularis, H. nana).**
11. Visceral larva migrans is due to: **Toxacara canis and cutaneous larvae migrans is caused by Ancylostoma brasilensis, strongyloides stercoralis.**
12. **P. falciparum** the no. of cycles, the parasite undergoes in the liver if: **1 and recrudescence is seen and relapse is seen in plasmodium vivax and ovale due to hypnozoites.**
13. **Casoni test** is positive in: **Echinococcus granulosus (Dog tapeworm) (Type I Hypersensitivity).**
14. Non-sheathed microfilaria are: **Mansonella ozzardi, Mansonella Streptocerca and microfilaria with tail tip free of nuclei seen in Wuchereria bancrofti and terminal two nuclei is seen in Brugyiamalayi.**
15. **Meningoencephalitis** caused by which amoeba: **Naegleria (Brain eating Amoeba).**
16. **Sabin feldman** test (Complement fixation test) is used in: **Toxoplasmosis –** It is a serologic test to diagnose for toxoplasmosis. The test is based on the presence of certain antibodies that prevent methylene blue dye from entering the cytoplasm of Toxoplasma organisms blue Patient serum is treated with Toxoplasma trophozoites and complements as activator, and then incubated. After incubation, methylene blue is added. If antitoxo antibodies are present in the serum, because these antibodies are activated by complements and lyse the parasite membrane, Toxoplasma trophozoites are not stained (positive result); if there are no antibodies, trophozoites with intact membrane are stained and appear blue under microscope (negative result).
17. Infective forms of Toxoplasma gondii: **Sporulated oocyst, Tachyzoites, Bradyzoites.**
18. **Leishman Donovan bodies** are seen in: **Human spleen (Amastigote form), Promastigote is infective stage. Promastigote is cultured on NNN media, Scheinder liquid medium.**
19. Ascaris lumbricoides is: Small intestinal **Nematode (infective stage – Embryonated egg), loefflers syndrome is seen but ascaris not associated with Malabsorption.**
20. The intermediate host for T. Saginata is: **Cow and for Taeniasolium is pig. Taenia saginata is longer than taenia-solium, eggs of Taeniasps are not distinguished as they look similar in appearance.**
21. The **largest** protozoan infection is: **Balantidium coli, micronucleus and macronucleus present, Rotatory motility seen.**

22. Toxoplasmosis is: **Teratogenicity is maximum in first trimester of pregnancy, least in third trimester of pregnancy. Chorioretinitis is seen in congenital toxoplasmosis.**
23. **Hepatitis–B:** HbsAg +ve and IgMHBcAg–Acute Hep B and > 6 months HBsAg +ve – chronic hepatitis.
24. Mycocardium involvement is seen in: **Trichinella.**
25. Cryptococcal neoformans is most common cause of meningitis in HIV positive patients.
26. Primary amoebic meningitis is caused by: **Naegleria fowleri, also known as Brain eating amoeba, Abundant neutrophils are seen in CSF whereas acanthamoeba is also free living amoeba which leads to Contact lens keratitis and granulomatous encephalitis. Abundant lymphocytes are seen.**
27. **Trichinella spiralis:** Cannot cause pulmonary eosinophilia. PE is caused by Ancylostomaduodenale.
28. **Ascaris lumbricodes** does not cause malabsorption, Loefflers syndrome is associated.
29. **FATEH** – Fertilised egg of ascaris, ancylostoma duodenale, Trichuris trichiura, Enterobius vermicularis, H. nana float on saturated salt solution.

PRACTICE QUESTIONS

1. **Which of the following is not a cestode?**
   (a) Diphylobothrium latum
   (b) Taenia saginata
   (c) Schistosoma mansonia
   (d) Echinococcus granulosus

2. **Nematodes are differentiated from other worms by:**
   (a) Segmentation absent
   (b) Separate celomic cavity
   (c) Sexes separate
   (d) They are cylindrical
   (e) GIT is formed completely

3. **Which one of the following statements is false?**
   (a) The presence of ingested erythrocytes is seen only in Entamoeba histolytica
   (b) Young adult male of low socioeconomic status are most commonly affected by invasive amoebiasis
   (c) A low iron content in the diet predisposes to invasive amoebiasis
   (d) The pathogenic and non-pathogenic strains of E. histolytica can be differentiated by the electrophoretic study of zymodemes

4. **True about amoebic colitis is:**
   (a) Caused by E histolytica
   (b) Cyst contains eight nuclei
   (c) Flask-shaped ulcers are present
   (d) Cecum is most commonly affected
   (e) Premalignant

5. **E. Histocytica. True are:**
   (a) Mostly symptomatic
   (b) Differentiated morphologically from E. dispar
   (c) Antigenically different from E. dispar
   (d) None of the above

6. **Acute Primary Amoebic meningoencephalitis true is:**
   (a) Meningitis caused by acanthamoeba species is acute in nature
   (b) Diagnosis is by demonstration of trophozoite in CSF
   (c) Caused by feco-oral transmission
   (d) More common in tropical climate

7. **Eosinophilic meningoencephalitis is caused by:**
   (a) Gnathostoma spinigeum
   (b) Naegleria
   (c) Toxocara canis
   (d) Angiostrongylus cantonensis

8. **The patbogenecity of Entamoeba histolytica is indicated by:**
   (a) Zymodeme pattern
   (b) Size
   (c) Nuclear pattern
   (d) ELISA test

9. **Chronic amoebic keratitis is seen in:**
   (a) E. histolytica
   (b) Acanthamoeba
   (c) Naegleria
   (d) Haemoflagellates

10. **Which of the following infestation leads to malabsorption?**
    (a) Giardia lamblia
    (b) Ascaris lumbricoides
    (c) Necater Americana
    (d) Ancylostoma duodenale

11. Which of the following is true with Giardia lamblia?

(a) Malabsorption commonly seen
(b) Trophozoite forms is binucleate
(c) Diarrhea is seen
(d) Jejunal wash fluid is diagnostic

12. The following tests help in laboratory diagnosis of Kala Azar except:

(a) Bone marrow examination
(b) Immobilisation test
(c) Blood smear examination
(d) Aldehyde test

13. Leishmania is cultured in media:

(a) Chocolate agar
(b) NNN
(c) Tellurite
(d) Sabourauds

14. Stages seen in peripheral smear of falciparum malaria:

(a) Schizonts
(b) Gametocytes
(c) Accole
(d) Ring form

15. RBC's are enlarged in infection with:

(a) P. vivax
(b) P. malariae
(c) P. ovale
(d) P. falciparum

16. Senescent RBC's are mainly attacked in:

(a) Vivax malaria
(b) Ovale malaria
(c) Falciparum malaria
(d) Quartan malaria

17. Chronic complication of malaria:

(a) Splenomegally
(b) Nephrotic syndrome
(c) Pneumonia
(d) Hodgkin's disease

18. P.F. causes:

(a) Thrombocytopenia
(b) DIC
(c) Hemolysis
(d) Haematemesis

19. Which one of the following is detected by the antigen detection test used for the diagnosis of P. falciparum malaria?

(a) Circum-sporozoite protein
(b) Merozoite surface antigen
(c) Histidine-Rich-Protein I (HRP-I)
(d) Histidine-Rich-Protein II (HRP-II)

20. Infectious stage of plasmodium is:

(a) Trophozoite
(b) Cryptozoite
(c) Sporozoite
(d) Merozoite

21. True about toxoplasmosis:

(a) Due to ingestion of sporocyst with meat
(b) Due to ingestion of oocyst from cat's faeces
(c) Spiramycin given in pregnancy
(d) Due to bite of anopheles mosquito

22. Cysticercosis is caused by:

(a) T. Solium
(b) T. Saginata
(c) A. Duodenale
(d) E. Granulosus
(e) E. Multilocularis

23. The following regarding cysticercosis are true except:
(a) Most common sites are meninges and cerebral ventricle
(b) Calcification is common
(c) Causes focal neurological complication
(d) Found in subcutaneous tissues

24. Neurocysticerosis, following are true except:
(a) Not acquired by eating contaminated vegetables
(b) Caused by regurgitation of larva
(c) Acquired by orofaecal route
(d) Acquired by eating pork

25. Which of the following is the most common location of intracranial neurocysticercosis?
(a) Brain parenchyma
(b) Subarachnoid space
(c) Spinal cord
(d) Orbit

26. Most common parasite of CNS in India is:
(a) Schistosomiasis
(b) Cysticercosis
(c) Trichenella-spiralis
(d) Hydatid cyst

27. Which of the following is the most common central nervous system parasitic infection?
(a) Echinococcosis
(b) Sparganosis
(c) Paragonimiasis
(d) Neurocysticercosis

28. The egg which of the following parasites consist of polar filaments arising from either end of the ambrophore?
(a) Taenia saginata
(b) Taenia solium
(c) Echinococcus granulosus
(d) Hymenolepis nana
(e) Diphyllobothrium latum

29. Ascariasis causes:
(a) Appendicitis
(b) Intestinal obstruction
(c) Bile duct obstruction
(d) All of the above

30. Specific diagnosis of ascaris is made by:
(a) Adult worm in stool
(b) Egg detection
(c) Antigen detection
(d) Antibody detection
(e) Skin test

31. The organism most commonly causing genital filariasis in most part of Bihar and easteran U.P. is:
(a) Wuchereria bancrofti
(b) Brugia malayi
(c) Onchocerca volvulus
(d) Dirofilaria

32. False regarding filariasis is:
(a) Morbidity increase with age in endemic areas
(b) Humoral immunity plays dominant role
(c) Usually unilateral
(d) Man is the only host for filariasis

33. In which stage of filariasis are microfilaria seen in peripheral blood?
(a) Tropical eosinophilia
(b) Early adenolymphangitis stage
(c) Late adenolymphangitis stage
(d) Elephantiasis

34. Kallu, a 30 years old man, presented with subcutaneous itchy nodules over the left iliac crest. On examination they are firm, non-tender and mobile. Skin scrapping contains microfilaria and adult worms of:

(a) Loa Loa
(b) Onchocerca volvulus
(c) Brugia malayi
(d) Mansonella persutans

35. Chronic dysentery, abdominal pain, and rectal prolapse in children is caused by:

(a) Enterobius vermicularis
(b) Ascariasis
(c) Trichuris trichiura
(d) Trichinella spiralis

36. Parasites causing lung infestation are:

(a) H. nana
(b) Paragonimus westermanii
(c) Taenia saginata
(d) E. granulosus
(e) E. multilocülaris

37. Pulmonary eosinophilia is seen in the following parasitic infections except:

(a) Babesiosis
(b) Hookworm infection
(c) Strongyloidiasis
(d) Visceral larva migrans

38. Parasite causing encephalitis is/are:

(a) E. histolytica
(b) T. gondii
(c) Angiostrongyloid cantonensis
(d) T. cruzi

39. Fish acts as intermediate host in:

(a) D. latum
(b) Clonorchis sinensis
(c) H. Diminuta
(d) H. Nana

40. Bile duct Ca is caused by:

(a) Fasciola
(b) Clonorchis
(c) Paragonimus
(d) None

41. Cholangiocarcinoma is caused by:

(a) Fasciola infestation
(b) Clonorchis infestation
(c) Paragonimus infestation
(d) Ascaris infestation

42. Which of the following is true with microsporidia?

(a) It is fungus
(b) It is a protozoa
(c) It is a bacteria
(d) It is associated with diarrhoea in HIV

43. Which of the following is viviparous?

(a) Strongyloides stercoralis
(b) Trichinella spiralis
(c) Enterobius
(d) Ascaris

44. Skin snip is used in the diagnosis of:

(a) Trichinosis
(b) Strongyloidosis
(c) Schistosomiasis
(d) Onchocerciasis

45. Intracellular parasite is A/E:

(a) Babesia
(b) Toxoplasma
(c) Giardia
(d) Leishmania

46. Malabsorption is caused by A/E:
(a) Ascaris lumbricoides
(b) Giardiasis
(c) Strongyloides
(d) Capillaria phillipinesis

47. Acute Primary Amoebic meningoencephalitis true is:
(a) Meningitis caused by acanthamoeba species is acute in nature
(b) Diagnosis is by demonstration of trophozoite in CSF
(c) Caused by feco-oral transmission
(d) More common in tropical climate

48. Which of the following is not a cestode?
(a) Diphylobothrium latum
(b) Taenia saginata
(c) Schistosoma mansonia
(d) Echinococcus granulosus

49. Giardiasis is associated with:
(a) Common variable immunodeficiency
(b) C1 esterase deficiency
(c) C8 deficiency
(d) Anaemia

50. A patient presents with diarrhea. Analysis of stool on wet mount shows mobile protozoa without RBCs and pus cells. The diagnosis is:
(a) Balantidium coli
(b) Giardiasis
(c) Trichomonas hominis
(d) Entamoeba histolytica

51. Winter bottoms sign in sleeping sickness refers to:
(a) Unilateral conjunctivitis
(b) Posterior cervical lymphadenopathy
(c) Narcolepsy
(d) Transient erythema

52. Painless terminal hematuria is seen as one of the manifestations in the infection caused by:
(a) Schistosoma Japonicum
(b) Schistosoma mansoni
(c) Schistosoma haematobium
(d) Plasmodium falciparum

53. Schistosoma Japonicum resides in:
(a) Vesical Plexus
(b) Ileocaecal plexus
(c) Systemic Circulation
(d) Gallbladder

54. Parasites penetrating through skin for entry into the body are:
(a) Ankylostoma duodenale
(b) Strongyloides
(c) Round worm
(d) Trichuris trichiura

55. Sputum examination is not useful in diagnosis of:
(a) Trichuris trichiura
(b) Ankylostoma duodenale
(c) Paragomniasis
(d) Strongyloides

56. Parasitic Encephalitis is caused by:
(a) Naegleria
(b) Acanthamoeba
(c) Balamuthia
(d) Gnathostoma
(e) All of the above

57. Which of the following have their transmission by fish?
(a) *Clonorchis sinensis*
(b) *Schistosoma japonicum*
(c) *Diphylobothrium latum*
(d) *Paragonimus westermani*

58. Chronic complication of malaria:
(a) Splenomegaly
(b) Nephrotic syndrome
(c) Pneumonia
(d) Hodgkin's disease

ANSWERS AND EXPLANATIONS

Ans. 1 (c)

Cestodes can be classified according to their habitat into:

1. **Pseudophyllidean Cestodes:** Possessing false or slit like grooves, include Dophyllobothrium latum (fish tapeworm), Sporganum mansoni, Sporganum proliferum.
2. **Cyclophyllidean Cestodes:** Possessing cup-like and round suckers (acetabula) and includes:
   a. **Adult worms in intestines:** Taenia saginata (beef tapeworm), Taenia solium (pork tapeworm), Hymenolepis nana (dwarf tapeworm), Hymenolepis diminuta (rat tapeworm), Dipylidium caninum (double pored dog tapeworm).
   b. **Larval stages in man:** Echinococcus granulosus (dog tapeworm), Echinococcus multilocularis, Cysticercus cellulosae of T.solium, genus Multiceps.

   Schistosoma mansonia comes under Trematodes or flukes. It is a blood fluke found in the mesenteric veins of the sigmoidorectal area and in the branches of the portal vein of the liver.

(Ref: Parasitology–Protozoology and Helminthology by K.D.Chatterjee, 13th edition)

Ans. 2 (a),(c),(d)

Ans. 3 (c)

Entamoeba histolytica is the only species which contains RBCs, leucocytes and tissue debris. The other species donot contain any ingested RBCs. World Health Organization estimates that every year more than 70,000 people die because of amoebiasis. E. histolytica is common in developing countries and in persons of lower socio-economic status due to poor hygiene. **A low iron content in the diet do not predispose to invasive amoebiasis**. Zymodemes are used to analyze the various pathogenic strains of E. histolytica. The various zymodeme distribution pattern can be analysed by isoenzyme electrophoresis.

(Ref: Medical Parasitology by D.R. Arora and B. Arora, 2nd edition)

Ans. 4 (a),(c),(d)

The only member of the subphylum Sarcodina that is pathogenic to humans and causes intestinal amoebiasis E. histolytica. It is found worldwide.

It has 3 morphological stages:

1. **Trophozoite**–growing or feeding stage – has a clear translucent ectoplasm and a granular endoplasm. RBCs, leucocytes and tissue debris are found in the endoplasm. It contains a single large nucleus.
2. **Precystic Stage–10 to 20 mcg.**
3. **Cystic Stage**–surrounded by a cyst wall, quadrinucleate.

   The intestinal lesions of amoebic dysentery are amoebic ulcers confined to the large intestines and mostly found in the ileocaecal region. They are typically described as flask shaped ulcers. The margin of the ulcer is ragged and undermined and the base is formed by the muscular coat and is filled up by necrotic material, yellowish or blackish slough.

(Ref: Parasitology–Protozoology and Helminthology by K.D.Chatterjee, 13th edition)

Ans. 5 (c)

The clinical features of E. histolytica can vary from an asymptomatic carrier state to acute colitis and chronic colitis.

E.dispar has been designated as the non-invasive non-pathogenic species. **E. histolytica and E. dispar are morphologically identical**. Trophozoites containing ingested RBCs can be identified as E. histolytica but the cysts cannot be differentiated microscopically. They can be differentiated isoenzyme analysis.

(Ref: Medical Parasitology by D.R.Arora and B. Arora, 2nd edition)

Ans. 6 (b)

Primary Amoebic Meningoencephalitis is caused by the free-living amoebae of the genus Naegleria which are found in fresh water, mud, moist soil, polluted warm lake water, streams, ponds, indoor swimming pool. Most of the human infections are caused by Naegleria fowleri. Human infections probably occur either from nasopharyngeal contamination during swimming. The incubation period is 5-7 days. The amoebae are specifically neurotropic and cerebral invasion takes place through the olfactory nerves. The disease is characterized by acute onset of Upper respiratory tract infection followed by symptoms and signs of meningitis.

Fresh unstained CSF preparations are essential to detect motile trophozoites. CSF can be stained by Wright or Giemsa. Fluorescent antibody staining of CSF can also be done.

(Ref: Parasitology–Protozoology and Helminthology by K.D.Chatterjee, 13th edition)

Ans. 7 (a),(d)

The syndrome Eosinophilic meningoencephalitis is most commonly caused by **Angiostrongylus cantonensis.** It is prevalent in several areas including Pacific islands and south east Asia. The signs and symptoms of Eosinophilic meningoencephalitis include intense headache, fever, neck stiffness, convulsions and paralysis. Complications like optic neuritis and sixth cranial nerve palsy are associated with it.

Thus in the Pacific a patient who develops signs of meningitis along with peripheral eosinophilia and the CSF shows eosinophilic pleocytosis (50-70%) should be suspected to be a case of angiostrongyliasis. Other helminthic parasites which may cause this syndrome are cerebral gnathostomiasis, cerebral cysticercosis, cerebral echinococcosis, cerebral schistosomiasis and toxocara.

(Ref: Parasitology–Protozoology and Helminthology by K.D.Chatterjee, 13th edition)

Ans. 8 (a)

Zymodemes are used to analyze the various pathogenic strains of E. histolytica. The various zymodeme distribution pattern can be analysed by isoenzyme electrophoresis. There are various zyodemes that have been studied which describe the pathogenicity of the strain.

(Ref: Parasitology–Protozoology and Helminthology by K.D.Chatterjee, 13th edition)

Ans. 9 (b)

Acanthamoeba spp have been linked to several clinical conditions, including, Granulomatous amoebic encephalitis, cutaneous infections and amoebic keratitis. The primary group at risk for developing this condition is individuals you wear contact lenses especially the soft and extended wear type. The organism enters through a corneal trauma and there is subsequent colonization. It produces a protein which causes cell Lysis thus causing clinical symptoms of keratitis.

Ans. 10 (a)

Giardia lamblia is a cosmopolitan parasite, more prevalent in children than adults and more common in warm than in cool climates. It inhabits the deudenum and upper part of the jejunum. The presence of G.lamblia in the glandular crypts of duodenal-jejunal mucosa may not cause any pathology. These flagellates do not invade the tissues, but feed on mucous secretions. With the sucking disc it attaches to the surface of the epithelial cells. Patient may complain of dull epigastric pain, flatulence and chronic diarrhea of steatorrhoea type. The stool is voluminous, foul smelling and contains large amount of mucus and fat but no blood. This is due to malabsorption since the parasites are coated on the mucosa, thus absorption suffers. Patient loses weight due to the malabsorption.

(Ref: Parasitology–Protozoology and Helminthology by K.D.Chatterjee, 13th edition)

Ans. 11 (a),(b)

G. lamblia is a cosmopolitan parasite, more prevalent in children than adults and more common in warm than in cool climates. It exists in 2 forms–trophozoite (bilaterally symmetrical, binucleate, 4 pairs of flagella, 2 pairs of blepharoplasts, 2 axonemes, typical motility – falling leaf like) and cyst (2 pairs of nuclei).

It inhabits the duodenum and upper part of the jejunum. The presence of G.lamblia in the glandular crypts of duodenal-jejunal mucosa may not cause any pathology. These flagellates do not invade the tissues, but feed on mucous secretions.

With the sucking disc it attaches to the surface of the epithelial cells. Patient may complain of dull epigastric pain, flatulence and chronic diarrhea of **steatorrhoea** type. The stool is voluminous, foul smelling and contains large amount of mucus and fat but no blood. This is due to malabsorption since the parasites are coated on the mucosa, thus absorption suffers. **Patient loses weight due to the malabsorption**.

(Ref: Parasitology–Protozoology and Helminthology by K.D.Chatterjee, 13th edition)

Ans. 12 (b)

The various methods for laboratory diagnosis of Kala Azar include:

1. **Direct evidence (demonstration of L. donovani)**
   - A. Peripheral blood by thick film – Amastigote form
   - B. Blood culture in NNN medium–Promastigote form
   - C. Biopsy from lymph node, bone marrow (sternal or iliac crest), splenic puncture
2. **Indirect evidence**
   - A. Blood count – leucopenia and raised ESR
   - B. Serum tests:
     - I. Aldehyde test
     - II. Antimony test
     - III. Complement fixation test with WKK antigen
     - IV. Demonstration of antibodies (ELISA, DAT, IHA, IFA with specific antigens)

(Ref: Parasitology–Protozoology and Helminthology by K.D.Chatterjee, 13th edition)

Ans. 13 (b)

Blood culture is a less sensitive method for diagnosis of Leishmania. It is a slow method and takes a long time (about 1 month). About 1-2 ml of blood is taken aseptically from a vein and diluted in 10 ml of citrated saline solution. The cells are then either allowed to settle at 22°C in an incubator overnight or centrifuged. The cellular deposit is then inoculated into the water of condensation of NNN medium and incubated at 22°C for 1 to 4 weeks. At the end of each week, a drop of condensation fluid is examined for promastigote forms.

Ans. 14 (b),(c),(d)

The blood smear for diagnosis of malaria should be collected during the febrile paroxysms. All erythrocytic stages and gametocytes can be seen in the peripheral blood in infection of P. vivax, P. malariae and P.ovale but in P.falciparum infection, only the ring forms and crescent shaped gametocytes can be seen. Late trophozoite and schizont stages of P.falciparum are usually confined to the internal organs and appear in the peripheral blood only in severe or pernicious malaria. The occurrence of multiple rings in an individual RBC with accole forms is diagnostic of falciparum infection.

Ans. 15 (a),(c)

Alterations in the infected RBC:

P.vivax–enlarged, pale and the portion of the cytoplasm not occupied by the parasite shows a dotted or stippled appearance, called Schuffner's dots.

P.falciparum–normal size and possess 6-12 Maurer's dots.

P. malariae–normal size and occasionally show fine stippling.

P.ovale–enlarged, pale, James' dots.

Ans. 16 (d)

Age of the RBC invaded:

P.vivax–young

P.falciparum–all ages (young and old)

P.malariae (Quartan fever)–old or senescent

P. ovale–young

Ans. 17 (a),(b)

Various clinical features and complications of malaria are:

Febrile paroxysm

Anaemia

Splenomegaly

Pernicious malaria (cerebral malaria, algid malaria, septicemic malaria)

Blackwater fever

Ans. 18 (a),(c)

Ans. 19 (d)

Antigens targeted by the rapid diagnostic tests:

1. Histidine Rich Protein II–produced by P. falciparum
2. Parasite lactate dehydrogenase (p-LDH)–produced by all 4 plasmodium species

(Ref: Medical Parasitology by D.R.Arora and B. Arora, 2nd edition)

Ans. 20 (c)

Malaria parasites exhibit a complex life cycle involving alternating cycles of asexual division (schizogony) occurring in man (intermediate host) and sexual development (sporogony) in mosquito (definitive host). Thus, malaria exhibits alteration of generation. **The sporozoite is the infective stage found in the salivary gland of the female mosquito.**

(Ref: Medical Parasitology by D.R.Arora and B. Arora, 2nd edition)

Ans. 21 (b),(c)

Toxoplasma gondii is of worldwide distribution. It is an obligate intracellular parasite. The various morphological forms are – tachyzoites, tissue cysts and oocysts. All the stages are infectious to man.

Modes of infection:

1. Congenital
2. Acquired – by ingestion, inhalation or by inoculation

Treatment–Pyrimethamine or sulphadiazine or Spiramycin

(Ref: Medical Parasitology by D.R.Arora and B. Arora, 2nd edition andParasitology–Protozoology and Helminthology by K.D.Chatterjee, 13th edition)

Ans. 22 (a)

Cysticercosis is caused by T.solium. The larval forms of T. saginata are not found in man but those of T. solium may occasionally be found. Man, occasionally serving as the larval host of T.solium, becomes infected in the same was as the pig, i.e., either by drinking contaminated water or by eating uncooked vegetables infected with eggs. Besides this, a man harbouring the adult worm may auto infect himself either unclean or unhygienic personal habits, or by reversal of peristaltic movements. The distribution of these cysticerci is usually in the subcutaneous tissues and muscles causing palpable or visible nodules.

(Ref: 2nd edition and Parasitology–Protozoology and Helminthology by K.D.Chatterjee, 13th edition)

Ans. 23 (a)

Cysticercosis is caused by T.solium. The larval forms of T.saginata are not found in man but those of T.solium may occasionally be found. Man, occasionally serving as the larval host of T.solium, becomes infected in the same was as the pig, i.e., either by drinking contaminated water or by eating uncooked vegetables infected with eggs. Besides this, a man harbouring the adult worm may auto infect himself either unclean or unhygienic personal habits, or by reversal of peristaltic movements. The distribution of these cysticerci is usually in the subcutaneous tissues and muscles causing palpable or visible nodules. It may develop in brain leading to epileptic attacks and in anterior and vitreous chambers in the eye. In India, it is regarded as the second most important cause of intracranial space occupying lesions following tuberculosis and the most common cause of epilepsy.

(Ref: Medical Parasitology by D.R.Arora and B. Arora, 2nd edition and Parasitology–Protozoology and Helminthology by K.D.Chatterjee, 13th edition)

Ans. 24 (a),(b)

Cysticercosis is caused by T.solium. The larval forms of T.saginata are not found in man but those of T.solium may occasionally be found. Man, occasionally serving as the larval host of T.solium, becomes infected in the same was as the pig, i.e., either by drinking contaminated water or by eating uncooked vegetables infected with eggs. Besides this, a man harbouring the adult worm may auto infect himself either unclean or unhygienic personal habits, or by reversal of peristaltic movements. The distribution of these cysticerci is usually in the subcutaneous tissues and muscles causing palpable or visible nodules.

(Ref: 2nd edition and Parasitology–Protozoology and Helminthology by K.D.Chatterjee, 13th edition)

Ans. 25 (b)

Most common location for brain is Subarachnoid followed by Brain parenchyma. Cysticercosis is caused by T.solium. The larval forms of T.saginata are not found in man but those of T.solium may occasionally be found. Man, occasionally serving as the larval host of T.solium, becomes infected in the same was as the pig, i.e., either by drinking contaminated water or by eating uncooked vegetables infected with eggs. Besides this, a man harbouring the adult worm may auto infect himself either unclean or unhygienic personal habits, or by reversal of peristaltic movements. The distribution of these cysticerci is usually in the subcutaneous tissues and muscles causing palpable or visible nodules. It may develop in brain leading to epileptic attacks and in anterior and vitreous chambers in the eye. In India, it is regarded as the second most important cause of intracranial space occupying lesions following tuberculosis and the most common cause of epilepsy.

(Ref: Medical Parasitology by D.R.Arora and B. Arora, 2nd edition and Parasitology–Protozoology and Helminthology by K.D.Chatterjee, 13th edition)

Ans. 26 (b)

The distribution of these cysticerci is usually in the subcutaneous tissues and muscles causing palpable or visible nodules. It may develop in brain leading to epileptic attacks and in anterior and vitreous chambers in the eye. In India, it is regarded as the second most important cause of intracranial space occupying lesions following tuberculosis and the most common cause of epilepsy.

(Ref: Parasitology–Protozoology and Helminthology by K.D.Chatterjee, 13th edition)

Ans. 27 (d)

The distribution of these cysticerci is usually in the subcutaneous tissues and muscles causing palpable or visible nodules. It may develop in brain leading to epileptic attacks and in anterior and vitreous chambers in the eye. In India, it is regarded as the second most important cause of intracranial space occupying lesions following tuberculosis and the most common cause of epilepsy.

(Ref: Parasitology–Protozoology and Helminthology by K.D.Chatterjee, 13th edition)

Ans. 28 (d)

Eggs of:

(a) **H.nana**–spherical or oval, two distinct membranes–outer: thin and colorless, inner embryophore encloses an oncosphere with 3 pairs of lancet shaped hooklets. **There are polar filaments emanating from little knobs at either end of embryophore, float in saturated solution of common salt. It is nonbile stained.**

(b) **T. saginata and T.solium** – bile stained, thin outer transparent shell, inner embryophore is brown, thick walled and radially striated. Contains an oncosphere with 3 pairs of hooklets, does not float in saturated solution of common salt.

(c) **Echinococcus granulosus** – ovoid and resembles other eggs of Taenia, contains hexacanth embryo with 3 pairs of eggs.

(d) **Diphyllobothrium latum** – bile stained, contains abundant yolk granules and unsegmented ovum, inconspicuous operculum, does not float in saturated solution of common salt.

Ans. 29 (d)

The worm inhabits the upper part of the small intestine. Pathogenic effect are:

Spoliative action: robbing the host of its nutrition.

Toxic action: may give rise to typhoid like fever, responsible for allergic reactions urticarial, oedema of the face, conjunctivitis and irritation of the upper respiratory tract.

Mechanical effects–can cause intussusception, can penetrate through the ulcers of the alimentary canal, intestinal obstruction.

Ectopic Ascariasis.

(Ref: Parasitology–Protozoology and Helminthology by K.D.Chatterjee, 13th edition)

Ans. 30 (a),(b),(d)

Methods for laboratory diagnosis:

1. **Parasitis diagnosis:**
   i. Demonstration of adult worm–the worm passed through anus, mouth, nose
   ii. Demonstration of larvae–detected in sputum during the migration
   iii. Demonstration of fertilized and unfertilized egg: detected by direct microscopy or concentration of the faeces by salt floatation or formalin ether concentration method.
2. **Serodiagnosis:** Antibody can be detected by indirect Haemagglutination (IHA) and immunofluoroscence antibody (IFA).
3. **Eosinophilia.**

Ans. 31 (a)

The organism most commonly causing genital filariasis in most part of Bihar and easteran U.P. is Wuchereria bancrofti. It causes lymphangitis, lymphadenitis, filarial fever, hydrocele, elephantiasis.

B. malayi causes lymphangitis and elephantiasis. It is characterized by absence of chyluria and rarity of scrotal swelling

O.volvulus causes formation of subcutaneous fibrous nodules and ocular lesions

Dirofilaria rarely causes human zoonosis.

Ans. 32 (b)

Infection caused by Wuchereria bancrofti is called wuchereriasis or bancroftian fever. It occurs in Asia, Africa, Australia, pacific and south America. Adult male and female reside in the lymph nodes and lymphatic vessels of man. The microfilariae are found in the blood. Humans are the only reservoir hosts. The lymphatic nodes are one of the essential elements of the reticuloendothelial system in which the adult worm localizes.

Ans. 33 (b)

The biological incubation period of Wuchereria bancrofti is 1 year. During this period the third stage infective larvae grows to adult form which becomes sexually mature and fertilise the female producing microfilariae in the peripheral blood. The microfilariae circulating in the blood are not known to cause any pathogenic effect except in occult filariasis. The injurious influence excited by the adult worm and developing larva on its host is an inflammatory reaction of the lymphatic system, lymphangitis, which is the classic lesion.

Ans. 34 (b)

O.volvulus–causes onchocerciasis in man. The worms develop in the subcutaneous tissue often encapsulated in dense fibrous nodules. The nodules occur over anatomic sites where the bone is superficial such as knees, hips, iliac crests, elbow, ribs, scalp etc. The nodules are movable. The microfilariae live in the superficial layers of the skin causing itching and in heavy chronic infections, gross thickening of the skin.

***Loa loa*–causes loiasis. The adult worms live in subcutaneous connective tissues and wander round the body causing, usually painless, oedematous swellings known as fugitive or calabar swellings.**

B. malayi causes lymphangitis and elephantiasis. It is characterized by absence of chyluria and rarity of scrotal swelling.

Mansonella perstans–live adults appear to produce little or no host reaction, however, eosinophilia is common. Pruritis, abdominal pain, urticaria and **calabar like swellings occur.**

Ans. 35 (c)

The **immature T.trichiura buries its entire body in the epithelium of the large intestine forming a tunnel. As the worm matures, its posterior portion is extruded or ruptures from the tunnel and hangs in the intestinal lumen.** Intimate contact of T.trichiura with the mucosa of large intestine leads to inflammation of mucosa. Depending upon the intensity of the infection, the inflammation may extend from the distal part of small intestine to the rectum. The mucosa may be oedematous and friable. **The surface tissue of the rectum becomes extremely oedematous and when the patient strains to defecate, rectal prolapse may occur. Rectal bleeding (whipworm dysentery) with abdominal cramps and severe rectal tenesmus are seen in massive infections.Q**

Ans. 36 (b),(d)

Parasites residing in lungs:

(a) Trematodes–Paragonimus westermanii

(b) Nematodes–Capillaria aerophilia, Dirofilaria immitis

(c) Cestodes–Echinococcus granulosus

Ans. 37 (a)

The parasites causing Pulmonary eosinophilia are: Strongyloides, Ascaris, Toxocara and Ancylostoma

Ans. 38 (b),(c),(d)

Parasite causing encephalitis is/are:

T. gondii, Angiostrongylos cantonensis, T. cruzi, Echinococcus spp, Gnathostoma, Spirometra spp, Paragonimus, Schistosoma, Naegleria fowleri, Acanthamoeba and Balamuthia

Ans. 39 (a),(b)

Intermediate host in:

D. latum – 1st intermediate host–cylops, 2nd intermediate host–fresh water fish

Clonorchis sinensis–fish

H. Diminuta – various arthropods

H. Nana – only cestode that can complete life cycle in a single host

Ans. 40 (b) Clonorchis sinensis strongly corelates with bile duct carcinoma

Ans. 41 (b)

Clonorchis lives on protein and glucose of blood in peribiliary plexus. It can be found in the gallbladder and pancreatic duct. The worm causes blocking of the biliary passage causing stagnation of bile. Complications arising include–cholangitis, intra hepatic calculi formation, and cholangiocarcinoma and aplastic carcinoma.

Ans. 42 (b),(d)

Microsporidia are unicellular obligate intracellular protozoan parasites. They have been increasing reported as pathogens in patients with HIV. **Intestinal microsporidiasis is the most common infection mainly caused by E.bieneusi. In AIDS patients ocular involvement is often the presenting sign.**

Ans. 43 (b)

Viviparous nematodes:

Dracunculus medinensis

Wuchereria bancrofti

Brugia malayi

B.timori

Trichinella spiralis

Ans. 44 (d)

Skin biopsy is a diagnostic method for:

Dermal leshmania, espundia, Onchocerciasis

Ans. 45 (c)

Some of the intracellular parasites are:

Babesia

Toxoplasma

Leishmania

Plasmodium

Ans. 46 (a)

Ascaris typically inhabits the upper part of the small intestine. Pathogenic effect are:

Spoliative action: robbing the host of its nutrition, thus causing malnutrition and not malabsorption

Toxic action: may give rise to typhoid like fever, responsible for allergic reactions urticarial, oedema of the face, conjunctivitis and irritation of the upper respiratory tract

Mechanical effects–can cause intussuception, can penetrate through the ulcers of the alimentary canal, intestinal obstruction.

Ectopic Ascariasis

Pathogenic parasites detected in patients with malabsorption are: Giardia lamblia, E. histolytica / dispar, Ancylostoma duodenale, H. nana, Cyclospora cayetanensis Cryptosporidium and Isospora belli.

Ans. 47 (b)

Primary Amoebic Meningoencephalitis is caused by the free-living amoebae of the genus Naegleria which are found in fresh water, mud, moist soil, polluted warm lake water, streams, ponds, indoor swimming pool. Most of the human infections are caused by Naegleria fowleri. Human infections probably occur either from nasopharyngeal contamination during swimming. The incubation period is 5-7 days. The amoebae are specifically neurotropic and cerebral invasion takes place through the olfactory nerves. The disease is characterized by acute onset of Upper respiratory tract infection followed by symptoms and signs of meningitis.

Fresh unstained CSF prepartions are essential to detect motile trophozoites. CSF can be stained by Wright or Giemsa. Fluorescent antibody staining of CSF can also be done.

(Ref: Parasitology–Protozoology and Helminthology by K.D.Chatterjee, 13th edition)

Ans. 48 (c)

Cestodes can be classified according to their habitat into:

(a) **Pseudophyllidean Cestodes:** Possessing false or slit like grooves, include Dophyllobothrium latum (fish tapeworm), Sporganum mansoni, Sporganum proliferum.

(b) **Cyclophyllidean Cestodes:** Possessing cup-like and round suckers (acetabula) and includes:

(c) **Adult Worms in Intestines:** Taenia saginata (beef tapeworm), Taenia solium (pork tapeworm), Hymenolepis nana (dwarf tapeworm), Hymenolepis diminuta (rat tapeworm), Dipylidium caninum (double pored dog tapeworm).

(d) **Larval Stages in Man:** Echinococcus granulosus (dog tapeworm), Echinococcus multilocularis, Cysticercus cellulosae of T.solium, genus Multiceps.

Schistosoma mansonia comes under Trematodes or flukes. It is a blood fluke found in the mesenteric veins of the sigmoido-rectal area and in the branches of the portal vein of the liver.

(Ref: Parasitology–Protozoology and Helminthology by K.D.Chatterjee, 13th edition)

Ans. 49 (a)

Both humoral and cell mediated immunity are essential for clearance of giardia. The disease usually affects IgA deficient persons and anti IgA antibody can be detected on the surface of giardia trophozoites.

Ans. 50 (b)

G. lamblia is a cosmopolitan parasite, more prevalent in children than adults and more common in warm than in cool climates. It exists in 2 forms–trophozoite (bilaterally symmetrical, binucleate, 4 pairs of flagella, 2 pairs of blepharoplasts, 2 axonemes, typical motility – falling leaf like) and cyst (2 pairs of nuclei).

It inhabits the duodenum and upper part of the jejunum. The presence of G.lamblia in the glandular crypts of duodenal-jejunal mucosa may not cause any pathology. These flagellates do not invade the tissues, but feed on mucous secretions. With the sucking disc it attaches to the surface of the epithelial cells. Patient may complain of dull epigastric pain, flatulence and chronic diarrhea of steatorrhoea type. The stool is voluminous, foul smelling and contains large amount of mucus and fat but no blood. This is due to malabsorption since the parasites are coated on the mucosa, thus absorption suffers. Patient loses weight due to the malabsorption.

A microscopic examination of a freshly passed stool shows motile trophozoites without RBC and pus cells.

Engulfed RBCs and cell debris are found in the cytoplasm of E.histolytica.

(Ref: Parasitology–Protozoology and Helminthology by K.D.Chatterjee, 13th edition)

Ans. 51 (b)

Trypanosoma brucei gambiense causes African sleeping sickness.

The trypomastigotes spread throughout the body. They move through the blood and lymph vessels and rapidly multiply. Patient first experience intermittent recurring fever associated with lymphadenopathy. **Lymph nodes in the posterior cervical region are often involved producing a lesion called Winterbottom's sign.** Hepatosplenomegaly is evident during the early stage of infection.

Ans. 52 (c)

Schistosoma Japonicum and Schistosoma mansoni – inhabit the rectal venous plexus and portal venous system.

Schistosoma haematobium – inhabits the vesical venous plexus.

In infection with Schistosoma haematobium recurrent painless haematuria results from ulcers of the bladder. A burning sensation while micturition and/or suprapubic discomfort may be associated with it. It is associated with bladder cancer.

Ans. 53 (b)

Schistosoma Japonicum and Schistosoma mansoni – inhabit the rectal venous plexus and portal venous system.

Schistosoma haematobium – inhabits the vesical venous plexus.

Ans. 54 (a),(b)

Parasites entering directly through the skin:

- Ancylostoma duodenale
- A. brazilienses
- A. caninum
- Necator americanus
- Strongyloides stercoralis
- Acanthamoeba sp

- Schistosoma mansoni
- S. japonicum
- S. haematobium

Ans. 55 (a)

Parasites found in sputum:

- Paragonimus westermani
- Capillaria aerophila
- Entamoeba histolytica
- Ascaris lumbricoides
- Strongyloides stercoralis
- Ancylostoma duodenale
- Necator americanus

Ans. 56 (e)

Parasite causing encephalitis is/are:

T. gondii, Angiostrongylois cantonensis, T. cruzi, Echinococcus spp, Gnathostoma, Spirometra spp, Paragonimus, Schistosoma, Naegleria fowlerii, Acanthamoeba and Balmuthia.

Ans. 57 (a),(c),(d)

Fish are the source of:

- **Freshwater fish:**
  - i. Diphyllobothrium latum
  - ii. Clonorchis sinensis
  - iii. Capillaria philippinensis
  - iv. Dioctophyma renale
  - v. Metagonimus yokogawai
  - vi. Heterophyes heterophyes
  - vii. Gnathostoma spinigerum
- **Marine water fish:**
  - i. Anisakis simplex
- **Crab and crayfishes:**
  - i. Paragonimus westermani
  - ii. Angiostrongylus cantonensis

Ans. 58 (a),(b)

Various clinical features and complications of malaria are:

Febrile paroxysm
Anaemia
Splenomegaly
Pernicious malaria (cerebral malaria, algid malaria, septicemic malaria)
Blackwater fever

Chapter 8

VIROLOGY

GENERAL PROPERTIES

- **Obligate intracellular parasites.**
- Viruses are the smallest infectious agents (ranging from **about 20 to 300 nm in diameter**) and contain only one kind of nucleic acid (RNA or DNA) as their genome.
- The nucleic acid is encased in a **protein shell (capsid),** which may be surrounded by a lipid-containing membrane. The entire infectious unit is termed a virion.
- Viruses **have no metabolic activity outside susceptible host cells.** They do not possess protein-synthesizing apparatus therefore, cannot multiply in inanimate media but only inside living cells where it takes over the host protein-synthesizing machinery to synthesize new virus particles.

STRUCTURE AND CHEMICAL COMPOSITION OF VIRUSES

Viral Proteins

- Proteins which are a part of the **virion are called as structural proteins** (capsid, surface glycoprotein, enzymes (in some viruses).
- Functions of **structural proteins**
  - Facilitate **transfer of viral nucleic acid** from one host cell to another.
  - Protect the **viral genome** from nucleases.
  - Promote **attachment** of the virus particle to susceptible cell.
  - Provide **structural symmetry** to the virus particle.
- **Capsid**
  - Composed of repeating protein units called as **capsomeres.**
  - Capsid with enclosed nucleic acid is called as **nucleocapsid.**
- **Capsid shows three types of symmetry:**
  - **Icosahedral/cubic symmetry:** Capsomeres are arranged in such a way that the capsid appears as an icosahedron having 20 facets and 12 vertices, e.g., adenoviruses. There is a possibility of formation of some empty particles devoid of nucleic acid.
  - **Helical symmetry:** The nucleic acid and capsomeres are wound together in the form of a helix, e.g., orthomyxo-viruses. It is not possible for empty helical particles to form.
  - **Complex symmetry:** Viruses, which do not show either icosahedral or helical symmetry but are more complicated in structure, e.g., poxviruses).

VIRAL NUCLEIC ACID

- Viruses contain a single kind of nucleic acid, either DNA or RNA.
- The genome may be single-stranded or double-stranded, circular or linear and segmented or unsegmented.
- It is the major characteristic used for classification of the viruses.

Remember – **All DNA viruses** are Double stranded except Parvo virus (SS DNA).
All RNA viruses are Single stranded except Reo virus (DS RNA).

Note that: Some viruses carry enzymes, which are essential for the initiation of the viral replicative cycle when a virion enters the host cell. For, e.g., **RNA polymerase carried by the viruses with negative sense RNA genomes (orthomyxoviruses, rhabdoviruses).**

LIPID ENVELOPE

- A number of viruses contain lipid envelope.

  The lipid is acquired when the viral nucleocapsid buds through a cellular membrane (cytoplasmic or nuclear membrane) in the course of maturation.
- **Budding occurs only at sites** where virus-specific proteins have been inserted in the host membrane.
- **Enveloped viruses are sensitive to treatment with ether and other organic solvents.Q**

SURFACE GLYCOPROTEINS

- **Viral envelope contains glycoproteins (peplomers),** which project as spikes from the outer surface of the envelope. In contrast to the lipids in the viral membranes, the envelope glycoproteins are virus encoded.**Q** For e.g., **Hemagglutinin and Neuraminidase in influenza virus.**
- **Functions:**
  - **Mediate attachment of the virus to the host cell receptor.**
  - Some attach to receptors on the red blood cells leading to haemagglutination.
  - Some cleave neuraminic acid from the host cell glycoproteins **(neuraminidase/receptor destroying enzyme).** This process is known as **Elution.**

SUSCEPTIBILITY TO PHYSICAL AND CHEMICAL AGENTS

- **Heat and cold:** Enveloped viruses are heat labile as compared to non-enveloped viruses. Viral infectivity is generally destroyed by heating at 56°C with the exception of hepatitis B virus, papovaviruses and scrapie agent.
- **PH:** Some viruses (e.g., enteroviruses) are resistant to acidic conditions. All viruses are destroyed by alkaline conditions.
- **Ether susceptibility:** Enveloped viruses are susceptible to ether while non-enveloped viruses are resistant.
- **Chlorine:** Larger concentrations of chlorine are required to kill viruses than to destroy bacteria.

FAMILIES OF VIRUSES THAT INFECT HUMANS

Nucleic acid core	Capsid symmetry	Enveloped/naked	Physical type of nucleic acid	Virus family
DNA	Icosahedral	Naked	ss ds circular ds	Parvoviridae Papovaviridae Adenoviridae
		Enveloped	ds circular ds	Hepadenaviridae Herpesviridae
	Complex	Complex coat	ds	Poxviridae
RNA	Icosahedral	Naked	ss ss ss ds segmented	Picornaviridae Astroviridae Caliciviridae Reoviridae
		Enveloped	ss	Togaviridae
	Unknown or complex	Enveloped	ss ss segmented ss ss diploid	Flaviviridae Arenaviridae Coronaviridae Retroviridae
	Helical	Enveloped	ss segmented ss segmented ss ss ss	Bunyaviridae Orthomyxoviridae Paramyxoviridae Rhabdoviridae Filoviridae

REPLICATION OF VIRUSES

Learn These Steps by

A PUB MR

Attachment

Mediated by binding of virion surface structures (ligands) to receptors on the cell surface therefore the attachment is specific.

Virus	Receptor
HIV	CD4
Rhinoviruses	ICAM 1
Epstein-Barr virus	CD 21/complement receptor 2 (CR2) Q
Measles virus	CD 2
Rabies virus	Acetylcholine receptors

Penetration

- After binding, the virus particle is taken up inside the cell.
- **Receptor mediated endocytosis.Q**
- In some viruses **(especially non-enveloped) there is receptor-mediated endocytosis,** with uptake of ingested virus particles within endosomes.
- Fusion of viral envelope with the plasma membrane.
- This **requires the interaction of viral fusion protein with a second cellular receptor (e.g., chemokine receptors for HIV).**

Uncoating

- Occurs concomitantly or shortly after penetration.
- **It is the physical separation of the viral nucleic acid from the outer structural components of the virion such that it can function.**
- **Infectivity of the parental virus is lost at the uncoating stage.Q**
- Expression of viral genome and synthesis of viral components.
- **Specific mRNAs are transcribed from the viral nucleic acid.**
- Some viruses **(negative sense RNA viruses) carry their own RNA polymerases to synthesize mRNA (conventionally designated positive sense).**
- Viruses then use the cell components to translate the mRNA.
- **Initially early or non-structural proteins are synthesized,** there are enzymes which initiate the synthesis of viral components and induce the shutdown of host protein and nucleic acid synthesis.

This is **followed by replication of viral nucleic acid. Finally there is synthesis of late or structural proteins which constitute daughter virion capsids.**

Morphogenesis

- Newly synthesized viral genomes and capsid polypeptides assemble together to form progeny viruses.

Release

- **Non-enveloped viruses** lyse the infected cells and are released, e.g., poliovirus.
- **Enveloped viruses are released by the process of budding** through the special areas of the host cell membrane, where virus encoded glycoproteins have been inserted.

  Note: Enveloped viruses are not infectious until they have acquired their envelopes.

Eclipse Phase

- Between the **stages of penetration to the release of daughter virion the infective virion is disrupted and its measurable infectivity is lost.** This phase is called as **eclipse phase.**

VIRUS ISOLATION

Laboratory Animals

- **Suckling mice for isolation of arboviruses and coxsackieviruses.Q**
- Primates for hepatitis viruses.

Chick Embryos

Process of inoculating in Embryonated egg is called CandlingQ

- **Chorioallantoic membrane: P**oxviruses, **H**erpes simplex virus.
- **Amniotic cavity:** Primary isolation of influenza virus, mumps virus.
- **Allantoic cavity: Influenza virus** (for serial passages, vaccine production).
- **Yolk sac:** Japanese B encephalitis virus, West Nile virus.

Cell Culture

Most commonly used method for cultivation of viruses.

- **Primary cell culture:** These are normal cells freshly taken from the body and cultured.

  Capable of **limited growth (5-10 divisions).** Preferred for cultivating viruses for vaccine production, **e.g., Rhesus monkey kidney cell culture, Human amnion cell culture, Chick embryo fibroblast cell culture.Q**
- **Semicontinuous/diploid cell strains:** These are the cell of a single type which that have retained their normal diploid chromosome number and karyotype. They can be passaged 10-50 times before the cells die off. Used for isolation of viruses and production of viral vaccines.

  E.g., Human embryonic lung cell strain.
- **Continuous cell lines:** These are cells of a single type capable of indefinite propagation in vitro. They are derived from malignant tissue therefore have irregular chromosome numbers.

  E.g., HeLa (human carcinoma cervix), **Hep-2** (human epithelioma of larynx), **Kb** (human carcinoma of nasopharynx).

DETECTION OF GROWTH IN CELL CULTURE

Cytopathic Effect

Many viruses produce morphological changes in the cells in which they grow. These are called as cytopathic effects.

- **Rounding and degeneration of cells:** Picornaviruses.
- **Rounding and aggregation of cells (Grape like clusters):** Adenoviruses.
- **Synctium formation:** Measles virus, RSV.
- **Cytoplasmic vacuolation:** SV-40.
- **Complete degeneration of cell sheet:** Enterovirus.
- **Inclusion bodies: Intracellular or intranuclear aggregates of products of viral replication.**

Nucleus: Cowdry Type **A** – (Remember by H**A**Y) – Herpes and Yellow fever.
Cowdry type **B** – (Rememeber by **B**AP) – Adeno and Polio virus.

Cytoplasmic: **Mollusum bodies (Henderson Patterson) –** Molluscum contagiosum.Q
Paschen bodies – Variola.
Guarneri bodies – Vaccinia.
Negri bodies – Rabies.Q

Both: Measles virus.Q

Intranuclear and Intracytoplasmic

Haemadsorption

- Some Orthomyxoviruses and Paramyxoviruses code for red cell agglutinins that are incorporated in the host cell membrane during infection. When erythrocytes are added to the infected cell layer, they adhere to the surface of the infected cells. This is called as **Haemadsorption.**

Immunofluorescence

- Cells from **virus infected cultures can be staining with fluorescent-conjugated antiserum and examined under UV light for detection of viral antigen.**

Interference

- The growth of the noncytopathogenic virus in cell culture can be detected by subsequent challenge with a known cytopathogenic virus. The growth of the first virus will inhibit the infection with the second virus by interference. **It is seen in Rubella and Polio virus.**

Transformation

- Oncogenic viruses induce cell transformation, so that growth of cells appears in **the piled up fashion due to the formation of microtumors.**

VIRAL GENETICS

Mutation

- **Random, undirected, heritable variation.**

  Frequency in viruses: 10^{-4}–10^{-8}.
- **Conditional lethal mutants:** Mutants that multiply in susceptible cells under permissive conditions but cannot grow under non-permissive conditions. **E.g., temperature-sensitive mutants: grow at low temperatures (31-35°C) but not at high temperatures (38°C-42°C).**

Recombination

- **When two different viruses infect same cell, genetic recombination can take place.**

Reassortment

- Occurs in viruses having **segmented genome** (Arenaviridae, Bunyaviridae, Influenza A virus, Rota virus). In a **single cell infected by two related viruses** there is exchage of segments with the production of reassortants.

NON-GENETIC INTERACTIONS

Phenotypic Mixing

When two different viruses such as influenza virus and a paramyxovirus infect the same cell, some mixup may take place during the assembly so that progeny genome of one virus is surrounded by the capsid belonging entirely or partly to other virus. This is called as phenotypic mixing.

Polyploidy

Viruses that mature by budding (e.g., **Paramyxoviruses**) from the plasma membrane, several nucleocapsids may be enclosed within a single envelope. This is called as **polyploidy.**

Complementation

Protein encoded by one virus allows a different virus to replicate in doubly infected cells, e.g., HDV (defective virus) and HBV (helper virus).Q

SMALLPOX, VACCINIA AND OTHER POXVIRUSES

Poxviruses

Characterized by brick shaped morphology:

- Double stranded DNA genome.
- **Only DNA viruses that replicate in cytoplasm** where viral particles accumulate to form **Eosinophilic inclusions, or Guarnieri bodies,** visible by light microscope.

Poxviruses associated with human diseases

1. Variola.
2. Vaccinia.
3. Molluscum contagiosum.

Poxviruses associated with zoonotic infection: Monkey Pox.

Smallpox

- Last case reported in 1977 in Somalia.
- **WHO officially declared in 1980 that small pox has been eradicated completely.**
- **Factors contributing to this accomplishment:**
  1. Universal interest in eliminating this costly disease with high mortality and morbidity.
  2. **Infection's long incubation** and low communicability.
  3. **Ease of diagnosis of skin lesions by histology or antigen detection.**
  4. Human – sole reservoir of infection.
  5. No carrier state.
  6. Availability of live virus vaccine: which was resistant to temperature changes and drying.
- Transmission requires **close contact.**
- **IP: 12 days and C/F: Fever, macular rash – progressing to typical vesicular and pustular lesion over 1-2 weeks.**

Variola Virus: Existed in 2 strains

- Variola Major (Smallpox) [Case mortality – 20-50%].
- Variola Minor (Alastrim) [Milder form of smallpox case mortality less than 1%].

Vaccinia Virus

- **Virus used for vaccination** against smallpox.
- Probably derived from cowpox, variola virus or hybrid of the two.
- **Now a laboratory virus, no natural host.**
- Per cutaneous administration of vaccinia virus vaccine results in protective cellular and humoral immune response in more than 95% of primary vaccine.

Monkey Pox Viruses

- Infect non-human primates.
- Humans infected if come in direct contact with infected animal.

MOLLUSCUM CONTAGIOSUM

Benign disease characterized by:

- **Pearly, flesh coloured umbilicated skin lesions 2-5 mm in diameter.**
- Infection transmitted by **close contact including sexual intercourse.**
- Can occur anywhere, but **mainly genital region; palmes and soles spared.**

- **Disease self-limited**, no systemic complication.
- **Associated with advanced stages of HIV infection.** Disease more generalized, severe and persistent in AIDS patients. **Involves face and upper body.**
- **Diagnosis:** By Histological demonstration of cytoplasmic eosinophilic inclusions **(Molluscum bodies/Henderson Patterson bodies).**
- **The virus has not been cultured so far.Q**
- **Virus identification by** Electron microscopy and molecular methods.
- **Treatment:** No specific systemic treatment.

Other Pox Viruses

Cause localized vesicular lesion when human come in direct contact with infected animal (zoonotic infection).

1. Cowpox virus.
2. Pseudocowpox virus (Milker's nodule).Q
3. Buffalopox.
4. Bovine papular stomatitis virus.
5. Orf virus (contagious pustular dermatitis).Q

PARVOVIRUSES

Parvoviruses group includes several species-specific viruses of animals.

Parvo B–19–It is a human pathogen – Named so after code number of human serum in which it was discovered.

- Icosahedral, Nonenveloped.
- **Single stranded DNA virus** with outer caspid made of two structural proteins.
- **Individual virus particles contain DNA strands** of +ve and -ve polarity.
- **Fails to grow in conventional cell culture lines and animal model.**
- **Only replicates in vitro in erythroid progenitor cells** derived from human bone marrow, umbilical cord, peripheral blood or fetal liver.

Remember: B19 binds specifically to cellular receptors, erythrocyte P antigen, therefore, explains the tropism of B19 for erythroid precursor cells particularly pronormoblast and normoblasts.Q

Clinical Manifestation

Erythema Infectiosum: Most common manifestation of parvovirus B19 infection also **called Fifth disease/erythema infectiosum.**

Clinical Features: A mild illness, facial rash (typical presentation) with a **"Slapped cheek" appearance preceded by low grade fever.** Rash – on arms, legs and has lacy, reticular, erythematous appearance.

Arthropathy

Most common manifestation in adults, Arthralgia and Arthritis.

Arthritis: Symmetrical, peripheral involving wrists, hands, knees most frequently.

- Usually resolves in 3 weeks, non-destructive, may last for many months even years.

Transient Aplastic Crisis

Parvovirus B19 causes transient aplastic crisis in patients with chronic hemolytic disease.

- B19 can cause aplastic crisis in all hemolytic conditions, e.g., sickle cell disease, hereditary spherocytosis, thalassemias etc.

Chronic anemia in Immunodeficient patients: Unable to eliminate B19 infection due to inadequate production of IgG antibodies thus persistence of infection.

Fetal and congenital infections: Maternal B19 infections generally do not adversely affect the fetus.

Diagnosis

- **Parvovirus B19 specifies IgM and IgG antibodies.**
- Acute infection **shows raised IgM.**
- **Bone marrow biopsy:** Giant pronormablast and Hyperplasia.
- **Fetal infection:** Presence of B19 DNA in amniotic fluid or Fetal blood.

Treatment

- **Erythema infectiosum:** Self immunity.
- **Arthritis and Arthropathy:** NSAIDS.
- **Aplastic crisis:** Erythrocyte transfusion.
- **Immunodeficient patient:** I/V Ig contain anti Parvovirus IgG.
- **No vaccine for Parvovirus B19 is currently available: A baculo virus infected insect cell line that expresses noninfectious immunogenic B19 caspid proteins is being evaluated as a vaccine candidate.**

ADENO VIRUS

- **DNA virus:** Double stranded DNA, non-enveloped, icosahedral symmetry.
- 47 distinct antigenic types have been isolated from humans.
- Human adenoviruses are divided into six groups (A-F) based on their physical, chemical and biological properties.
- **Pathogenesis:**
  - Adenoviruses infect and replicate in the epithelial cells of respiratory tract, eye, gastrointestinal tract, urinary bladder and liver.
- **Clinical Features:**

Group	Principal types	Disease
B	3,7,14	Pharyngoconjunctival fever **(swimming pool conjunctivitis)**
	3,7,14,21	Acute respiratory disease
	3,7	Pneumonia, acute febrile pharyngitis in small children
	11,21	**Acute hemorrhagic cystitis**
	34,35	Pneumonia with dissemination (AIDS patients)
D	8,19,37	**Epidemic keratoconjunctivitis (ship yard eye)**
F	40,41	Infantile gastroenteritis (difficult to cultivate)

- **Laboratory Diagnosis:**
  - **Culture:** Primary human embryonic kidney cells, Hep-2, HeLa.
    Rounding and clustering of swollen cells.
  - **Antigen detection:** Immunofluorescence, ELISA, latex agglutination, electron microscopy.
  - **Antibody detection:** CT, Nt, HAI.
  - **Treatment:** Symptomatic.
  - **Vaccine:** Live attenuated/killed, for prevention of acute respiratory disease, useful for military recruits.

HERPES VIRUSES

- Spherical ds DNA virus, 120-200 nm in diameter.
- Comprise four structural elements: **Envelope, tegument, capsid and core.**
- **Envelope is outer most; tegument is present between envelope and capsid. Inner to tegument is icosahedral capsid, which contains double stranded DNA.**
- These groups of viruses establish latent infections which get reactivated in immunosuppressed hosts.

CLASSIFICATION OF HUMAN HERPESVIRUSES					
Subfamily	**Growth cycle**	**Cytopathology**	**Site of latent infection**	**Official name**	**Common name**
Alpha-herpesvirinae	Short	Cytolytic	Neurons	HHV1 HHV2 HHV3	HSV1 HSV2 Varicella zoster virus
Beta-herpesvirinae	Long	Cytomegalic	Glands, kidneys	HHV5	CMV
		Lympho-proliferative	Lymphoid tissue (T-cells)	HHV6 HHV7	HHV6 HHV7
Gamma-herpesvirinae	Variable	Lympho-proliferative	Lymphoid tissue (B-cells)	HHV4 HHV8	EBV Kaposi's sarcoma associated herpes virus

HERPES SIMPLEX VIRUS

Two types HSV1 and HSV2:

- **HSV1:** Infects **mouth, eye, CNS** (regions above the waste), but is also responsible for few cases of genital herpes.
- **HSV2:** Infects **genital and anal regions**

  Infections caused by herpes simplex can be divided into primary infection, latent infection and reactivation.
- **Primary infections:** Transmitted by contact through damaged skin or mucosa, classic lesion is a vesicle.
- **HSV1 cause following primary infections:**
  - Acute gingivostomatitis.
  - Herpetic whitlow seen in doctors and nurses. Herpetic gladiatorum seen in wrestlers.
  - Keratoconjunctivitis – Steroid are contraindicated.
  - Eczema herpeticum.
  - **Encephalitis (involves temporal lobes) and Mollarets meningitis associate with it.**
  - Generalized infections.
- **HSV2 causes following primary infections:**
  - **Genital herpes** (painful vesicles, fever, malaise, swollen lymph nodes).
  - **Aseptic meningitis**
  - **Neonatal infection:** Acquired during passage of the baby through infected birth canal. Disseminated disease: mortality rate: 80%.
  - Encephalitis.
  - Localized infection (skin, eye, mouth).
- **Latent Infection**
  - HSV1: **Cranial (trigeminal) ganglia.**
  - HSV2: **Sacral ganglia.**
  - Within the sensory ganglia, viral DNA exists as a free circular episome.
    - Virions migrate back to the nerve endings, where infection of the epithelial cells results in cluster of vesicles commonly found at the mucocutaneous junctions of the lips, nose, eyes.

- **Laboratory Diagnosis**
  - **Direct examination:** Electron microscopy (virions), fluorescence microscopy (viral antigens), **Light microscopy (Tzank smear: multinucleated giant cells with faceted nuclei, homogeneously stained ground glass chromatin with eosinophilic intranulear inclusions).Q**
  - **Culture: Human fibroblast/vero cell line,** swollen rounded cells (CPE), immunofluorescent staining of the infected cells.
  - **Serological tests:** CFT, Nt, Immunofluorescence, ELISA.

  Treatment: Acyclovir.
- **Reactivation**
  - Provoked by various stimuli like common cold, fever, stress etc.

VARICELLA ZOSTER

- 2 distinct clinical entities:

Varicella/Chickenpox

- **Mode of infection:** Respiratory route.
- **Vesicles:** Corium + dermis – ballooning, multinucleated giant cells, Eosinophilic intranuclear IB.
- **Involve blood vessels of skin:** Necrosis + epidermal hemorrhage.

Pulmonary Involvement:

- Interstitial pneumonitis.
  - **CNS involvement:** Perivascular cuffing.

Chickenpox

- Humans are only reservoir for VZV.
- **Secondary attack rate: 90%** (70-90%).
- Late winter + Early spring.
- Age: 5-9 years, **I.P. 10-21 days.**
- **Infectious: 48 hours prior to onset of vesicular rash, during the period of vesicular formation (4-5 days) and until all vesicles are erupted.**
- **Skin lesions: Maculopapules/vesicles/scabs.**
- **Immunocompromised patients:** Have more lesions and greater risk of visceral complications (30-50%) and fatal (15%).
- **Most common, infectious complication** – S. pyogenes/S. aureus.
- **Most common extracutaneous site involved:** CNS (acute cerebellar ataxia + meningeal irritation).

CSF: Increased protein + lymphocytes, other CNS manifestations: aseptic meningitis, Reye's syndrome, GBS and transverse Myositis.

- **Varicella pneumonia** is serious complication, more common in adults.
- **Perinatal varicella:** ↑mortality, if maternal disease 5 days before delivery or 48 hours thereafter (Mortality – 30%), Immunoglobulins is to be given within 96 hours to child.
- **Congenital Varicella Syndrome:** Limb hypoplasia, cicatricial skin lesions, Microcephaly.

Herpes Zoster

- 6th – 8th decade.
- T3 – L3, if ophthalmic division of trigeminal nerve: Herpes Zoster ophthalamicus.
- **Zoster associated pain:** Continuation of pain from onset to resolution.
- **1st dermatomal pain (48–72 hours), then rash (3–5 days).**

In Ramsay Hunt Syndrome:

- **Pain and vesicles in external auditory canal.**
- **Loss of taste in anterior 2/3rd of tongue and develop ipsilateral facial palsy (Geniculate ganglion of sensory branch of VII nerve involved).**
- **Most debilitating complication:** Pain associated with neuritis and post herpetic neuralgia.
- **Patient with Hodgkin's, non-Hodgkin's lymphoma and bone marrow transplant are at increased risk of HZV.**

Laboratory Investigation:

1. TZANCK smear.Q
2. Isolation of VZV in susceptible tissue culture cell.
3. Demonstration of seroconversion.
   Demonstration of a 4 fold/greater rise in antibody titre between convalescent and acute phase sera by ELISA, CFT, Nt, IFA.
4. PCR.

Prophylaxis:

- **VZIG and ZIG: Within 96 hours (pref. 72 hours).**
- **Vaccine: OKA strain (Live attenuated vaccine).**

Treatment:

- Acyclovir, vidarabine, valacyclovir.
- **Acute Neuritis/Neuralgia:** Analgesics/Glucocorticoids.

CYTOMEGALOVIRUS

- Beta herpes virus group.
- ds DNA, Protein capsid, Lipoprotein envelope, Icosahedral symmetry.
- Virus **replicates in epithelial cells in salivary glands, kidneys and respiratory epithelium.**
- Virus may be present in milk, saliva, faeces and urine.

Transmission

- Infection is transmitted by close contact between individuals.
- Blood transfusion.
- Vertical transmission (prenatal, perinatal and postnatal).
- Once infected, an individual probably carries the virus for life.
- The infection usually remains latent.
- Lab abnormalities in decreasing order of frequency
  - Serum IgM level > 20 mg/dl.
  - **Atypical lymphocytosis.**
  - Elevated liver aminotransferases.
  - Thrombocytopenia.
  - Hyperbilirubinemia.
  - CSF protein level > 20 mg/dl.

Perinatal CMV Infection:

Acquired either from **infected maternal genital secretions** or from breast milk.

Postnatal Infection:

Acquired by kissing, sexual intercourse, blood transfusion or organ transplantation, Generally subclinical.

CMV Mononucleosis:

- Most often involves sexually active young adults.
- **I.P. 20–60 days.**
- Illness lasts for 2–6 weeks.
- **Characteristic laboratory abnormality: Relative lymphocytosis in peripheral blood with > 10% atypical lymphocytes.**

CMV Infection in Immunocompromised Host

- Most common and important viral pathogen complicating organ transplantation.
- Period of maximum risk between 1 and 4 months after transplantation.
- **Patients with CD4 + T cell count below 100/µl are highly susceptible to CMV.**
- CMV reactivation syndromes develop frequently when T-lymphocyte mediated immunity is compromised.

Pathology: Cytomegalic cells in vivo, **"Owl's Eye"** appearance.

CLINICAL MANIFESTATIONS

Prenatal CMV infection:

- **Most common agent responsible** for intrauterine infection.
- Primary maternal infection or reactivation during pregnancy.
- **Most common presenting features: Growth retardation, Hepatosplenomegaly (Most common)Q (jaundice, thrombocytopenia, microcephaly, encephalitis, chorioretinitis, deafness, mental retardation.**

Laboratory Diagnosis:

- **Direct detection:** Inclusion bodies, viral antigen (immunofluorescence), virus (electron microscopy).

  Culture: Virus grows slowly taking 1-2 weeks for appearance of cytologic changes (multinucleate giant cells with perinuclear cytoplasmic and intranuclear inclusions).

  - Nucleic acid detection: DNA probe, PCR.
  - Serology: Nt, CF, IFA, RIA.

  Treatment: Drug of choice **ganciclovir for CMV RETINITIS.**

EPSTEIN-BARR VIRUS

- Family Herpesviridae, double stranded DNA virus.
- **EBV replicates in epithelial cells of nasopharynx and salivary glands.**
- Latent infection is established in B cells (EBV receptor: **CD21 on surface of B cells).**
- **Infection acquired through kissing or contaminated utensils.**

  It is associated with following diseases:

  1. **Heterophile +ve infectious mononucleosis.**
  2. **Burkitt's lymphoma** (equatorial Africa, children).
  3. **Hodgkin's disease** (mixed cellularity).
  4. **Primary B cell lymphomas** (in immunocompromised).
  5. **Oral hairy leukoplakia.**
  6. **X-linked lymphoproliferative syndrome** (DUNCAN'S DISEASE).
  7. **Anaplastic nasopharyngeal carcinoma** (southern provinces of China, adults).

Bimodal Peak

1. Early childhood (asymptomatic).
2. Late adolescence (symptomatic, infectious mononucleosis of glandular fever).

Pathogenesis: Infects epithelium of orophraynx and salivary glands, Proliferation of EBV infected B-cell, reactive T cell, enlargement of lymphoid tissue, Inverted CD4+/CD8+ T cell ratio.

Clinical Manifestation: I.P.: 4-6 weeks, patient presents with sore throat, generalized lymphadenopathy, fever, malaise, myalgia.

Complications: Most cases of IM self-limited but few develop GBS, Bells palsy, meningoencephalitis, transverse myelitis, thrombocytopenia, carditis, nephritis, pneumonia, splenic rupture.

Laboratory Diagnosis:

1. WBC – 10,000–20,000/μl.
2. Lymphocytosis with > 10% atypical lymphocytes.
3. Neutropenia and thrombocytopenia.

Serological Testing:

- **Isolation** by immortalisation of normal human lymphocytes.
- **Nucleic acid detection:** DNA hybridization, PCR.
- Antibody detection.
- Early in the acute disease, a transient rise in IgM antibodies to viral capsid antigen occurs, replaced within weeks by IgG antibodies to this antigen, which persist for life. Slightly later, antibodies to the early antigen develop and persist for several months. **Several weeks later, antibodies to EB nuclear antigen (EBNA) and the membrane antigen arise and persist throughout life.**

  IgM anti-viral capsid antigen: Current infection.
  - **IgG anti-viral capsid antigen:** Past infection and immunity.
  - **Heterophile antibody test (Paul Bunnel test): Agglutination of sheep RBCs (less specific).**

Treatment:

1. **Patients of IM:** Supportive measures with rest and analgesics.
2. Prednisolone (40-60 mg/d) in complicated IM like airway obstruction, autoimmune haemolytic anemia or severe thrombocytopenia.
3. **Acyclovir:** Decreases shedding from oropharynx, no effect on symptoms of IM.

Human Herpes Virus 6

Infect CD4+ T cells.

- **Exanthem subitum/roseola infantum/sixth disease:** Mild facial rash occurring between 6 months to 3 years of age with fever.

Human Herpes Virus 7

Like HHV 6, it may also cause roseola infantum.

Human Herpes Virus 8

Also called as **Kaposi's sarcoma associated herpes virus.**

Detected in over 90% of Kaposi's sarcomas.

ORTHOMYXOVIRIDAE

- Spherical, pleomorphic, 80-120 nm.
- **Single stranded RNA, negative sense, segmented (A,B: 8 segments, C: 7 segments),** Enveloped.
- Influenza virus A, B and C.

INFLUENZA VIRUS

- Affects both upper and lower respiratory tracts.
- Outbreaks in winter.

Etiological Agents:

- **Orthomyxoviridae family.**
- Divided into A, B and C depending on antigenic characteristics of nucleoprotein (NP) and Matrix (M).
- **Influenza A** further divided on the basis of **Hemagglutinin (H) and neuramidase (N).**
- Virions are irregularly spherical, 80-120 nm in diameter and contain lipid envelope, from the surface of which H and N glycoprotein projects.
- **Hemagglutinin** is the site at which **virus binds to cell receptor.** Antibodies to H Ag are major determinants of immunity to Influenza virus.
- **Neuraminidase degrades the receptor** and also causes release of virus from infected cells. Antibodies to N Ag limits viral spread, process known as Elution.
- **M protein present on surface of lipid envelope** causes virus **assembly and stabilizes lipid envelope.**
- **Genome is 8, single stranded RNA segments.**
- **Segmentation of genome leads to increased chances of genetic reassortment.Q**

Epidemiology:

- Localized epidemics occur every 1-3 years.
- Pandemics occur every 10-15 years.
- Epidemics occur mainly due to Influenza A virus due to Antigenic variation in H and N Ag.
- **Antigenic Shift:** Major antigenic variation, due to genetic reassortment. They are associated with pandemics and are restricted to Influenza A.
- **Antigenic drift:** Minor antigenic variations due to point mutation.
- Influenza B causes less severe outbreaks.

Clinical Features:

- Abrupt onset of symptoms.
- Moderate fever, sore throat, myalgia.
- **Ocular signs,** e.g., Photophobia and burning of eyes.
- Mild cervical lymphadenopathy.
- Acute illness lasts for 2–5 days.

Pathogenesis:

- Infection spreads by aerosols.
- Virus multiplies mainly in ciliated columnar respiratory epithelium. Virus is not found in any extrapulmonary site.
- Severity of illness is related to quantity of virus shed in secretions. Virus shedding lasts for 2-5 days after appearance of symptoms.
- **Incubation period 18-72 hours.**
- Serum antibodies appear after 2 weeks of primary infection.
- IgA antibodies are found in respiratory secretions.

Complications:

1. **Pneumonia:** Most common complication.
    - Primary viral pneumonia is severe with scanty sputum production. Secondary bacterial pneumonia is commonly caused by Streptococcus pneumoniae, Staphylococcus aureus and Hemophilus influenzae.
    - Mixed bacterial and viral pneumonia commonly occurs.

2. **Worsening of COPD and exacerbation of chronic bronchitis and asthma.**
3. **Reye's Syndrome:** Mainly associated with Influenza 'B', especially with the use of aspirin for viral infection.
4. **Myositis, myoglobinuria, rhabdomyolysis**
   - Myositis leads to increase in CPK and aldolase.
   - Myoglobinuria may cause renal failure.
5. **Pericarditis, Myocarditis.**

Laboratory Diagnosis:

- **Demonstration of viral antigen:** Immunofluorescence staining.
- **Virus is isolated from throat swabs, nasopharyngeal washes or sputum through tissue culture or amniotic cavity of chick embryo within 48-72 hours of inoculation.**
- **Antibody detection:** CFT, HAI, Nt.

Treatment:

- Salicylates and acetaminophen are used for symptomatic relief.
- Amantadine and Rimantadine are active only against influenza A.
- **Ribavarin is effective against both Influenza A and Influenza B.**

Prophylaxis:

- Vaccines against Influenza A and B are effective in 50-80% cases.
- Live attenuated vaccine against Influenza A is given **intranasally.**
- **Commercially available vaccine** is the killed vaccine.

SEQUENTIAL CHANGES IN INFLUENZA A VIRUS ANTIGENS DUE TO ANTIGENIC DRIFT

Year	Subtype
1890	H2N2
1900	H3N8
1918	H1N1 Spanish influenza
1957	H2N2 Asian influenza
1968	H3N2 Hong Kong influenza
1977	H3N2 and H1N1 Russian influenza
1990	H3N2 and H1N1

PARAMYXOVIRIDAE

- Spherical, pleomorphic, 150-300 nm.
- Single stranded RNA, linear, nonsegmented, negative sense.
- **Enveloped,** contains two different transmembrane glycoproteins.

  HN/H: May possess both **haemagglutinin and neuraminidase acitivities.**

  F: Membrane fusion and hemolysin activities.

CHARACTERISTICS OF GENERA IN THE SUBFAMILIES OF THE FAMILY PARAMYXOVIRIDAE

Property	Paramyxovirinae			Pneumovirinae
	Paramyxovirus	Rubulavirus	Morbillivirus	Pneumovirus
	Parainfluenza 1,3	Mumps, parainfluenza 2,4	Measles	RSV
Serotypes	4	1	1	1
Dia. of nucleocapsid (nm)	18	18	18	13

Contd.

Contd.

F protein	+	+	+	+
Hemolysin	+	+	+	-
Hemagglutinin	HN	HN	H	-
Hemadsorption	+	+	+	-
Neuraminidase	HN	HN	-	-
Inclusions	C	C	N,C	C

PARA INFLUENZA VIRUS

- **Infection acquired by droplets.**
- All parainfluenza viruses produce respiratory tract infections.
- **In infants and children:** Lower respiratory tract infection, pneumonia.
- **In older children** (6 months to 5 years): Mainly type 1 and in some cases type 2 cause **laryngotracheobronchitis or croup.**
- Fever, cough, respiratory distress, emergency tracheostomy.

Laboratory Diagnosis

- **Demonstration of viral antigen:** Immunofluorescence staining.
- Virus is isolated from throat swabs, nasopharyngeal washes or sputum through tissue culture, viral growth detected by immunofluorescent staining.
- **Antibody detection:** CFT, HAI, Nt, ELISA.

MUMPS

- Disease of childhood.
- Transmitted **by respiratory secretions.**

Virus multiplies in the upper respiratory tract and local lymph nodes, viraemia occurs and virus spreads to many organs.

Major manifestation: Painful swelling of one or both salivary glands (Bilateral parotitis) 14-18 days after exposure.

Complications: Meningoencephalitis, orchitis, oophritis, pancreatitis, arthritis, myocarditis, renal dysfunction.

Laboratory Diagnosis:

- **Isolation:** Tissue culture.
- **Serology:** ELISA, IgM antibody detection.
- **Prophylaxis:** Live attenuated vaccine **(Jeryll–lynn strain).**

MEASLES (RUBEOLA) VIRUS

- Contagious childhood disease **spread by respiratory secretions.**

Pathogenesis

Virus gains access through respiratory route → multiplies locally → spreads to the regional lymph nodes → **primary viraemia → dissemination of virus → multiplies in reticuloendothelial system → secondary viraemia → seeds epithelial surfaces of the body (skin, respiratory tract, conjunctiva).**

Clinical Features

- **Incubation period: 10-12 days.**
- **Upper respiratory tract infection,** fever, rhinitis, cough, conjunctivitis.

- **Koplik's spots:** Small, 1-3 mm diameter, bluish white spots surrounded by erythema seen on buccal mucosa **opposite lower 2nd molar.**
- After 1-2 days symptoms decline with the appearance of maculopapular rash which appears first on the cheek and then spreads to the rest of the body. In next 10-14 days rash fades with the desquamation of the skin.

  4 days before Rash and 5 days after, patient remains infective.Q

Complications

- Secondary bacterial infections.
- **Giant cell pneumonia (Hechts pneumonia)** in patients with impaired cell mediated immunity.
- **Acute post infectious encephalitis** (1/1000 cases of measles).
- **Subacute sclerosing panencephalitis** (1/300,000 cases of measles)–It occurs 5-15 years after an attack of measles. Progressive mental deterioration, involuntary movements, muscular rigidity, coma. Invariably fatal. High titres of measles antibody in CSF, defective measles virus in brain cells.

Laboratory Diagnosis

- **Direct detection:** Multinucleated giant cells, antigen (immunofluorescence) in nasopharyngeal aspirates.
- **Isolation:** Tissue culture, multinucleated giant cells containing eosinophilic inclusions in cytoplasm and nucleus, detection of growth by immunofluorescence.
- **Serology:** IgM antibody by ELISA, CFT.

Prophylaxis

- Live attenuated vaccine, **Edmonston-Zagreb strain.**

RESPIRATORY SYNCYTIAL VIRUS

- Lacks both **haemagglutinin and neuraminidase activities.**
- Contains **fusion (F) protein** that results in the formation of **multinucleated synctia.**
- Responsible for 50% cases of bronchiolitis and 25% cases of pneumonia during first few months of life.
- Infection is spread through respiratory secretions–Lower respiratory infection (bronchiolitis, pneumonia) in infants less than 6 months of age.

  Upper respiratory tract infection (cold) in older children and adults.

  Immunocompromised transplant recipients, it may cause severe pneumonia.

Laboratory Diagnosis

- **Detection of antigen:** In nasopharyngeal aspirates by immunofluorescence, ELISA.
- **Isolation:** Tissue culture, synctia formed in 2-10 days, definitive identification by immunofluorescence.
- **Serology:** Immunofluorescence, ELISA, CFT, Nt.

  Treatment: Supportive care, Ribavirin.

RUBELLA VIRUS

- **German measles/3-day measles.**
- **Genus: Rubivirus.**
- Belongs to Togaviridae family not a paramyxovirus.
- Spherical, 70 nm diameter, positive sense, single stranded RNA, enveloped.
- **Not transmitted by arthropods.Q**
- Mild child hood fever.
- May also be acquired congenitally or postnatally.

Postnatal Rubella

- Virus excreted in oropharyngeal secretions and infection is acquired by inhalation.
- Virus multiplies locally in upper respiratory tract and cervical lymph nodes → viraemia, dissemination throughout the body.
- **Incubation period: 2-3 weeks,** fine pink macules first appearing on the face and then spreading to involve trunk and limbs.
- Enlargement of postauricular, suboccipital, posterior cervical lymph nodes.
- Recovery within 3-4 days of appearance of rash.

  Complications: Polyarthritis (adult women, thrombocytopenic purpura, encephalopathy, panencephalitis).

Congenital Rubella

- Virus can cross the placental barrier and infect the fetus.
- **Congenital anomalies/death of the fetus.**

Classical triad is CHD – Cataract, Heart disease (Patent ductus arteriosus) and DeafnessQ

- **Congenital defects:** Deafness, cataract, glaucoma, microphthalmia, retinopathy, congenital heart disease (patent ductus arteriosus, pulmonary artery stenosis), microcephaly, mental retardation, thrombocytopenic purpura, hepato-splenomegaly.

Laboratory Diagnosis

- **Isolation:** Tissue culture, detection by immunofluorescence, immunoperoxidase staining.
- **Serology:** IgM antibodies, ELISA, RIA.

Prophylaxis

- Live attenuated vaccine, **RA 27/3 strain.**

PICORNAVIRIDAE

- Icosahedral, 28-30 nm (small size), single stranded RNA, linear positive sense, nonenveloped.
- Three genera containing viruses infecting humans.

Genus	Species
Enterovirus	Polio virus 1-3 Coxsackieviruses A1-24 except 23 Coxsackieviruses B1-6 Echoviruses 1-34 except 10 and 28 Enteroviruses 68-71
Rhinovirus	Rhinoviruses 1-100
Hepatovirus	**Hepatitis A virus (earlier called as Enterovirus 72)**

DIFFERENCES BETWEEN COXCASCKIE A abd B VIRUSES		
	A	B
Pathological changes induced by inoculation of suckling mice	Generalised myositis Flaccid paralysis Death within one week	Patchy focal myositis Spastic paralysis Localized lesions in the liver, pancreas, myocardium
Number of types	23 (1-24 except 23)	6 (1-6)

Contd.

Contd.

	Acute haemorrhagic conjunctivitis is caused by Coxsackie virus A 24	Bornholms disease (Acute pleurodynia)
	Herpangina (Acute vesicular pharyngitis)	Diabetes mellitus (B4)

POLIOVIRUSES

Consists of three types (1-3) based on neutralization tests.

Type 1: Epidemic.

Type 2: Endemic infections (Mostly antigenic).

Type 3: Vaccine associated paralysis.

Natural infections occurs only in man.

Spread by faeco-oral route and droplet infection.

Pathogenesis

Virus multiplies in the tonsils and peyer's patches → spread to regional lymph nodes (cervical, mesenteric) → viraemia → disseminated throughout the body including spinal cord and brain.

Clinical Features

- **Inapparent infection:** 90-95% of individuals.
- **Minor illness/abortive poliomyelitis:** Influenza like illness, 4-8%.
- **Non-paralytic poliomyelitis:** Headache, neck stiffness, back pain, complete recovery; 1-2%.
- **Paralytic poliomyelitis:** Flaccid paralysis, may be spinal, bulbar or bulbospinal; <1%.Q

Laboratory Diagnosis

Isolation: Tissue culture, CPE: cell retraction, cytoplasmic granularity, nuclear pyknosis.

Prophylaxis

Inactivated polio (Salk) vaccine.

Live attenuated polio (Sabin) vaccine.

RHINOVIRUSES

- Differentiated from the enteroviruses by their acid lability (therefore not able to infect intestinal tract) and their optimal temperature for replication (33°C).
- **Consist of more than 100 serotypes.**
- Most important cause of common cold (>50% of common colds).
- Infection transmitted by droplet infection.

RHABDOVIRIDAE

- **Bullet shaped,** 75 × 180 nm, single stranded RNA, linear, non-segmented, negative-sense, enveloped.
- Two genera:
  - **Vesiculovirus:** Infections in animals.
  - **Lyssavirus: Rabies virus.**

RABIES VIRUS

- Pathogenesis.
- Rabies is a natural infection of dogs, foxes, wolves etc.

ANIMAL SUSCEPTIBILITY TO RABIES			
Very high	**High**	**Moderate**	**Low**
Foxes Jackals Wolves	Hamsters Raccoons Cats Bats Rabbits Cattle	Dogs Sheeps Goats Horses Nonhuman primates	Opossums

- **Man acquires infection** by the bite of the rabid dog or other animals.
- Rarely infection can occur following licks on abraded skin and intact mucosa.

Pathogenesis

- Bite of the animal results in deposition of rabies infected saliva in the muscle → virus replicates at the local site → infects peripheral nerves → **within the nerve fibers it travels along the axon towards the central nervous system (speed of 3 mm per hour)Q** → in central nervous system it multiplies and produces encephalitis → **virus then spreads outwards along the nerve trunks to various parts of the body including salivary glands** → **shed in saliva.**

Clinical Features

- **Incubation period: 1-2 months,** shorter in children and then in adults, shorter in persons bitten on the face or head than those bitten on the legs (related to the distance virus has to travel to reach brain).
- **Malaise, headche, fever, paraesthesia at the site of bite followed by anxiety, hyperactivity, aggression, convulsions, hydrophobia. Finally patient develops coma and death.**
- Disease once developed is always fatal in about 4-14 days.
- Virus is secreted in saliva, urine and other secretions; human to human transmission rare.

Immune Response

- **Rabies virus ascends to the brain along the nerves and does not come in contact with immune system. It is only after virus spreads from the CNS to different parts of the body that antibodies are formed.** By this time it is too late as irreversible damage of the neurons have already occurred.
- **Antibody is protective if it is present before exposure (pre-exposure vaccination) or after exposure (post-exposure vaccination or passive immunisation) thereby preventing the binding of the virus to the nerve fibres at the site of inoculation.**

Laboratory Diagnosis

- **Demonstration of Negri bodies (intracytoplasmic, round, oval, eosinophilic with basophilic inner granules) by Seller's stain.** Mainly found in **pyramidal cells of ammon's horn, purkinje cells of hippocampus, brainstem, and cerebellum.Q**
- Demonstration of antigen by direct immunofluorescence.

  Antemortem diagnosis: Salivary, corneal smears, skin biopsy from nape of the neck.

  Postmortem diagnosis: Impression smears of cut surface of salivary glands, hippocampus, brainstem and cerebellum.

  - Detection of genomic RNA or viral mRNA: PCR, DNA probes.
  - **Virus isolation:** Mouse inoculation: Suckling mouse.
  - **Cell culture:** No CPE, detection by fluorescent antibody staining.
  - **Serology:** In CSF and serum by CFT, ELISA.

RABIES VACCINES

- **Neural vaccines**
  - Pasteur vaccine.
  - Fermi vaccine.
  - Semple vaccine.
  - Beta-propiolactone vaccine.
  - Suckling mouse brain vaccine.
- **Non-neural vaccine**
  - Duck egg vaccine.
  - Cell culture vaccine.
  - **First generation vaccine.**

    Human diploid cell vaccine (HDCV).
  - **Second generation vaccine:**

    Purified chick embryo cell vaccine (PCEC).

    Purified vero cell rabies vaccine (PVRV).

ARBOVIRUSES: TOGAVIRIDAE, FLAVIVIRIDAE, BUNYAVIRIDAE

Family	Genus	Important species
Togaviridae	Alpha virus	Chikungunya, Western equine encephalitis, eastern equine encephalitis
Flaviviridae	Flavivirus	Japanese encephalitis, Dengue, Yellow fever, KFD
Bunyaviridae	Bunyavirus	California encephalitis virus
	Nairo	Crimean congo haemorrhagic fever, Ganjam virus
	Hanta virus	Hantaan, seoul, Puumala virus
Reoviridae	Orbivirus	Colorado tick fever

Aedes aegypti	Yellow fever, Dengue, Rift valley fever, Chikungunya.
Culex	Bancroftian filariasis, Enecephalitis, West Nile fever, Arthritis like feature.
Tick	KFD, Crimean congo haemorrhagic fever, Colorado tick fever.
Sand fly	Sandfly fever, Rift valley fever.

JAPANESE ENCEPHALITIS

- Discovered in Japan and named Japanese 'B' encephalitis.
- Russia, Japan, China, India (Gorakhpur district, West Bengal, Bihar) are affected.

  Transmitted by Culex tritaeniorhynchus C. vishnui–India
- All ages; children in highly endemic areas.
- **Clinical features:** Abrupt onset and symptoms of fever, headache and vomiting. After 1-6 days encephalitis characterised by neck rigidity, convulsions, altered sensorium and coma appear.
- Cases fatality rate: 20–50%.
- Reservoir: Adreid (wading) birds.
- Amplifying hosts: Pigs (abortion), bats, horses (encephalitis).
- Incidental hosts: Humans, others.

  Killed vaccine **(Nakayama)** is employed to provide immunisation.

DENGUE

- DEN 4 serotypes: 1,2,3,4.
- Aedes aegypti mosquito: Vector.
- **Mixed infection: Antibody dependent enhancement (ADE).Q**
  1. **Dengue fever (DF):** Biphasic (Saddle back), Breakbone fever, LN↑Maculopapular rash.
  2. Dengue Hemorrhagic Fever (DHF).
  3. Dengue Shock Syndrome (DSS).

Factors Determining the Outcome

- Presence of enhancing and non-neutralizing antibodies:
  - Nutritional status—Malnutrition is protective.
  - **Sequence of infection**—For example, serotype 1 followed by serotype 2 seems to be more dangerous.
  - **Infecting serotype**—Type 2 is apparently more dangerous.

Criteria for Diagnosis of Dengue Hemorrhagic Fever (DHF)

- **Fever**–Acute, high, continuous for 2-7 days.
- **Positive Tourniquest test**–Petechial spot >20 per square inch in cubital.
- Enlargement of liver.
- **Laboratory evidence:**
  - Thrombocytopenia (< 100,000/mm^3).
  - Haemoconcentration (Haematocrit raised by >20%).
- **Criteria for diagnosis of Dengue Shock Syndrome (DSS):**

  All the above criteria of DHF, plus
- **Shock**–Manifested with rapid and weak pulse with narrow pulse pressure (<20 mm Hg) or hypotension with presence of cold, clammy skin and restlessness.

Yellow Fever Virus

- Endemic–West Africa and Central South America.
- Reservoir:
  - Forest–Monkey and forest mosquito (other Aedes spp).
  - Urban–Cases urban mosquito Aedes aegypti.

Don't Exist In India–because:

- Aedes aegypti is present in East coast area in India (whereas YF is endemic in West Africa).
- Strict vigilance and Quarantine for the travellers.
- Cross reacting Dengue antibody provides protection.

Incubation period–*3-6 days.*

- Clinical feature–Hemorrhages, Fever, Platelet dysfunction, Relative bradycardia, Jaundice.
- ***Torres*** bodies (intranuclear inclusion body).
- 17D Live attenuated vaccine:
  - Prepared in India (CRI, Kasauli).
  - Chick embryo, no risk of encephalitis.
  - Cholera and YF vaccine shouldn't be given together **(REMEMBER).**

  Now: Life long validity of vaccine.
- **Measures in airport:**
  - Unprotected travelers – 6 days quarantine.
  - Aedes aegypti index <1 400 mt surrounding airport.Q

Kyasanur Forest Disease

- Hemorrhagic fever, sudden onset headache, vomiting with severe prostration.
- Case fatality is around 5%.
- Tick borne (Haemaphysalis spinigera).
- Discovered in Kyasanur Forest in Shimoga District, Karnataka as a fatal epizootic affecting monkeys.

CHIKUNGUNYA

- ("that which bends up"), rural areas of Africa and Asia (India).
- Adults: Fever, rash (trunk and limbs), LN↑, Migratory polyarthritis.
- Differ from Dengue:
  - Hemorrhagic manifestations rare.
  - Chikungunya outbreaks are shorter.
- Vector: Aedes aegypti.
- 1964 outbreak: Africa, India (Vellore, Pondicherry, Chennai).
- 1973-2005: No outbreaks.

Re-emerged in 2005 – Hyderabad, Karnataka, Maharashtra.

Hemorrhagic Virus (Non Arthropod Borne)

Hantavirus leads to:

- HF with renal syndrome.
- Hanta pulmonary syndrome.
- Both of these are Rodent borne (Most common route–inhalation from rodent excreta).Q

RETROVIRIDAE

- Spherical, 80-100 nm, cylindric core, single stranded RNA, linear, positive sense, diploid, enveloped. Reverse transcriptase enzyme makes DNA copy from genomic RNA.

HUMAN RETROVIRUSES			
Subfamily	**Genus**	**Virus**	**Disease**
Oncovirinae	Retrovirus	HTLV1	Adult T cell leukemia
		HTLV2	Infection in intravenous drug users, not associated with any disease
Lentivirinae	Lentivirus	HIV1 HIV2	AIDS AIDS
Spumavirinae	Spumavirus	Human foamy virus	Not associated with any disease

HUMAN IMMUNODEFICIENCY VIRUSES

Two Antigenic Types HIV1 and HIV2

DIFFERENCES BETWEEN HIV1 AND HIV2		
	HIV1	HIV2
Related to	Chimpanzee simian immunodeficiency virus	Sooty mangabay simian immunodeficiency virus
Geographical distribution	Worldwide	West Africa
Virulence	More virulent	Less virulent
Envelope antigens • Spike antigen • Transmembrane pedicle antigen	 gp120 gp 41	 gp140 gp 36
Matrix protein antigen	p17	p16
Capsid protein antigen	p24	p26
Groups and subtypes	Divided into three groups: M (major), N (new), O (outlier) M comprises 8 subtypes or clades (A,B,C,D,F,H,J) O comprises 9 subtypes India most common: C Western countries: B	5 subtypes (A-E)

- The genome of HIV contains three major genes:
  - **Gag** (group-specific antigen): Codes for capsid and matrix proteins.
  - **Pol** (polymerase): Codes for reverse transcriptase.
  - **Env** (envelope): Codes for envelope peplomer and transmembrane protein.

Modes of Transmission:

ROUTE	EFFICACY
Blood transfusion	>90%
Perinatal	30%
Sexual intercourse • Anal • Vaginal	(0.1% to 1%) 1% per episode 0.1% per episode
Needle stick injury	0.5-1%

- **In India most common mode of transmission is by heterosexual route.**

Pathogenesis

AIDS is a unique sexually transmitted disease without local genital manifestations at any time during the infection but with grave systemic manifestations.

Infection of resident macrophages and submucosal lymphocytes in the genital tract or rectum → virus transported to draining lymph nodes → replication → after 2-3 weeks viraemia → fall in CD4+ T cells, glandular like fever → within one month viraemia declines and illness subsides → followed by long asymptomatic period, average 10 years → low titres present in blood, but high level in lymph nodes → slow destruction of CD4+ T cells → when count falls below 400/μl, person becomes susceptible to opportunistic infections and cancers → death due to opportunistic infections and malignancy.

OPPORTUNISTIC INFECTIONS AND MALIGNANCIES ASSOCIATED WITH HIV INFECTION
Bacterial M. tuberculosis (disseminated/extrapulmonary), M. avium complex Salmonella (recurrent septicaemia)
Viral Cytomegalovirus, Herpes simplex virus, Varicella-zoster virus, Epstein-Barr virus, Human herpes virus 6, Human herpes virus 8
Fungal Candidiasis, Cryptococcosis, Aspergillosis, Pneumocystis carinii pneumonia
Parasitic Toxoplasmosis, Cryptosporidiosis, Isosporiasis, Microsporidiosis, Generalized strongyloidiasis
Malignancies Kaposi's sarcoma, B cell lymphoma, Non-Hodgkin's lymphoma

Laboratory Diagnosis

- **Screening (E/R/S) tests**
  - ELISA.
  - Rapid tests: Time less than 30 minutes, donot require expensive equipment, but more expensive per test than ELISA.
  - Dot blot assay.
  - HIV spot and Coomb test.
  - * **Simple tests:** Time 1-2 hours, donot require expensive equipment.
- **Supplemental tests:**
  - Western blot assay.
  - Immunofluorescence test.
- **Confirmatory tests:**
  - Virus isolation.
  - Detection of p24 antigen.
  - Detection of viral nucleic acid: In situ hybridization, PCR.

Strategies for HIV Testing

Strategy I: The serum is tested with one E/R/S test and if reactive, sample is considered positive and if nonreactive it is considered negative. Used for testing blood for transfusion.

Strategy II: The serum reactive with one E/R/S test is retested with a second E/R/S test based on **different antigen or different test principle.** If found reactive on second test it is reported as positive, otherwise negative. Used for **HIV surveillance.**

Strategy III: The serum reactive with two E/R/S tests is retested with third E/R/S. The third test should be of different antigen system and of different principle. A serum reactive in all three tests is considered as positive while serum sample non-reactive in third E/R/S test is considered equivocal/borderline. **Such individuals should be retested after three weeks.** Used for diagnosis of HIV infection in an individual case.

HEPATITIS VIRUSES

- Cause systemic disease primarily involving liver.

Caused by

- Hepatitis A virus.
- Hepatitis B virus.
- Hepatitis C virus.
- Hepatitis D virus.
- Hepatitis E virus.

Other viruses that can cause sporadic hepatitis are:

- Yellow fever virus.
- Cytomegalovirus.
- Epstein-Barr virus.
- Herpes simplex virus.
- Enteroviruses.

HEPATITIS VIRUSES

Feature	HAV	HBV	HCV	HDV	HEV
Incubation (days)	15-45, mean 30 days	30-180, mean 60-90 days	15-160, mean 50 days	30-180, mean 60-90 days	14-60, mean 40 days
Onset	Acute	Insidious or acute	Insidious	Insidious or acute	Acute
Age preference	Children, young adults	Young adults (sexual and percutaneous), babies toddlers	Any age, but more common in adults	Any age (similar to HBV)	Young adults (20-40 years)
Transmission					
Feco-oral	+++	-	-	-	+++
Percutaneous	Unusual	+++	+++	+++	-
Perinatal	-	+++	±	+	-
Sexual	±	++	±	++	-
Clinical					
Severity	Mild	Occasionally severe	Moderate	Occasionally severe	Mild

Contd.

Fulminant	0.1%	0.1-1%	0.1%	5-20%	1-2%
Progression to chronicity	None	Occasional (1-10%) (90% of neonates)	Common (85%)	Common	None
Carrier	None	0.1-30%	1.5-3.2%	Variable	None
Cancer	None	+ (Neonatal infection)	+	±	None
Prognosis	Excellent	Worse with age, debility	Moderate	Acute-good chronic - poor	Good
Prophylaxis	IG, inactivated vaccine	HBIG, recombinant vaccine	None	HBV vaccine (none for HBV carriers)	Vaccine
Therapy	None	Interferon Lamivudine Adefovir Pegylated interferon Entecavir	Pegylated interferon Plus ribavirin Teleprevir Boceprevir	Infection ±	None

HEPATITIS A VIRUS

- Member of **Picornaviridae.**
- Previously classified **as Enterovirus 72.**
- Now assigned to new genus Hepatovirus. 27 nm, icosahedral, linear, single stranded RNA, linear, positive polarity, non-enveloped.
- Only one serotype exists.
- One of the most stable viruses infecting humans.
- Only one of the human hepatitis viruses that can be cultivated in vitro.Q

Pathogenesis

- Virus is shed in the stools of infected persons.
- Infection is transmitted by faeco-oral route.Q
- First multiplies in the intestinal epithelial cells → spreads to the liver via blood.
- Accounts for 25% of acute hepatitis cases worldwide.

Clinical Features

- Acute self-limiting disease, I.P.: 2-6 weeks.Q
- Abrupt onset with fever, malaise, anorexia, nausea, lethargy followed by jaundice and hepatomegaly.
- Less than 0.1% cases develop fulminant hepatitis.Q
- Complete recovery in 8-12 weeks.
- Severity of the disease varies with the age:
  - 5% children < 3 years develop jaundice.
  - >50% of the adults develop jaundice.
- No extra hepatic manifestation, no carrier state.
- Not associated with cirrhosis/heptaocellular carcinoma.

Laboratory Diagnosis

- Raised AST and ALT.
- Demonstration of virus particles: Immunoelectron microscopy.
- Antigen detection: ELISA.
- Serology: IgM antibodies, ELISA.
- Isolation: Tissue culture.
- Nucleic acid detection: PCR.

Prophylaxis: Killed vaccine available.

HEPATITIS B VIRUS

- Family: Hepadnaviridae.
- Consists of Hepatitis viruses of humans (HBV) and animals.

Morphology

Hepatitis B virus/Dane particle: 42 nm, envelop contains hepatitis B surface antigen (HBsAg). It encloses an inner icosahedral 27 nm nucleocapsid.

It contains Hepatitis B core antigen. Inside the core is the genome of HBV and DNA-dependent DNA-polymerase.

HBV genome: 3.2 Kbp molecule of circular dsDNA. The plus strand is incomplete leaving 15-50% of the molecule single stranded. The minus strand is complete and contains four overlapping open reading frames.

HBV has four genes S,C,P and X

P gene: Codes for DNA polymerase. It has three distinct enzymatic activities:

- DNA polymerase.
- Reverse transcriptase.
- RNaseH.

S gene: Codes for protein which occurs in three forms:

- Large protein: Translated from pre-S1, pre-S2 and S region; present in the infectious virion.
- Middle sized protein: Translated from pre-S2 and S region.
- Small sized protein: Translated from S region (most commonly found). Basic constituent of non-infectious HBsAg particles.

C gene: Has two initiation sites that divide it into a pre-C and C region producing two distinct proteins HBe Ag (secreted from the virus) and HbcAg (not secreted) respectively.Q

X gene codes for HBxAg, it may be involved in carcinogenesis.

Morphological Forms

- **Mature infectious virion**/Dane particle: 47 nm diameter.
- **Spherical particle:** 22 nm diameter composed of HBsAg, non-infectious (Most common).
- **Elongated tubules:** 22 nm diameter, length variable, composed of HBsAg, non-infectious.

Antigenic Structure

- **Group specific antigen 'a'.**
- **Two type specific antigens: d or y/w or r.**
- **Four antigenic types: adw, adr, ayw, ayr.**
- Most common subtype in India: **ayw;** Western countries: **adw.**

Cultivation: HBV has not been cultivated in the laboratory.Q

Pathogenesis

Three main modes of transmission:

- **Parenteral**
  - Accidental inoculation of body fluids during medical, surgical, dental procedures, intravenous drug abusers, blood transfusion.
- **Perinatal**
  - Prenatal: Transplacental.
  - Perinatal: Contamination of mucous membranes of the baby with maternal blood.
  - Post natal: Breastfeeding.
  - 90% of the babies infected at birth become chronic carriers as compared to 10% of those infected after the age of 6 years.
- **Sexual.**

Clinical Features

- **Prodromal (preicteric phase): I.P.:** 6 weeks to 6 months. Malaise, anorexia, nausea, vomiting.
- **Icteric phase: 2 days to 2 weeks** after prodromal phase. Jaundice, pale stools, dark urine.
- Convalescent phase: Malaise and fatigue lasting for several weeks.

Outcome of Infection:

- **<1% of icteric cases develop fulminant hepatitis.**
- **90-95% recover without sequelae.**
- **5-10% develops chronic hepatitis which can lead to development of cirrhosis and hepatocellular carcinoma.**
  Carriers: Persistence of HBsAg in the serum for more than six months.

Chronic Active Hepatitis	Chronic Persistent Hepatitis
Replicative phase	Non-replicative phase
HbeAg+	HbeAg-
Anti-HbeAg-	Anti-HBeAg-
DNA exists in the free form in the hepatocyte	DNA integrated into host genome
Intact virions presenting the circulation	No intact virions present in the circulation
More infectious	Less infectious

Laboratory Diagnosis

- Elevated AST, ALT.
- Raised serum bilirubin.

SEROLOGICAL MARKERS OF HEPATITIS B INFECTION

HBsAg	Anti-HBsAg	HBeAg	Anti-HbeAg	Anti-HBcAg		Interpretation
				IgM	IgG	
+	-	+	-	-	-	Incubation period
+	-	+	-	+	-	Acute hepatitis
+	-	+	-	-	+	Chronic active hepatitis
+	-	-	+	-	+	Chronic persistent hepatitis
-	+	-	-	-	+	Past infection
-	+	-	-	-	-	Vaccination

- Epidemiological marker of HBV infection: IgG-Anti-HbcAg.
- Surrogate marker of HBV replication: HbeAg.

Prophylaxis

- Passive immunization: HBIG.
- Active immunization:
  - Plasma derived hepatitis B vaccine.
  - Recombinant yeast derived hepatitis B vaccine.
  - Recombinant Chinese hamster ovary cell hepatitis vaccine.

  Schedule is (0,1 and 6 months) and dose is 0.5 ml and for above 20 years dose is 1 ml.

HEPATITIS C VIRUS

- Belongs to **family Flaviviridae.**
- Placed in separate genus: Hepacivirus.
- 30-60 nm, spherical, single standed RNA, positive sense, enveloped.
- Classified into 11 genotypes based on heterogeneity of nucleotide sequence.

Pathogenesis

Three main modes of transmission:

- **Parenteral**
  - Accidental inoculation of body fluids during medical, surgical, dental procedures, intravenous drug abusers, blood transfusion.
- **Perinatal**
  - Prenatal: Transplacental.
  - Perinatal: Contamination of mucous membranes of the baby with maternal blood.
  - Post natal: Breastfeeding.
- **Sexual.**

Clinical Features

- Incubation period: 15-150 days.
- About 75% infections sub-clinical.
- Acute infection as compared to HBV infection is less severe, shorter duration of prodromal phase, milder symptoms. >85% cases of acute infection develop chronic disease.Q
- Fulminant infection: 0.1%.
- Patients with chronic disease **may later on develop cirrhosis and hepatocellular carcinoma.**

Prophylaxis

- No vaccine available currently.

HEPATITIS D VIRUS

- Defective virus requiring help from HBV (HBV necessary for the production of HDV virions) Spherical, 36-38 nm, HBsAg coat, HDAg nucleocapsid, single, circular RNA, minus strand.
- Genus: Delta virus.

Pathogenesis

- Parenteral.
- Perinatal.
- Sexual.

Two Types of Infection

- **Coinfection:** Simultaneous infection with HBV, HDV. Most commonly results from parenteral transmission. Infection more severe than HBV alone. IgM-Anti-HBcAg+.
- **Super infection:** Infection of HBV carrier with HDV. **Commoner and more serious** than coinfection (as liver function already compromised by HBV infection). Develops into fulminant infection. IgG-Anti-HBcAg+, IgM Anti HDV.

Laboratory Diagnosis

- HDAg detection: ELISA.
- HDV RNA detection: PCR.
- IgM Anti-HDV detection: ELISA.

Prophylaxis

- Prevention of infection with HBV.

HEPATITIS E VIRUS

- Belongs to **Family Caliciviridae.**
- Spherical, 27-38 nm, single stranded, positive sense RNA.

Pathogenesis

Ingestion of contaminated drinking water.

Virus first identified in New Delhi, India in 1955.

Clinical Features

- **I.P.: 2-8 weeks.**
- Disease resembles that produced by Hepatitis A virus.

  Fulminant infection: 1-2% in general population; 10-20% in pregnant women.

  Does not progress to chronic infection, cirrhosis or hepatocellular carcinoma.

Laboratory Diagnosis

- Demonstration of virus particles: **Immunoelectron microscopy.**
- **Antigen detection:** ELISA.
- **Serology:** IgM antibodies, ELISA.
- Nucleic acid detection: PCR.

FILOVIRIDAE

- Long filamentous virus 80 nm × 1000 nm, enveloped, single stranded, **negative sense RNA.**
  - Marburg virus.
  - Ebola virus.

Pathogenesis

Highly virulent infection, invariably fatal.

Transmitted to man from primates by aerosols rarely, direct contact with blood, body fluids etc.Q

Clinical Features

- **I.P.:** 3-15 days, patient develops headache, fever, myalgia, severe haemorrhages and hypotension.

Laboratory Diagnosis

- Demonstration of virus: Electron microscopy.

- Isolation.
- Serology: Immunofluorescence.

ARENAVIRIDAE

- **Sandy appearance on electron microscopy** (Arena means sand), due to the incorporation of the host cell ribosomes during assembly.
- 10-130 nm, pleomorphic, **single strand RNA, negative sense,** two segments, enveloped.
  Natural hosts are the rodents in which they cause persistent infection with viraemia. Virus is shed in the urine.

DISEASES CAUSE BY VIRUSES IN THE FAMILY ARENAVIRIDAE		
Virus	**Geographical distribution**	**Human disease**
Lymphocytic choriomeningitis	Worldwide	Influenza-like illness, aseptic meningitis, rarely encephalomyelitis
Lassa	West Africa	Hemorrhagic fever
Junin	Argentina	Argentine hemorrhagic fever
Machupo	Bolivia	Bolivian hemorrhagic fever
Guanarito	Venezuela	Venezuelan hemorrhagic fever

REOVIRIDAE

- Spherical virions, nonenveloped, segmented (10-12 segments), ds DNA.
- Medically important genera
  - Orthoreovirus: 10 segments.
  - Orbivirus: 10 segments.
  - Rotavirus: 11 segments.
  - Coltivirus: 12 segments.

COLTIVIRUS

- 2 serotypes.
- Causes **Colorado tick fever.**
- Transmitted by ticks.
- **I.P.:** 3-6 days; myalgia, headache, leucopenia, rash.
- **Complications:** Meningoencephalitis, haemorrhagic fever.

ORBIVIRUS

- 100 serotypes.
- Infections in animals; mild fevers in humans.

ORTHOREOVIRUS

- 3 serotypes.
- May be associated with enteritis in infants and children; upper respiratory tract infections, neonatal biliary atresia.

ROTAVIRUS

- **Divided into six groups (A-F) and 14 serotypes (9 human, 5 animal).**
- Most common cause of gastroenteritis in children below 2 years of age.
- Infection is transmitted by contaminated water and food.
- **I.P.: 1-2 days,** vomiting, diarrhea, dehydration.

Laboratory Diagnosis

- Antigen detection: Latex agglutination, passive haemagglutination, ELISA.Q
- Detection of virus: Electron microscopy, immunoelectron microscopy.

VIRUSES ASSOCIATED WITH ACUTE GASTEROENTERITIS IN HUMANS	
Rotavirus	
Group A	Single most important cause (viral or bacterial) of endemic severe diarrheal illness in infants and young children worldwide
Group B	Outbreaks of diarrheal illness in adults and children in China
Group C	Outbreaks of diarrheal illness in children
Enteric adenoviruses	Second most important viral agent of endemic diarrheal illness in infants and young children worldwide
Norwalk virus and Norwalk like viruses 27 nm, single stranded RNA, positive sense, non-enveloped	Important cause of outbreaks of vomiting and diarrheal illness in older children and adults in families, communities, institutions; frequently associated with ingestion of food
Calciviruses 27-38 nm, single stranded RNA, positive sense, non-enveloped	Sporadic cases and outbreaks of diarrheal illness in infants, young children and adults
Astroviruses 30 nm, nonenvelped, RNA viruses	Sporadic cases and outbreaks of diarrheal illness in infants, young children and adults

ONCOGENIC VIRUSES

ONCOGENIC VIRUSES ASSOCIATED WITH HUMAN NEOPLASIA		
DNA viruses		
Papovaviridae	Human papilloma virus	Genital tumors, sqamous cell carcinoma
Herpesviridae	Epstein-Barr virus	Nasopharyngeal carcinoma Burkitt's lymphoma B cells lymphoma Hodgkin's disease
	Herpes Simplex Virus 1 and 2	
	Cytomegalovirus	
	Human Herpes Virus 8	Kaposi's sarcoma
Hepadnaviridae	HBV	Hepatocellular carcinoma
Poxviridae	Molluscipoxvirus	Molluscum contagiosum
RNA viruses		
Retroviridae	HTLV1	Adult T cell leukaemia
Flaviviridae	HCV	Hepatocellular carcinoma

Viral Carcinogenesis

1. Viruses can cause cancer in animals and humans.
2. Tumor viruses frequently establish persistent infections in natural hosts.
3. Host factors are important determinants of virus-induced tumorigenesis.
4. Viruses are seldom complete carcinogens.
5. Virus infections are more common than virus-related tumor formation.
6. Long latent periods usually elapse between initial virus infection and tumor appearance.
7. Viral strains may differ in oncogenic potential.
8. Viruses may be either direct- or indirect-acting carcinogenic agents.

9. Oncogenic viruses modulate growth control pathways in cells.
10. Animal models may reveal mechanisms of viral carcinogenesis.
11. Viral markers are usually present in tumor cells.
12. One virus may be associated with more than one type of tumor.

PRIONS

- Proteinaceous infectious particles.

Diseases of Humans

• **K**uru. • **C**reutzfeldt-Jacob disease. • **G**erstmann-Straussler-Scheinker syndrome. • **F**amilial fatal insomnia.	KFC gaya

Diseases of Animals

• **S**crapie of sheep and goats. • **B**ovine spongiform encephalopathy of cattle. • **M**ink and feline encephalopathy. • **W**asting disease of deer.	Scrap BMW

MCQs

General Virology

1. Virus quantification is done by: *(Recent MCQ)*
(a) Egg inoculation (b) Hemadsorption
(c) Plaque assay (d) Electron microscopy

2. Human fibroblast cell line is used for cultivation of: *(Recent MCQ)*
(a) Adeno (b) Polio
(c) CMV (d) Measles

3. Both intranuclear and cytoplasmic inclusion is seen in: *(Recent MCQ)*
(a) Pox virus (b) Herpes virus
(c) Measles virus (d) Mumps virus

4. Live attenuated vaccine are all *except*: *(Recent MCQ)*
(a) Measles (b) Rabies
(c) Oral polio (d) Yellow fever
(e) Influenza

5. Viral infection that is least transmitted transplacentally: *(Recent MCQ)*
(a) Hepatitis B (b) Rubella
(c) Herpes simplex (d) HIV

6. Latency seen in viral infections of: *(PGI Dec 2008)*
(a) HSV-II (b) CMV
(c) Rotavirus (d) HIV
(e) EBV

7. **All the following vaccines are developed from embryonated eggs *except*:**
   (a) Influenza (b) Hepatitis A
   (c) Yellow fever (d) Rabies
   (e) CMV
8. **DNA covering material in a virus is called as:** *(PGI 96)*
   (a) Capsomere (b) Capsid
   (c) Nucleocapsid (d) Envelop
9. **All of the following are general properties of viruses *except*:** *(AI 94)*
   (a) May contain both DNA and RNA (b) Form extracellular infectious particles
   (c) Heat labile (d) Not affected by antibodies
10. **Bollinger bodies are seen in:** *(NEET 13)*
   (a) Chickenpox (b) Cowpox
   (c) Fowlpox (d) Smallpox
11. **Appearance of cowdry type A inclusion bodies:** *(NEET 13)*
   (a) Granular (b) Circumscribed
   (c) In Polio (d) None
12. **All of the following are having lipid envelop *except*:** *(AMU 09)*
   (a) HIV (b) Rabies
   (c) Varicella (d) Enterovirus
13. **Lipid envelop is found in which virus?** *(PGI 2000)*
   (a) Reo (b) Herpes
   (c) Picorna (d) All of the above
14. **In which of the following has genome double standard nucleic acid?** *(PGI 10)*
   (a) Orthomyxovirures (b) Poxviruses
   (c) Parvoviruses (d) Reoviruses
15. **HPV belongs to:** *(NEET 12)*
   (a) Papovavirus (b) Parvovirus
   (c) Herpesvirus (d) Poxvirus
16. **Which of the following is not an RNA virus?** *(AIIMS 08)*
   (a) Ebola (b) Simian 40
   (c) Rabies (d) Vesicular stomatitis virus
17. **Non enveloped ss-RNA virus is:** *(NEET 12)*
   (a) Picornavirus (b) Poxvirus
   (c) Retrovirus (d) Bunyavirus
18. **Negative sense Nucleic acid genome is found in:** *(PGI 10)*
   (a) Poliovirus (b) Rabies
   (c) Measles (d) Picornavirus
   (e) Influenza
19. **Which of the following does not possess both RNA and DNA?** *(Kerala 99)*
   (a) Bacteria (b) Fungus
   (c) Virus (d) Spirochetes
20. **Segmented genome is found in:** *(AIIMS 98)*
   (a) Retrovirus (b) Rotavirus
   (c) Poliovirus (d) Rhabdovirus

21. Virus can be isolated from clinical samples by cultivation in the following *except*: *(AI 05)*

(a) Tissue culture
(b) Embryonated eggs
(c) Animals
(d) Defined media

22. Which of the following is a primary cell culture? *(NEET 13)*

(a) Chicken fibroblast (b) HeLa
(c) HEP-2 (d) HL-8

23. Which is not a cytopathic effective of virus? *(JIPMER 10)*

(a) Syncytium formation (b) Budding
(c) Ballooning and floating (d) Focal degeneration

24. Pocks on chick embryo are formed by all *except*: *(AIIMS 96)*

(a) Variola (b) Vaccinia
(c) Chickenpox (d) Cowpox

25. Lab diagnosis of viral respiratory tract infection can be established by all of the tests *except*: *(AI 10)*

(a) Detection of virus specific IgM Abs in single serum specimen
(b) Demonstration of viral Ag by indirect immunofluorescence assay in nasopharyngeal washing
(c) Isolation of virus using centrifugation enhanced culture
(d) Detection of viral Hemagglutination inhibiting (HAI) Abs in a single specimen

26. Reverse transcriptase PCR can aid in diagnostics of all of the following viral infections *except*: *(AI 09)*

(a) Adenovirus (b) Astrovirus
(c) Rotavirus (d) Poliovirus

27. Vaccine preparation requires which virus as vector? *(PGI 08)*

(a) Rhinovirus (b) Vaccinia
(c) Adenovirus (d) Ebola
(e) Hepatitis B

28. Susceptible cultured cells infected with which of the following viruses would exhibit hemadsorption with the appropriate erythrocyte? *(AIIMS 15)*

(a) Sindbis virus (b) Rabies virus
(c) Measles virus (d) Respiratory syn. virus

29. Property of elution is found in:

(a) Myxovirus (b) Togavirus
(c) Parvovirus (d) Adenovirus

30. One virus particle prevents multiplication of second virus, this phenomena is: *(UP 12)*

(a) Viral interference (b) Mutation
(c) Supervision (d) Permutation

31. Von Magnus phenomenon: *(MP 10)*

(a) Is a normal replicative cycle
(b) Virus yield has low Hemagglutination
(c) Virus has high infectivity
(d) Virus yields has high Hemagglutination low infectivity

32. Animal reservoir for swine influenza virus is: *(Karnataka 10)*

(a) Field mice (b) Urban rats
(c) Pigs (d) Calomys callosus

33. Basophilic inclusion bodies are seen in: *(JIPMER 10)*

(a) Adenovirus
(b) Polio virus
(c) Measles virus
(d) Herpesvirus

34. Coxsackie A virus causes all *except*: *(JIPMER 11)*

(a) Aseptic meningitis
(b) Herpangina
(c) Foot and mouth disease
(d) Bornbolm disease

35. Prions are killed by: *(DNB 12)*

(a) Autoclave
(b) Ethylene dioxide
(c) Gamma radiation
(d) Autoclave and NaOH

36. True about viroid is: *(DNB 13)*

(a) Cause tumors in animals
(b) Lack envelop like covering
(c) Have only genetic material
(d) Visible on light microscope

37. Bacteriophages are mostly needed for: *(AIIMS 97)*

(a) Bacterial identification
(b) Epidemiologically
(c) As antibacterial agent
(d) Conversion property in bacteria

38. All of the following statements are true about bacteriophages, *except*: *(AIIMS 08)*

(a) It is a virus which infect bacteria
(b) It helps in transduction of bacteria
(c) It imparts toxigenicity to bacteria
(d) It transfers only chromosomal gene

39. Phage typing is useful as an epidemiological tool in all, *except*: *(JIPMER 15)*

(a) Salmonella
(b) Staph aureus
(c) V. Cholerae
(d) Shigella dysenteriae

40. Phage typing is widely used for the intraspecies classification of one of the following bacteria:

(a) Staphylococci
(b) E. coli
(c) Kleb. pneumoniae
(d) Pseudomonas aeruginosa

ANSWERS AND EXPLANATIONS

General Virology

1. **Ans. is 'c'** i.e., Plaque assay (***Ref:*** *Ananthanarayan, 9th/e, p. 437, 8th/e, p. 436*)
   Assay of Infectivity of Viruses:
   - Quantal assay – End point biologic assay.
   - Quantitative infective assay – Plaque assay – Most widely used for infectious virus.
   - Monolayer of host cells are inoculated with suitable dilutions of virus, each infectious viral particle gives rise to localized focus of infected cells known as plaques.
2. **Ans. is 'c'** i.e., CMV (***Ref:*** *Ananthanarayan, 9th/e, p. 434, 8th/e, p. 433*)
   Human fibroblast cell line is used for cultivation of CMV.
3. **Ans. is 'c'** i.e., Measles virus (***Ref:*** *Ananthanarayan, 9th/e, p. 452*)
   Both intranuclear and cytoplasmic inclusions is seen in – Measles and CMV.
4. **Ans. is 'b'** i.e., Rabies (***Ref:*** *Ananthanarayan, 9th/e, p. 452*)
   Rabies (both neural and nonneural vaccine is an inactivated vaccine).
5. **Ans. is 'a'** i.e., Hepatitis B (***Ref:*** *Arora Microbiology, 3rd/e, p. 702*)
   Rubella and HSV are teratogenic virus, so their transplacental transmission is expected to be high, HIV have 30% transplacental transmission but HBV is least transmitted transpalcentally.
6. **Ans. are 'a', 'b', 'd'** and **'e'** i.e., HSVII, CMV, HIV, EBV
   Latent infections – defined as a state of infection in which the virus is not replicating, no demonstrable infectious virus between episodes of recurrent disease.

7. Ans. are 'b' and 'e' i.e., Hepatitis A, CMV (***Ref:*** *Ananthanarayan, 9th/e, p. 428, 442*)

Vaccine prepared in embryonated egg is (Yellow fever, Influenza and Rabies) and site of inoculation for all these vaccines is Allantoic sac.

DNA Viruses

All DNA viruses are **double-stranded** (except parvovirus); are **icosahedral** (except poxvirus which is a brick-shaped "complex"); and **replicate their DNA in the nucleus** (except poxvirus).

Virus Family	DNA type	Virion-Associated Polymerase	Envelope	DNA Replicates in	Major Viruses
Parvovirus	ssDNA	No	Naked	Nucleus	B19
Papillomavirus Polyomavirus	Ds DNA, circular	No	Naked	Nucleus	Papilloma, Polyoma
Adenovirus	dsDNA, linear	No	Naked	Nucleus	Adenoviruses
Hepadnavirus	Partially ds DNA, circular	Yes***	Enveloped	Nucleus, RNA intermediate	Hepatitis B
Herpes virus	dsDNA, linear	No	Enveloped (nuclear)	Nucleus; virus assembled in nucleus	HSV, Varicella-zoster, Epstein-Barr, Cytomega-lovirus
Poxvirus	dsDNA, linear	Yes**	Enveloped	Cytoplasm	Variola, Vaccinia, Mollus-cum contagionsum

* Mnemonic: Pardon Papa As He Has Pox

** Poxviruses have a virion-associated transcriptase (DNA dependent RNA polymerase), so it can transcribe its own DNA in the cytoplasm and make all of the enzymes and factors necessary for replication of the poxvirus DNA in the cytoplasm.

*** Hepadnaviruses: DNA viruses that carry a DNA polymerase with reverse transcriptase activity to synthesize an RNA intermediate that is then used to make the genomic DNA. Hepatitis B is partially double-stranded with one complete strand.

RNA Viruses (+ Stranded)

Virus Family	RNA Structure	Virion-Associated Polymerase	Envelope	Shape	Multiplies in	Major Viruses
Calicivirus	ss(+) RNA Linear	No polymerase	Naked	Icosahedral	Cytoplasm	Norwalk agent Noro-like virus
Hepesvirus	ss(+) RNA linear	No polymerase	Naked	Icosahedral	Cytoplasm	Hepatitis E
Picornavirus	ss(+) RNA Linear	No polymerase	Naked	Icosahedral	Cytoplasm	Pollo** ECHO Enteroviruses Rhino Coxsackie Hepatitis A
Flavivirus	ss(+) RNA Linear	No polymerase	Enveloped	Icosahedral	Cytoplasm	Yello fever Dengue St. Louis encephalitis Hepatitis C West Nile virus
Togavirus	ss(+) RNA Linear	No polymerase	Enveloped	Icosahedral	Cytoplasm	Rubella WEE, EEE Venezuelan encephalitis
Coronavirus	ss(+) Linear	No polymerase	Enveloped	Helical	Cytoplasm	Coronaviruses SARS-CoV
Retrovirus	Diploid ss(+) RNA Linear	RNA dep. DNA polymerase	Enveloped	Icosahedral or truncated conical	Nucleus	HIV HTLV Sarcoma

* Mnemonic: (+) RNA Viruses: **C**all **H**enry **P**ico and **Flo** **To** **Co**me **R**ightaway

** Mnemonic: Picornaviruses: **PEE Co Rn A** Viruses
Polio, **E**ntero, **E**cho, **Co**xsackie, **R**hi**n**o, Hep **A**

RNA Viruses (- Stranded)

Virus	RNA Structure	Virion-Associated Polymerase	Envelope	Shape	Multiplies in	Major Viruses
Paramyxovirus	ss(–) RNA Linear Non-segmented	Yes	Yes	Helical	Cytoplasm	Mumps Measles Respiratory syncytial Parainfluenza
Rhabdovirus	ss(–) RNA Linear Non-segmented	Yes	Yes	Helical, bullet-shaped	Cytoplasm	Rabies Vesicular stomatitis
Filovirus	ss(–) RNA Linear Non-segmented	Yes	Yes	Helical	Cytoplasm	Merburg Ebola
Orthomyxovirus	ss(–) RNA Linear 8 segmented	Yes	Yes	Helical	Cytoplasm and nucleus	Influenza
Bunyavirus	ss(–) RNA Pseudocircular, 3 segments, 1 is ambisense	Yes	Yes	Helical	Cytoplasm	California encephalitis La Crosse encephalitis Hantavirus
Arenavirus	ss(–) RNA Circular 2 segments 1 (–) sense 1 ambisense	Yes	Yes	Helical	Cytoplasm	Lymphocytic choriomeningitis Lassa fever

Mnemonic for ss(–) RNA viruses: Pain Results From Our Bunions Always. Gives them in order or size. Remember that these are the negative ones because pain is a negative thing. Another one: Bring a polymerase or fall replication.

Note that all are enveloped, all have virion-associated polymerase, and all have helical nucleocapsids. The oddballs are the last three:

- The orthomyxoviruses are linear (Ortho) but with 8 (ortho/octo) segments, which is one of the reasons they can genetically "mix" it up. The orthomyxoviruses are also odd in that they replicate in both the nucleus and cytoplasm.
- The bunyaviruses are somewhat contortionists (circular): California playboy bunnies in a ménage a trois?
- The arenaviruses have one negative sense and one ambisense strand of RNA.

8. **Ans. is 'b'** i.e., Capsid

   All viruses have a protein coat called a capsid that covers the genome. The capsid is composed of repeating subunits called capsomers. In some viruses, the capsid is the outer surface, but in other viruses, the capsid is covered with a lipoprotein envelope that becomes the outer surface. The structure composed of the nucleic acid genome and the capsid proteins is called the nucleocapsid.

9. **Ans. is 'a'** i.e., May contain both DNA and RNA

   Viruses contain either DNA or RNA, but not both.

10. **Ans. is 'c'** i.e., Fowlpox

    In fowlpox virus-infected epithelial cells, the large intracytoplasmic inclusion bodies are called Bollinger bodies and contain smaller elementary bodies (Borrel bodies). The inclusions appear red, are approximately 0.2–0.3 m in size and can be demonstrated in section of cutaneous lesions.

11. **Ans. is 'a'** i.e., Granular

    Inclusion bodies are aggregates of stainable substances in the nucleus or cytoplasm.

    Cowdry inclusion bodies are classified into two groups called type A and B.

    Type A included those (a) which were granular and (b) which produced a severe reaction in the cell leading to death.

    Type B were those (a) which were amorphous irregular masses or hyaline spheres and (b) which produced only mild reactions in the cell.

Viral inclusion bodies:

Intracytoplasmic:

1. Henderson-Peterson bodies in Molluscum Contagiosum.
2. Negri bodies in Rabies.
3. Guarnieri bodies (B type inclusion bodies) in Smallpox.

Intranuclear:

1. **Acidophilic**
    - Cowdry Type A.
        - Varicella Zoster Virus.
        - Herpes Simplex Virus.
        - Yellow Fever Virus (Torres bodies).
    - Cowdry Type B
        - Polio.
2. **Basophilic**
    1. Cowdry Type B – Adenovirus.
    2. Cytomegalovirus – Owl eye.

Intranuclear and Intracytoplasmic: Measles virus.

Inclusion Bodies in Red Blood Cells:

1. **Developmental**
    - Howell Jolly Bodies.
    - Basophilic Stipplings.
    - Pappenheimer Bodies.
    - Cabot Rings.
    - Polychromatophilic Red Cells.
2. **Hemoglobin Precipitates**
    - Heinz bodies.
    - Hemoglobin H inclusions.
3. **Protozoal**
    - Malaria.
    - Babesia.

Inclusion Bodies in Skin Conditions:

1. Asteroid bodies - Sporotrichosis.
2. Cowdry A - Herpes Simplex.
3. Donovan bodies - Granuloma Inguinale.
4. Dutcher bodies - Multiple Myeloma, Primary cutaneous marginal zone lymphoma.
5. Pustulo-ovoid bodies - Granular cell tumor.
6. Medlar bodies - Chromoblastomycosis.
7. Michaelis - Gutmann bodies - Malakoplakia.
8. Rocha Lima bodies - Verruga peruana.
9. Russell bodies - Multiple myeloma.
10. Rhinoscleroma bodies.
11. Verocay bodies - Schwannoma.
12. Virchow bodies - Leprosy.

Councilman Bodies:

Eosinophilic bodies found in the liver in the following cases:

1. Yellow Fever.
2. Acute Viral Hepatitis.
3. Viral Hemorrhagic Fever.

Dohle Bodies:

Dohle bodies are basophilic inclusions found in cytoplasm of neutrophils and are thought to be remnants of rough endoplasmic reticulum.

Dohle bodies are seen in:

1. Burns.
2. Infections.
3. Physical trauma.
4. Neoplastic diseases.
5. Wissler's disease.
6. May-Hegglin anomaly.
7. Chédiak-Steinbrinck-Higashi's syndrome.

12. Ans. is 'd' i.e.,Enterovirus

Already explained.

13. Ans. is 'b' i.e., Herpes

Already explained.

14. Ans. are 'b, d'

Poxviruses have genome consisting dsDNA (linear) and Viruses in the family **Reoviridae** have **genomes** consisting of segmented, double-stranded RNA (dsRNA).

15. Ans. is 'a' i.e., Papovavirus

A Papovavirus is any member of the former virus family of Papovaviridae. They are mainly associated with various neoplasms in mammals. The family of Papovaviridae is no longer used in recent taxonomy, but is split into the Papillomaviridae and the Polyomaviridae.

16. Ans. is 'b' i.e., Simian 40

SV40 is an abbreviation for Simian vacuolating virus 40 or Simian virus 40, a polyomavirus (DNA virus) that is found in both monkeys and humans.

17. Ans. is 'a' i.e., Picornavirus

Already explained.

18. Ans. are 'b, c, e'

Already explained.

19. Ans. is 'c' i.e., Virus

Already explained.

20. Ans. is 'b' i.e., Rotavirus

Rotavirus has segmented linear dsRNA genome.

Virus having segmented genome – (Mnemonic - **PARBO** virus)

P – Picornavirus

A – Arenaviridae

R – Reoviridae

B – Bunyaviridae

O – Orthomyxoviridae

21. Ans. is 'd' i.e., Defined media

Virus cannot be isolated or cultured on cell free media like Defined media. Defined media is used for culturing bacteria from clinical samples.

22. Ans. is 'a' i.e., Chicken fibroblast

The source of primary cultures is excised animal tissue that is cultured either as an explant culture, suspension or as monolayer and maintained in vitro. The excised tissue is subjected to enzyme treatment and the dissociated cells are cultured under the appropriate conditions in culture medium until they reach adequate numbers

The most popular primary cells used in research are epithelial cells, **fibroblasts**, keratinocytes, melanocytes, endothelial cells, muscle cells, hematopoietic and mesenchymal stem cells. The cultures are initially heterogeneous (represents a mixture of cell types present in the tissue) and can be maintained in vitro only for a limited period of time.

23. Ans. is 'b' i.e., Budding

Budding is not cytopathic effect; **it's a method of reproduction in yeast** like Cryptococcus species and candida species.

24. Ans. is 'c' i.e., Chickenpox

Quantitative assay of infectivity: Quantitative assay is used to estimate the presence of actual **number of viable infectious viral particles in the inoculum**. Two methods are available for the purpose, which include **plaque assay in monolayer cell culture** and **pock assay on chick embryo CAM.**

(a) **Plaque assay:** This is based on the principle that each infectious viral particle gives rise to a localized focus of infected cells that can be visualized by the naked eye. **Such foci are called *plaques,* and each plaque indicates an infectious virus. The test is performed by adding a viral inoculum to a monolayer of culture cells in a bottle or Petri dish.** After sometime, this allows adsorption of viruses.

(b) **Pock assay:** Viruses that form pocks on CAM can be assayed by counting the number of pocks formed on the inoculated CAM. Each pock on CAM arises from a single virus particle. This is known as pock assay. **Vaccinia and variola viruses can be assayed by pock assay.**

25. Ans. is 'd' i.e., Detection of viral Hemagglutination inhibiting (HAI) Abs in a single specimen

The nucleic acids of various viruses encode surface proteins that agglutinate the red blood cells (RBC) of a variety of species. For example; Influenza virus particles have an envelope protein called the hemagglutinin, or HA, which binds to erythrocytes, causing the formation of a lattice. This property is called **hemagglutination**.

Hemagglutination phenomenon is almost commonly used for diagnosis of infection produced by Orthomyxoviruses, paramyxoviruses, and the abroviruses-togaviruses (including rubella), flaviviruses and bunyaviruses.

The presence of virus in infected cell cultures can be detected by hemagglutination; the identity of the virus or of antibodies in a patient's serum can be determined by specific inhibition of that hemagglutination. Although influenza viruses can be detected by hemadsorption test, typing of the isolate is done most efficiently by hemagglutination inhibition (HAI). Reagents and conditions for the test vary by virus.

26. Ans. is 'a' i.e., Adenovirus

Adenoviruses are medium-sized, nonenveloped viruses with an icosahedral nucleocapsid containing a double stranded DNA genome. Their name derives from their initial isolation from human adenoids in 1953.

Reverse transcriptase PCR is used in detection of RNA viruses for various clinical specimens.

27. Ans. are 'b, c'

Vaccinia virus, a member of the poxvirus family, is a large, complex, enveloped virus. The virus is traditionally used for the smallpox vaccine, and its efficacy and safety have been demonstrated. During vaccine development, highly attenuated vaccinia virus strains have been generated, including replication-competent (LC16m8) and replication-deficient (NYVAC, ALVAC, TROVAC and MVA) strains. These strains are most frequently used for vaccinia virus vector production, although numerous strains of vaccinia virus exist in humans and animals.

Approximately 50 human adenovirus (Ad) serotypes have been identified. Among them, human Ad serotype 5 (Ad5) has been widely investigated as a gene delivery vector because it can be easily produced in high titers. **Recombinant Ad vectors are widely used** because of their high transduction efficiency, high level of transgene expression, and broad range of viral tropism. They can infect both dividing and non-dividing cells.

https://www.ncbi.nlm.nih.gov/pmc/articles/PMC4494222/

https://www.ncbi.nlm.nih.gov/pmc/articles/PMC3710930/

28. Ans. are 'b, c'

Hemadsorption is the process of adsorption of erythrocytes to the surfaces of infected cells which serves as an indirect measurement of viral protein synthesis. Viruses, such as **influenza virus, parainfluenza virus, mumps**

virus, Measles and Togavirus, when infect cell lines code for the expression of red cell agglutinins, which are expressed on the infected cell membrane during infections. These hemagglutinins bind some erythrocytes to the infected cell surface. Sometimes, viruses can be detected by agglutination of erythrocytes in the culture medium.

Chicken embryo cells infected with the HEP Flury strain of rabies virus adapted to tissue culture produced a hemadsorption (HAD) phenomenon by using goose erythrocytes. Used for determining virus and neutralizing antibody titers of rabies.

29. **Ans. is 'a'** i.e., Myxovirus

Property of elution (reversal of hemagglutinin due to presence of neuraminidase that destroys receptor) is shown by Myxovirus.

30. **Ans. is 'a'** i.e., Viral interference

Interference denotes inhibition of growth of one virus in a host cell when it is simultaneously infected with another virus. Interferon is the most important mediator of interference. Autointerference is another type of interference, in which a high multiplicity of infection inhibits production of infectious progeny. **In contrast, mixed infections sometimes increase the yield of one virus and produce well-marked cytopathic effects in the cell lines. This phenomenon is called enhancement.**

31. **Ans. is 'd'** i.e., Virus yields has high Hemagglutination low infectivity

Incomplete viruses: Due to defect during assembly of viral components, some of the daughter virions that are produced may not be infective. Example of such incomplete virus is the influenza virus that shows a high Hemagglutination titer but with a low infectivity. This is known as **von Magnus phenomenon.**

32. **Ans. is 'c'** i.e., Pig

Pigs can be infected with both human and avian influenza viruses in addition to swine influenza viruses. Infected pigs exhibit signs of illness similar to humans, such as cough, fever and runny nose. Because pigs are susceptible to avian, human and swine influenza viruses, they potentially may be infected with influenza viruses from different species (e.g., ducks and humans) at the same time. If this happens, it is possible for the genes of these viruses to mix and create a new virus.

33. **Ans. is 'a'** i.e., Adenovirus

Already explained in Ans. No. 11.

34. **Ans. is 'd'** i.e., Bornholm disease

Bornholm disease or epidemic pleurodynia, Devils grip or epidemic myalgia is a disease caused by the Coxsackie B virus or other viruses.

The **main symptom of Bornholm disease** is severe stabbing chest pain, which is often made worse by deep breathing, coughing, or sudden movements. The pain tends to come and go, with episodes lasting 15-30 minutes. Bornholm disease sometimes also causes tummy pain, fever, headache, sore throat and muscle pain.

35. **Ans. is 'd'** i.e., Autoclave and NaOH

Prions can be destroyed by one of these four options:

Option 1. Autoclave at 134°C for 18 minutes in a prevacuum sterilizer.

Option 2. Autoclave at 132°C for 1 hour in a gravity displacement sterilizer.

Option 3. Immerse in 1 N NaOH (1 N NaOH is a solution of 40 g NaOH in 1 L water) for 1 hour; remove and rinse in water, then transfer to an open pan and autoclave (121°C gravity displacement sterilizer or 134°C porous prevacuum sterilizer) for 1 hour.

Option 4. Immerse in 1 N NaOH for 1 hour and heat in a gravity displacement sterilizer at 121°C for 30 minutes, then clean and subject to routine sterilization.

36. **Ans. are 'b, c'**

Already explained.

37. **Ans. is 'a'** i.e., Bacterial identification

Bacteriophages are mostly needed for Bacterial identification by phage typing.

38. **Ans. is 'd'** i.e., It transfers only chromosomal gene

Already explained.

39. **Ans. is 'd'** i.e., Shigella dysenteriae

40. **Ans. is 'a'** i.e., Staphylococci

Staphylococcus strains are further differentiated into subspecies level on the basis of their bacteriophage susceptibility.

DNA VIRUSES

Poxviruses

1. **Man is the primary host for which poxvirus?** *(Recent MCQ)*
   (a) Monkey pox (b) Orf
   (c) Tanapox (d) Molluscum contagiosum
2. **Which virus cannot be cultivated?** *(Recent MCQ)*
   (a) Vaccinia (b) Variola
   (c) Molluscum contagiosum (d) Cowpox
3. **Most common molluscum virus:** *(Recent MCQ)*
   (a) 1 (b) 2 (c) 3 (d) 4
4. **Smallpox belongs to which class of poxviruses?** *(Recent MCQ)*
   (a) Parapoxvirus (b) Capripoxvirus
   (c) Leporipox virus (d) Orthopoxvirus

Herpesviruses

5. **HHV-6B causes:**
   (a) Carcinoma cervix (b) Carcinoma endometrium
   (c) Clear cell carcinoma (d) Focal encephalitis
6. **Kaposi sarcoma is caused by:** *(NBE Based AI 2013-14 Pattern)*
   (a) Human herpesvirus-2 (b) Human herpesvirus-4
   (c) Human herpesvirus-6 (d) Human herpesvirus-8
7. **Varicella are classified under:** *(AI 96)*
   (a) Enterovirus (b) Retrovirus
   (c) Poxvirus (d) Herpesvirus
8. **Varicella zoster attacks:** *(Recent MCQ)*
   (a) B-cell (b) T
   (c) NK (d) Neurons

Herpes Simplex Virus

9. **Herpes simplex virus is:** *(Recent MCQ)*
   (a) Single stranded DNA (b) Double stranded DNA
   (c) Single stranded RNA (d) Double stranded RNA

Clinical Features

10. **All of the following are true about Herpes group virus *except*:** *(AI 98)*
    (a) Ether sensitive (b) May cause malignancy
    (c) HSV II involves below diaphragm (d) Burkitt's lymphoma involves T cells
11. **Herpes simplex virus causes all *except*:** *(Recent MCQ)*
    (a) Encephalitis (b) Pharyngitis
    (c) IMN (d) Whitlow
12. **The most common cause of sporadic viral encephalitis is:** *(AI 09)*
    (a) Japanese B encephalitis (b) Herpes simplex encephalitis
    (c) HW encephalitis (d) Rubeola encephalitis

13. True about varicella is following *except*: *(AIIMS 08)*
- (a) One stage of rash is seen at one time
- (b) Humans are the only known reservoir
- (c) Children between 5-10 years old are most commonly affected
- (d) Patients are infectious–48 hours before onset of the vesicular rash and until all vesicles are crusted

14. Varicella zoster remains latent in: *(AI 10)*
- (a) Lymphocytes
- (b) Monocytes
- (c) Trigeminal ganglion
- (d) Plasma cells

15. Infectivity of chickenpox last for: *(AI 02)*
- (a) Till the last scab falls off
- (b) 6 days after onset of rash
- (c) 3 days after onset of rash
- (d) Till the fever subsides

16. Treatment of Herpes zoster: *(Recent MCQ)*
- (a) Zidovudin
- (b) Valacyclovir
- (c) Ribavarin
- (d) Nevirapine

Epstein-Barr Virus

17. Paul Bunnell antibodies are reactive in all *except*: *(AI 2007)*
- (a) Ox
- (b) Sheep
- (c) Dog
- (d) Horse

18. All are associated with EBV *except*: *(Recent MCQ)*
- (a) Infectious mononucleosis
- (b) Nasopharyngeal carcinoma
- (c) Oral hairy leukoplakia
- (d) Epidermodysplasia

Cytomegalovirus

19. Owl eye intranuclear inclusion body is seen in: *(DNB Aug 13 Pattern)*
- (a) Herpes zoster
- (b) Herpes simplex
- (c) CMV
- (d) EBV

20. The most common presentation of congenital CMV infection is: *(PGI 94)*
- (a) Hepatosplenomegaly
- (b) Microcephaly
- (c) Cerebral calcification
- (d) Chorioretinitis

Adenoviruses

21. Pharyngoconjunctival fever is caused by: *(Recent MCQ)*
- (a) Adenovirus 3 and 7
- (b) Adenovirus 11, 21
- (c) Adenovirus 40, 41
- (d) Adenovirus 8, 19

22. Adenovirus causes all *except*: *(Recent MCQ)*
- (a) Hemorrhagic cystitis
- (b) Diarrhea
- (c) Respiratory tract infection
- (d) IMN

Human Papilloma Virus

23. HPV vaccine is: *(AIIMS Nov 09)*
- (a) Monovalent
- (b) Bivalent
- (c) Quadrivalent
- (d) Both bivalent and quadrivalent

24. Most common tumor caused by virus is: *(AIIMS Dec 97)*
- (a) Warts
- (b) Carcinoma cervix
- (c) Nasopharyngeal carcinoma
- (d) Lymphoma

25. Which of the following clinical specimen for detection of BK polyomavirus by electron microscopy?

(a) Brain tissues
(b) Urine
(c) Blood
(d) None of the above

Parvovirus

26. One of the following is not a cultivable virus: *(Manipal 10)*

(a) Papova
(b) Parvovirus B19
(c) Herpes
(d) Adenovirus

27. In parvovirus infection what is common in adult? *(APPG 07)*

(a) Bone marrow aplasia
(b) PRCA
(c) Erythema infectiosum
(d) Arthropathy

28. All of the following statements about parvovirus B-19 are true *except*: *(AI 09)*

(a) DNA virus
(b) Crosses placenta in only < 10% of cases
(c) Can cause severe anemia
(d) Can cause aplastic crisis

ANSWERS AND EXPLANATIONS

Poxviruses

1. **Ans. is 'd'** i.e., Molluscum contagiosum (***Ref:*** *Ananthanarayan, 8th/e, p. 461*)
   - Pox viruses affecting primarily human are Variola,Vaccinia and Molluscum contagiosum.
   - Monkey pox – Its primary host are rodents.
   - Orf – Its primary host is Sheep – Human infections are rare.
   - Tanapox – Its primary host are Monkeys – Human infections are rare.
2. **Ans. is 'c'** i.e., Molluscum contagiosum (***Ref:*** *Ananthanarayan, 9th/e, p. 465 and 8th/e, p. 465*)
   - Humans are the only susceptible host. This disease is caused by molluscum contagiosum belongs to poxvirus. It is an enveloped, dsDNA-containing virus with complex symmetry. This is a **noncultivable virus.**
   - The infection is sexually transmitted and manifests as **umbilicated fleshy lesions.** The infection is diagnosed by demonstrating intracytoplasmic inclusions called as **molluscum bodies or Henderson-Peterson bodies.**
   - Cell cultures can be used for virus isolation, though culture of variola virus is only attempted in **Biosafety Level 4 facilities.** The orthopoxviruses grow well in cultured cells; parapoxviruses and tanapoxvirus grow less well, and molluscum contagiosum virus cannot be cultured.
3. **Ans. is 'a'** i.e., 1 (***Ref:*** *Essentials of Dermatology, p. 127*)
   - There are four types of Molluscum contagiosum virus, MCV – 1 to MCV – 4.
   - MCV – 1 is the most prevalent.
   - MCV – 2 is seen usually in adults and often sexually transmitted.
4. **Ans. is 'd'** i.e., Orthopoxvirus (***Ref:*** *Ananthanarayan, 9th/e, p. 461 and 8th/e, p. 461*)
   - **Orthopoxvirus:** These are mammalian pox viruses that tend to cause generalized infection with rash. Examples are variola (smallpox virus), vaccinia, cowpox, monkeypox, rabbitpox, buffalopox, camelpox, mousepox.

Herpesviruses

5. **Ans. is 'd'** i.e., Focal encephalitis (***Ref:*** *Ananthanarayan, 9th/e, p. 477 and 8th/e, p. 477*)
   - HHV – 6 has two variants → 'A' and 'B'
   - HHV – 6 'B' causes:
     (i) In children → Exanthem subitum (roseola infantum or sixth disease)
     (ii) In older age groups → Infectious mononucleosis, focal encephalitis
     (iii) In immunodeficient → Pneumonia, Disseminated disease
   - Whereas variant 6A has much less clear disease association.

6. **Ans. is 'd'** i.e., Human herpesvirus – 8 (***Ref:*** *Essentials of Medical Microbiology, p. 412*)
   - HHV – 8 (KSHV) is associated with Kaposi sarcoma.
   - KSHV (Kaposi's sarcoma–associated herpesvirus) is the cause of Kaposi sarcomas, vascular tumors of mixed cellular composition, and is involved in the pathogenesis of body cavity-based lymphomas occurring in AIDS patients and of multicentric Castleman disease (Primary effusion lymphoma).
7. **Ans. is 'd'** i.e., Herpesvirus (***Ref:*** *Ananthanarayan, 9th/e, p. 467 and 8th/e, p. 467*)
   - VZV is HSV – 3 belong to Alpha subfamily.
8. **Ans. is 'd'** i.e., Neurons (***Ref:*** *Ananthanarayan, 8th/e, p. 467-468*)
   - Among herpesviruses, alpha subfamily (HSV – 1, HSV – 2, VZV) affects neurons.

Site of latent infection	Official name	Common name
Neurons	HHV1 HHV2 HHV3	HSV1 HSV2 Varicella zoster virus
Glands, kidneys	HHV5	CMV
Lymphoid tissue (T-cells)	HHV6 HHV7	HHV6 HHV7
Lymphoid tissue (B-cells)	HHV4 HHV8	EBV Kaposi's sarcoma associated herpesvirus

9. **Ans. is 'b'** i.e., Double standard DNA (***Ref:*** *Ananthanarayan, 9th/e, p. 466 and 8th/e, p. 468*)
   - HSV belongs to herpesvirus family.
   - They are enveloped DNA (ds DNA) viruses.

Clinical Features

10. **Ans. is 'd'** i.e., Burkitt's lymphoma involves T cells
    - Burkitt's lymphoma is caused by EBV and Burkitt lymphoma is a B cell lymphoma commonly presenting as a tumor of the jaw in African children and young adults.
11. **Ans. is 'c'** i.e., IMN (***Ref:*** *Harrison, 18th/e, p. 1455-1460; Ananthanarayan, 8th/e, p. 470*)
    - IMN (Infectious Mononucleosis)/Glandular fever is caused by EBV.
    - Encephalitis, Pharyngitis and Whitlow are caused by HSV.
12. **Ans. is 'b'** i.e., Herpes simplex encephalitis (***Ref:*** *David Greenwood, 18th/e, p. 424*)
    - Encephalitis caused by HSV-1 is a rare condition but it is the most common cause of sporadic fatal encephalitis in developed countries (1-2 cases per million population annually).
    - The disease carries a high mortality rate, and those who survive often have residual neurologic defects. About half of patients with HSV encephalitis appear to have primary infections, and the rest appear to have recurrent infection.
13. **Ans. is 'a'** i.e., One stage of rash is seen at one time (***Ref:*** *David Greenwood, 18th/e, p. 428*)
    - The skin lesions of chickenpox VZV–**the hallmark of the infection**–include **maculopapules, vesicles, and scabs in various stages of evolution. These lesions, which evolve from maculopapules to vesicles over hours to days,** appear on the trunk and face and rapidly spread to involve other areas of the body. Most are small and have an erythematous base with a diameter of 5-10 mm. Successive crops appear over a 2- to 4-day period.
14. **Ans. is 'c'** i.e., Trigeminal ganglion (***Ref:*** *Ananthanarayan, 9th/e, p. 472 and 8th/e, p. 473*)
    - Trigeminal ganglion is involved in **herpes zoster ophthalmicus and follows Hutchinson rule and dermatomal involvement is present (T3-L3).**

15. **Ans. is 'b'** i.e., 6 days after onset of rash
    - Person is infective -2 days to rash to 6 days after the rash and some sources quote till the scab falls but better answer is 5-6 days after the rash.

16. **Ans. is 'b'** i.e., Valacyclovir (***Ref:*** *Jawetz, 27th/e, p. 470*)
    - **Famcyclovir or valacyclovir are the DOC for Herpes Zoster.**
    - Several antiviral compounds provide effective therapy for varicella, including acyclovir, valacyclovir, famciclovir and foscarnet. Acyclovir can prevent the development of systemic disease in varicella-infected immunosuppressed patients and can halt the progression of herpes zoster in adults. Acyclovir does not appear to prevent postherpetic neuralgia.

Epstein-Barr Virus

17. **Ans. is 'a'** i.e., Ox
    (***Ref:*** *Ananthanarayan, 9th/e, p. 109, 476 and 8th/e, p. 108, 477; Harrison, 18th/e, p. 1469, 1470; 19th/e, p. 1189*)
    - In infectious mononucleosis, **Paul Bunnel heterophile antibodies are produced.**
    - These IgM class antibodies have an affinity for sheep, horse and bovine erythrocyte and a titre of >40 is diagnostic of acute EBV infection.
    - Because these heterophile antibodies are adsorbed by ox red cells, they are not reactive in Ox (Ox red cells remove these antibodies).
    - **Monospot test is more sensitive and specific than Paul Bunnel test.**
    - **EBV specific antibody testing is used for patients, Titers of IgM and IgG abs to Viral capsid antigen (VCA) are elevated in 90% of patients at the onset of disease.**
    - Abs against EBNA are also demonstrated. EA – D abs are found in severe disease by EBV.
    - Nowadays **EBV DNA are demonstrated by PCR.**

18. **Ans. is 'd'** i.e., Epidermodysplasia
    (***Ref:*** *Ananthanarayan, 8th/e, p. 472, 473; Harrison, 18th/e, p. 1467-1470; 19th/e, p. 1189*)
    - Important diseases caused by EBV are **IMN, nasopharyngeal carcinoma, Burkitt's lymphoma (c myc translocation) (NHL), Hodgkin's lymphoma (mixed cellularity), gastric carcinoma, oral hairy leukoplakia and chronic fatigue syndrome, X-linked lymphoproliferative syndrome.**
    - Higher level of Abs before the onset of disease is more common in persons with multiple sclerosis than in the general population.

Cytomegalovirus

19. **Ans. is 'c'** i.e., CMV (***Ref:*** *Jawetz, 27th/e, p. 440*)
    - Human fibroblasts are used for virus isolation attempts. The virus can be recovered most readily from tissues, body fluids, throat washings and urine. **In cultures, 2–3 weeks are usually needed for the appearance of cytologic changes, consisting of small foci of swollen, translucent cells with large intranuclear inclusions resembling an 'owl's eye'.**
    - Shell vial cultures allow for detection of CMV antigen using fluorescent antibodies prior to development of cytopathic effect for a more rapid diagnosis.
    - PCR is used for definitive and rapid diagnosis.

20. **Ans. is 'a'** i.e., Hepatosplenomegaly (***Ref:*** *Harrison, 18th/e, p. 1473; 17th/e, p. 1110*)
    - **Most common presentation of congenital CMV infection is petechial lesions, hepatosplenomegaly and jaundice.** "About 50% all renal transplant recipient presenting with fever 1 to 4 months after transplantation have evidence of CMV disease; CMV itself accounts for the fever in more than two-third of cases.

Adenoviruses

21. **Ans. is 'a'** i.e., Adenovirus 3 and 7
    (***Ref:*** *Harrison, 18th/e, p. 1491; Ananthanarayan, 9th/e, p. 482; 8th/e, p. 480-481; Clinical Ophthalmology, p. 486*)

- **Pharyngoconjunctival fever is caused most commonly by serotypes 3 and 7,** but serotypes 2, 4 and 14 also have been documented as etiologic agents.

22. Ans. is 'd' i.e., IMN (***Ref:*** *Harrison, 18th/e, p. 1491; Ananthanarayan, 9th/e, p. 482 and 8th/e, p. 480-481*)

- Hemorrhagic cystitis – Adenovirus serotype 11, 22.
- Diarrhea and vomiting – Adenovirus serotype 40, 41.
- Respiratory tract infection – Adenovirus serotype 1 to 7, 14, 14a, 21.

Human Papilloma Virus

23. Ans. is 'd' i.e., Both bivalent and quadrivalent (***Ref:*** *Harrison, 18th/e, p. 1483; 17th/e, p. 1119*)

- There are two types of HPV vaccines:
  - (i) *Quadrivalent:* Containing HPV types 6, 11, 16, 18.
  - (ii) *Bivalent:* Containing HPV types 16, 18.
- Both vaccine proved to be safe and highly efficacious in clinical trials, providing almost complete protection from high grade cervical disease associated with HPV-16 and HPV-18 (both vaccine) and from genital warts (quadrivalent vaccine).

24. Ans. is 'c' i.e., 16, 18 (***Ref:*** *Harrison, 18th/e, p. 1482*)

- HPV DNA of oncogenic types (high risk) in HPV-16, 18, 31, 33 and 45 associated with cervical cancer.

25. Ans. is 'b' i.e., Urine (***Ref:*** *Dr D.R. Arora, 3rd/e, p. 552*)

- BK virus was isolated from urine of a renal transplant recipient, causes subclinical infection of children before the age of 10; virus persists for throughout life in kidneys. Reactivation may occur in last trimester of pregnancy and following immunosuppression for organ transplantation.

Parvovirus

26. Ans. is 'b' i.e., Parvovirus B19 (***Ref:*** *Harrison, 18th/e, p. 1478; 16th/e, p. 1055*)

- **Parvovirus is not cultivable properly but can be cultured in cells from human bone marrow of foetal liver by presence of erythropoietin and interleukin 3.**
- Parvoviruses including B19 are the smallest viruses known to infect and cause human disease.

27. Ans. is 'd' i.e., Arthopathy (***Ref:*** *Harrison, 18th/e, p. 1478; 16th/e, p. 1055*)

- **Parvovirus infection in adult commonly causes acute arthralgia and arthritis.**

28. Ans. is 'b' i.e., Crosses placenta in only < 10% of cases (***Ref:*** *Jawetz, 24th/e, p. 414, 417*)

- Maternal infection with B19 virus may pose a serious risk to the fetus, resulting in hydrops fetalis and fetal death due to severe anemia. Fetal loss occurs in fewer than 10% of primary maternal infections and **death occurs most commonly before the 20th week of pregnancy.** Although there is frequent intrauterine transmission of human parvovirus **(with estimates of vertical transmission rates of 30% or higher).**

RNA VIRUS

Picornaviruses

1. All belong to Picornaviruses *except*: *(PGI 98)*

(a) Enterovirus 70
(b) Coxsackievirus
(c) Rhinovirus
(d) Chickenpox virus

Enterovirus

2. Coxsackie A virus does not cause: *(Recent MCQ)*

(a) Herpangina
(b) Hand, foot and mouth disease (HFM)
(c) Laryngotracheobronchitis
(d) Aseptic meningitis

3. **Coxsackie group A commonly cause:** *(Manipal 10)*
   (a) Conjunctivitis
   (b) Aseptic meningitis
   (c) Hepatitis
   (d) Myocarditis
4. **Acute hemorrhagic conjunctivitis is caused by:** *(AI 97)*
   (a) Enterovirus 70
   (b) Adenovirus
   (c) Poliovirus
   (d) Hepadnavirus
5. **Enterovirus causes all *except*:** *(AIIMS Nov 01, AI 09)*
   (a) Haemorrhagic fever
   (b) Pleurodynia
   (c) Herpangina
   (d) Aseptic meningitis
6. **Mode of spread of Enterovirus is:** *(Recent MCQ)*
   (a) Vector mediated
   (b) Droplet infection
   (c) Faeco oral route
   (d) Skin contact

Poliovirus

7. **True about Polio is:** *(AI 11)*
   (a) Paralytic polio is most common
   (b) Only one type exists
   (c) Increased muscular activity and IM injections leads to increased paralysis
   (d) Polio drops given only in <3 years

Clinical Features and Lab Diagnosis

8. **False about polio:** *(Recent MCQ)*
   (a) Descending paralysis
   (b) Bilateral symmetrical paralysis
   (c) Non-progressive
   (d) LMN type paralysis
9. **All are true about polio, *except*:** *(Recent MCQ)*
   (a) 99% non-paralytic
   (b) Flaccid paralysis
   (c) Exaggerated tendon reflexes
   (d) Aseptic meningitis

MISCELLANEOUS

Myxoviruses

10. **Myxoviruses include:** *(PGI Nov 14)*
    (a) Orthomyxovirus
    (b) Parainfluenzae
    (c) Measles
    (d) Polio
    (e) HSV

Orthomyxovirus (Influenza)

11. **Influenza virus has:** *(Recent MCQ)*
    (a) 5 segments of ss RNA
    (b) 8 segments of ds DNA
    (c) 8 segments of ss DNA
    (d) 8 segments of ss RNA

Antigenic Structure and Antigenic Variations

12. **False about antigen drift:** *(Recent MCQ)*
    (a) Causes pandemic
    (b) Occurs due to mutation
    (c) Occurs more frequently
    (d) Affected by previous antibodies

Avian Flu

13. H5N1 is a strain of: *(AI 08)*

(a) Avian flu
(b) New vaccine against AIDS
(c) Agent for Japanese encephalitis
(d) Causes Chikungunya fever

PARAMYXOVIRUSES

Measles

14. Which of the following is the "Least Common Chronic" complication of measles? *(AI 98)*

(a) Diarrhoea
(b) Pneumonia
(c) Otitis media
(d) SSPE

15. Giant cell (Hecht's) pneumonia is due to: *(PGI Dec 98)*

(a) CMV
(b) Measles
(c) Malaria
(d) P. carinii

Mumps

16. With reference to mumps which of the following is true? *(AI 06)*

(a) Meningoencephalitis can precede parotitis
(b) Salivary gland involvement is limited to the parotid
(c) The patient is not infectious prior to clinical parotid enlargement
(d) Mumps orchitis frequently leads to infertility

17. Most common complication of mumps is: *(AI 00)*

(a) Orchitis and oophritis
(b) Encephalitis
(c) Pneumonia
(d) Myocarditis

R.S.V.

18. Most common cause of viral pneumonia in infant is: *(Recent MCQ)*

(a) Rhinovirus
(b) RSV
(c) Reovirus
(d) CMV

Rubella

19. All of the following statements are true about congenital rubella *except*: *(AI 05)*

(a) It is diagnosed when the infant has IgM antibodies at birth
(b) It is diagnosed when IgG antibodies persist for more than 6 months
(c) Most common congenital defects are deafness, cardiac malformation and cataract
(d) Infection after 16 weeks of gestation results in major congenital defects

Extra Practice Questions

20. Coxsackievirus is: *(Recent MCQ)*

(a) Herpesvirus
(b) Poxvirus
(c) Enterovirus
(d) Myxovirus

21. Suckling mice is used for isolation of: *(Recent MCQ)*

(a) Coxsackievirus
(b) Poxvirus
(c) Herpes
(d) Adenovirus

22. All are included in picorna group of viruses *except*: *(Kerala 04)*

(a) ECHO virus
(b) HEV
(c) Foot and mouth virus
(d) Poliovirus

23. Epidemic hemorrhagic conjunctivitis is caused by: *(Delhi 09)*

(a) HSV
(b) HZV
(c) HIV
(d) Picornavirus

24. Which of the following virus is shed in stool? *(AI 04)*

(a) Herpangina
(b) Influenza
(c) Varicella
(d) Smallpox

25. Herpangina is caused by: *(Recent MCQ)*

(a) Enterovirus
(b) Rhinovirus
(c) Myxovirus
(d) Rabies virus

26. Conjunctivitis is caused by *except*: *(AIIMS)*

(a) CMV
(b) Enterovirus 70
(c) Coxsackie A 24
(d) Adenovirus

27. Enterovirus 72 is: *(Recent MCQ)*

(a) Hepatitis A
(b) Hepatitis E
(c) Hepatitis G
(d) Hepatitis C

28. Enterovirus causes: *(Bihar 09)*

(a) Acute hemorrhagic conjunctivitis
(b) Acute follicular conjunctivitis
(c) Posterior follicular conjunctivitis
(d) Epidemic keratoconjunctivitis

29. Enterovirus causes all, *except*: *(Manipal 05)*

(a) Hemorrhagic fever
(b) Pleurodynia
(c) Herpangina
(d) Aseptic meningitis

30. Coxsackie B virus causes all *except*: *(JIPMER 11)*

(a) Aseptic meningitis
(b) Herpangina
(c) Myocarditis
(d) Bornholm diseases

31. All are true about poliovirus, *except*: *(AIIMS 02)*

(a) Type 1 is responsible for most epidemics
(b) Very difficult to eliminate type 1
(c) Type 1 is responsible for vaccine paralytic poliomyelitis
(d) Type 1 most commonly responsible with paralysis

32. Death in Poliomyelitis is due to: *(Orissa 09)*

(a) Infection
(b) Neurogenic shock
(c) Cardiac failure
(d) Respiratory paralysis

33. All of the following statements are true regarding poliovirus, *except*: *(AI 10)*

(a) It is transmitted by feco-oral route
(b) Asymptomatic infections are common in children
(c) There is a single serotype causing infection
(d) Live attenuated vaccine produces herd immunity

34. The most definitive method for laboratory diagnosis of poliomyelitis are A/E: *(Recent MCQ)*

(a) Virus isolation from blood
(b) Virus isolation from CSF
(c) Virus isolation from faces or throat
(d) Serological diagnosis

35. Diagnosis of polio: *(Manipal 06)*

(a) Detection of virus in stool
(b) Serology
(c) Limb wasting
(d) AFP

36. Portal of entry of poliovirus in mainly: *(PGI 01)*

(a) GIT
(b) Nasal mucosa
(c) Lung
(d) Skin

37. The virus, which spreads by both hematogenous and neural route is:

(a) Rabies virus
(b) VZV
(c) Poliovirus
(d) EBV

38. Which of the following statement is/are true of all paramyxovirus? *(PGI)*

(a) They contain a single stranded RNA genome of negative polarity
(b) Envelope is derived from the host cells plasma membrane
(c) They have a cytoplasmic site of replication
(d) They enter the body by the respiratory route

39. Reye's syndrome following influenza is most commonly associated with: *(AIIMS)*

(a) Type A
(b) Type B
(c) Type C
(d) All of the above

40. Influenza vaccines is administered: *(Recent MCQ)*

(a) Subcutaneously
(b) Intradermal
(c) Nasal drops
(d) Intrathecal

41. True statement about influenza A is: *(AI 99)*

(a) It has a double stranded segmented RNA
(b) Pandemic are caused by antigenic drift
(c) Nucleocapsid Ab is not specific
(d) Hemagglutinin and Neuraminidase is strain specific

42. False about antigenic drift: *(AIIMS 04)*

(a) Occur under pressure for immunity
(b) Responsible for epidemics of Influenza
(c) Occurs only in Influenza A
(d) Occur every 10-12 years

43. Antigenic shift: *(Recent MCQ)*

(a) Occurs every 2-3 years
(b) Gradual change over time
(c) Results from genetic recombination
(d) Occurs in all influenza viruses

44. Not true regarding influenza virus is: *(AIIMS)*

(a) All types do not exhibit antigenic shift
(b) Only type A shows antigenic drift
(c) Drift is accumulation of point mutations
(d) None of the above

45. Antigenic variation seen in which of the following: *(PGI)*

(a) Influenza virus
(b) Hepatitis virus
(c) Yellow fever virus
(d) Leptospira

46. Causes of antigenic drift in influenza viral infections: *(Manipal 07)*

(a) Small mutations in neuraminidase and hemagglutinin
(b) Large mutations in hemagglutinin only
(c) Step mutations in viral genome
(d) None of the above

47. Which of the following is true regarding influenza? *(MP 09)*

(a) It is caused by an enveloped DNA virus
(b) Lab studies may show neutropenia early in the course of disease
(c) Primary infectious pneumonia is less common than secondary bacterial pneumonia
(d) Antiviral agents given early prevents complications

48. Swine flu is caused by: *(DNB 12)*

(a) H1N1
(b) H5N1
(c) H3N1
(d) H3N3

49. Croup is most commonly due to: *(Recent MCQ 13)*

(a) Respiratory syncytial virus
(b) Parainfluenza virus 1,2
(c) Adenovirus
(d) Coronavirus

50. Avian influenza is: *(Recent MCQ 13)*

(a) H1N1
(b) H3N2
(c) H5N1
(d) None

51. Paramyxovirus includes: *(Recent MCQ)*

(a) Retrovirus
(b) Poliovirus
(c) Parainfluenza virus
(d) Rabies

52. Measles virus is: *(PGI)*

(a) Paramyxovirus
(b) Orthomyxovirus
(c) Poxvirus
(d) Picornavirus

53. Which one of the following virus produces both intranuclear and intracytoplasmic inclusion bodies? *(Comed 09)*

(a) Chicken pox
(b) Rabies
(c) Small pox
(d) Measles

54. Most common complication of mumps is: *(AI 2000)*

(a) Orchitis and Oophritis
(b) Encephalitis
(c) Pneumonia
(d) Myocardium

55. Most common agent responsible for bronchiolitis is: *(AI 04)*

(a) RSV
(b) Adenovirus
(c) Herpesvirus
(d) Influenza virus

56. Virus lacking hemagglutinin and neuraminidase but having membrane fusion protein is: *(Recent MCQ)*

(a) RSV
(b) CMV
(c) HSV
(d) EBV

57. Incubation period of rubella is: *(AI 05)*

(a) 18-72 hours
(b) 2-3 weeks
(c) 1-3 months
(d) >1 year

58. Risk of the damage to fetus by maternal rubella is maximum if mother gets infected in: *(AIIMS)*

(a) 6-12 weeks of pregnancy
(b) 20-24 weeks of pregnancy
(c) 24-28 weeks of pregnancy
(d) 32-36 weeks of pregnancy

59. Classic triad of congenital rubella includes all except? *(Recent MCQ)*

(a) Cataract
(b) Deafness
(c) Retinitis
(d) CHD (congenital heart disease)

60. The congenital rubella syndrome: *(Delhi 08)*

(a) May be prevented by vaccination in early pregnancy
(b) Causes IUGR
(c) Causes cataract
(d) Causes deafness only if acquired only if acquired before 16 weeks of gestation

ANSWERS AND EXPLANATIONS

Picorna Viruses

1. **Ans. is 'd'** i.e., Chickenpox virus (***Ref:*** *Ananthanarayan, 9th/e, p. 485 and 8th/e, p. 483, 484*)
   - Chickenpox or varicella zoster belongs to herpesvirus group (HHV3). Other three are Picornaviruses.
   - **REMEMBER** – Chickenpox is not a **poxvirus.**
   - The first five groups contain important human pathogens. Rhinoviruses historically were placed in a separate genus but are now considered to be members of the enterovirus genus.
2. **Ans. is 'c'** i.e., Laryngotracheobronchitis (***Ref:*** *Greenwood, 10th/e, p. 459*)

Coxsackievirus Group	Type	Clinical illness
A	1-24	• **Aseptic meningitis** • **Febrile illness** • **Herpangina** • **Hand, foot and mouth disease**

3. **Ans. is 'b'** i.e., Aseptic meningitis (***Ref:*** *Jawetz, 23rd/e, p. 495*)
   - Aseptic meningitis is caused by all types group B Coxsackieviruses and by many **Group 'A' Coxsackie-viruses most commonly A7 and A9.**

   ABOUT OTHER OPTIONS
   - Acute hemorrhagic conjunctivitis can be caused **by Coxsackievirus A-24 and Enterovirus – 70** but not so common.
   - **Myocarditis and hepatitis are mainly caused by Coxsackievirus group B along with Bornholms disease.**
4. **Ans. is 'a'** i.e., Enterovirus 70 (***Ref:*** *Ananthanarayan, 9th/e, p. 491 and 8th/e, p. 490*)
   - Enterovirus 70 causes → Acute hemorrhagic conjunctivitisQ
   - Coxsackie A-24 causes → Acute hemorrhagic conjunctivitisQ
   - Adenovirus causes → Epidemic keratoconjunctivitis
     Acute follicular conjunctivitis
     Pharyngoconjunctival feverQ
5. **Ans. is 'a'** i.e., Hemorrhagic fever (***Ref:*** *Ananthanarayan, 9th/e, p. 491 and 8th/e, p. 489*)
   - Enteroviruses are the most common cause of **aseptic meningitis.***
   - Herpangina and Hand, foot and mouth disease is caused particularly by → **Coxsackie A virus.***
   - Cardiac and muscular disease (Pleurodynia, myocarditis and pericarditis) caused particularly by → Coxsackie B virus.*

   Hemorrhagic fever is not caused by Enteroviruses.Q
6. **Ans. is 'c'** i.e., Faeco oral route (***Ref:*** *Jawetz, 27th/e, p. 515*)
   - Humans are the only known reservoir for members of the human Enterovirus group. These viruses are generally shed for longer periods of time in stools than in secretions from the upper alimentary tract. Thus, **fecal contamination (hands, utensils, food and water) is main source followed by respiratory droplets via inhalation or rarely by conjunctival contact.**
7. **Ans. is 'c'** i.e., IM injections and increased muscular activity lead to increased paralysis
   (***Ref:*** *Jawetz, 27th/e, p. 518*)
   - Intramuscular injection and strenuous physical exercise (increased muscular activity) increase the risk for paralytic polio.
   - **Mild Disease –** This is the **most common form** of disease. The patient has only a minor illness, characterized by fever, malaise, drowsiness, headache, nausea, vomiting, constipation, and sore throat in various combinations. Recovery occurs in a few days.
   - Poliovirus types 1–3 causes polio.

8. **Ans. is 'b'** i.e., Bilateral symmetrical paralysis (***Ref:** Jawetz, 27th/e, p. 516*)
   - There is flaccid paralysis which is not symmetrical.
   - There are absent tendon reflexes (not exaggerated).
   - Paralytic polio occurs in only 1% cases (that means 99% is non-paralytic).
   - Aseptic meningitis occurs in 1% of cases.
   - **Bilateral symmetrical paralysis is caused by West nile virus.**

9. **Ans. is 'c'** i.e., Exaggerated tendon reflexes

   Explained in above Question.

Orthomyxovirus

10. **Ans. is 'a'** i.e., Orthomyxovirus; **'b'** i.e., Influenza; **'c'** i.e., Measles

    (***Ref:** Ananthanarayan, 9th/e, p. 496 and 8th/e, p. 504*)
    - Myxovirus are divided into two important families:
      - (i) Orthomyxovirus → Influenza
      - (ii) Paramyxovirus → Mumps, measles, RSV, Parainfluenza virus

11. **Ans. is 'd'** i.e., 8 segments of ssRNA (***Ref:** Ananthanarayan, 8th/e, p. 498*)
    - Influenza virus contains single stranded RNA which is segmented → 8 pieces.
    - **Outstanding characteristics:** Genetic reassortment common among members of the same genus and Influenza viruses cause worldwide epidemics.

12. **Ans. is 'a'** i.e., Cause pandemic (***Ref:** Ananthanarayan, 9th/e, p. 499 and 8th/e, p. 496*)
    - **Antigenic shift** is responsible for **pandemic (Abrupt, drastic and discontinuous).**
    - **Antigenic drift** occurs due to **point mutation.**
    - Antigenic drift occurs more frequently (2-3 years) than antigenic shift (10-15 years).
    - Antigenic drift is influenced by the presence of antibodies to the predecessor strains in the host population (Single point mutation continuous in nature).

13. **Ans. is 'a'** i.e., Avian flu (***Ref:** Park, 22nd/e, p. 145*)
    - At present three types of influenza viruses are circulating in the world: A (H_1N_1), A (H_3N_2) and B viruses.
    - WHO global surveillance activities have identified human infection with a new influenza virus called A (H_5N_1) in Hong Kong in mid 1997. However, the possibility that the outbreak heralded a global influenza pandemic did not materialize and it is transmitted to man only from birds, requires close respiratory contact.

14. **Ans. is 'd'** i.e., SSPE (***Ref:** PSM Park, 19th/e, p. 128*)
    - Subacute sclerosing panencephalitis (SSPE) is a rare complication (1 in 300000) of measles, which develops many years after the initial infection.
    - SSPE belongs to **group C slow virus infection, caused by a defective Measles virus.**

15. **Ans. is 'b'** i.e., Measles (***Ref:** Harrison, 19th/e, p. 1297*)
    - **Primary giant cell or Hecht's pneumonia** is seen in case of measles. It is a complication of measles and is seen in immunocompromised and malnourished patients.
    - It is a serious complication in children and adults with deficiencies in cell-mediated immunity and it is believed to be caused by unrestrained viral replication and has a high fatality rate.

16. **Ans. is 'a'** i.e., Meningoencephalitis can precede parotitis (***Ref:** Harrison, 19th/e, p. 1298*)

    "Aseptic meningitis may develop before, during, after, or in the absence of parotitis."

    ABOUT OTHER OPTIONS:
    - Mainly parotid glands are involved, but sublingual and submaxillary glands may also be involved.

- Patient is infectious 4-6 days before the onset of swelling.
- Sterility after mumps orchitis is rare.Q

17. Ans. is 'a' i.e., Orchitis and oophritis (***Ref:*** *Harrison, 18th/e, p. 1609; 19th/e, p. 1298*)

- Epididymoorchitis is the most common manifestation of mumps among postpubertal males (15-30%).
- Aseptic meningitis (<10%), which may develop before, during, after, or in the absence of parotitis.
- Oophritis (5%) and Pancreatitis (4%).

18. Ans. is 'b' i.e., RSV (***Ref:*** *Jawetz, 27th/e, p. 587*)

- RSV is the most common cause of pneumonia and bronchilitis in infants.
- In adults, influenza is the most common cause of viral pneumonia.

19. Ans. is 'd' i.e., Infection after 16 weeks of gestation results in major congenital defects (***Ref:*** *Harrison, 18th/e, p. 1606; 19th/e, p. 1300*)

- The most important factor in the pathogenicity of Rubella virus for the fetus is **gestational age** at the time of infection.
- "In general, the earlier in pregnancy infection occurs, the greater the damage to the fetus. Maximum damage to the fetus occurs when infection acquired in the first trimester of pregnancy."
- Risk of damage to fetus by maternal rubella during pregnancy.
- Birth defects are uncommon if maternal infection occurs after the 20th week of gestation.

20. Ans. is 'c' i.e., Enterovirus

Human enteroviruses consist of at least 72 serotypes, which include poliovirus types 1–3, coxsackieviruses A types 1–24, coxsackieviruses B types 1–6, echoviruses types 1–34, and enteroviruses 68–71. Originally hepatitis A virus (enterovirus 72) was included in this group but has been reclassified as a hepatovirus in the genus Hepatovirus.

21. Ans. is 'a' i.e., Coxsackievirus

Intracerebral inoculation of coxsackie virus into suckling mice – In suckling mice, signs of illness appear usually within 1–2 weeks.

Coxsackie- A virus produces Flaccid paralysis.

Coxsackie- B virus produces Spastic paralysis.

22. Ans. is 'b' i.e., HEV

HAV – Picornaviridae family.

HEV – Caliciviridae family.

23. Ans. is 'd' i.e., Picornavirus

Acute hemorrhagic conjunctivitis (AHC) is an **epidemic** form of highly contagious conjunctivitis and is characterized by sudden onset of painful, swollen, red eyes, with conjunctival hemorrhaging and excessive tearing. AHC typically is caused by one of two enteroviruses (Coxsackie A24 or Enterovirus 70). This disease is transmitted person-to-person usually through contact with contaminated hands or through sharing of contaminated personal-care items. No specific treatment is available for AHC; however, the illness is self-limiting, and severe complications are rare. Nonetheless, because of its extremely contagious nature, AHC can disrupt the local economy and require substantial health care resources.

Reference: https://www.cdc.gov/mmwr/preview/mmwrhtml/mm5328a2.htm

24. Ans. is 'a' i.e., Herpangina

Herpangina (acute vesicular pharyngitis) is an acute febrile illness associated with small vesicular or ulcerative lesions on the posterior oropharyngeal structures (**enanthem**). Herpangina typically occurs during the summer and usually develops in children, occasionally occurring in newborns, adolescents, and young adults. It is caused by Coxsackie- A and Enteroviruses are transmitted by feco-oral route. Coxsackie virus comes under enterovirus.

25. Ans. is 'a' i.e., Enterovirus

Already explained.

26. Ans. is 'a' i.e., CMV

Conjunctivitis is not caused by CMV.

27. Ans. is 'a' i.e., Hepatitis A

HAV is earlier called as Enterovirus 72.

28. Ans. is 'a' i.e., Acute hemorrhagic conjunctivitis

Already explained.

29. Ans. is 'a' i.e., Hemorrhagic fever

Pleurodynia, Herpangina and Aseptic meningitis are caused by coxsackievirus.

30. Ans. is 'b' i.e., Herpangina

Already explained in Ans No. 24.

31. Ans. is 'c' i.e., Type 1 is responsible for vaccine paralytic poliomyelitis

Sabin strain type 1, 2, 3 are associated with Vaccine-associated paralytic polio (VAPP) and Vaccine derived poliovirus (VDPV).

Reference:http://www.who.int/immunization/diseases/poliomyelitis/endgame_objective2/oral_polio_vaccine/VAP-PandcVDPVFactSheet-Feb2015.pdf

32. Ans. is 'd' i.e., Respiratory paralysis

Paralytic polio: About 1 percent of polio cases can develop into paralytic polio. Paralytic polio leads to paralysis in the spinal cord (spinal polio), brainstem (bulbar polio), or both (bulbospinal polio). It's rare for full paralysis to develop. Less than 1 percent of all polio cases will result in permanent paralysis. In 5–10 percent of the polio paralysis cases, the virus will attack the muscles that help you breathe and cause death.

33. Ans. is 'c' i.e., There is a single serotype causing infection

There are 3 types of poliovirus which are associated with infection.

34. Ans. is 'd' i.e., Serological diagnosis

- Isolation of viruses from clinical specimen by tissue culture is the most specific method in the diagnosis of poliomyelitis.
- PCR is a highly sensitive and specific test for diagnosis of poliomyelitis. The test, however, is not widely available in the developing countries.

35. Ans. is 'a' i.e., Detection of virus in stool

Virus isolation from feces and throat swab is carried out by cultivation on monkey kidney, human amnion, HeLa, Hep-2, Buffalo green monkey (BGM), MRC-5 and other cell cultures.

36. Ans. is 'a' i.e., GIT

Pathogenesis of poliomyelitis: On entering the body, the virus infects and multiplies in the tonsils and Peyer's patch of the ileum. It then spreads to regional lymph nodes and enters the blood, causing a primary viremia. On continued infection and multiplication of virus in the reticuloendothelial cells, it invades the **blood** stream again and causes secondary viremia. During this period of viremia, the poliovirus crosses the blood–brain barrier or gains access to the brain by infecting skeletal muscle and **travelling up on the nerves** to the brain as in rabies virus.

37. Ans. is 'c' i.e., Poliovirus

Already explained.

38. Ans. are 'a, b, c, d'

Measles and Human parainfluenza viruses replicates in the cell cytoplasm.

39. Ans. is 'b' i.e., Type B

Reye syndrome is an acute encephalopathy of children and adolescents, usually between 2 and 16 years of age. The mortality rate is high (10–40%). The cause of Reye syndrome is unknown, but **it is a recognized rare complication of influenza B**, influenza A and varicella zoster infections. There is a possible relationship between salicylate use and subsequent development of Reye syndrome.

40. Ans. are 'a, c'

- Inactivated vaccines are administered by IM or subcutaneously.
- Live attenuated cold adapted influenza vaccine is administered by nasal spray.

41. Ans. is 'd' i.e., Hemagglutinin and Neuraminidase is strain specific

All the strains of influenza A, B and C share the common internal proteins, such as nucleoproteins and membrane proteins. They, however, differ in their surface proteins, such as HAs and NAs. Antigenic variation is a unique feature of influenza virus. The surface antigens HA and NA show variations and are primarily responsible for antigenic variations exhibited by influenza viruses. The internal RNP antigen and M protein are stable, hence do not contribute to the antigenic variations. Antigenic variations are of two types: antigenic shift and antigenic drift.

42. Ans. is 'c' i.e., Occurs only in influenza A

Antigenic drift: The gradual, sequential, regular antigenic change in influenza virus is known as antigenic drift. This occurs due to minor antigenic changes due to point mutations in the HA or NA occurring at frequent intervals. This is caused even by a single mutation affecting HA glycoprotein. The antigenic drift is characterized by changes in certain epitopes in the HA, while others are being conserved.

43. Ans. is 'c' i.e., Results from genetic recombination

Antigenic shift: A major change in one or both of the surface antigens, a change that yields an antigen showing no serologic relationship with the antigen of the strains prevailing at the time is called antigenic shift. **Antigenic shift has been demonstrated in type A influenza virus only.**

44. Ans. is 'b' i.e., Only Type A shows Antigenic drift

Antigenic shift reflects drastic changes in the sequence of a viral surface protein, caused by genetic reassortment between human, swine and avian influenza viruses. Influenza B and C viruses do not exhibit antigenic shift because few related viruses exist in animals.

45. Ans. is 'a' i.e., Influenza virus

46. Ans. is 'a' i.e., Small mutations in neuraminidase and hemagglutinin

Already explained in Answer No. 42.

47. Ans. is 'c' i.e., Primary infectious pneumonia is less common than secondary bacterial pneumonia

Secondary bacterial infections: Life-threatening influenza is often caused by secondary bacterial infections with staphylococci, pneumococci and haemophilus influenzae. Pneumonia may develop as a complication and may be fatal, particularly (a) in elderly persons above 60 years with underlying chronic disease, (b) in people with impaired resistance (chronic cardiorespiratory disease, renal disease, etc.) and (c) in pregnant women.

48. Ans. is 'a' i.e., H1N1

Swine flu is caused by H1N1 and H3N2.

49. Ans. is 'b' i.e., Parainfluenza virus

Croup or laryngotracheobronchitis is a heterogeneous group of illnesses that affects the larynx, trachea and bronchi. The condition manifests as fever, cough, laryngeal obstruction and expiratory stridor. Type1,2 causes croup while type 3 causes LRTI.

50. Ans. is 'c' i.e., H5N1

The H5N1 bird flu, caused by an avian subtype influenza virus, which has been associated with bird flu in the domesticated birds, can be transmitted from birds to humans. The H5N1 was first described in Hong Kong in 1997.

An epidemic of bird flu occurred in domesticated birds in Southeast Asia, primarily Vietnam, in January 2004. More than 240 human cases have been documented and more than 140 persons have died due to the poultry outbreaks and bird-to-human transmission. Most deaths have been reported in Vietnam and Indonesia. Sporadic outbreaks have continued to occur since the 2004 outbreak even outside Southeast Asia, including Turkey.

51. Ans. is 'c' i.e., Parainfluenza

Paramyxovirus includes – RSV, Parainfluenza virus, Mumps and Measles.

52. Ans. is 'a' i.e., Paramyxovirus

Already explained.

53. Ans. is 'd' i.e., Measles

It produced multinucleated giant cell lines (Warthin-Finkeldy cells) containing both intracellular and intracytoplasmic inclusion bodies.

54. Ans. is 'a' i.e., Orchitis and Oophritis

Complications of mumps: Meningoencephalitis is the most frequent complication of mumps in childhood. Other rare complications include oophritis, mastitis, pancreatitis, thyroiditis, arteritis, thrombocytopenia and pneumonia. Death due to mumps is rare.

55. Ans. is 'a' i.e., RSV

In infants, **RSV causes a more severe lower respiratory tract illness, resulting in bronchiolitis or pneumonia.** Clinically, the condition presents as cough, coryza, wheezing, rales, and low-grade fever (< 101°F). Bronchiolitis is usually self-limiting, but may cause a serious disease in premature infants, in immunocompromised hosts, and in individuals with underlying lung diseases. Reinfection with the virus occurs throughout the life. However, with advancing age and recurrent infection, the RSV infection is confined more to the upper respiratory tract than the lower respiratory tract.

56. Ans. is 'a' i.e., RSV

The viral envelope contains a surface **glycoprotein G**, by which it is attached to the cell surface of the host cells. **It contains F protein but lacks both H and N proteins**. The F protein induces the fusion of the infected cells with adjoining cells, resulting in the formation of large multinucleated syncytia, from which the virus derives its name.

57. Ans. is 'b' i.e., 2-3 weeks

Incubation period is about 14 days (12-23 days).

58. Ans. is 'a' i.e., 6-12 weeks of pregnancy

In the first trimester, 80% of the infants would be affected, and severity of the disease depends on how early the infection occurs.

59. Ans. is 'c' i.e., Retinitis

The classic triad for congenital rubella syndrome is: Sensorineural deafness (58% of patients), Eye abnormalities—especially retinopathy, cataract, and microphthalmia (43% of patients), Congenital heart disease—especially pulmonary artery stenosis and patent ductus arteriosus (50% of patients).

60. Ans is 'c' i.e., Causes cataract

Cataract, mental retardation, and deafness are the most common manifestations of congenital rubella infection.

ARBOVIRUSES

Classification and Transmission

1. Hemorrhagic fever is not caused by: *(Recent MCQ)*

(a) Yellow fever
(b) KFD
(c) Japanese encephalitis
(d) Dengue fever

2. Which of the following is not common in India? *(Recent MCQ)*

(a) Japanese B encephalitis
(b) Lassa fever
(c) KFD
(d) Dengue

3. Which of the following statements is true regarding Arboviruses? *(AI 04)*

(a) Yellow fever is endemic in India
(b) Dengue virus has only one serotype
(c) Kyasanur forest disease (KFD) is transmitted by ticks
(d) Mosquito of culex visnoi-complex is the vector of Dengue fever

4. Viruses causing hemorrhagic fever are: *(PGI Nov 14)*

(a) Lassa fever virus
(b) Yellow fever virus
(c) West Nile virus
(d) Crimean Congo virus
(e) Ross river virus

Hantavirus

5. All are true regarding Hantavirus *except*: *(AIIMS Sept 96)*
- (a) DNA virus
- (b) Carried by rodents
- (c) Causes recurrent respiratory infection
- (d) Hemorrhagic manifestation may occur

Kyasanur Forest Disease

6. Following are true of Kyasanur forest disease *except*: *(AI 94)*
- (a) Transmitted by soft tick
- (b) Caused by retrovirus
- (c) Incubation period is 3-8 days
- (d) Killed vaccine available

Japanese Encephalitis

7. In Japanese Encephalitis, pig acts as: *(PGI 2000)*
- (a) Amplifier
- (b) Definitive host
- (c) Intermediate host
- (d) Any of the above

Dengue Fever

8. Most virulent dengue fever strain is: *(Recent MCQ)*
- (a) 1
- (b) 2
- (c) 3
- (d) 4

9. Most sensitive diagnostic test for dengue is: *(AIIMS Nov 08)*
- (a) IgM ELISA
- (b) Complement fixation test
- (c) Reverse transcriptase PCR
- (d) Electron microscopy

10. Following are arboviral diseases: *(PGI)*
- (a) KFD
- (b) West Nile fever
- (c) Ganjam virus
- (d) RSV
- (e) Puumala virus

11. Hemorrhagic fever is caused by: *(Recent MCQ)*
- (a) West Nile fever
- (b) Sandfly fever
- (c) Ebola virus
- (d) All of the above

12. Fever and hemorrhagic rash are seen in all *except*: *(PGI 11)*
- (a) Dengue fever
- (b) Lassa fever
- (c) Rift Valley fever
- (d) Sandfly fever
- (e) Yellow fever

13. Which of the following is/are arboviral diseases? *(PGI 09)*
- (a) JE
- (b) Dengue
- (c) Yellow fever
- (d) Hand-foot-mouth disease
- (e) Rocky montain spotted fever

14. Group B (flavivirus) arbovirus is/are: *(PGI 06)*
- (a) Dengue fever
- (b) Rift valley fever
- (c) Chikungunya fever
- (d) JE
- (e) Yellow fever

15. The vector of JE virus is: *(Recent MCQ)*
- (a) Anopheles mosquito
- (b) Culex mosquito
- (c) Aedes mosquito
- (d) All of the above

16. In India, human infection has been reported with dengue virus type: *(AI 04)*

(a) 1, 2
(b) 1, 3
(c) 2, 4
(d) All 4 types

17. Break bone fever is caused by: *(Recent MCQ)*

(a) Variola
(b) Coxsackie
(c) Dengue
(d) Adenovirus

18. Which of the following flavivirus is closely related to Russian spring summer encephalitis causing virus? *(APPGE 04)*

(a) Dengue
(b) Chickungunya
(c) KFD
(d) West Nile fever

19. Which of the following is true about arboviruses? *(AI 08)*

(a) They are non-enveloped icosahedral viruses
(b) Produce papilloma and warts in humans
(c) RNA virus
(d) Oncogenic virus

20. Which of the following is true? *(AIIMS 08)*

(a) Hanta virus pulmonary syndrome is caused by inhalation of rodent urine and feces
(b) KFD is caused by bite of wild animal
(c) Lyssa virus is transmitted by tick
(d) Dengue virus has 3 serotypes

21. Which of the following are true regarding KFD? *(PGI)*

(a) It is zoonosis
(b) Affects monkeys
(c) Caused by bacteria
(d) Caused by rickettsia

22. Amplifier host is: *(Recent MCQ)*

(a) Pig in JE
(b) Dog in rabies
(c) Man in JE
(d) Cattle in JE

23. Dengue hemorrhagic fever is caused by: *(Recent MCQ)*

(a) Type 1 dengue virus
(b) Reinfection with same serotype of dengue virus
(c) Reinfection with a different serotype of dengue virus
(d) Infection in an immunocompromised host

RHABDOVIRUS (RABIES)

Morphology and Strains

24. Which antigen of rabies virus stimulates antibody production?

(a) Lipoprotein
(b) Glycoprotein
(c) Phosphoprotein
(d) Intranuclear protein

25. Which of the following statements is true about rabies virus? *(AI 03)*

(a) It is double stranded RNA virus
(b) Contains a DNA-dependent RNA polymerase
(c) RNA has a negative polarity
(d) Affects motor neurons

Pathological Manifestations

26. In rabies the characteristic pathological manifestationis: *(AI 97)*

(a) Ventriculitis
(b) Brainstem encephalitis
(c) Basal ganglia affection
(d) Meningitis

27. Regarding rabies, true is: *(AI 00)*

(a) Incubation period depends on the site of bite
(b) Diagnosis is by eosinophilic intranuclear inclusion
(c) It is a DNA virus
(d) Caused only by dogs

Diagnosis of Rabies

28. A 15 years old girl was admitted to the infectious disease hospital with a provisional diagnosis of rabies. The most suitable clinical sample that can confirm the antemortem diagnosis is: *(AIIMS Nov 04)*

(a) Serum for anti-rabies IgG antibody
(b) Corneal impression smear for immunofluorescence stain
(c) CSF sample for viral culture
(d) Giemsa stain on smear prepared from salivary secretions

Prophylaxis of Rabies

29. Which anti-rabies vaccine has been recommended by WHO? *(AI 10)*

(a) Duck cell vaccine
(b) Chick fibroblast vaccine
(c) HDCV
(d) Sheep brain vaccine

30. The schedule of HDCV in rabies is: *(AI 96)*

(a) 0, 3, 7, 10, 14, 28
(b) 0, 3, 10, 30
(c) 3, 7, 14, 16, 18
(d) 0, 7, 14, 16, 18

31. Schedule of intradermal rabies vaccine is: *(AI 09)*

(a) 2-2-0-1-0-1
(b) 8-0-4-0-1-1
(c) 8-4-4-1-0-1
(d) 2-0-2-0-1-1

32. All of the following rabies vaccines are commercially available *except*: *(AIIMS 2011)*

(a) Killed sheep brain vaccine
(b) Human diploid cell vaccine
(c) Vero continuous cell vaccine
(d) Recombinant glycoprotein

Rotavirus

33. Viral enterotoxin is detected as a possible of mechanism pathogenesis in: *(Manipal 11)*

(a) Adenovirus
(b) Calcivirus
(c) Rotavirus
(d) Astrovirus

34. Rotavirus infections is diagnosed by the presence of: *(AI 10)*

(a) Antigen in stool
(b) Virus in stool
(c) Antigen in blood
(d) Antibody in stool

35. Best vaccine for rotavirus infection is: *(AI 98)*

(a) Asymptomatic neonatal vaccine
(b) DNA vaccine
(c) Genetic reassortment
(d) Capsular component vaccine

ANSWERS AND EXPLANATIONS

ARBOVIRUSES

Classification and Transmission

1. **Ans. is 'c'** i.e., Japanese encephalitis (***Ref:*** *Jawetz, 27th/e, p. 548*)
   - JE is not a hemorrhagic group arboviral disease.

- Japanese B encephalitis is the leading cause of viral encephalitis in Asia. The mortality rate can exceed 30%. A high percentage of survivors (up to 50%) are left with neurologic and psychiatric sequelae. Infections during the first and second trimesters of pregnancy have reportedly led to fetal death.

2. **Ans. is 'b'** i.e., Lassa fever (***Ref:*** *PSM Park, 19th/e, p. 238*)
   - Lassa fever is an acute viral haemorrhagic illness of 2-21 days duration that occurs in West Africa. Lassa fever is a zoonotic disease and transmitted to human via contact with food or household items contaminated with rodent (multimammate rats) urine or feces.

Some Arboviruses Known to be Prevalent in India

Group A	Group B
(Alphaviruses)	(Flaviviruses)
Sindbis	**Dengue**
Chikungunya	**KFD**
	JE
	West Nile

3. **Ans. is 'c'** i.e., Kyasanur forest disease is transmitted by tick
   (***Ref:*** *Ananthanarayan, 9th/e, p. 522, 523 and 8th/e, p. 520*)
   - **KFD is mainly transmitted by Hard tick, but soft tick can also transmit the disease and reservoirs are monkeys and rats.**
   - Dengue virus has **four serotypes.**
   - **Yellow fever is not endemic in India;** it is distributed in Africa and South America.
   - Dengue fever is transmitted by **Aedes mosquito.**
4. **Ans. are 'b' and 'd'** i.e., Yellow fever virus, Crimean Congo virus
   (***Ref:*** *Ananthanarayan, 9th/e, p. 522, 523 and 8th/e, p. 520*)
   - Group B arboviruses are JE, Dengue, Westnile virus,Yellow fever and KFD.
   - Other Viruses causing hemorrhagic fever are – Kyasanur forest disease virus, Omsk hemorrhagic fever virus, Crimean Congo hemorrhagic fever virus.

Hantavirus

5. **Ans. is 'a'** i.e., DNA virus (***Ref:*** *Ananthanarayan, 9th/e, p. 527 and 8th/e, p. 522*)
   - It is a RNA virus belonging to family Bunyaviridae.
   - **Transmission is from rodent to rodent and rodent to human is primarily respiratory, by inhalation of the virus contained in dried excreta.**
   - Hantavirus species are natural pathogens of rodents – field mice being the major host.
   - Disease caused by Hantaviruses:
     - Milder epidemic nephritis.
     - Serious epidemic hemorrhagic fever.
     - Hantavirus pulmonary syndrome.

Kyasanur Forest Disease

6. **Ans. is 'b'** i.e., Caused by retrovirus (***Ref:*** *Ananthanarayan, 9th/e, p. 524 and 8th/e, p. 520*)
   - **KFD is a febrile disease associated with haemorrhages.**
   - **Caused by an arbovirus flavivirus (group B Togavirus).**
   - **Mode of transmission → Tick bite.**
   - **Incubation period → 3-8 days.**
   - For population at risk, killed KFD vaccine is available.

Japanese Encephalitis

7. **Ans. is 'a'** i.e., Amplifier (***Ref:*** *Park, 22nd/e, p. 260*)
   - JE virus multiplies exponentially in pigs without causing any manifestation so considered as the amplifier host.
   - The natural cycles of JE virus are:
     (a) Pigs → Mosquito (Culex) → Pigs.
     (b) Ardeid bird → Mosquito (Culex) → Ardeid bird

Dengue Fever

8. **Ans. is 'b'** i.e., 2 (***Ref:*** *Quick Review Series: Microbiology, p. 280*)
   "Dengue type-2 strain is being considered to be more virulent strain". – *Quick Review Series: Microbiology*
   "Strains of the virus in the type-2 serotype are often more virulent than those of other serotypes".
   – *Principles of Clinical Virology*
9. **Ans. is 'c'** i.e., RT-PCR (***Ref:*** *Ananthanarayan, 9th/e, p. 523 and 7th/e, p. 137; Harper, 27th/e, p. 604*)
   - **Reverse transcriptase PCR (RT-PCR)-based methods** are available for rapid identification and serotyping of dengue virus in acute-phase serum, roughly during the period of fever. Isolation of the virus is difficult.
   - Neutralizing and Hemagglutination inhibiting antibodies appear within a week after the onset of dengue fever. Analysis of paired acute and convalescent sera to show a significant rise in antibody titer is the most reliable evidence of an active dengue infection.
10. **Ans. are 'a, b, c, e'**
    Respiratory syncytial virus, or RSV, is a common respiratory virus that usually causes mild, cold-like symptoms, it cause acute bronchiolitis and it is not arboviral disease. Treatment of same is Ribavarin.
11. **Ans. is 'c'** i.e., Ebola virus
    Symptoms of Ebola virus disease: The incubation period, that is, the time interval from infection with the virus to onset of symptoms is 2 to 21 days. Humans are not infectious until they develop symptoms. First symptoms are the sudden onset of fever fatigue, muscle pain, headache and sore throat. This is followed by vomiting, diarrhoea, rash, symptoms of impaired kidney and liver function, and in some cases, both internal and external bleeding (e.g., oozing from the gums, blood in the stools). Laboratory findings include low white blood cell and platelet counts and elevated liver enzymes.
12. **Ans. is 'd'** i.e., Sandfly fever
    Sandfly fever (Genus - Phlebovirus): It is transmitted by Phlebotomus pappatasi. It is a febrile illness presenting with chills malaise. In India, it has been reported from Aurangabad.
13. **Ans. are 'a, b, c'**
    Already explained.
14. **Ans. is 'a, d, e'**
    Rift valley fever is a member of Bunyaviridae family.
    Chikungunya fever is a member of Togaviridae family.
15. **Ans. is 'b'** i.e., Culex mosquito
    Culex tritaeniorhynchus is the major vector worldwide including India and Culex vishnui is the next common vector found in India.
16. **Ans. is 'd'** i.e., All 4 types
    All 4 serotypes have been isolated from India.
17. **Ans. is 'c'** i.e., Dengue
    The dengue virus causes classic dengue or breakbone fever characterized by fever, muscle and joint pain, lymph-adenopathy and rash. In addition, it also causes dengue hemorrhagic fever, i.e., a much more severe disease than classic dengue fever with a high fatality rate.

18. Ans. is 'c' i.e., KFD

Tick-borne encephalitis, or TBE, is a human viral infectious disease involving the central nervous system. TBE is caused by the tick-borne encephalitis virus (TBEV), a member of the family Flaviviridae, and was initially isolated in 1937. Three virus sub-types are described: **European or Western tick-borne encephalitis virus, Siberian tick-borne encephalitis virus, and Far eastern tick-borne encephalitis virus (formerly known as Russian Spring Summer Encephalitis Virus, RSSEV).**

The family Flaviviridae includes several tick-borne viruses affecting humans. These viruses are closely related to TBEV and Far-eastern TBE, and include Omsk hemorrhagic fever virus in Siberia, Kyasanur Forest disease virus in India and its close relative, Alkhurma virus in Saudi Arabia. Louping ill virus (United Kingdom) is also a member of this family; it causes disease primarily in sheep and has been reported as the cause of a TBE-like illness in laboratory workers and persons with contact to sick sheep (e.g., veterinarians, butchers). In the USA and Russia, another tick-borne flavivirus, Powassan virus, is responsible of encephalitis in human.

https://www.cdc.gov/vhf/tbe/index.html

19. Ans. is 'c' i.e., RNA virus

20. Ans. is 'a' i.e., Hanta virus pulmonary syndrome is caused by inhalation of rodent urine and feces

21. Ans. is 'a, b'

22. Ans. is 'a' i.e., Pig in JE

Pigs are the amplifying hosts, because they have persistent, high-grade viremia and help in transmission of the virus in humans living close to the pig-rearing areas.

23. Ans. is 'c' i.e., Reinfection with a different serotype of dengue virus

Dengue hemorrhagic fever is a most severe manifestation of the disease. The initial classic phase of dengue hemorrhagic fever is similar to that of dengue fever and other febrile viral illnesses. But, subsequently, the condition of the patient suddenly worsens with shock and hemorrhage, especially into the gastrointestinal tract and skin. The hemorrhagic manifestations include bleeding from nose, melena and hematemesis. This condition shows a high fatality rate as high as 10%. It occurs in children with passively acquired maternal antibodies. It may also occur in a person previously infected with a different serotype of the virus, showing non-neutralizing heterologous antibodies in the serum.

RHABDOVIRUS (RABIES)

Morphology and Strains

24. Ans. is 'b' i.e., Glycoprotein (***Ref:*** *Ananthanarayan, 9th/e, p. 510, 533 and 8th/e, p. 525-527*)

- **Glycoprotein G (on surface spikes) induces protective antibodies.**
- The G glycoprotein is a major factor in rabies virus neuroinvasiveness and pathogenicity. **A substitution at amino acid position 333 of the glycoprotein results in loss of virulence,** indicating some essential role for that site of the protein in disease pathogenesis. Purified spikes containing the viral glycoprotein elicit neutralizing antibody in animals.

25. Ans. is 'c' i.e., RNA has negative polarity (***Ref:*** *Ananthanarayan, 9th/e, p. 510, 532 and 8th/e, p. 525*)

- It is an **enveloped, RNA (negative sense ss RNA) virus.**
- **It has RNA dependent RNA polymerase.Q**
- Rabies virus multiplies in muscle or connective tissue at the site of inoculation and then enters peripheral nerves at neuromuscular junctions and spreads up the nerves to the central nervous system. It multiplies in the central nervous system and progressive encephalitis develops. The virus then spreads through peripheral nerves to the salivary glands and other tissues.

26. Ans. is 'b' i.e., Brainstem encephalitis (***Ref:*** *Robbin's 7th/e, p. 1375*)

- Rabies is severe encephalitis, mainly involves. Rhombencephalon (Brainstem), Basal ganglia, Spinal Cord, Dorsal root ganglia.

27. Ans. is 'a' i.e., Incubation period depends on the site of bite (***Ref:*** *PSM Park, 19th/e, p. 228*)

Variability of Incubation Period

- **Incubation period of rabies depends on:**

- The site of bite.
- Number of wounds.
- Species of biting animal.
- Severity of bite.
- Amount of virus injected.
- Protection provided by clothing and treatment undertaken.

ABOUT OTHER OPTIONS

- Pathognomonic **Negri bodies are intracytoplasmic (not intranuclear) eosinophilic inclusion bodies.Q**
- Rabies virus is a RNA virus.
- It can be caused by many wild animals (not only by dogs).

28. Ans. is 'b' i.e., Corneal impression smear for immunofluorescence stain

(***Ref:*** *Ananthanarayan, 9th/e, p. 533 and 8th/e, p. 529*)

- The diagnosis of rabies is usually made by the **detection of rabies virus antigens by immunofluorescence.**
- Tissues infected with rabies virus are currently identified most rapidly and accurately by means of immunofluorescence or immunoperoxidase staining using antirabies monoclonal antibodies. A biopsy specimen is usually taken from the skin of the neck at the hairline. Impression preparations of brain or cornea tissue may be used.

Prophylaxis of Rabies

29. Ans. is 'b' i.e., Chick fibroblast vaccine (***Ref:*** *Park, 19th/e, p. 229*)

- Because of their potency and low cost, second generation tissue culture vaccines (chick embryo fibroblast, vero continuous cell line) are preferred.
- This vaccine is prepared from the fixed rabies virus strain **Flury LEP grown in chicken fibroblasts.** It is inactivated with β-propiolactone.

30. Ans. is 'a' i.e., 0, 3, 7, 10, 14, 28 (***Ref:*** *Park, 20th/e, p. 243*)

Schedules of vaccination for post exposure prophylaxis

A. Intramuscular schedules

(i) Routine schedule → **6 doses** on 0, 3, 7, 14 and 28 days with a booster on day 90.

(ii) Abbreviated multisite schedule → **2-1-1 regimen** one dose is given in the right arm and one in left arm on day 0 after that one dose is given on day 7 and 21.

31. Ans. is 'b' i.e., 8-0-4-0-1-1 (***Ref:*** *Jawetz, 27th/e, p. 613*)

- To enumerate doses of different schedule, one should remember the routine days → 0, 3, 7, 14, 28 and 90.
- For example, in intradermal 2-sites schedule, injections are given at 2 sites on day 0, 3, 7 and 28.
- Thus, enumeration will be as follows:

Days→	0	3	7	14	28	90
	↑	↑	↑	↑	↑	↑
	2 sites	2 sites	2 sites	No injection	2 sites	No injection

- **This is written as 2-2-2-0-2-0.Q**
- **Similarly, 8 sites intradermal schedule is written as 8-0-4-0-1-1.Q**

32. Ans. is 'a' i.e., Killed sheep brain vaccine

(***Ref:*** *Ananthanarayan, 9th/e, p. 535 and 8th/e, p. 530-531; PSM Park, 19th/e, p. 230, 231*)

- Neural Vaccines especially (Semple Vaccine – derived from infected sheep brain) are encephalitogenic, poor immunogenic and can cause serious neurological complications. So they are no longer in use since 2004 and have been replaced by non-neural vaccines.

ROTAVIRUS

33. Ans. is 'c' i.e., Rotavirus (***Ref:*** *Harrison, 18th/e, p. 1591; 16th/e, p. 1142, Jawetz, 27th/e, p. 535*)

- Rotavirus produces **enterotoxin.**
- Rotaviruses infect cells in the **villi of the small intestine** (gastric and colonic mucosa are spared). They multiply in the cytoplasm of enterocytes and damage their transport mechanisms. **One of the rotavirus-encoded proteins, NSP4, is a viral enterotoxin and induces secretion by triggering a calcium dependent signal transduction pathway.** Damaged cells may slough into the lumen of the intestine and release large quantities of virus, which appear in the stool **(up to 10^{12} particles per gram of faeces).**

34. Ans. is 'a' i.e., Antigen is stool by ELISA

(***Ref:*** *Harrison, 18th/e, p. 1591, 1592; 16th/e, p. 1142; Greenwood, 16th/e, p. 525*)

- Because Rotavirus is shed in large amounts is stool, detection is relatively easy. Most commonly used are commercial immunoassays to detect rotavirus antigen in fecal specimen.
- Also see Ans. No. 19.

35. Ans. is 'c' i.e., Genetic reassortment (***Ref:*** *Harrison, 18th/e, p. 1590; 17th/e, p. 1206*)

- **The segmented genome of rotavirus allows genetic reassortment during coinfection – a property that may play a role in viral evolution** and has been utilized in the development of reassortment animal – human rotavirus – based vaccines.
- An **oral live attenuated pentavalent human–bovine** reassortant rotavirus vaccine was licensed in the United States, followed by licensing of an **oral live attenuated monovalent human rotavirus vaccine** in 2008. Both vaccines are safe and effective, and neither is associated with intussusception.

HUMAN IMMUNODEFICIENCY VIRUS

1. When was HIV virus discovered? *(AIIMS May 14)*

(a) 1983 (b) 1976 (c) 1969 (d) 1992

Structure and Genome

2. Subtype of HIV most common in India: *(Pattern MCQ)*

(a) A (b) B (c) C (d) D

3. Nef gene in HIV is for use: *(Recent MCQ)*

(a) Enhancing the expression of genes
(b) Enhancing viral replication
(c) Decreasing viral replication
(d) Maturation

4. HIV virus contains: *(AI 02)*

(a) Single stranded DNA
(b) Single stranded RNA
(c) Double stranded DNA
(d) Double stranded RNA

Transmission of HIV

5. Mother to child transmission of HIV: *(Recent MCQ)*

(a) 25% (b) 50% (c) 60% (d) 75%

6. The chance that a health worker gets HIV from an accidental needle prick is: *(PGI June 99)*

(a) 1% (b) 10% (c) 95% (d) 100%

7. True about HIV: *(PGI 2000)*

(a) Not transmitted through semen
(b) More chances of transmission during LSCS than normal labour
(c) More infectious than hepatitis B
(d) Male to female transmitted > female to male

Replication and Spread of HIV

8. Regarding HIV which of the following is not true? *(AI 02)*

(a) It is a DNA retrovirus
(b) Contains Reverse Transcriptase
(c) May infect host CD_4 cells other than T lymphocytes
(d) Causes a reduction in host CD_4 cells at late stage of disease

9. HIV infects most commonly: *(AIIMS Jun 00, AI 09)*

(a) CD4+helper cells
(b) CD8+cells
(c) Macrophage
(d) Neutrophil

10. AIDS involves: *(AI 98)*

(a) T-helper cells
(b) T-suppressor cells
(c) T-cytotoxic
(d) B. cells

11. The receptor through which M-tropic HIV strains bind? *(Recent MCQ)*

(a) CCR5
(b) CXR4
(c) CXCR5
(d) Any of the above

12. What is the sequence which a retrovirus follows onentering a host cell? *(AI 2K)*

(a) RNA-DNA-RNA
(b) RNA-DNA
(c) DNA-RNA
(d) DNA-RNA-DNA

13. Regarding HIV infection, not true is: *(AI 01)*

(a) p24 is used for early diagnosis
(b) Lysis of infected CD4 cells is seen
(c) Dendritic cells do not support replication
(d) Macrophage is a reservoir for the virus

Clinical Spectrum of HIV Infection

14. CMV retinitis in HIV occurs when the CD4 counts falls below: *(AI 02)*

(a) 50
(b) 100
(c) 200
(d) 150

15. An HIV patient complains of visual disturbances. Fundal examination shows bilateral retinal exudates and perivascular hemorrhages. Which of the following viruses are most likely to be responsible for this retinitis? *(AI 04)*

(a) Herpes simplex
(b) Varicella zoster
(c) Cytomegalovirus
(d) EBV

16. The most common organism amongst the following that causes acute meningitis in an AIDS patient is a: *(AI 05)*

(a) Streptococcus pneumoniae
(b) Streptococcus agalactiae
(c) Cryptococcus neoformans
(d) Listeria monocytogenes

17. Which of the following lesions is associated with HIV infection? *(AIIMS May 04)*

(a) Hairy leukoplakia
(b) Erythroplakia
(c) Oral lichen planus
(d) Bullous pemphigoid

18. Oral hairy leukoplakia is caused by: *(Recent MCQ)*

(a) HSV
(b) EBV
(c) CMV
(d) HPV

19. In a patient having HIV infections, oral ulcer is most commonly due to: *(Orissa 05)*

(a) Candida
(b) Cryptococcosis
(c) Histoplasma
(d) Trichophyton

20. Most common genital lesion in HIV patient is: *(AI 10)*

(a) Chlamydia (b) Herpes
(c) Syphilis (d) Candida

21. Most common helminthic infection in AIDS is: *(AI 99)*

(a) Trichuris trichiura (b) Strongyloides stercoralis
(c) Enterobius vermicularis (d) Nector-americanus

22. Which of the following is not seen in HIV patient with CD count less than 100 per micro litre, who has non productive cough? *(AIIMS June 99)*

(a) Mycobacterium tuberculosis (b) Pneumocystis carinii
(c) Mycoplasma pneumoniae (d) Cryptococcal infection

23. The tissue of origin of the Kaposi's sarcoma is: *(AIIMS May 05)*

(a) Lymphoid (b) Vascular
(c) Neural (d) Muscular

24. Multifocal tumor of vascular origin in a patient of AIDS: *(AI 00)*

(a) Kaposi sarcoma (b) Astrocytoma
(c) Gastric carcinoma (d) Primary CNS lymphoma

25. A patient with HIV has diarrhoea with AFB (+)ve organism in stool. The most likely organism is: *(AI 00)*

(a) Mycobacterium avium intracellulare (b) Mycobacterium TB
(c) Mycobacterium leprae (d) Mycoplasma

26. True about HIV all *except*: *(Recent MCQ)*

(a) PML caused by JC virus
(b) CNS lymphoma is the most common CNS tumor
(c) CMV is the most common cause of retinitis
(d) Most common cause of seizure is candida

27. Most common agent causing tuberculosis in AIDS patient in tropical countries is: *(AI 97)*

(a) Mycobacterium tuberculosis (b) Mycobacterium intracellulare
(c) Mycobacterium parvum (d) Mycobacterium atypical

28. In India most common cause of T. B. in HIV: *(PGI 2000)*

(a) Myco. Tuberculosis (b) Myco. Avium intracelluare
(c) M. bovis (d) M. scrofulaceum

Lab Diagnosis of HIV Infection

29. ELISA test when compared to western blot technique is: *(AI 93, 96)*

(a) Less sensitive, less specific (b) More sensitive, more specific
(c) Less sensitive, more specific (d) More sensitive, less specific

30. Most sensitive test for HIV infection: *(Recent MCQ)*

(a) Western blot (b) ELISA
(c) Agglutination test (d) CFT

31. Following is the marker of HIV infection in blood: *(AIIMS 94)*

(a) Reverse transcriptase (b) DNA polymerase
(c) RNA polymerase (d) None

32. A patient comes to hospital with a history of sore throat, diarrhea and sexual contact 2 weeks before. The best investigation to rule out HIV is: *(AI 00)*

(a) P24 antigen assay (b) ELISA
(c) Western blot (d) Lymph node biopsy

33. False about p24 is: *(NBE Based AI 2012-13)*

(a) Seen after 3 weeks of infection (b) Can't be seen in first week
(c) Can't be detected after seroconversion (d) Detected by ELISA

34. In HIV window period indicates: *(AIIMS Nov 07)*

(a) Time period between infection and onset of first symptoms
(b) Time period between infection and detection of antibodies against HIV
(c) Time period between infection and minimum multiplication of the organism
(d) Time period between infection and maximum multiplication of the organism

35. HIV can be detected and confirmed by: *(AI 05)*

(a) Polymerase Chain Reaction (PCR) (b) Reverse Transcriptase – PCR
(c) Real Time PCR (d) Mimic PCR

Oncogenic Viruses

36. RNA oncogenic virus amongst the following is: *(DNB Aug 13 Pattern)*

(a) HIV (b) HTLV
(c) HBV (d) Cytomegalovirus

37. Oncogenic virus is: *(Recent MCQ)*

(a) CMV (b) VZV
(c) Polio virus (d) EBV

38. HTLV extra gene segment is: *(Recent MCQ)*

(a) Gag (b) Pol (c) Env (d) Px

39. HTLV-1 causes which of the following? *(Recent MCQ)*

(a) Tropical spastic paraparesis (b) Familial Mediterranian fever
(c) Cutaneous T cell lymphoma (d) Burkitt's lymphoma

40. All oncogenic viruses containing RNA belongs to: *(Recent MCQ)*

(a) Picornaviridae (b) Herpesviridae
(c) Retroviridae (d) Bunyaviridae

41. Most common oncogenic RNA virus: *(Recent MCQ)*

(a) Retrovirus (b) Picornavirus
(c) Orthomyxovirus (d) Paramyxovirus

42. All of the following are DNA oncogenic virus *except*: *(Recent MCQ)*

(a) EBV
(b) HBV
(c) Adult T cell leukemia/Lymphoma virus
(d) Kaposi sarcoma virus

43. The following viruses has been associated with oncogenic *except*: *(Recent MCQ)*

(a) HPV (b) EBV
(c) Human T cell leukemia virus (d) Varicella Zoster virus

44. Which of the following oncogenic virus is so far not shown to be (oncogenic) in man: *(PGI)*

(a) HBV (b) EBV
(c) HSV 2 (d) Adenovirus
(e) HTLV

45. The only oncogenic virus whose pathogenicity has been proved without doubt is:

(a) HTLV - I
(b) HTLV - II
(c) HTLV - III
(d) HTLV - IV

46. All are associated with EBV *except*: *(Recent MCQ)*

(a) Infectious mononucleosis
(b) Nasopharyngeal carcinoma
(c) Oral hairy leukoplakia
(d) Epidermodysplasia

Slow Viral Diseases

47. Which of the following is not considered to be a slow virus disease? *(PGI)*

(a) Kuru
(b) Scrapie
(c) Creutzfeldt Jakob disease
(d) Maedi
(e) Sarcoidosis

48. True about prion protein disease is all, *except*: *(AIIMS 01)*

(a) Myoclonus is seen in 10% of the patients
(b) Caused by infectious protein
(c) Brain biopsy is diagnostic
(d) Commonly manifests as dementia

49. Prions are: *(AI 08)*

(a) Made up of bacterial and viral particles
(b) Immunogenic
(c) Infectious
(d) RNA particles

50. Prions consists of: *(AIIMS 07)*

(a) DNA and RNA
(b) DNA, RNA and Protein
(c) RNA and Protein
(d) Only Protein

51. Regarding prion which of the following statements is true? *(AIIMS 08)*

(a) It is protein product coded in viral DNA
(b) It catalyzes abnormal folding of other protein
(c) It protects disulfide bond from oxidation
(d) It cleaves normal proteins

52. True about prions is: *(AI 11)*

(a) Encoded by viral genome
(b) Associated with misfolding of protein
(c) Non infectious
(d) Immunogenic

53. Mad cow diseases (Bovine Spongiform disease) is similar in man to: *(AIIMS 06)*

(a) Alzheimer's disease
(b) Creutzfeldt Jakob diseases
(c) Huntington's chorea
(d) Picks diseases

54. Fatal familial insomnia is associated with:

(a) Prion disease
(b) Degenerative diseases
(c) Neoplastic diseases
(d) Vascular diseases

ANSWERS AND EXPLANATIONS

Human Immunodeficiency Virus

1. **Ans. is 'a'** i.e., 1983 (***Ref:*** *Harrison, 18th/e, p. 3146*)
   - In 1983, human immunodeficiency virus (HIV) was isolated from a patient with lymphadenopathy, and by 1984 it was demonstrated clearly to the causative agent of AIDS.

Structure and Genome

2. **Ans. is 'c'** i.e., C (***Ref:*** *Jawetz, 27th/e, p. 639*)
   - Subtype A is most prevalent worldwide (common in West Africa).

- Subtype B is predominant in Europe, America, Japan and Australia.
- **Subtype C is most prevalent in India and China.Q**

3. **Ans. is 'c'** i.e., Decreasing viral replication (***Ref:*** *Ananthanarayan, 9th/e, p. 572 and 8th/e, p. 571*)

   Nef (Negative factor gene): Downregulating viral replication.Q

   The Nef protein increases viral infectivity, facilitates activation of resting T cells, and downregulates expression of CD4 and MHC class I. The Nef gene is necessary for simian immunodeficiency virus (SIV) to be pathogenic in monkeys. (Jawetz)

4. **Ans. is 'b'** i.e., Single stranded RNA (***Ref:*** *Ananthanarayan, 9th/e, p. 571 and 8th/e, p. 570*)
   - The genome in HIV is diploid, composed of two identical single stranded positive sense RNA copies.

Transmission of HIV

5. **Ans. is 'a'** i.e., 25% (***Ref:*** *Jawetz, 27th/e, p. 651*)
   - Probability of transmission of HIV from mother to infant/fetus ranges from 15 to 25% in industrialized countries and from 25 to 40% in developing countries.
   - Mother-to-infant transmission rates vary from 13% to 40% in untreated women. Infants can become infected in utero, during the birth process, or through breastfeeding. In the absence of breastfeeding, about 30% of infections occur in utero and 70% during delivery. **Data indicate that from one third to one-half of perinatal HIV infections in Africa are due to breastfeeding. Transmission during breastfeeding usually occurs early (by 6 months). High maternal viral loads are a risk factor for transmission.**

6. **Ans. is 'a'** i.e., 1% (***Ref:*** *Ananthanarayan, 9th/e, p. 582 and 8th/e, p. 581*)
   - Risk of transmission after different route varies, i.e., chances of transmission of HIV per exposure: Blood and blood products have highest risk (> 90%) > tissue and organ donation (50-90%) > mother to child transmission (30%) > Needle and sharp instruments (0.5-1%) > sexual intercourse (0.1-1%).

7. **Ans. is. 'd'** i.e., Male to female transmission > female to male transmission

   (***Ref:*** *Harrison, 18th/e, p. 1510, 1512, 1515; 17th/e, p. 1143*)
   - **Male to female transmission is approximately eight times more efficient than female to male transmission.**
   - Seminal fluid (Semen) and vaginal fluid can transmit the infection.
   - Caesarean section (LSCS) results in decreased transmission from mother to infant.
   - After percutaneous injury Hepatitis B virus is more infectious than HIV.

     HBV – 6 to 30% chance of transmission.

     HCV – 1.8%.

     HIV – 0.3%.

Replication and Spread of HIV

8. **Ans. is 'a'** i.e., It is a DNA retrovirus (***Ref:*** *Ananthanarayan, 9th/e, p. 571, 574 and 8th/e, p. 570*)
   - HIV is a RNA virus (not DNA).
   - It contains reverse transcriptase enzyme, which is a characteristics feature of retroviruses.
   - The receptor for the virus is the CD4 antigen on surface. The cells affected are:
     - CD4 T Cells (major target).
     - B lymphocytes.
     - Monocytes and macrophages.
     - Langerhans cells in dermis.
     - Glial cells and microglia in the CNS.
     - **Follicular dendritic cells from tonsils can be infected by HIV** without the involvement of CD4.
   - CD4 T cells are reduced and T4:T8 Cell ratio is reversed.

9. **Ans. is 'a'** i.e., CD4 Helper cells (*See above question*)
CD4 (T-cells) are the major target.

10. **Ans. is 'a'** i.e., Helper T Cells (***Ref:*** *Ananthanarayan, 9th/e, p. 574, and 8th/e, p. 572*)
CD4 (T-cells) are the major target.
Already explained.

11. **Ans. is 'a'** i.e., CCR5 (***Ref:*** *Chemokines in Disease, 4th/e, p. 136*)
- **Macrophage (M-tropic) strains of HIV-1, or non-synctia-inducing strains (NSI) use the beta-chemokine receptor CCR5 for entry and are thus able to replicate in macrophages and CD4+ T-cells.** These strains **are now called R5 viruses.**
- The normal ligands for this receptor, **RANTES,** macrophage inflammatory protein (MIP)-1-beta and MIP-1-alpha, are able to suppress HIV-1 infection in vitro. This CCR5 coreceptor is used by almost all primary HIV-1 isolates of viral genetic subtype.
- **T-tropic isolates or synctia-inducing (SI) strains** replicate in primary CD4+ T-cells as well as in macrophages and use the alpha-chemokine receptor, CXCR4, for entry.

12. **Ans. is 'a'** i.e., RNA - DNA - RNA (***Ref:*** *Ananthanarayan, 9th/e, p. 574 and 8th/e, p. 570*)
- When HIV infects a cell, the viral RNA is transcribed by reverse transcriptase, first into single stranded DNA and then to double stranded DNA (Provirus).
- Provirus is integrated into host cell chromosome.
- This provirus initiates viral replication by directing synthesis of viral RNA, in response to viral promoters.

13. **Ans. is 'c'** i.e., Dendritic cells do not support replication
(***Ref:*** *Ananthanarayan, 9th/e, p. 574, 577 and 8th/e, p. 573; Harrison, 18th/e, p. 1531; 17th/e, p. 1159*)
- Follicular dendritic cells from tonsil can be infected by HIV without the involvement of CD4.
- Dendritic cells play an important role in the initiation of HIV infection.
- "Complexes of infected CD4+T Cells and dendritic cells provide an optimal microenvironment for virus replication." – *Harrison, 16th ed., p. 1095*

Clinical Spectrum of HIV Infection

14. **Ans. is 'a'** i.e., 50 (***Ref:*** *Harrison, 18th/e, p. 1563; 17th/e, p. 1185*)
- The majority of cases of CMV retinitis occur in patients with CD4+T cell count < 50/ml.

15. **Ans. is 'c'** i.e., Cytomegalovirus (***Ref:*** *Harrison, 18th/e, p. 1563; 17th/e, p. 1185*)
- **Perivascular hemorrhage and exudate are characteristic of CMV retinitis.**
- CMV infection – Other organ infection excluding liver, spleen and lymph nodes.
- Other viral opportunistic infections – Chronic HSV infection, Progressive multifocal leukoencephalopathy, varicella-zoster virus, adenovirus, polyomavirus JC virus, hepatitis B virus, hepatitis C virus.

16. **Ans. is 'c'** i.e., Cryptococcus neoformans (***Ref:*** *Harrison, 18th/e, p. 1559, 1560; 17th/e, p. 1182*)
- Most common cause of **seizures** → Toxoplasma
- Most common cause of **meningitis** → Cryptococcus
- Most common cause of **focal neurological deficit** → Toxoplasma

17. **Ans. is 'a'** i.e., Hairy leukoplakia (***Ref:*** *Harrison, 18th/e, p. 1549, 1550; 17th/e, p. 1174*)
Oral lesions in AIDS include:
   1. Hairy leukoplakia (caused by EBV).
   2. Thrush (caused by candida).
   3. Aphthous ulcer.

18. **Ans. is 'b'** i.e., EBV (***Ref:*** *Harrison, 18th/e, p. 1549, 1550*)
- Oral hairy leukoplakia is seen in AIDS patients and is caused by EBV.

19. Ans. is 'a' i.e., Candida (***Ref:*** *Harrison, 18th/e, p. 1549, 1550; 17th/e, p. 1174*)

- Amongst the given options, only candida causes oral lesion in AIDS patient.

20. Ans. is 'b' i.e., Herpes (***Ref:*** *Reference with text*)

- Herpes simplex (in the developed world) and chancroid (in Africa) are the most common cause of genital ulceration in HIV infected patients.
- Herpesvirus infections are common in AIDS patients, and multiple herpesviruses are frequently detected being shed in saliva. Cytomegalovirus retinitis is the most common severe ocular complication of AIDS.

21. Ans. is 'b' i.e., Strongyloides stercoralis (***Ref:*** *Paniker Parasitology, 6th/e, p. 173*)

- Amongst the given options only stongyloides causes opportunistic infection in AIDS.
- Generalised strongyloidosis may be seen in AIDS.
- Protozoa causing opportunistic infection are: Toxoplasma gondii, Isospora belli, Cryptosporidium species.

22. Ans. is 'c' i.e., Mycoplasma pneumonia (***Ref:*** *Harrison, 18th/e, p. 1546, 1547; 17th/e, p. 1171*)

- Mycoplasma pneumoniae is not among the opportunistic organisms causing pneumonia in a patient with AIDS.

23. Ans. is 'b' i.e., Vascular

(***Ref:*** *Harrison, 18th/e, p. 1565; 17th/e, p. 1186; Robbins,7th/e, p. 54, 550; Ananthanarayan, 9th/e, p. 576 and 8th/e, p. 575*)

- Kaposi sarcoma is an **intermediate grade, multicentric vascular tumour.**
- It is caused by HHV-8. **It is a cancer that develops from the cells that line lymph or blood vessels. This type of Kaposi sarcoma develops in people who are infected with HIV. Most visual signs of this sarcoma are lesions on the skin (flat, painless spots that are red or purple on white skin and bluish, brownish or black on dark skin).** It affects 8 times more men than women.

24. Ans. is 'a' i.e., Kaposi sarcoma (***Ref:*** *Harrison, 18th/e, p. 1565; 17th/e, p. 1186*)

25. Ans. is 'a' i.e., Mycobacterium avium intracellulare

(***Ref:*** *Ananthanarayan, 9th/e, p. 576; Harrison, 18th/e, p. 1548; 17th/e, 1173*)

- MAC infection is a late complication of HIV infection, occurs when CD4 < 50/ml, in contrast to T.B. which occurs early even with CD4 > 300/ml.
- **Clinical Features:**
  - Disseminated disease with fever, weight loss and night sweats (most common).
  - Abdominal pain.
  - Diarrhoea.
  - Lymphadenopathy.
- Diagnosis is made by demonstration of AFB positive mycobacteria in sputum, stool, blood or bone narrow.

26. Ans. is 'd' i.e., Most common cause of seizure is candida (***Ref:*** *Harrison, 18th/e, p. 1559, 1560*)

- Most common cause of seizure in the HIV infected patient is toxoplasma.
- Progressive multifocal leukoencephalopathy (PML) is a common CNS lesion in HIV infected patients. It is caused by a papovavirus called JC virus.
- Primary CNS lymphoma is one of the most common brain tumor in HIV infected patients.
- CMV is the most common cause of retinitis in HIV infected patients.

27. Ans. is 'a' i.e., Mycobacterium tuberculosis (***Ref:*** *Ananthanarayan, 9th/e, p. 576 and 8th/e, p. 575*)

Common pathogens causing T.B. in AIDS patients are M. tuberculosis and M. avium intracellulare. In developing countries, the most important pathogen is M. tuberculosis, with many strain being multidrug resistant.

28. Ans. is 'a' i.e., Myco tuberculosis (***Ref:*** *Ananthanarayan, 9th/e, p. 574, 576 and 8th/e, p. 575*)

- In developing countries, the most important pathogen is M. tuberculosis.

Lab Diagnosis of HIV Infection

29. Ans. is 'd' i.e., More sensitive, less specific (***Ref:*** *Harrison, 18th/e, p. 1538; 17th/e, p. 1165*)

- ELISA is an extremely good screening test with a sensitivity of > 99.5%.
- While ELISA is an extremely sensitive test, it is not optimal with regard to specificity.

30. Ans. is 'b' i.e., ELISA (***Ref:*** *Harrison, 18th/e, p. 1538*)

- Most sensitive test → ELISA
- Most specific test → HIV RNA PCR, Western blot

31. Ans. is 'a', i.e., Reverse transcriptase (***Ref:*** *Harrison, 18th/e, p. 1539, 1540; 19th/e, p. 1219*)

- Plasma level HIV RNA can be measured by reverse – transcriptase polymerase chain reaction (RT-PCR) or branched DNA assay (b DNA).
- Other markers of HIV infection:
  - p24 antigen.
  - Double stranded DNA.

32. Ans. is 'a' i.e., p. 24 antigen assay (***Ref:*** *Ananthanarayan, 9th/e, p. 577-578 and 8th/e, p. 576*)

- P-24 antigen is the earliest virus marker to appear in blood and is the one tested for.
- It may be detectable in blood after about 2 weeks.

Remember: Nucleic acid tests (RT-PCR, BONA, PCR) are the earliest test to become positive (even before p-24 antigen detection).

Test	Positive after infection
Nucleic acid test	12 days
P - 24 antigen test	16 days
Antibodies test	22 days

33. Ans. is 'a > c' i.e., Seen after 3 weeks of infection > Can't be detected after seroconversion

(***Ref:*** *Harrison, 18th/e, p. 1538-1540*)

Antigen Detection in HIV

- Following a single massive infection, as by blood transfusion, the virus antigens may be detectable in blood after about two weeks. **The major core antigen, p24 is the earliest virus marker to appear in the blood and is the one tested for. IgM antibodies appear in about 4-6 weeks, to be following by IgG antibodies.**
- If the infecting dose is small, as following a needle-stick injury, the process may be considerably delayed.
- The appearance of p24 antigenemia and viremia, followed by IgM antibody response, coincides with acute or seroconversion illness. Afterwards, free p24 antigen disappears from circulation and remains absent during the long asymptomatic phase, to reappear only when severe clinical disease sets in.
- The test is most useful in persons recently exposed to risk of infection, in whom the antibody test is negative.

34. Ans. is 'b' i.e., Time period between infection and detection of antibodies against HIV

(***Ref:*** *Ananthanarayan, 9th/e, p. 579 and 8th/e, p. 578*)

- It takes 2-8 weeks to months for antibodies to appear after infection. This period, from infection to appearance of antibodies is called as window period.
- During this period patients is seronegative, i.e., serological tests (ELISA and Western blot) are negative.
- The individual may be highly infectious during this period.

35. Ans. is 'b' i.e., Reverse transcriptase PCR (***Ref:*** *Greenwood, 18th/e, p. 532*)

"Both direct and indirect diagnostic methods are available to make a laboratory diagnosis of HIV infection. Of these the most important sensitive assay, is **reverse transcriptase PCR for viral nucleic acid,** which can detect a single copy of RNA or proviral DNA from infected cells." (***Ref:*** *Greenwood, 16th/e, p. 532*)

ONCOGENIC VIRUSES

36. Ans. is 'a' i.e., HIV and **'b'** i.e., HTLV (***Ref:*** *Harrison's 18th/e, Chapter 226; Jawetz, 27th/e, p. 619*)

- Retroviruses contain an RNA genome and an RNA-directed DNA polymerase (reverse transcriptase). Both HIV and HTLV are oncogenic retrovirus.

37. Ans. is 'd' i.e., EBV (***Ref:*** *Ananthanarayan, 9th/e, p. 565 and 8th/e, p. 563*)

- EBV has been implicated in causation of Nasopharyngeal carcinoma and Burkitt's lymphoma.

38. Ans. is 'd' i.e., Px (***Ref:*** *Jawetz, 27th/e*)

- The HTLV-1 genome contains Gag, pol and env genes in that order like other retroviruses and **an extra gene called TAX** in Px region.
- Some viruses, exemplified by the human retroviruses (Delta retrovirus and Lentivirus), contain additional genes downstream from the env gene. One is a transactivating regulatory gene (tax or tat) that encodes a nonstructural protein that alters the transcription or translational efficiency of other viral genes. (*Jawetz*)

39. Ans. is 'a' i.e., Tropical spastic paraparesis (***Ref:*** *Jawetz, 24th/e, Chapter 43*)

- HTLV-1 has been established as the causative agent of adult T cell leukemia-lymphomas (ATL) as well as a nervous system degenerative disorder called Tropical spastic paraparesis.
- HTLV-1 may also play a role in infective dermatitis and uveitis syndromes.

40. Ans. is 'c' i.e., Retroviridae (***Ref:*** *Ananthanarayan, 9th/e, p. 565 and 8th/e, p. 563*)

- All Oncogenic RNA viruses belong to family Retroviridae (HTLV-1 and HIV) and Flaviviridae (HCV).
- All oncogenic DNA viruses belong to family Papillomaviridae, Herpesviridae (EBV, HHV-8) and Hepadnaviridae (HBV).

41. Ans. is 'a' i.e., Retrovirus (***Ref:*** *Ananthanarayan, 9th/e, p. 565 and 8th/e, p. 563, 565*)

Already explained.

42. Ans. is 'c' i.e., Adult T cell leukemia / Lymphoma virus

Already explained in book text.

43. Ans. is 'd' i.e., Varicella zoster virus

Already explained in book text.

44. Ans. is 'd' i.e., Adenovirus

Adenoviruses most commonly cause respiratory illness. The illnesses can range from the common cold to pneumonia croup and bronchitis. Depending on the type, adenoviruses can cause other illnesses such as gastroenteritis, conjunctivitis, cystitis, and, less commonly, neurological disease.

45. Ans. is 'a' i.e., HTLV-I

HTLV-1 has been established as the causative agent of adult T-cell leukemia-lymphomas (ATL) as well as a nervous system degenerative disorder called tropical spastic paraparesis. It does not carry an oncogene. The human lymphotropic viruses have a marked affinity for mature T cells. HTLV-1 is expressed at very low levels in infected individuals. It appears that the viral promoter enhancer sequences in the long terminal repeat may be responsive to signals associated with the activation and proliferation of T cells. If so, the replication of the viruses may be linked to the replication of the host cells—a strategy that would ensure efficient propagation of the virus.

46. Ans. is 'd' i.e., Epidermodysplasia

Epidermodysplasia verruciformis is a rare, heritable disease characterized by an unusual susceptibility to infection with specific types of human papillomavirus and a propensity for developing malignant skin tumours.

47. Ans. is 'e' i.e., Sarcoidosis

Sarcoidosis is a rare condition that causes small patches of red and swollen tissue, called granulomas, to develop in the organs of the body. It usually affects the lungs and skin. It's thought that sarcoidosis happens because the immune system has gone into "overdrive", where the body starts to attack its own tissues and organs. The resulting inflammation then causes granulomas to develop in the organs.

48. Ans. is 'a' i.e., Myoclonus is seen in 10% of the patients

CJD is the most common prion disease responsible for nearly 85% of all human prion diseases. **Creutzfeldt–Jakob disease is a subacute progressive encephalopathy characterized by a rapidly progressive dementia, associated with myoclonic jerks**. Memory loss, behavioral changes, and confusion are the common clinical manifestations. The condition is also associated with ataxia, aphasia, visual loss and hemiparesis. The condition progresses and in the terminal stage of the disease, the patient becomes mute and comatose. **The condition is associated with extensive cortical spongiosis, gliosis and neural loss**. The condition is invariably fatal and death occurs in about 8 months.

49. Ans. is 'c' i.e., Infectious

Prions are **small protein-containing infectious particles with no detectable nucleic acid**. They were suspected to be viruses but otherwise do not conform to the standard definition of viruses. They differ from the viruses in their many properties. **The prions show following characteristics:**

1. Prions like viruses are filterable.
2. They apparently lack any virion structure or genome.
3. Unlike viruses, they are unusually resistant to inactivation by heat, disinfectants and radiation.
4. They do not elicit any specific immune response in the infected host.

50. Ans. is 'd' i.e., Only Protein

Already explained.

51. Ans. is 'b' i.e., It catalyzes abnormal folding of other protein

Already explained.

52. Ans. is 'b' i.e., Associated with misfolding of protein

Already explained.

53. Ans. is 'b' i.e.,Creutzfeldt Jakob diseases

54. Ans. is 'a' i.e., Prion disease

Fatal familial insomnia: Patients with this illness present with intractable insomnia, dysautonomia, dementia and motor paralysis. Death occurs within 6 months to 3 years following presentation. The clinical presentation of the disease, however, varies widely; **hence definitive diagnosis of the condition is made by genotyping.**

HEPATITIS VIRUSES

1. Incubation period of HBV is: *(Recent MCQ)*

(a) 45 to 180 days (b) 6 to 60 days
(c) 10 days (d) 10 hours

2. Carrier state does not exist for: *(AIIMS 07)*

(a) Hepatitis B virus (b) Hepatitis A virus
(c) Non A Non B Hepatitis (d) Delta agent

3. Acute liver failure is caused by A: *(Recent MCQ)*

(a) Hepatitis A (b) Hepatitis B
(c) Hepatitis E (d) Hepatitis C

4. HCV is: *(PGI Dec 05, June 08)*

(a) Enveloped RNA (b) Nonenveloped RNA
(c) Nonenveloped positive strand RNA (d) Enveloped negative strand RNA
(e) DNA virus

HEPATITIS A VIRUS

5. Transmission of hepatitis A virus occurs: *(PGI 99)*

(a) One week before and one week after onset of symptom
(b) 2 weeks before onset of symptoms
(c) 2 weeks after onset of symptoms
(d) 1 week after onset of symptoms

6. True about hepatitis A virus: *(Recent MCQ)*

(a) Causes cirrhosis (b) Helps HDV replication
(c) Common cause of hepatitis (d) Causes chronic hepatitis

7. Hepatitis A virus is best diagnosed by: *(AI 01)*

(a) IgM antibodies in serum
(b) Isolation from stool
(c) Culture from blood
(d) Isolation from bile

HEPATITIS B VIRUS

8. Reverse transcriptase of HBV is coded on following gene: *(AI 00)*

(a) C gene
(b) S gene
(c) P gene
(d) X gene

9. Which is the longest DNA of hepatitis B virus? *(Recent MCQ)*

(a) P gene
(b) X gene
(c) S gene
(d) C gene

10. Which is not true about hepatitis B virus? *(Recent MCQ)*

(a) DNA virus
(b) Transmitted by faeco-oral route
(c) Can be transmitted from mother to child (Perinatal transmission)
(d) Contains reverse transcriptase

11. All of the following are components of Dane Particle *except*: *(AIIMS 98)*

(a) Surface antigen
(b) Core antigen
(c) C-antigen
(d) Delta antigen

Complications of HBV

12. HBV is associated with all of the following *except*: *(Recent MCQ)*

(a) Hepatic cancer
(b) Chronic hepatitis
(c) Hepatic adenoma
(d) Cirrhosis

13. HBV all true, *except*: *(PGI 98)*

(a) It is a DNA virus
(b) Spreads by blood transfusions
(c) HBsAg marker of infection
(d) Least chance of chronicity

Serological Markers and Lab Diagnosis

14. Which of the following antigen is found within the nuclei of infected hepatocytes and not usually in the peripheral circulation in Hepatitis 'B' infection? *(Recent MCQ)*

(a) HBeAg
(b) HBcAg
(c) Anti-HBc
(d) HBsAg

15. A thirty-year-man presented with nausea, fever and jaundice of 5 days duration. The biochemical tests revealed a bilirubin of 6.7 mg/dl (conjugated 5.0 mg/dl) with SGOT/SGPT (AST/ALT) 1230/900 IU/ml. The serological tests showed presence of HBsAg, IgM anti HBc and HBeAg. The most likely diagnosis: *(AIIMS 02)*

(a) Chronic hepatitis B infection with high infectivity
(b) Acute hepatitis B infection with high infectivity
(c) Chronic hepatitis B infection with low infectivity
(d) Acute hepatitis B infection with low infectivity

16. Recent hepatitis infection is best diagnosed by: *(AIIMS Nov 01)*

(a) Hbs Ag
(b) IgG Anti HBe abs
(c) Anti HBs Ag abs
(d) IgM anti HBc abs

17. Anti HBsAb indicates: *(AIIMS 93)*

(a) Resistance to Hepatitis B
(b) Acute infection
(c) Good prognosis
(d) Hepatocellular carcinoma

18. A 30-year-old patient presented with history of jaundice for 10 days. His liver function tests showed bilirubin of 10 mg/dl, SGOT/SGPT – 1100/1450, serum alkaline phosphatase – 240 IU. He was positive for Hbs Ag. What should be the confirmatory test to establish acute hepatitis B infection? *(AIIMS 06)*

(a) IgM anti-HBc antibody
(b) Hbe Ag
(c) HBV DNV by PCR
(d) Anti-HBc antibody

19. In a patient only anti HBsAg is positive in serum, all other markers are negative. This indicates: *(AIIMS 01)*

(a) Acute hepatitis
(b) Chronic active hepatitis
(c) Persistent carrier
(d) Hepatitis B vaccination

20. Hepatitis B vaccination is given to a patient. His serum will reveal: *(AIIMS May 02)*

(a) HBsAg
(b) Anti-HBsAg
(c) IgM Anti-HBcAg and HBsAg
(d) IgM and IgG Anti-HBcAg

Prophylaxis

21. Best means of giving hepatitis B vaccine is: *(Recent MCQ)*

(a) Subcutaneous
(b) Intradermal
(c) Intramuscular deltoid
(d) Intramuscular gluteal

22. A blood donor is not considered for safe transfusion, if he has: *(AI 12)*

(a) Anti HBsAg +ve
(b) Anti HBsAg and HBcAg (+)ve
(c) HBsAg + ve and IgM anti HBc +ve
(d) Anti HBc +ve

HEPATITIS C VIRUS

23. Hepatitis C virus TRUE finding is: *(AIIMS Dec 98)*

(a) Spreads along feco oral route
(b) Antibody to HCV may not be seen in acute stage
(c) Does not cause chronic hepatitis
(d) It cannot be cultured

24. Most common hepatotropic virus causing increased chronic carrier state is: *(Recent MCQ)*

(a) HEV
(b) HAV
(c) HBV
(d) HCV

25. Which of the following statements about Hepatitis 'C' is true? *(AI 09)*

(a) DNA virus
(b) Most common indication for liver transplant
(c) Does not cause liver cancer
(d) Does not cause coinfection with hepatitis B

26. Hepatitis C virus is a: *(Recent MCQ)*

(a) Togavirus
(b) Flavivirus
(c) Filovirus
(d) Retrovirus

27. Max. Hepatitis C virus transmission to foetus in pregnancy depends on: *(PGI 2000)*

(a) Duration of illness
(b) Time of infection
(c) Route of delivery
(d) HIV infection
(e) High level of HCV RNA

HEPATITIS E VIRUS

28. A young pregnant woman presents with fulminant hepatic failure. The most likely aetiological agent is: *(AI 04)*

(a) Hepatitis B virus
(b) Hepatitis C virus
(c) Hepatitis E virus
(d) Hepatitis A virus

29. Regarding Hepatitis E true is: *(AIIMS 98)*

(a) Occurs with Hepatitis B
(b) Single stranded DNA virus
(c) Occurs along with HIV
(d) Mortality increased in pregnancy

30. Which of the following is Calcivirus? *(AIIMS Nov 01)*

(a) Hepatitis E
(b) Hepatitis B
(c) Hepatitis C
(d) Hepatitis A

HEPATITIS D VIRUS

31. HBV and HDV false is: *(New Pattern MCQ)*

(a) Both can infect simultaneously
(b) HDV causes more serious infection due to superinfection
(c) HDV cannot infect in absence of HBV
(d) DNA viruses

32. HDV is: *(NBE Based AI 2014-15 Pattern)*

(a) SS-RNA virus
(b) SS-DNA virus
(c) DS-RNA virus
(d) DS-DNA virus

ANSWERS AND EXPLANATIONS

HEPATITIS VIRUSES

1. **Ans. is 'a'** i.e., 45 to 180 days (***Ref:*** *Harrison, 18th/e, p. 2546; 19th/e, p. 2006*)

Remember:

Enterically transmitted non-A, non-B (NANB) virus → HEV.

Parenterally transmitted NANB → HCV.

Hepatitis Virus		**Incubation period**
HAV	→	15-45 days (mean 30 days)
HBV	→	30-180 days
HCV	→	15-160 days (mean 50 days)
HDV	→	30-180 days
HEV	→	14-60 days (mean 40 days)

2. **Ans. is 'b'** i.e., Hepatitis A virus (***Ref:*** *Harrison, 18th/e, p. 2546; 19th/e, p. 2006*)

Carrier

- **Present**: HBV, HCV, HDV (only with HBV)
- **Absent**: HAV, HEV

Remember: Non A, Non B hepatitis is HCV.

3. **Ans. is 'd'** i.e., Hepatitis C (***Ref:*** *Handbook of Liver Disease, p. 712*)

- Among hepatitis viruses, hepatitis A, B and E are common causes of acute liver failure.
- Among these, HBV is the most common cause.

Note: Hepatitis C can also cause acute liver failure, but it is very rare.

4. **Ans. is 'a'** i.e., Enveloped RNA (***Ref:*** *Ananthanarayan, 9th/e, p. 549 and 8th/e, p. 545*)

Virus	Family
1. Hepatitis A	Enterovirus (Picornavirus), non-enveloped RNA virus
2. Hepatitis B	Hepadna virus, DNA virus
3. Hepatitis C	Flavivirus, enveloped RNA virus
4. Hepatitis D	Defective RNA virus resembling viroids
5. Hepatitis E	Calcivirus, non-enveloped RNA virus

HEPATITIS A VIRUS

5. **Ans. is 'b'** i.e., 2 weeks before onset of symptoms; **'d'** i.e., 1 week after onset of symptoms

   (***Ref:*** *PSM Park, 19th/e, p. 174*)

   - The risk of transmission of HAV is greatest from 2 weeks before to 1 week after the onset of jaundice.
   - **Infectivity falls rapidly with onset of jaundice.**
   - HAV is excreted in faeces for about 2 weeks before the onset of jaundice and for up to one week thereafter.

6. **Ans. is 'c'** i.e., Common cause of hepatitis in children (***Ref:*** *Ananthanarayan, 8th/e, p. 537*)

   - HAV the most common cause of hepatitis in children.
   - HAV does not cause chronic hepatitis or cirrhosis.
   - HBV (no HAV) helps in HDV replication.

7. **Ans. is 'a'** i.e., IgM antibodies in serum (***Ref:*** *19th/e, Harrison, 2004*)

   "Detection of IgM-specific anti-HAV in the blood of an acutely infected patient confirms the diagnosis of hepatitis A." HAV is the **only cultivable** hepatitis virus. Diagnosis is based on IgM detection due to the early presence of these antibodies in patient serum, in fact so early that a lack of hepatitis A antibodies at the onset of clinical manifestations excludes hepatitis A.

HEPATITIS B VIRUS

8. **Ans. is 'c'** i.e., P gene (***Ref:*** *Ananthanarayan, 9th/e, p. 544 and 8th/e, p. 540*)

   P gene of HBV codes for DNA polymerase which has 3 activities: (i) DNA dependent DNA polymerase, (ii) Reverse transcriptase activity, (iii) RNase H activity.

9. **Ans. is 'a'** i.e., P gene (***Ref:*** *Ananthanarayan, 8th/e, p. 540*)

   P gene is the largest gene.

10. **Ans. is 'b'** i.e., Transmitted by faeco-oral route (***Ref:*** *Harrison, 18th/e, p. 2547; 17th/e, p. 1939*)

    - Hep B is partially double stranded DNA virus, amongst the hepatitis viruses, HBV has maximum risk of perinatal transmission.

Perinatal transmission				
HAV	HBV	HCV	HDV	HEV
-	+++	±	+	-

11. **Ans. is 'd'** i.e., Delta antigen (***Ref:*** *Ananthanarayan, 9th/e, p. 543 and 8th/e, p. 539*)

    Dane particle contains:

    1. Core antigen (C antigen – HBc Ag).
    2. Surface antigen (HBsAg).
    3. Hepatitis B 'e' antigen (HBeAg).

COMPLICATIONS OF HBV

12. **Ans. is 'c'** i.e., Hepatic adenoma (***Ref:*** *Harrison, 18th/e, p. 2552; 17th/e, p. 1944, 1945*)
    - Hepatic complications of HBV infection are acute hepatitis, chronic hepatitis, fulminant hepatitis, cirrhosis and HCC.
13. **Ans. is 'd'** i.e., Least chance of chronicity (***Ref:*** *Harrison, 18th/e, p. 2546; 17th/e, p. 1939*)
    - Least chances of chronicity are with HAV and HEV.
    - Maximum chance of chronicity is with HCV.
    - 90% of infants infected with HBV, become chronically infected.

    Remember: By definition, HBV chronic carriers are those in whom HBs Ag persists for more than 6 months.

Serological Markers and Lab Diagnosis

14. **Ans. is 'b'** i.e., HBcAg (***Ref:*** *Ananthanarayan, 8th/e, p. 373*)
    - HBcAg is not demonstrable in the circulation because it is enclosed within the HBs Ag coat.
    - HBcAg remains in the hepatocyte, where it can readily be detectable by immunohistochemical staining.
15. **Ans. is 'b'** i.e., Acute hepatitis B infection with high infectivity (***Ref:*** *Ananthanarayan, 9th/e, p. 548 and 8th/e, p. 544*)
    - Presence of HBsAg, IgM anti HBc and HBeAg suggest the diagnosis of acute hepatitis B with high infectivity.

	HBs Ag	Anti HBs Ag	HBe Ag	Anti HBe Ag	Anti HBc Ag
Acute HBV (high infectivity)	+	-	+		IgM
Acute HBV (low infectivity)	+	-		+	IgM
Chronic HBV (high infectivity)	+	-	+		IgG
Chronic HBV (low infectivity)	+	-		+	IgG
Recovery	-	+	-	+	IgG
Immunized	-	+		-	

16. **Ans. is 'd'** i.e., IgM anti HBc abs (***Ref:*** *Ananthanarayan, 9th/e, p. 548 and 8th/e, p. 544*)
    - **HBsAg is the first marker to be elevated and Anti HBc-IgM** appears within 1-2 weeks after the appearance of HBsAg and lasts for 3-6 months.
    - Diagnostic tests in recent hepatitis B infection are HBsAg detection and HBc-IgM and overall best is to look out for IgM anti HBc.
17. **Ans. is 'a'** i.e., Resistance to hepatitis B (***Ref:*** *Harrison, 18th/e, p. 2550; 17th/e, p. 1935*)
    - Persons with anti-HBs in serum are protected against infection with HBV.
    - Anti-HBs Ag is the protective antibody.
    - It is present either after recovery from hepatitis B or after immunization.
18. **Ans. is 'a'** i.e., IgM anti-HBc antibody (***Ref:*** *Ananthanarayan, 9th/e, p. 548 and 8th/e, p. 543-544*)
    - Has been explained.
    - IgM anti-HBc antibody is the marker of acute or recent HBV infection.
19. **Ans. is 'd'** i.e., Hepatitis B vaccination (***Ref:*** *Ananthanarayan, 9th/e, p. 548 and 8th/e, p. 544*)
    - The surface Ag (HBsAg) is used in vaccine preparation which is prepared in Baker's yeast (Saccharomyces cerevisiae) by DNA recombination technology by cloning the S gene into the yeast chromosome and **Anti-HBsAg titer should be more than 10 IU/ml to be considered as protective titer.Q**
20. **Ans. is 'b'** i.e., Anti HBsAg (***Ref:*** *Ananthanarayan, 9th/e, p. 548 and 8th/e, p. 543*)
    - Anti HBs Ag is protective antibody.
    - It is the only serological marker, present after immunization.

Prophylaxis

21. **Ans. is 'c'** i.e., Intramuscular Deltoid (***Ref:*** *Ananthanarayan, 9th/e, p. 548 and 8th/e, p. 544*)
    - Vaccine is given intramuscular into the deltoid or in infants into the anterolateral aspect of thigh. Gluteal injection is not recommended as it may result in poor immune response.
22. **Ans. is 'c'** i.e., HBs Ag + ve and IgM anti HBc +ve (***Ref:*** *Ananthanarayan, 9th/e, p. 547-548 and 8th/e, p. 544-545*)
    - HBs Ag (+) ve and IgM anti HBc (+) ve indicate acute HBV infection, which is a contraindication of blood tranfusion.

ABOUT OTHER OPTIONS

Option a

- Anti HBs Ag antibody may be (+) ve either after immunization or after recovery from HBV infection. In both the conditions, blood can be transfused.

Option b

- HBc Ag cannot be (+) ve as it does not appear in blood.

Option c

- When Anti HBe is (+) ve blood can be transfused if other markers of infection are also negative, e.g., HBsAg, HBV DNA, IgM anti HBC.

HEPATITIS C VIRUS

23. **Ans. is 'b and d'** i.e., Antibody to HCV may not be seen in acute stage and it cannot be cultured

    (***Ref:*** *Ananthanarayan, 9th/e, p. 548-549 and 8th/e, p. 545; Harrison, 18th/e, p. 2551; 17th/e, p. 1943*)
    - A specific serological diagnosis of hepatitis 'C' can be made by the presence of anti HCV in the serum. This antibody may never become detectable in 5 to 10% of patients with acute Hepatitis 'C'.
    - HCV cannot be grown in culture. It can only be cloned in E coli.Q
    - **The only Hepatitis virus, which can be cultivated is HAV.**
24. **Ans. is 'd'** i.e., HCV (***Ref:*** *Harrison, 18th/e, p. 2546; 17th/e, p. 1939*)

    Most common cause of chronic carrier state is HCV. About 50-70% of patients progress to chronic hepatitis.

    Chronicity → HCV > HDV > HBV.
25. **Ans. is 'b'** i.e., Most common indication for liver transplantation (***Ref:*** *Harrison, 17th/e, p. 1984, 1983, 1939*)
    - **The most common indication for liver transplantation currently is cirrhosis due to chronic hepatitis 'C' infection.**

    ABOUT OTHER OPTIONS
    - HCV is an RNA virus; the only hepatitis virus which has DNA is HBV.
    - HCV can cause liver carcinoma.
    - HCV may cause coinfection with HBV and coinfection of HCV with HBV increases the rate of development of cirrhosis and the risk of HCC compared with infection with either virus alone.
26. **Ans. 'b'** i.e., Flavivirus

    (***Ref:*** *Ananthanarayan, 9th/e, p. 549 and 8th/e, p. 547; Harrison, 18th/e, p. 2542; 17th/e, p. 1936*)
    - The hepatitis 'C' virus has been classified as a new genus Hepacivirus in the family flaviviridae.
27. **Ans. is 'e'** i.e., High level of HCV RNA (***Ref:*** *Jawetz, 27th/e, p. 503*)
    - Transmission appears to be a function of the degree of maternal viremia which is detected by PCR for HCV RNA.
    - The virus can be transmitted from mother to infant, although not as frequently as for HBV. Estimates of mother-to-child vertical transmission vary from 3% to 10%. Mothers with higher HCV viral loads or coinfection with HIV more frequently transmit HCV. No risk of transmission has been associated with breastfeeding.

HEPATITIS E VIRUS

28. Ans. is 'c' i.e., Hepatitis E virus (***Ref:*** *Ananthanarayan, 9th/e, p. 550 and 8th/e, p. 546*)

- Fulminant hepatitis may occur rarely in 1-2% of cases, except for the pregnant women who are particularly at higher risk (20%) of developing fulminant hepatitis.

29. Ans. is 'd' i.e., Mortality increased in pregnancy (***Ref:*** *Ananthanarayan, 9th/e, p. 550 and 8th/e, p. 546*)

- A unique feature of hepatitis E is high case fatality rate of 20-40% in pregnant women, especially in the last trimester of pregnancy.

30. Ans. is 'a' i.e., Hepatitis E (***Ref:*** *Ananthanarayan, 9th/e, p. 550 and 8th/e, p. 546*)

- HEV is Classified the genus Herpesvirus under the family Calciviridae.
- Type E hepatitis was previously mistaken for hepatitis A because of clinical and epidemiological similarities.
- Both have acute onset with mild illness.
- Both are transmitted by fecal oral route.
- **Differences are:**
  - **Hep. A is more common in children, while Hep. E is more common in young adults.**
  - **Hepatitis E can cause fulminant hepatitis in pregnant women (not HAV).**
  - **Secondary attack rate of HEV is very low (2–3%) as against 10-20% in HAV.**

HEPATITIS D VIRUS

31. Ans. is 'd' i.e., DNA virus (***Ref:*** *Ananthanarayan, 9th/e, p. 549 and 8th/e, p. 549*)

- HDV and HBV can infect simultaneously **(coinfection).**
- HDV superinfection on HBV has more serious infection than coinfection.
- HDV infection causes hepatitis only in persons with acute or chronic HBV infection; the HDV cannot produce infection in the absence of HBsAg.
- HDV is an RNA virus, while HBV is a DNA virus.

32. Ans. is 'a' i.e., SS-RNA virus (***Ref:*** *Ananthanarayan, 9th/e, p. 549 and 8th/e, p. 549*)

- HDV is a single-stranded RNA (ss-RNA) virus.

RED ALERT POINTS

1. The intracytoplasmic inclusion Negri bodies are diagnostic of: **Rabies (Most common site – Hippocampus).**
2. HIV virus has predilection for infecting: **CD4 + T-cells and coreceptors like CXCR4 and CCR5 are present which helps in attachment to T cells and macrophages.**
3. **Torres bodies and Cowdry type A inclusion bodies** are seen in: **Yellow fever, first viral disease discovered, 17 D vaccine is used, which is a Live attenuated vaccine can be given in pregnant females.**
4. HIV can be detected and confirmed by: **Reverse transcriptase – PCR, most sensitive is ELISA and most specific commonly used is Western blot.**
5. **Dengue** virus belongs to the family of: **Flaviviridae, 4 serotypes are present, Serotype 2 is most dangerous, serotype 1 followed by serotype 2 most likely go to Dengue shock syndrome. NS1 antigen and IgM ELISA test are used for early diagnosis and confirmed by PCR.**
6. **Prions** is: **Defect in folding of proteins PrPc (rich in alpha helix) changes to PrPsc (rich in beta structure).**
7. **Simian virus 40, Polyoma virus, BK virus** are **DNA viruses belonging to Papovaviridae.**
8. **Measles** pathognomic feature is Koplik spot, with ICP is 10 days, warthin finkeldey giant cell is a feature.
9. Only hepatitis virus which can be cultured is: **HAV, vaccines are available for hepatitis A and B show high efficacy. Carrier rate is highest in HepB, chronicity is a feature of Hep C.**
10. The best antirabies vaccine is: **HDC vaccine, Post exposure prophylaxis is PCEC (0, 3, 7, 14, 28 and 90 days).**
11. **Chronic hepatitis** is most common in infection with: **Hepatitis C (85%) (Flavivirus), Transfusion mediated hepatitis and Quasi species is seen.**
12. Infection Not transmitted transplacentally is: **Polio.**
13. Route of transmission of **Hepatitis E and Hep A** virus is: **Faeco-oral.**
14. Carrier state in liver disease is due to infection with: **HBV (0.1-30%).**
15. **Hepatitis A virus** is not transmitted through blood in serum.
16. **EBV** causes: **Nasopharyngeal carcinoma, Burkitts lymphoma, Non Hodgkin's lymphoma, Duncan syndrome and Infectious mononucleosis.**
17. **Pocks on CAM** are produced by: HSV smallpox (variola), vaccinia, camelpox, cowpox, monkey pox. Quantitative assay of viral infectivity: Plaque assay, pock assay.
18. **Most sensitive serological test for IMN;** Monospot test. Lymphocytosis with atypical lymphocytes is caused by: EBV (in IMN). **Most common presentation of congenital CMV infection:** Petechie, hepatosplenomegaly, jaundice. **Most sensitive diagnostic test** for CMV retinitis: Nucleic acid detection (by PCR) in intraocular fluid.

    Most common CMV disease after bone marrow transplantation: pneumonia. Owl eye intranuclear inclusions are seen in: CMV.
19. **Rabies virus has:** Single stranded RNA with negative polarity (SS negative sense RNA). **Rabies virus contains:** DNA dependent RNA polymerase. **Speed of rabies virus** in axons: 3 mm per hour.
20. **Routine intramuscular schedule for post exposure praphylaxis of rabies:** 6 doses on O, 3, 7,14, 28 days with booster on 90th day. **Schedule for intradermal (8 sites)** rabies vaccine: 8-0-4-0-1-1. **Number of doses of rabies vaccine for pre-exposure** prophylaxis: Three doses on days 0, 7 and 21 or 28. **Schedule of post-exposure prophylaxis in previously immunized person:** Two doses on day 0 and day 3.
21. **Incubation period of HBV:** 45-180 days.

    Components of dane particle: Core (C) antigen (HBcAg), surface antigen (HBs Ag), 'e' antigen (HBeAg). Reverse tanscriptase of HBV is encoded by: p gene.

    Largest gene of HBV: P gene. Reverse transcriptase is encoded by: Pol.

    Gene encoding for core of HIV: Gag.

    Gag gene encodes for: Core and shell. Nef gene in HIV is used for: Downregulating viral replication.

22. AIDS patients having diarrhea with AFB (+)ve bacilii in stool: Mycobacterium avium intracellulare. Progressive multi-focal leukoencephalopathy in HIV infected patients is caused by: JC virus (a Papovavirus).
23. Antigenic variation is not seen in: **Type C, maximum in Type A and Type B strain infected patient is prone for Reye's syndrome development.**
24. HSV 1 and HSV 2 causes infection above the waist and below the waist respectively. It is diagnosed with the help of Tzank smear, same is done for human herpes virus 3 (chickenpox).
25. Hepatitis B have highest carrier rate and Hepatitis C have Maximum chronicity.
26. Escape mutants are those who unable to form HBsAg -ve (S gene mutation), seen in infants born to HBe Ag +ve mother, seen in Liver transplant receiving combined HBV vaccine + Immunoglobulin.
27. Dane particle (42 nm), complete particle, infectious form, present in active replicating phase of virus. Most common form of Hepatitis B is spherical, another is tubular.
28. **Ante mortem diagnosis of Rabies is made** by RT PCR – Most sensitive and specific, sample is saliva, **CSF and skin.**
29. **NACO guidelines to prevent neonatal HIV** – Single dose of Nevirapine to mother during labor and to the baby within 72 hours after birth.

PRACTICE QUESTIONS

Herpes Virus

1. **The following diseases are associated with Epstein-Barr virus infection, *except*:**
   (a) Infectious mononucleosis
   (b) Epidermodysplasia verruciformis
   (c) Nasopharyngeal carcinoma
   (d) Oral hairy leukoplakia
2. **Epstein-Barr virus has been implicated in the following malignancies *except*:**
   (a) Hodgkin's disease
   (b) Non-Hodgkin's lymphoma
   (c) Nasopharyngeal carcinoma
   (d) Multiple myeloma
3. **Infectivity of chickenpox lasts for:**
   (a) Till the last scab falls off
   (b) 6 days after the onset of rash
   (c) 3 days after the onset of rash
   (d) Till the fever subsides
4. **A patient with sore throat has a positive Paul Bunnel test. The causative organism is:**
   (a) EBV
   (b) Herpesvirus
   (c) Adenovirus
   (d) Cytomegalic virus
5. **The most common cause of sporadic viral encephalitis is:**
   (a) Japanese B encephalitis
   (b) Herpes simplex encephalitis
   (c) HW encephalitis
   (d) Rubeola encephalitis
6. **A 40-year-old man underwent kidney transplantation. Two months later, he developed fever and features suggestive of bilateral diffuse interstitial pneumonia. Which of the following is most likely etiologic agent of the following?**
   (a) Herpes simplex virus
   (b) Cytomegalovirus
   (c) Epstein-Barr virus
   (d) Varicella zoster virus
7. **True about Herpesvirus *except*:**
   (a) HSV encephalopathy is treated with Acyclovir
   (b) Oropharynges involvement is common with HSV–I
   (c) Recurrent genital involvement is seen in HSV–II
   (d) Recurrence is rare in HSV–I
8. **Latent infection is seen in:**
   (a) Smallpox
   (b) Adenovirus
   (c) Chickenpox
   (d) Measles
9. **Genital Herpes simplex can be diagnosed by:**
   (a) Gram stain
   (b) Kotl preparation
   (c) Tzank smear
   (d) Acid-Fast stain
10. **Lipid envelop is found in which virus?**
    (a) Reo
    (b) Herpes
    (c) Picorna
    (d) Entero

Pox and Adenovirus

11. **Which of the following is not a Pox virus?**
    (a) Cowpox
    (b) Molluscum contagiosum
    (c) Smallpox
    (d) Chickenpox

12. Virus causing hemorrhagic cystitis, diarrhea and conjunctivitis is:
(a) RSV
(b) Rhino virus
(c) Adenovirus
(d) Rota virus
(e) Orthomyxo and Paramyxo viruses

13. H_5N1 is:
(a) Swine flu
(b) Avian flu
(c) An eradicated virus
(d) Paramyxovirus

14. The most common etiological agent for acute bronchiolitis in infancy is:
(a) Influenza virus
(b) Parainfulenza virus
(c) Rhinovirus
(d) Respiratory syncytial virus

15. All are true about congenital rubella *except*:
(a) It is diagnosed when infant has IgM antibodies at birth
(b) It is diagnosed when IgA antibodies persist for more than 6 months
(c) Most common congenital defects are deafness, cardiac malformation and cataract
(d) Infection after 16 weeks of gestation result in major congenital defects

16. Regarding mumps which is true?
(a) Causes SSPE
(b) Causes aseptic meningitis in children
(c) Sublingual gland is involved commonly
(d) All of the above

17. Segmented RNA is found in:
(a) Influenza virus
(b) Herpesvirus
(c) Rabies virus
(d) Measles virus

18. Strain used in measles vaccine is:
(a) Salk
(b) Sabin
(c) TAF
(d) Edmonston zagreb

19. Rubella vaccination is contraindicated in all *except*:
(a) Patient on immunosuppressant
(b) Girl with leukemia
(c) Girls between 11 and 14 years
(d) Pregnancy

Arboviruses

20. Which is true about Arboviral disease?
(a) Yellow fever is endemic in India
(b) Dengue viruses have only one sero types
(c) KFD is transmitted by tick
(d) Japanese encephalitis is transmitted by Aedes

21. In Japanese encephalitis pig act as:
(a) Amplifier
(b) Definitive host
(c) Intermediate host
(d) Any of the above

Rabies Viruses

22. Class II exposure in animal bites includes the following:
(a) Scratches without oozing of blood
(b) Licks on a fresh wound
(c) Scratch with oozing of blood on palm
(d) Bites from wild animals

23. Negri bodies are commonly seen in:
(a) Hippocampus
(b) Hypothalamus
(c) Cerebrum
(d) Pons

24. All are true of rabies *except*:

(a) 100% mortality
(b) Spreads from periphery
(c) Infects only the brain
(d) Prophylactic immunization of people at risk

25. The staining useful for antemortem diagnosis of rabies:

(a) Sellar (b) Machiavillo (c) Giemsa (d) Fluorescent

26. A vaccine for rabies was first developed by:

(a) Louis Pasteur
(b) Robert Koch
(c) Edward Jenner
(d) Landsteiner

Enteroviruses

27. Coxsackie group A commonly causes:

(a) Conjunctivitis
(b) Aseptic meningitis
(c) Hepatitis
(d) Myocarditis

28. True about polio:

(a) Paralytic polio is most common
(b) Only one type exists
(c) Increased muscular activity leads to increased paralysis
(d) Polio drops given only in <3 years

29. Acute epidemic keratoconjunctivitis caused by:

(a) Herpesvirus
(b) Echo–51
(c) Enterovirus–70
(d) Enterovirus–72

Hepatitis Viruses

30. Serology of a young man shows HBsAg, however HBeHg is negative with normal levels of AST and ALT. He is asymptomatic. What is the next line of management?

(a) Wait and watch
(b) Antivirals
(c) Immunoglobulins
(d) Liver transplant

31. A young pregnant woman presents with fulminant hepatic failure the most likely etiologic agent is:

(a) HBV (b) HCV (c) HEV (d) HAV

32. Chronic liver disease is caused commonly by:

(a) HBV (b) HCV (c) HAV (d) HEV

33. Reverse transcriptase of HBV is coded by:

(a) C gene (b) X gene (c) P gene (d) S gene

34. Acute infection with HBV is characterised by:

(a) HBsAg
(b) Anti-HBs Ag
(c) IgM anti–HBsAg and HBsAg
(d) Anti-HBc Ag

35. Which of the following viruses is cultivable?

(a) HAV (b) HBV (c) HDV (d) HEV

36. Hepatitis-C virus is a:

(a) Toga (b) Flavi (c) Filo (d) Retro

37. Best epidemiological tool for investigation of HBV is:

(a) Anti-HBs Ag
(b) Anti-HBc Ag
(c) Anti-HBe Ag
(d) HBc Ag

38. HBV present in India is:

(a) ADW (b) Ayx (c) Adr (d) Ayr

39. Which of the following is not present in DANE particle?

(a) Core antigen
(b) Surface antigen
(c) P-53
(d) None of the above

HIV

40. HIV can be detected and confirmed by:

(a) Polymerase chain reaction
(b) Reverse transcriptase – PCR
(c) Real time PCR
(d) Mimic PCR

41. An HIV patient complains of visual disturbances. Fundal examination shows bilateral retinal exudates and perivascular hemorrhages. Which of the following viruses are most likely to be responsible for this?

(a) Herpes simplex virus
(b) Varicella Zoster virus
(c) Cytomegalovirus
(d) EBV

42. Which of the following is true regarding HIV infection?

(a) Following needle stick injury infectivity is reduced by
(b) Administration of nucleoside analogues
(c) CD4 counts are best predictors of disease progression
(d) Infected T cells survive for a month in infected patients
(e) In latent phase HIV has minimal replication

43. HIV virus has:

(a) Single Stranded DNA
(b) Single Stranded RNA
(c) Double Stranded DNA
(d) Double Stranded RNA

44. Reverse transcriptase sequence in HIV is best described as:

(a) RNA → DNA → RNA
(b) DNA → RNA
(c) DNA → RNA→DNA
(d) RNA → DNA

45. A patient with HIV has diarrhea with acid fast organism in stool. The most likely organism is:

(a) M. avium intracellulare
(b) MTB (M. Tuberculosis)
(c) M.leprae
(d) Mycoplasma

46. A patient comes to hospital with history of sore throat, diarrhea and sexual contact 2 weeks before. The best investigation to rule out HIV is:

(a) P – 24 Antigen assay
(b) ELISA
(c) Western blot
(d) Lymph node biopsy

47. The chances of acquiring HIV infection following needle prick is:

(a) 0.3% (b) 0.003% (c) 0-30% (d) 3%

Miscellaneous Viruses

48. Prions consist of:

(a) DNA and RNA
(b) DNA, RNA and Proteins
(c) Only Proteins
(d) RNA and Proteins

49. True about prions:

(a) Are virus coded
(b) Cause misfolding of protein
(c) Cleave protein
(d) Defect in synthesis of protein

50. Which of the following is not a Prion associated disease?

(a) Scrapie
(b) Kuru
(c) Creutzfeldt-Jakob disease
(d) Alzheimer's disease

51. Rotavirus is responsible for:

(a) Acute non-bacterial GE in adults
(b) Infantile diarrhea
(c) Teratogenic effects
(d) Respiratory tract infection in immunocompromised

52. True about Ebola virus:

(a) Belongs to family filoviridae
(b) Transmission may occur from dead bodies
(c) Transmitted by sexual contact
(d) Incubation period is less than 48 hours
(e) Contain single stranded RNA

ANSWERS

1.	(b)	2.	(d)	3.	(b)	4.	(a)	5.	(b)	6.	(b)	7.	(d)	8.	(c)
9.	(c)	10.	(b)	11.	(d)	12.	(c)	13.	(b)	14.	(d)	15.	(d)	16.	(b)
17.	(a)	18.	(d)	19.	(c)	20.	(c)	21.	(a)	22.	(a)	23.	(a)	24.	(c)
25.	(d)	26.	(a)	27.	(b)	28.	(c)	29.	(c)	30.	(a)	31.	(c)	32.	(b)
33.	(c)	34.	(c)	35.	(a)	36.	(b)	37.	(b)	38.	(c)	39.	(c)	40.	(b)
41.	(c)	42.	(a)	43.	(b)	44.	(a)	45.	(a)	46.	(a)	47.	(a)	48.	(c)
49.	(b)	50.	(d)	51.	(b)	52.	(a,b, c,e)								

Chapter 9

IMMUNOLOGY

Resistance Offered by Host Against Offenders of the Body

Immunity can be broadly classified into two types: Innate Immunity and Acquired Immunity.

Innate Immunity – Resistance that an individual possess by birth.

It is determined by **Species, Racial and Individual levels (SIR).**

Components of Innate Immunity – Phagocyte (Monocyte, macrophage, neutrophils), Natural killer cells, Alternate complement pathway, acute phase protein (CRP, Mannose binding protein, Serum amyloid protein), Normal resident flora, Inflammation, fever, skin and mucosal barrier.

Adaptive/Acquired Immunity – Resistance acquired by an individual during life time.

Components of Acquired Immunity – B cell, T cell, Antigen presenting cells and Classical complement pathway.

Active immunity	Passive immunity
• **Natural**	**Natural**
Clinical infection	Ab (IgG) acquired through Placenta
Subclinical infection	Ab (IgA) acquired through Breast milk
• **Artificial**	**Artificial**
Vaccination	Immune cells
Live	Immune serum containing Abs
Killed	(Rabies immunoglobulin)

Local Immunity

- Produced at mucosal surfaces – GIT or respiratory mucosa.
- Provided by IgA antibody.
- Induced by infection or by live vaccination.

Adoptive Immunity:

- It is acquired by injection of immunologically competent lymphocytes known as **Transfer factor.**
- Used for treatment when the CMI is low, e.g., Lepromatous leprosy.

Herd Immunity:

- Overall immunity of a community to a pathogen.
- If Herd immunity is good–chance of epidemic is less.
- Eradication of a communicable disease–depends on good Herd immunity.
- Provided by mass vaccination by live vaccination to all individual at same time.

ANTIGEN

Stimulate Immune Response

- **Immunogenicity:** Ability to stimulate immune response.
- **React specifically**
  - Effector molecules (Antibodies).
  - Effector cells (Lymphocytes).
- Antigenicity: Proteins > Carbohydrates > Lipids > Nucleic acid.
- Antigenic determinant/Epitopes bind to paratope on the antibody/T-cell receptors.

Incomplete Antigen/Hapten

1. Low, molecular weight.
2. Cannot induce immune response.
3. Single epitope.
4. Carrier molecular required.

Determinants of Antigenicity

1. Size.
2. Foreignness.
3. Chemical nature (proteins and polysaccharides).
4. Susceptibility to tissue enzymes.

SPECIES SPECIFICITY

- **Iso-specificity**
  1. Found in some but not all members of a species.
  2. A, B, AB, O Blood groups.
- **Histocompatibility antigens**
  1. Present on the cells of each individual of species.
  2. Graft rejection.
  3. MHC (Short arm Chromosome 6).Q
- **Auto specificity**
  1. Normally non-antigenic.
  2. Hidden/sequestered antigens.
  3. Lens protein/spermatozoa.

Organ specificity – Some organs (brain, kidney, lens protein) of different species share same antigen–it is the basis of neuroparalytic complication following anti-rabies vaccine.

Heterogenetic (Heterophile) Specificity

- **Paul bunnel** – EBV with sheep RBC. Q
- **Weil-Felix** – Proteus OX2, OX19, OX K with Rickettsial polysaccharide.Q
- **Cold Agglutination test** – Mycoplasma with human O+ve RBC at 4°C.Q
- **Streptococcus MG** with Mycoplasma.Q
- **Forssman antigen** – Lipid-CHO complex, present all except rabbit.Q

Superantigen

- Receptor for Superantigen is – **Vβ** of TCR (Lateral aspect of TCR).Q

- **Do not require antigen presentation by macrophage**, directly stimulate non-specific T-cells–Leads to massive release of cytokines and polyclonal B cell activation → increase production of non-specific Abs.
- **Examples:**
  1. Staphylococcus – TSST, Exfoliative toxin, Enterotoxins.
  2. Streptococcus – Str pyrogenic exotoxin A, C.
  3. Fungus – Malassezia furfur.
  4. Mycoplasma arthritidis.
  5. Yersinia enterocolitica.
  6. Virus – EBV, CMV, HIV, Rabies nucleocapsid.

T Independent Ag	T Dependent Ag
• Simple–LPS, capsule, flagella	• Complex
• Dose dependent	• Immunogenic over wide range of dose
• IgM and IgG3	• All Ab raise
• No memory	• Memory present
• No macrophage processing	• Macrophage processing needed
• Directly acts on B cell causing polyclonal B cell activation	• Rapidly metabolized
• Slowly metabolized	

Note: T cell independent: Develop after 3-4 years, so Pneumococcal and meningococcal vaccine not effective <2 years.

ANTIBODY

- Abs are glycoprotein (γ globulin) which protects us from microbial infection. They are produced by the plasma cells following antigenic stimulation of the immune system.
- Consists – 2 Heavy and 2 Light chain.
- Heavy chains – μ, gamma, α, epsilon, δ and Light chain – kappa/lambda.
- Depending upon the type of H chain present, Igs are divided into 5 major classes – IgA, IgG, IgD, IgM, IgE.
- Fc – Biological function complement binding, NK, monocyte adherence
  - Fab – Hypervariable – CDR – (Complementarity determinant region) – N-terminal.Q
  - Hinge – Cysteine, proline.

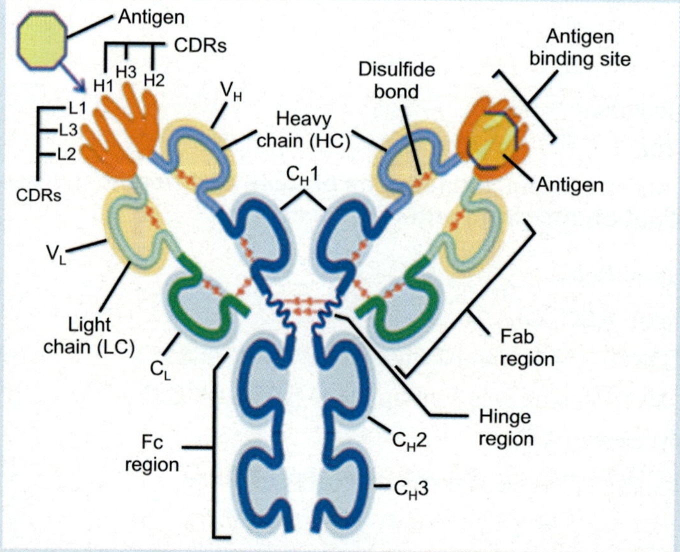

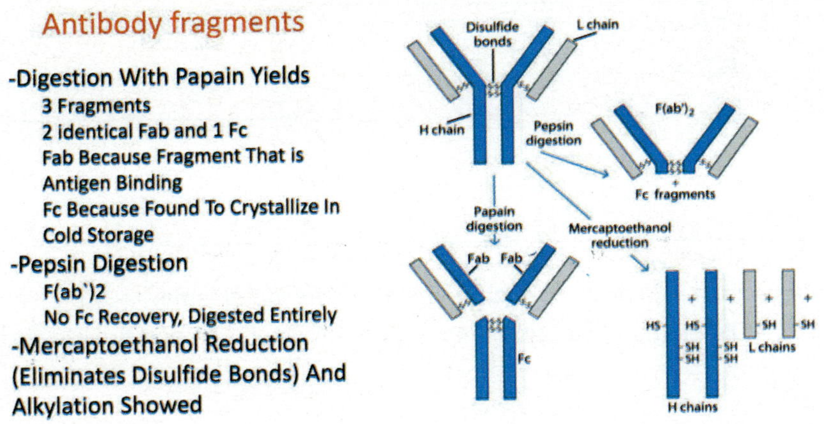

Bence Jones Protein/BJP (Abnormal Ig)Q:

- Coagulated when Heated at 50°C, dissolved at 70°C.
- **Multiple myeloma** – In theory, multiple myeloma can produce all classes of immunoglobulin, but **IgG** paraproteins are most common, followed by **IgA** and **IgM. IgD** and **IgE** myeloma are very rare. In addition, **light** and or **heavy chains** (the building blocks of **antibodies**) may be secreted in isolation: κ- or λ-light chains or any of the five types of heavy chains (α-, γ-, δ-, ε- or μ-heavy chains).
- Kappa or lambda (Kappa: Lambda = 2:1).Q

Properties of Various Immunoglobulins

Property	IgG	IgA	IgM	IgD	IgE
Usual form	Monomer	Monomer, dimer	Monomer, pentamer	Monomer	Monomer
Valency	2	2 or 4	2 or 10	2	2
Other chains	None	J chain, secretory component	J chain	None	None
Subclasses	G1, G2, G3, G4	A1, A2	None	None	None
Molecular weight (kDa)	150	150-600	900	150	190
Serum level (mg/mL)	9.5-12.5	IgA 1-3.0 IgA 2-0.5	1.5	0.03	0.0003
% of total serum Ig	75-85%	10-15%	5-10%	0.3%	0.019%
Half-life, days	23*	6	5	3	2.5
Daily production (mg/kg)	34	24	3.3	0.4	0.0023
Intravascular distribution (%)	45	42	80	75	50
Sedimentation coefficient	7	7	19	7	8
Complement activation					
Classical	++(IgG3>1>2)	-	+++	-	-
Alternate	-	+	-	-	-
Binds of Fc receptors of phagocytes	++	-	?**	-	-
Placental transfer	Yes (except IgG2)	-	-	-	-

Contd.

Contd.

Mediates coagglutination	Yes (except IgG3)	-	-	-	-
Mucosal transport	-	Yes	-	-	-
Mast cell degranulation	-	-	-	-	Yes
Marker for B cells	-	-	+	+	-
Heat stability	+	+	+	+	-

Waldenström Macroglobulinaemia – Multiple myeloma of IgM producing plasma.

- **Isotypic determinants** – Distinguish H chain classes (Ig G, A, M, D, E) and subclasses (Ig G1, G2 etc.) and k and λ Light chains.
- **Allotypic determinants**
  1. Distinct amino acid residues located primarily in (γ and α) H chains and k, λ chains.
  2. Possessed by some individuals of a particular species.
  3. Reflect genetic polymorphism of Igs.
- **Idiotypic determinants** – Located on V regions of L and H chains.

Ag-Ab Reaction

- Antigen and antibody combine specifically.
- Non-covalent interaction.
- **Bonds involved: Hydrophobic** > Vander waals > Electrostatic > Hydrogen bonding.
- Principle-Marrack's (Lattice) hypothesis
  - Prozone phenomenon (Zone of Ab excess).
  - Zone of equivalence.
  - Post zone phenomenon (Zone of antigen excess).

Types of Ab-Ag Reaction

1. **Precipitation Reaction**
   - Soluble Ag + Ab (in presence of electrocytes) at an optimal temperature → Insoluble precipitate band (gel)/ floccules (liquid).
     - (a) **Ring test** – Ascoli thermo ppt test (anthrax), Lancefield grouping (Streptococcus).
     - (b) **Slide test** – VDRL.
     - (c) **Tube test** – Kahn test, standardization of toxin.
     - (d) **Immunodiffusion** (In gel) – Visible band, preservation, differentiate between antigens – e.g., Elek gel ppt (C diphtheria toxigenicity testing), Eiken (E.coli). These are precipitation tests in gel immunodiffusion done in 1% agar gel.

       Various immunodiffusion test:
       - (1) Single diffusion in one dimension **(Oudin procedure).Q**
       - (2) Double diffusion in one dimension **(Oakley fulthorpe procedure).Q**
       - (3) Single diffusion in two dimensions **(Radial immunodiffusion).Q**
       - (4) Double diffusion in two dimensions **(Ouchterlony procedure).Q**
     - (e) **CIEP** – **α** Fetoprotein, Ag of Cryptococcus and Meningococcus.
     - (f) **Rocket electrophoresis.**
2. **Agglutination Reaction**
   - Insoluble (Particulate) Ag + Ab (in presence of electrolytes) at an optimal temperature → Particles are clumped or agglutinated.

Contd.

Contd.

(a) **Slide agglutination** (Slide Widal, Serotyping, blood grouping).
(b) **Tube agglutination** (Widal, Weil-Felix, Paul Bunnel, standard agg. test for Brucella, Cold agg. test for Mycoplasma pneumoniae).
(c) **Antiglobulin (Coomb's test)**
  (1) **Direct (baby)** – In vivo test.
  (2) **Indirect (mother)** – In vitro test.
(d) **Passive (indirect) agglutination**
  (1) Latex agglutination – Detection of ASO, RA, CRP and HCG.
  (2) Haemagglutination test for RA (Rose Waaler test).Q
(e) **Coagglutination** (Staphylococcus aureus Cowan 1 strain having protein A).

3. Blotting Techniques

Blot transfer is a technique used for visualization of specific DNA, RNA or proteins among the thousands of molecules. These are:

(i) Southern blot for DNA
(ii) Northern blot for RNA
(iii) Western blot (immunoblot for Proteins)
(iv) South western blot for protein-DNA interaction.

4. Complement Fixation Test (CFT)

(a) Wasserman test (Syphilis).
(b) CFT for viral diseases and other infectious disease.
(c) Other complement dependent serological tests:
- TPI, Sabin Feldman test (Toxoplasmosis).
- Cytocidal or cytolytic tests – Vibrio.
- Immunoadherence – Vibrio and T. pallidum.

5. Neutralization Test

(a) In vivo test
- Schick test – Diphtheria toxin.
- Toxigenicity testing.

(b) In vitro test
- ASO test (antistreptolysin test).
- Virus neutralization test.
- Naglers reaction.
- Bacteriophage – By Plaque inhibition test.

6. Opsonization

Means Enhanced phagocytosis.
- Enhanced phagocytosis.
- Mediated by Opsonins like C3b and Fc (IgG).Q

7. Immunofluorescence

(a) Direct immunofluorescence (e.g., Rabies).
(b) Indirect immunofluorescence (FTA-AB).

8. Newer Methods using on Labelled Molecules
- ELISA – enzyme tagged.
- RIA – radioimmunoassay.
- CLIA – chemiluminescent compound like acridinum.
- IFA – fluorescent dye labelled.

Contd.

Contd.

ELISA

- **Substrate** used are O-phenyldiamine dihydrochloride, p-nitrophenyl phosphate.Q
- **Enzyme** used are **Horse radish peroxidase, alkaline phosphatase.Q**
  - (a) Indirect.
  - (b) Competitive.
  - (c) Direct sandwich.
  - (d) Indirect sandwich.

9. Rapid Test

Immunochromatographic test for detection of HIV, HBsAg, Malaria, Dengue etc.

HYBRIDOMA TECHNOLOGY

Done for Mass Production of Monoclonal Antibody

Principle:

- A normal B cell is fused with a myeloma cell to produce hybridoma cell.
- Hybridoma cells have property of both B cell and myeloma cell (immortal), hence can be used to produce antibody in mass.

Procedure:

- Mouse is injected with desire antigen.
- Mouse spleen B cells (HGPRT+ and Ig+) are isolated and mixed with myeloma cells (HGPRT -ve and Ig –ve) and allowed to grow in HAT media.
- **3 Types of cells will be generated:**
  - **Unfused spleen cells** – can grow but don't survive long as they are not immortal.
  - **Unfused myeloma cells** – can't grow as they lack HGPRT.
  - **Hybrid cell (fused myeloma with spleen cells)** – can grow and survive long.

HAT medium – contains **Hypoxanthine, Aminopterine, Thymine**

- Purine synthesis in mammalian cell (spleen B cell) occurs by either de novo or salvage pathways.
- Aminopterine blocks the de novo or pathway so that the cell has to perform the salvage pathway to synthesis purines for its survival.
- **Salvage pathway requires HGPRT (hypoxanthine guanine phosphoribosyl phosphate) and thymine kinase.**
- So any cell that lacks HGPRT can't grow on HAT medium (e.g., Myeloma cell).

LYMPHOID SYSTEM

- **Cells involved in the immune response** into tissues and organs which are collectively referred as lymphoid system.
- Lymphoid tissue is divided into Primary and Secondary.
- **Primary (central)**
  - Sites of lymphoid development.
  - T cells: Thymus.
  - B cells: Bone marrow.
- **Secondary (peripheral)**
  - Provide environment where lymphocytes can interact with antigens.
  - Spleen, lymph nodes, mucosa associated lymphoid tissue.

CELLS OF IMMUNE SYSTEM

- **Lymphocytes**
  - 20-40% of leukocyte population in the blood.
  - T cells (CD 3)

- Helper T cells (CD 4).
- Cytotoxic T cells (CD8).

– B cells – 10 to 20%

Property	T Cell	B Cell
Antigen recognition receptor	T cell receptor	M Igs
Surface antigen	CD3	CD19
Receptor for Fc piece of Ig	-	+
Receptor for C3 component of complement	-	+
EAC rosette (C3 receptor, CR2, EBV receptor)	-	+
E rosette (CD2, measles receptor)	+	-
Thymus specific antigen	+	-
Blast transformation on treatment	PHA, Concavalin A	EB virus, Endotoxin

- **Null cells:** 5% lymphocytes, no T cell or B cell marker.
- **Killer cell:** Subpopulation of null cells, receptor for Fc part of IgG, responsible for ADCC.
- **Natural killer cells:** Subpopulation of null cells, also known **as large granular lyphocytes (LGL),** involved in allograft, tumor rejection, killing of virus transformed cells.
- **Plasma cells:** Derived from activated B cells, secrete antibodies.
- **Neutrophils:** 60% of circulating leukocytes, phagocytosis of foreign, dead cells, inflammation.
- **Eosinophils:** 3-5% of circulating leukocytes, numbers raised in allergic and parasitic conditions.
- **Basophils:** Less than 1% of circulating leukocytes, tissue counterparts are called as mast cells. Contain mediators of type I hypersensitivity reaction.

LOCATION OF B AND T CELLS IN LYMPHOID TISSUE

Thymus Dependent (T Cells Collection)

- **Spleen** – Periarterial lymphoid collection, Malphigian corpuscle in white pulp.
- **Lymph node** – Paracortical area.

Thymus Independent (B Cell Collection)

- **Spleen** – Perifollicular region, Mantle layer.
- **Lymph nodes** – Cortical follicles, Germinal centre, Medullary cords.

CELLS OF IMMUNE SYSTEM

T Cells

T cells precursors arise in bone marrow (also in yolk sac and liver before birth) and migrate to thymus. Maturity of T cells takes place in thymus.

A. Helper T cell (Inducer T cell)

These cells constitute 60% of total T cell have CD4 surface marker and bind to MHC-II (MHC class II restricted). These are following types of CD4 cells (Helper T cell).

1. **Effector cells** (Effector CD4 helper T cell)

   These are divided into:

   TH-1 cells – These are **activated by IFN-γ** and themselves produce IL-2, IFN-γ and IL-12. These are the primary cells involved in delayed hypersensitivity, cell mediated immunity, macrophage activation and killing of intracellular microbes (M. tuberculosis, M. leprae).

   These cells also induce destruction of target cells by activating T cells to become cytotoxic T cells and by activating NK cells.

TH-2 cells – These are **activated by IL-4** and themselves produce **IL-4,5,6,13,** these cells facilitate synthesis of all antibodies except IgG2b. These cells induce synthesis of IgE more efficiently and cause activation of mast cells and eosinophils. Therefore these cells provide defence against Helminthic parasites.

TH-17 cells – These cells are **powerful recruiters of neutrophils and monocytes** to play a role in severe inflammatory diseases. **These produce IL-17, IL-22** and chemokines which recruits neutrophils and monocytes.

2. **Memory (CD4 T cells)** – Provide memory, used as later effector cells during a second immune response **(CD4 T cells are master regulator of Immune system).Q**

B. Cytotoxic T Cells (Cytolytic T cells)

These cells constitute **30% of total T cells** and have **CD8 Surface marker and are MHC class I restricted.** They kill and lyse target cells including Tumor cells, virus infected cells and allograft **and participate in Type II hypersensitivity.** Ratio of CD4: CD8 T cells – 2:1.

C. Suppressor T cells

These cells have CD8 surface marker and they are MHC class I restricted, these cells downregulate the immune response.

TCR

It is a molecule found on T cells that is responsible for recognizing antigens bound to MHC molecules. It is a heterodimer made up of α and β chain (TCR α β) in 95% of cases recognizes antigens bound to MHC. TCR (γ δ) in 5% of cases binds to antigens without MHC involvement.

TCR diversity is generated by **somatic rearrangements of the genes** that **encode TCR** happens during development in Thymus. Hence, **the presence of TCR gene rearrangements demonstrated by molecular analysis is marker of T lineage cells.**

TCR Coreceptors

- **Helper T cell** coreceptor is CD4 that binds exclusively to class II MHC.
- **Cytotoxic T cell** coreceptor is CD8 that is specific for class I MHC.

TCR Costimulator

- **CD-28 on surface of T cell interacts with B7-1(CD-80) and B7-2(CD-86)** expressed on APC, so for activation of T cells, two signals are required.

  Signal 1 – via TCR, MHC, CD4/CD8 interactions.

  Signal 2 – CD-28, B7-1/B7-2 interactions.

B Cells

B cells are part of adaptive immunity. B cell constitutes 10-20% of the circulating peripheral lymphocytes. B cell recognize antigen via the B cell antigen receptor complex. IgM and IgD, present on the surface of all naïve B cells, constitute the antigen binding component of B cell receptor complex. After antigenic stimulation, B cells form plasma cells that secrete immunoglobulin.

Plasma Cell – It make an antibody of a single specificity, of a single immunoglobulin class and allotypes and of a single light chain type only. An exception is seen in the primary antibody response, when plasma cell producing IgM initially, may later be switched to IgG production (called Isotype switching or class switching).

- Lymphocytes, lymphoblasts and transitional cells also produce Immunoglobulin to some extent.Q

CLONAL SELECTION

An antigen interacts with B cells that show best fit by virtue of its BCR (IgM and IgD).

B cell is stimulated to divide and form a clone (Clonal selection). This clone of cells will become plasma cells that will secrete antibody of a particular specificity and same class. In contrast to TCR, BCR can be activated by antigens, without MHC involvement – so antigen processing and presentation by APC donot occur for B cells (in contrast to T cells).

Property	T Cell	B Cell
Antigen recognition receptor	T cell receptor	M Igs
Surface antigen	CD3	CD19
Receptor for Fc piece of Ig	-	+
Receptor for C3 component of compliment	-	+
EAC rosette (C3 receptor, CR2, EBV receptor)	-	+
E rosette (CD2, measles receptor)	+	-
Thymus specific antigen	+	-
Blast transformation on treatment with	**PHA, Concavalin A**	**EB virus, Endotoxin**

CELL MEDIATED IMMUNE RESPONSES

- Accomplished by effector T cells and macrophages rather than B cells and antibodies.
- Protects against fungi, virus, intracellular bacterial pathogens (M.leprae, M.tuberculosis, Brucella, Salmonella), parasites (leishmania, trypanosomes).
- Allograft rejection.
- Delayed hypersensitivity.
- Immunological surveillance.
- Immunity against cancer.
- **Primary immune response**
  - Initial contact with foreign Ag.
  - Ag presented by antigen presenting cells to T cell.
  - T cell receptor combines with foreign antigen along with self MHC molecule.
  - Proliferation of specific clones of effector T cells.
  - It is **SLOW, SLUGGISH and SHORT LIVED,** Main Immunoglobulin – IgM.
- **Secondary immune response**
  - More pronounced, more rapid.
  - Memory cells play a role
    - **PROMPT, POWERFUL and PROLONGED,** Predominant Ig – IgG.

T CELL DIFFERENTIATION

- **Processing of phagocytosed material, e.g., Bacteria.** The antigen is degraded and associated with class II molecules. The antigen MHC II complex then expressed on the surface of antigen presenting cells.
- Processing of antigens derived from within the cell (viral infection). Antigen MHC I complex expressed on cell surface.
- CD8+ T cells recognize Ag in association with self MHC I.
- CD4+ T cells recognize Ag in association with self MHC II.

Natural killer cell/null cell/large granular (LGL)/lymphokine activated cell (IL-2)

- **5-10%** of total lymphocyte.
- Indented nuclei and several granules.
- Not MHC restricted.
- **CD16 and CD 56 markers**
  ADCC – uses CD16 (FcR like).
- Cytotoxicity to virus infected cell and malignant cells.
- Attach to glycoprotein receptors and release perforins and granzyme which lyse the target cells.

Macrophages

Derived from the bone marrow and has role in: Phagocytosis, Secretion of cytokines, Antigen presentation.

Macrophages in various locations Peripheral blood called as **Monocytes** Liver – Kupffer cells Brain – Microglia Kidney – Mesangial cells Bone – Osteoclasts Lung – Alveolar macrophage – lung	Any solid tissue – Histiocyte Skin – Langerhans cell Inflammation site – Multinucleated cell and epitheloid cell **Kill cell by** – Phagocytosis and phagolysosome fusion and lysosomal degranulation and by oxygen free radical generation.

Dendritic Cell

APC during primary immune response, BM derived (separate lineage), Transport the presented Ag to lymph nodes. MHC II > I, also B7.

CYTOKINES

- **Soluble mediators** of host defense responses, both specific and non-specific.
- Same cytokine can be produced by multiple cell types and can have multiple effects on the same cell.
- Small proteins (8-80 KDa) usually acting in an autocrine or paracrine manner.

Name	Major Cell Source	Biological Effect
• **IFN α, β**	Phagocytes, fibroblasts	Antiviral, pyrogenic
• **IFN γ**	T cells, NK cells	Activates mononuclear phagocytes
• **TNF β**	T cells, β cells	Activates leucocytes, antitumor
• **TGF β**	T cells, Macrophages	Leuckocyte growth, angiogenesis
• **IL1**	Phagocytes (APCs)	Fever, Cachexia
• **IL2**	Th1 cells	T cell growth, Activation
• **IL3**	Th cell, NK, Mast cell	Hematopoesis
• **IL4**	Th2 cells	Isotype switching to IgE
• **IL5**	Th2 cells	Promote eosinophilic growth and differentiation
• **IL6**	Th2 cells	Lymphocyte Growth (IL-1, TNF like effects)
• **IL8**	Macrophages	Chemotactic to Neutrophils
• **IL10**	Th2 cells	Inhibits Macrophages, reduce cytokine production
• **IL12**	B cells, Macrophages	Activates TH1 cells and NK cells
• **GM-CSF**	T cells, Phagocytes Lineage	Hematopoiesis of Granulocyte, Monocyte
• **M-CSF**	Macrophage	Differentiation to Monocyte
• **G-CSF**	Macrophages	Differentiation to Granulocyte

CHEMOKINES

Chemoattractant Cytokines

Four major groups based on the cysteine structure near the amino terminus.

C (γ chemokines): Lymphotactin (Specific for lymphocytes).

C-C (Beta chemokine): Attract all leukocytes except neutrophil, **MIP α** (macrophage inflammatory protein 1a), **MCP-1** (monocyte chemoattractant protein) (Lymphocytes, monocytes, eosinophils, basophils), **RANTES** (Regulated and normal T cell expressed and secreted).

CXC (alpha chemokine) – IL-1, IL8 and TNF **(neutrophils).**

CX3 C: Fractalkine, Strong adhesion between monocytes and T cell (Neutrophils, monocytes, T cells).

INTERFERON

They are family of host coded proteins produced by cell on induction by viral and nonviral inducers.

Interferons are proteins either glycosylated or non-glycosylated.

IFN – Alpha – Non glycosylated (produced by **Leucocytes**).

IFN – Beta – Glycoprotein, produced by **Fibroblasts.**

IFN – γ – Glycoprotein, produced by **T lymphocytes.**

Mechanism of action – Cells produces a **protein TIP (Translation inhibiting protein)** which **selectively inhibits translation of mRNA.**

Properties of Interferon – Interferons are **species specific** not viral specific and Interferons are stable over a wide range of (PH 2-10) except IFN-γ, which is labile at PH 2.

C-Reactive Protein

It is nonspecific inflammatory acute phase protein.Q

Beta globulin produced in liver, production improved by infection, inflammation, malignancies and tissue destruction. Testing done by passive latex agglutination.

Precipitates with somatic C antigen of pneumococci but **it is not an antibody.Q**

C reactive protein binds to phosphorylcholine residues in cell wall of certain microorganisms. This complex is very effective in activating the classical complement pathway.

Note remember – Negative acute phase proteins are Albumin, prealbumin, transferrin, Transthyretin and retinal binding protein.Q

Positive acute phase protein – Alpha1 antitrypsin, Fibrinogen, Ferritin, Serum amyloid A, hapatoglobin, Ceruloplasmin and Alpha 2 microglobulin.

THE COMPLEMENT SYSTEM

• Nonspecific proteins • Not species specific • 5% of serum protein • Heat labile–56c for 30 min • Binds to Fc of Ab – IgM, IgG3, 1, 2.	**Site of Synthesis** • Intestinal epithelium — C1 • Macrophages — C2, C4 • Spleen — C5, C8 • Liver — C3, C6, C9 • Not known — C7

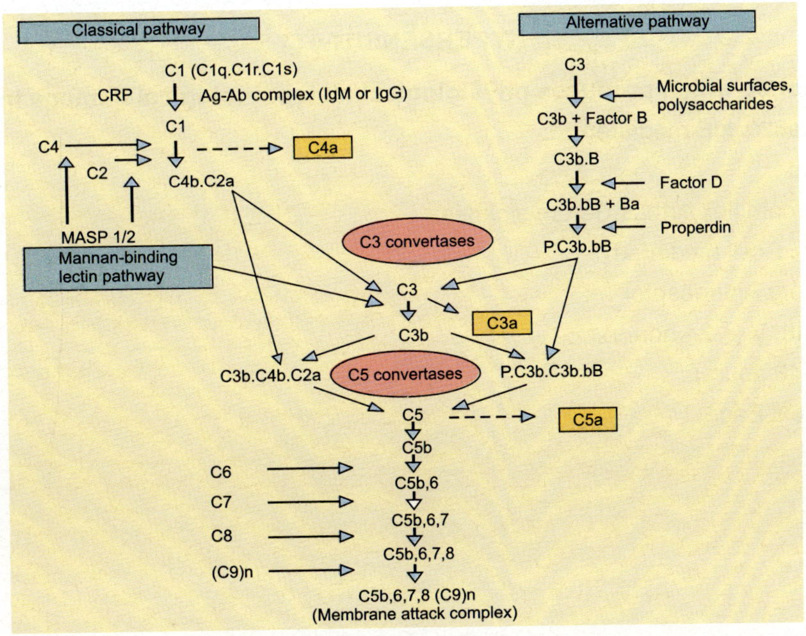

	Classical pathway	Alternate pathway	Lectin pathway
Activator	Antigen antibody complex	Zymosan, Endotoxin IgA, IgD, Cobra venom Nephritic factor	Carbohydrate residue of bacterial cell wall
1st complement activated	C1	C3b	C4
Component	Acquired immunity	Innate immunity	Innate immunity

REGULATION OF COMPLEMENT

Inhibitors	**Inactivators**
1. Bind to complement components and halt their further action 2. α Neuro aminoglycoprotein ↓ C1 esterase 3. S Protein ↓ C567	1. Destroy complement proteins 2. Factor I – ↓ C3 activation 3. Factor H binds to C3b 4. C4 binding protein 5. Anaphylotoxin inactivator degrades C3a, C4a, C5a.

Complement deficiency and diseases:	**Uses of Complement**
1. **Deficiency of early complements C2, 3, 4** causes immune complex diseases (e.g., SLE) and pyogenic infections. 2. **Deficiency of C3 and C3b** causes pyogenic infections. 3. **C5 – C9 complement deficiency** leads to recurrent Neisserial infections.	• Bacteriolysis/Cytolysis. • Amplification of inflammatory response (c3a, c5a). • Hypersensitivity reaction (type II, III). • Endotoxic shock • Immune adherence • Opsonisation (c3b) • Autoimmune diseases (SLE, RA)

Complement system is regulated by the following proteins:

- **Note** – Both **DAF** (CD55) and **MIRL** (CD 59) are anchored to cell membrane of blood cells by **GPI** (glycosylphosphatidylinositol).
- Thus deficiency of GPI causes deficiency of DAF and MIRL, which results in paroxysmal nocturnal hemoglobinuria (PNH).Q

HYPERSENSITIVITY

Abnormal immune response which produces physiological/histopathological damage in the host

1. Type I — Anaphylactic: IgE mediated
   Type II — Cytotoxic
   Type III — Immune complex Arthus/Serum sickness
   Type IV — Delayed: T-cell mediated
   Type V — Stimulatory/Antireceptor
2. Immediate type: I, II, III, V (< 24 hours).
3. Delayed type: IV (24-48 hours).

(See Figure on the Next Page)

	Type I	Type II		Type III	Type IV		
Immune reactant	IgE	IgG		IgG	T_H1 cells	T_H2 cells	CTL
Antigen	Soluble antigen	Cell- or matrix-associated antigen	Cell-surface receptor	Soluble antigen	Soluble antigen	Soluble antigen	Cell-associated antigen
Effector mechanism	Mast-cell activation	Complement, FcR^+ cells (phagocytes, NK cells)	Antibody alters signaling	Complement, phagocytes	Macrophage activation	IgE production, eosinophil activation, mastocytosis	Cytotoxicity
Example of hypersensitivity reaction	Allergic rhinitis, asthma, systemic anaphylaxis	Some drug allergies (e.g. penicillin)	Chronic urticaria (antibody against FCεRIα)	Serum sickness, Arthus reaction	Contact dermatitis, tuberculin reaction	Chronic asthma, chronic allergic rhinitis	Graft rejection

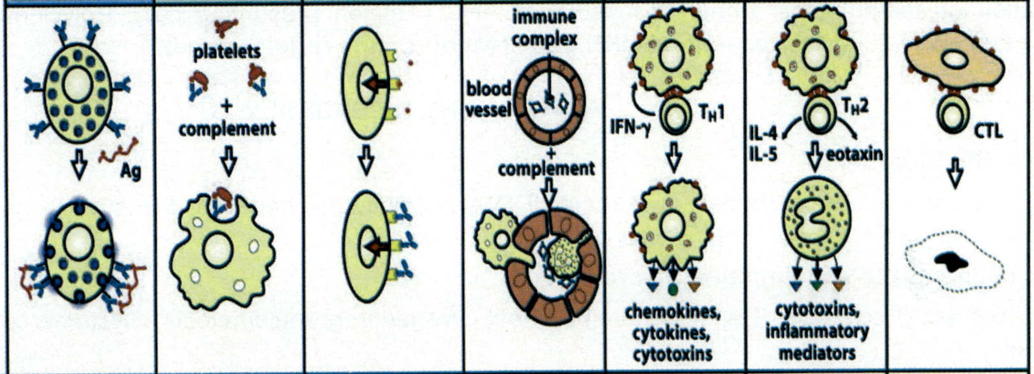

OTHER EXAMPLES OF HYPERSENSITIVITY REACTION

Type 1

Examples – Eczema, Hay fever, Atopy, Urticaria, Anaphylactic shock, acute dermatitis, Theobald Smith phenomenon, Casoni test.

Prausnitz – Kustner (PK) Reaction – Serum from allergic person into skin of normal person.

Anaphylaxis in vitro (Schultzdale) – Strips of smooth muscle contract in vitro following exposure to antigen.

Type 2

Examples – Blood transfusion reactions, Autoimmune hemolytic anaemia, Pemphigus vulgari, Good Pasteur syndrome, Acute rheumatic fever, Diabetes mellitus.

Type 3

Examples – Shick test, PAN, Rheumatoid arthritis, SLE.

Necrotizing vasculitis and fibrinoid necrosis is major pathological change which happens in type III hypersensitivity.Q

Type 4

Examples – Lepromin test, Fries test, Lepra type I, Tuberculin test.

Type 5

- Antibody mediated.
- Antibody reacts with a key surface component, e.g., hormone receptor and stimulates the cell.
- **Example** – In Graves' disease Ab has same effect As TSH.

AUTOIMMUNITY

- Reactivity of the body against self-antigen.
- Higher incidence is seen among females.
- **Central tolerance** – Premature lymphocytes which are self-reactive are killed in the central organs by Bone marrow and Thymus.
- **Peripheral tolerance** – Anergy, Suppression by T cells, Clonal deletion by activated cell death, Antigen sequestration, Cytokine activation.
- **Exogenous** – Mimicry, superantigenic stimulation.
- **Endogenous** – Altered Antigen presentation – Loss of immunologic privilege, presentation of cryptic epitopes, Alteration of self-antigens, Enhance function of APC (Antigen presenting cell), Polyclonal activation of B cell, Forbidden clones and **Expression of AIRE gene (Autoimmune regular gene).**

AUTOIMMUNE DISEASES

Organ Specific Disorder

Hashimoto's thyroiditis, Good Pasteur syndrome, IDDM, Autoimmune hepatitis, Myasthenia gravis, Graves' disease, Multiple sclerosis.

Systemic (Generalized Autoimmune Disorder)

SLE, RA, Systemic sclerosis, Reiter syndrome, PAN, Wegener granulomatosis, Systemic sclerosis, Inflammatory myopathies.

TRANSPLANTATION IMMUNITY

- **Autograft:** One part of body to another.
- **Isograft:** Between Genetically identical twins.
- **Allograft:** Between members of the **same species** but of different genetic constitution.
- **Xenograft:** Between members of **different species.**

Types of Graft Rejection

1. **Hyperacute Rejection**
   - Presence of antibodies against graft.
   - Prior blood transfusion, multiple pregnancies, previous transplant.
   - **Preformed antibodies** fix complement damaging endothelial lining of blood vessels (blockade) of micro-vasculature.
   - **Time:** Minutes to hours.
2. **Acute Rejection/Accelerated Rejection**
   - Days to weeks.
   - Primary Activation of T cells with Triggering of various effector mechanisms.
   - Transplant given to someone who has been presensitized → 2° Activation of T cells → Accelerated/second set rejection/white graft rejection (days).
3. **Chronic Rejection**
   - Months to years and walls of blood vessel thicken and eventually become blocked.
   - Exact cause:
     - Low grade cell mediated rejection.
     - Deposition of Ag – Ab complex.
     - Recurrence of original disease.
   - **Main Features:**
     - Proliferation of smooth muscle cells.
     - Interstitial fibrosis.

GRAFT VERSUS HOST REACTION

- Occurs in **Bone marrow transplantation.**
- Induced by immunologically competent T cells being transplanted into allogeneic recipients which are unable to reject them and due to lack of immunocompetence of host.
- Severe damage to skin and intestine.

Criteria is **Billingham's CriteriaQ**

- **Avoided by:** Careful typing, Removal of mature T cells from graft and use of immunosuppressive drugs.

Typing Methods

- ABO typing.
- HLA typing
  - Serological methods
    - Microcytotoxicity.
    - Mixed leukocyte reaction.
  - Molecular methods
    - Using DNA Probes.
    - PCR – RFLP.

MAJOR HISTOCOMPATIBILITY COMPLEX

- Genes Mediating graft rejection.
- **MICE:** Called as H Loci.
- **Humans: Human leukocyte antigen complex.**
- **Short arm of chromosome 6.**
- Codominantly expressed.
- 4 Loci of HLA: **A, B, C, D.**
- 3 classes of Genes in these HLA loci.

MHC CLASS I

- **HLA A, B, C loci.**
- Class I antigens.
- 2 poly peptide chains.
- Present **in virtually all nucleated cells** like Macrophages, neutrophils, langerhan cells, dendritic cell and platelets.
- CD8+ cells recognize Ag presented along with MHC I molecules.
- Causes **perforin granzyme dependent killing or Fas Fas ligand dependent killing and graft rejection.**

MHC CLASS II

- Encoded by **HLA-DP, HLA-DQ, HLA-DR.**
- Two polypeptide chains.
- B lymphocytes, macrophages, monocytes, activated T lymphocytes.
- Plays a role in **Graft versus host response and mixed leucocyte response.**

MHC CLASS III

- **Genes coding for complement components C2, C4, properdin, factor B, TNFα, TNFβ, Heat shock protein 70, Enzyme 21-hydroxylase.** It is involved in susceptibility to autoimmune disease.

IMMUNODEFICIENCY DISORDERS

Immunodeficiency diseases are broadly classified as primary and secondary. Primary immunodeficiency diseases results from inherited defects affecting immune system development and secondary immunodeficiency diseases are secondary to some other disease process that interferes with the proper functioning of the immune system (e.g., infection malnutrition, aging).

"T" Cell Deficiency

Category	Disease	Defect	Clinical Feature
Selective T cell deficiency	Digeorge Syndrome	Failure of formation of 3rd and 4th pharyngeal pouches, Thymic aplasia	Facial and cardiac abnormalities, hypoparathyroidism, decrease T cell response
	MHC I deficiency	Failure of TAP 1 molecules to transport peptides to Endoplasmic reticulum	CD8 decrease, CD4 normal, recurrent viral infections, normal delay type hypersensitivity and antibody response
	MHC II deficiency	Failure of MHC II expression defects in transcription factors	Deficient CD4 No GVHD ↓ Immunoglobulins
	*For graft versus Host deficiency. Graft goes through CD4 so if CD4 deficient then no GVHD.		

Disease	Molecular defect	Symptoms
1. Chronic Granulomatous Disease (CGD)	Deficiency of NADPH Failure to generate oxygen radicals	Recurrent infections with catalase positive bacteria and fungi
2. LAD syndrome	Absence of CD18, common β chains of integrins	Recurrent infections, failure to produce pus, inflammation around umbilicus but no pus (Omphalitis)
3. Chediak Higashi syndrome	Granule structural defect, absent Natural killer cells, Partial albinism	Recurrent infections, chemotactic and degranulation defects
4. Job syndrome	Th-17 deficiency	Coarse facies, cold abscess, increased IgE, Eczema
5. G6PD deficiency	Deficiency of enzymes in HMP shunt	CGD+Anaemia
6. MPO deficiency	Granule enzymes deficiency	Mild or none

DEFECTS OF PHAGOCYTOSIS

"B" Cell Disorders

Disease	Defect	Features	Treatment
1. Bruton's X linked agammaglobulinaemia	Deficiency of tyrosine kinase blocks B cell maturation	Decrease immunoglobulins of all classes, no circulating B cells, pre B cells in bone marrow normal, normal CMI	Monthly Gammaglobulins
2. X linked Hyper IgM syndrome	Deficiency of CD40L on activated T cells	Increase serum IgM, normal B and T cells	Antibiotics and Gammaglobulins
3. Selective IgA deficiency	Deficiency of IgA (most common)	Repeated sinopulmonary and GI infections	Antibiotics
4. Common variable hypogammaglobulinaemia	Unknown	Onset–late teenage, B cells present in blood, decreased immunoglobulins and increased autoimmunity	Antibiotics
5. Transient hypogammaglobulinaemia	Delayed onset of normal IgG synthesis	Detected in 5-6 months after birth, resolves by 2.6 years, infection with pyogenic bacteria	Antibiotics, Gammaglobulins replacement
Combined Partial B and T cell deficiency	Wiskott Aldrich syndrome	Defect in cytoskeletal glycoprotein, X-linked	↓ Response to bacterial polysacchride ↓IgM

Contd.

Contd.

	Ataxia telangiectasia	Defective in kinase involved in cell cycle	Functional – Ataxia Structural – telangiectasia Deficiency of IgA and IgE
Complete functional B and T cell deficiency	SCID	Defect in common gamma chain of IL-2 receptor Defect in receptor of IL-4,7,9,15, X-linked	Chronic diarrhea, skin mouth and throat lesion, unresponsive to mitogens
		Adenosine deaminase deficiency	As above features, opportunistic infections
		Rag 1 and Rag 2 gene, non-sense mutation	Total absence of B and T cells

MCQs

BASIC OF IMMUNE SYSTEM AND IMMUNITY

1. **Components of innate immunity are:** *(PGI 10)*
   (a) T lymphocytes (b) Complement system
   (c) B lymphocytes (d) NK cells
   (e) Integrins
2. **All are true about innate immunity *except*:** *(Recent MCQ)*
   (a) Non-specific (b) First line of defense
   (c) Not affected by genetic make up (d) Includes complement
3. **Which is concerned with cell mediated immunity?** *(AI 98)*
   (a) B-Lymphocytes (b) T-Lymphocytes
   (c) Eosinophils (d) Monocytes
4. **Adoptive immunity is by:** *(AI 2011)*
   (a) Infection (b) Injection of antibodies
   (c) Injection of lymphocytes (d) Immunization
5. **Active immunity is not acquired by:** *(Recent MCQ)*
   (a) Infection (b) Vaccination
   (c) Immunoglobulin transfer (d) Sub-clinical infection
6. **Lysozyme is present in the following secretions of the body *except*:** *(PGI 94)*
   (a) Lacrimal secretions (b) CSF
   (c) Saliva (d) Respiratory tract secretions
7. **First chemical barrier encountered by microorganism for common exposed sites:** *(AIIMS Nov 11)*
   (a) Lysozyme (b) Acidic pH
   (c) Skin (d) Lactose
8. **Vaccination is based on the principle of:** *(AI 12)*
   (a) Agglutination (b) Phagocytosis
   (c) Immunologic Memory (d) Clonal Detection
9. **NK Cell activity is enhanced by:** *(Recent MCQ)*
   (a) IL-1 (b) TNF (c) IL-2 (d) TGF-β
10. **Binary (secondary) exposure to an antigen results in sudden increase in:** *(AI 11)*
    (a) IgA (b) IgD (c) IgG (d) IgM

11. Immunoglobulin responsible for anamnestic response is: *(Manipal 11, RJ 04)*
(a) IgA (b) IgG (c) IgM (d) IgE

12. All are peripheral lymphoid organs *except*: *(Recent MCQ)*
(a) Lymph nodes (b) Spleen
(c) Mucosa associated lymphoid tissue (d) Thymus

13. Common between B and T cells: *(PGI Nov 14)*
(a) Origin from same cell lineage (b) Site differentiation
(c) Antigenic mark (d) Both humoral and cellular immunity
(e) Further differentiation seen

14. Neonatal thymectomy leads to: *(AI 02)*
(a) Decreased size of germinal center
(b) Decreased size of paracortical areas
(c) Increased antibody production by B cells
(d) Increased bone marrow production of lymphocytes

15. T cell dependent region is: *(PGI 98)*
(a) Corticle follicle of lymph nodes (b) Medullary cords
(c) Mantle layer (d) Paracortical layer

16. Apart from T and B lymphocytes, the other class of lymphocytes is: *(PGI 02)*
(a) Macrophages (b) Astrocytes
(c) NK cells (d) Langerhans cells

17. Memory T cells can be identified by using following marker: *(AI 96, 93)*
(a) CD45 RA (b) CD45RB
(c) CD45RC (d) CD45RO

18. All of these are antigen presenting cells *except*: *(PGI May 2014)*
(a) T cells (b) B cell
(c) Fibroblasts (d) Dendritic cell
(e) Langerhans cells

19. Plasma cells are derived from: *(AI 99)*
(a) T cells (b) B cells
(c) Macrophages (d) Neutrophils

20. IgE is secreted by: *(Recent MCQ)*
(a) Mast cell (b) Basophils
(c) Eosinophils (d) Plasma cells

21. Which one of the following immunoglobulins constitutes the antigen binding component of B-cells receptor? *(ICS 05)*
(a) IgA (b) IgD (c) IgM (d) IgG

22. Regarding NK cells, false statement is: *(AI 01)*
(a) It is activated by IL-2
(b) Expresses CD 3 receptor
(c) It is a variant of large lymphocyte
(d) There is antibody induced proliferation of NK cells

23. Virus infected cells killed by: *(Recent MCQ)*
(a) Natural killer cells (b) Plasma cells
(c) B cells (d) None

24. All are mononuclear-macrophages *except*: *(Recent MCQ)*
(a) Histiocytes (b) Microglia (c) Kupfer cells (d) B cells

25. All of these are antigen presenting cells (APC's) *except*: *(PGI May 14)*
(a) T cells
(b) B cells
(c) Fibroblasts
(d) Dendritic cells
(e) Langerhans cells

26. Most potent stimulator of naive T cells: *(AI 11, AIIMS Nov 08,05)*
(a) Mature dendritic cells
(b) Follicular dendritic cells
(c) Macrophages
(d) B cell

27. The function common to neutrophils, monocyte and macrophages is: *(UP 97)*
(a) Immune response
(b) Phagocytosis
(c) Liberation of histamine
(d) Destruction of old erythrocytes

28. Which cells cause rosette formation with sheep RBCs? *(AIIMS 05, AI 07)*
(a) T cells
(b) NK cells
(c) Monocytes
(d) B cells

29. What enhances multiplication of T cells in culture? *(AI 96, 93)*
(a) Phytohemagglutinin
(b) Chemotactic factor
(c) Leukotrienes
(d) Prostaglandins

30. Which of the following features is not shared between 'T cells' and 'B cells'? *(AIIMS Nov 12, AI 12)*
(a) Positive Selection during Development
(b) Class I MHC Expression
(c) Antigen Specific Receptors
(d) All of the above

31. The type of receptors present on T cells are: *(AI 96, 93)*
(a) IgG
(b) IgD
(c) CD4
(d) Prostaglandins

32. The role played by major histocompatibility complex proteins (MHC-1 and MHC-2) is to: *(AIIMS Nov 14, May 14, May 13)*
(a) Transduce the signals to T cells following antigen recognition
(b) Mediate immunoglobulin class-switching
(c) Present antigens for recognition by T cell antigen receptors
(d) Enhance the secretion of cytokines

33. HLA-I is present on: *(Recent MCQ)*
(a) All nucleated cells
(b) Only on cells of immune system
(c) Only on B cells
(d) Only on T cells

34. MHC II are presented by: *(PGI May 13, Nov 10)*
(a) Macrophage
(b) Dendritic cells
(c) Lymphocytes
(d) Eosinophils
(e) Platelets

35. Interleukin I primarily acts on: *(Recent MCQ)*
(a) T-lymphocytes
(b) B-lymphocytes
(c) Neutrophils
(d) Macrophages

36. IL-1 is produced by: *(PGI Nov 14)*
(a) Macrophage
(b) Helper T lymphocytes
(c) B cells
(d) Cytotoxic T cells

37. IL-2 is secreted by: *(AIIMS Feb 97, AI 2000, 97)*

(a) CD4 lymphocytes
(b) CD8 cells
(c) Macrophages
(d) Neutrophils

38. Perforins are produced by: *(PGI 01)*

(a) Cytotoxic T cells
(b) Suppressor T cells
(c) Memory helper T cells
(d) Plasma cells
(e) NK cells

39. About interferon true is: *(PGI 98)*

(a) It is a synthetic antiviral agent
(b) Inhibits viral replication in cells
(c) Is specific for a particular virus
(d) None

40. Acute phase reactants are all *except*: *(NBE Based AI 2013-14 Pattern)*

(a) C-reactive protein
(b) Haptaglobulin
(c) Endothelin
(d) Fibrinogen

41. C-reactive protein is: *(AIIMS 91)*

(a) Produced by pneumococcus
(b) A marker of Septicemia
(c) Raised in acute inflammation
(d) Low in Rheumatoid arthritis

42. C-reactive proteins are: *(PGI Dec 2000)*

(a) Alpha-I globulin
(b) Beta-1 globulin
(c) Alpha-2 globulin
(d) Non-specific inflammatory protein

ANTIBODIES-ANTIBODIES, AG-AB REACTION AND COMPLEMENT

43. A single immunoglobulin molecule contains: *(AI 95)*

(a) 1 light chain, 1 heavy chain
(b) 2 heavy chains, 1 light
(c) 2 light chains, 2 heavy chains
(d) 2 light chains, 1 heavy chain

44. Complement attaches to immunoglobulin at: *(Recent MCQ)*

(a) Aminoterminal
(b) Fab region
(c) Variable region
(d) Fc fragment

45. Which of the following class specific antigenic determinants of an immunoglobulin is associated with? *(AIIMS May 04)*

(a) L-chain
(b) H-chain
(c) J-chain
(d) Variable region

46. Variable portion of antibody molecule is: *(Recent MCQ)*

(a) C-Terminal
(b) N-Terminal
(c) CHO moiety
(d) None

47. Antigen binding site on antibody is: *(PGI Nov. 14)*

(a) Hinge region
(b) Constant region
(c) Variable region
(d) Hypervariable region
(e) Idiotype region

48. Idiotypic class of antibody is determined by: *(Recent MCQ)*

(a) Fc region
(b) Hinge region
(c) Carboxy end
(d) Amino end

49. Immunoglobulin isotype class switching is determined by: *(Recent MCQ)*

(a) Constant region of light chain
(b) Constant region of heavy chain
(c) Variable region of light chain
(d) Variable region of heavy chain

50. Which immunoglobulin is scarce in human serum? *(PGI June 05)*
(a) IgA (b) IgG (c) IgM (d) IgD
(e) IgE

51. Immunoglobulin inactive by heating and elevated in helminthic infections: *(Recent MCQ)*
(a) IgA (b) IgG (c) IgE (d) IgM

52. True of the following is/are: *(PGI June 01)*
(a) IgA crosses placenta
(b) Half-life of IgG is 23 days
(c) IgD is heat stable
(d) IgE has highest carbohydrate content
(e) IgG induces leukotrienes release during inflammation

53. Pentavalent immunoglobin is: *(AI 04)*
(a) IgA (b) IgG (c) IgM (d) IgE

54. Capacity of producing IgG starts at what age? *(Recent MCQ)*
(a) 6 months (b) 1 year (c) 2 years (d) 3 years

55. The secretory component of immunoglobulin molecule is: *(PGI June 01, AI 99)*
(a) Formed by epithelial cells of lining mucosa
(b) Formed by plasma cell
(c) Formed by epithelial cell and plasma cell
(d) Secreted by bone marrow

56. The serum concentration of which of the following human IgG subclass is maximum? *(AI 05)*
(a) IgG 1 (b) IgG 2 (c) IgG 3 (d) IgG 4

57. Which antibody deficiency causes recurrent infections by organisms with polysaccharide capsule? *(Recent MCQ)*
(a) IgA (b) IgG1 (c) IgG2 (d) IgM

58. Synthesis of an immunoglobulin in membrane bound or secretory form is determined by: *(AI 03)*
(a) One turn to two turn joining rule (b) Class switching
(c) Differential RNA processing (d) Allelic exclusion

59. The most avidly complement fixing antibody is: *(AIIMS May 02)*
(a) IgA (b) IgG (c) IgM (d) IgE

60. Which of the following immunoglobulin is responsible for opsonisation? *(Recent MCQ)*
(a) IgA (b) IgG (c) IgM (d) IgE

61. In respiratory and GIT infections, which is the most affected immunoglobulin? *(AI 94)*
(a) IgA (b) IgG (c) IgM (d) IgD

62. Which precipitates at 50 to 60°C but redissolve on heating? *(PGI 01)*
(a) Bence Jones protein (b) Heavy chain
(c) Both light and heavy chains (d) Light chains

63. PK reaction detects: *(Recent MCQ)*
(a) IgG (b) IgA (c) IgE (d) IgM

64. Antibody elevated in parasitic infection: *(Recent MCQ)*
(a) IgA (b) IgE (c) IgG (d) IgM

65. Bence Jones proteins are best described as: *(AI 96)*
(a) μ chains (b) γ chains
(c) Kappa and Lambda chains (d) Fibrin split products

66. Hybridoma technique is used to obtain: *(Recent MCQ)*
(a) Specific antigen (b) Complement
(c) Specific antibody (d) Interleukins

67. Which of the following statements is true about hapten? *(Recent MCQ, AI 04)*
(a) It induces brisk immune response
(b) It needs carrier to induce immune response
(c) It is a T-independent antigen
(d) It has no association with MHC

68. The exact part of the antigen that reacts with the immune system is called as: *(JIPMER 07)*
(a) Clone (b) Epitope
(c) Idiotope (d) Effector

69. Which part of bacteria is most antigenic? *(Recent MCQ)*
(a) Protein coat (b) Lipopolysaccharide
(c) Nucleic acid (d) Lipids

70. All of the following statements about carbohydrate antigen are true *except*: *(AI 11, AIIMS Nov 08)*
(a) It has lower immunogenicity (b) Memory response is seen
(c) Cause polyclonal B cell stimulation (d) Does require stimulation by T cells

71. The protection against small pox by previous infection with cowpox represents: *(AIIMS May 04)*
(a) Antigenic cross-reactivity (b) Antigenic specificity
(c) Passive immunity (d) Innate immunity

72. Superantigen causes: *(Recent MCQ)*
(a) Polyclonal activation of T-cells (b) Stimulation of B cells
(c) Enhancement of phagocytosis (d) Activation of complement

73. Superantigens are: *(PGI Nov. I4)*
(a) Erythrotoxin of Staph. Aureus (b) Cl. Difficile toxin
(c) Staphyloccocal toxic shock syndrome toxin (d) Cholera toxin

74. All of the following forces are involved in Antigen antibody reaction *except*: *(AI 98, AIIMS Sept. 96)*
(a) Vander Waal's forces (b) Electrostatic bond
(c) Hydrogen bond (d) Covalent bond

75. The reaction between antibody and soluble antigen is demonstrated by: *(AI 94)*
(a) Agglutination (b) Precipitation
(c) Complement fixation test (d) Hemagglutination test

76. VDRL is an example of: *(Recent MCQ)*
(a) Slide agglutination (b) Tube agglutination
(c) Slide flocculation (d) Tube flocculation

77. Which of the following is agglutination test? *(Recent MCQ)*
(a) Widal test (b) VDRL
(c) Ascoli's test (d) Kahn test

78. Skin test based on neutralization reaction is/are: *(PGI June 14)*
(a) Casoni test (b) Lepromin test
(c) Tuberculin test (d) Schick test

79. Nagler reaction is type of: *(Recent MCQ)*
(a) Neutralization reaction (b) CFT
(c) Precipitation (d) Agglutination

80. Coombs test is: *(Recent MCQ)*

(a) Precipitation test
(b) Agglutination test
(c) CFT
(d) Neutrilization test

81. Prozone phenomenon is due to: *(AI 96, PGI June 15)*

(a) Excess antigen
(b) Excess antibody
(c) Hyperimmune reaction
(d) Disproportionate antigen-antibody levels

82. DNA is detected by: *(Recent MCQ)*

(a) Southern blot
(b) Northern blot
(c) Western blot
(d) Eastern blot

83. Most sensitive test for antigen detection is: *(PGI 97)*

(a) RIA
(b) ELISA
(c) Immunofluorescence
(d) Passive hemagglutination

84. Which complement component is involved in both classical and alternative pathways? *(AI 11)*

(a) C1 (b) C2 (c) C3 (d) C4

85. Chemoattractant is: *(PGI 89)*

(a) C5a (b) C1 (c) C3 (d) C2

86. Recurrent Neisseria infections are predisposed by: *(Recent MCQ)*

(a) Early complement component deficiency
(b) Late complement component deficiency
(c) C1 esterase deficiency
(d) Properdin deficiency

87. Opsonization takes place through: *(Recent MCQ)*

(a) C3a (b) C3b (c) C5a (d) C5b

Hypersensitivity

88. Type I hypersensitivity is mediated by which of the following immunoglobulins? *(Recent MCQ)*

(a) IgA (b) IgG (c) IgM (d) IgE

89. The most important cells in type I hypersensitivity: *(AI 92)*

(a) Macrophages
(b) Mast cells
(c) Neutrophils
(d) Lymphocytes

90. True about type II hypersensitivity reaction is: *(Recent MCQ)*

(a) May be complement mediated
(b) Schultzdale phenomenin is a type 2 hypersensitivity
(c) Antibody independent
(d) Role of IgE

91. Graves' disease is an example of which type .... immunologic response? *(PGI Nov 14)*

(a) Type I
(b) Type II
(c) Type III
(d) Type IV
(e) Type V

92. Type III reaction is: *(AI 93)*

(a) Antibody mediated
(b) Immune complex mediated
(c) Cell mediated
(d) None

93. Delayed hypersensitivity involves: *(AIIMS 92)*

(a) Neutrophils
(b) Monocytes
(c) Eosinophils
(d) Lymphocytes

94. Which of the following is an example of Type IV hypersensitivity? *(Recent MCQ)*
(a) Arthus reaction (b) Serum sickness
(c) Shwartzman reaction (d) Granulomatous reaction

95. Which one of the following is False? *(AI 95)*
(a) Theobald-Smith phenomenon is a type I hypersensitivity reaction
(b) Serum sickness is a type II hypersensitivity reaction
(c) Allograft rejection is a type IV hypersensitivity reaction
(d) Transfusion reaction is a type II hypersensitivity reaction

96. Examples of type I hypersensitivity is: *(AI 98)*
(a) Lepromin test (b) Tuberculin
(c) Casoni's test (d) Arthus reaction

97. Which one of the following mast cell products is not preformed and therefore has to be newly synthesized? *(PGI 01)*
(a) Histamine (b) Prostaglandin D2
(c) Heparin (d) Neutral proteases
(e) Eosinophil chemotactic factor

98. Type I hypersensitivity includes all of the following *except*: *(PGI 2000)*
(a) Autoimmune hemolytic anemia (b) Anaphylaxis
(c) Extrinsic asthma (d) Hay fever

99. Myasthenia gravis is which type of hypersensitivity? *(Recent MCQ)*
(a) Type I (b) Type II (c) Type III (d) Type IV

100. The hypersensitivity reaction involved in the hyper acute rejection of renal transplant is: *(AIIMS May 05)*
(a) Type I (b) Type II (c) Type III (d) Type IV

101. In contact dermatitis which cells play major role? *(PGI June 08)*
(a) T cells (b) B cells
(c) Langhans cells (d) Macrophage

102. Autoimmunity can be caused due to all of the following *except*:
(a) Forbidden clones
(b) Expression of cryptic antigens
(c) Negative selection of T cells in thymus
(d) Inappropriate expression of MHC proteins

103. Which of the following is a non-organ-specific (systemic) autoimmune disease? *(Recent MCQ)*
(a) Myasthenia gravis (b) Systemic lupus erythematosus
(c) Hashimoto's thyroiditis (d) Pernicious anemia

104. All are true about autoimmune disease *except*: *(PGI May 10)*
(a) T cells recognize self-antigen (b) Hashimoto's thyroiditis is an example
(c) Higher incidence among males (d) Polyclonal B cell activation
(e) Costimulatory molecules involvement

105. Epstein Barr virus causes autoimmunity by: *(AI 12)*
(a) Molecular mimicry (b) Release of sequestrated antigen
(c) Inappropriate expression of MHC Class II molecules (d) Polyclonal B cell activation

106. A woman with infertility receives an ovary transplant from her sister who is an identical twin. What type of graft it is? *(AI 05)*

(a) Xenograft
(b) Autograft
(c) Allograft
(d) Isograft

107. Thomsen Friedensreich phenomenon: *(Recent MCQ)*

(a) Red cell infection by CMV
(b) Red cell agglutination by all blood group sera
(c) Hemolysis of transfused blood
(d) Due to B antigen

108. Graft versus Host reaction is caused by: *(PGI 86)*

(a) B-lymphocytes
(b) T-lymphocytes
(c) Macrophages
(d) Complement

109. Adenosine deaminase deficiency is seen in the following: *(AI 01, 05)*

(a) Common variable immunodeficiency
(b) Severe combined immunodeficiency
(c) Chronic granulomatous disease
(d) Nezelof syndrome

110. Which one of the following statements is correct regarding chronic granulomatous disease? *(AIIMS Nov 04)*

(a) It is an autosomal dominant disease
(b) It is characterized by abnormal bacterial phagocytosis
(c) Recurrent streptococcal infections are usual in this disease
(d) Nitroblue tetrazolium test is useful for screening

111. The NBT (nitroblue tetrazolium) reduction assay is used to: *(Recent MCQ)*

(a) Evaluate granulocyte function
(b) Evaluate T cell function
(c) Determine whether polymorphonuclear leucocytes can produce superoxide
(d) Stain B-lymphocytes

112. The most common primary immunodeficiency is: *(AI 94, PGI June 05)*

(a) Common variable immunodeficiency
(b) Isolated IgA immunodeficiency
(c) Wiskott-Aldrich syndrome
(d) AIDS

113. A child present with recurrent episodes of sinopulmonary infection by bacteria with polysaccharide rich capsule. Deficiency of which of the following immunoglobulin subclasses should be specifically investigated? *(AI 12, AIIMS May 12)*

(a) IgA
(b) IgG1
(c) IgG2
(d) IgA+IgG2

114. Chediak-Higashi syndrome, true is: *(Recent MCQ)*

(a) Defect in phagocytosis
(b) Neutropenia
(c) Agammaglobulinemia
(d) IgA deficiency

115. Which fungal infection is most common to occur in neutropenia? *(AIIMS June 99)*

(a) Candida
(b) Histoplasma
(c) Aspergillus niger
(d) Aspergillus fumigates

ANSWERS AND EXPLANATIONS

1. **Ans. are 'b, d, e'** (***Ref:*** *Harrison, 18th/e, p. 202-23; Robbin's 7th/e, p. 194-196*)
   Components of Innate immunity – Complement proteins, NK cells, integrins.
   Components of Adaptive immunity – T cells (T lymphocytes), B cells (B lymphocytes).
2. **Ans. is 'c'** i.e., Not affected by genetic make-up (***Ref:*** *Harrison, 18th/e, p. 2654-2656*)
   Every individual have different genetic make-up so immune response to particular disease also be different.
3. **Ans. is 'b'** i.e., T-Lymphocytes (***Ref:*** *Ananthanarayan, 9th/e, p. 152*)
   - Cellular (Cell mediated immunity) – T lymphocytes – defense against intracellular microbes.
   - Humoral immunity – B lymphocytes produces antibodies and convert into plasma cell which are responsible of immunogenic memory-defense against extracellular microbes and their toxins.
4. **Ans. is 'c'** i.e., Injection of lymphocytes (***Ref:*** *Jawetz, 27th/e, p. 130*)
   - An extract of immunologically competent T-lymphocytes, known as transfer factor can be used in the treatment of lepromatous leprosy when CMI is low.
5. **Ans. is 'c'** i.e., Immunoglobulin transfer (***Ref:*** *Ananthanarayan, 9th/e, p. 82-83 and 8th/e, p. 86, 87*)
   - Immunoglobulin transfer gives passive immunity.
   - Rest of the other options are examples of active immunity.
6. **Ans. is 'b'** i.e., CSF (***Ref:*** *Ananthanarayan, 9th/e, p. 80 and 8th/e, p. 85*)
   - Lysozyme is present in all secretions except CSF, sweat and urine.
7. **Ans. is 'b'** i.e., Acidic pH (***Ref:*** *Kuby Immunology, p. 5-8*)
   - Human body is protected due to acidic pH which creates the unfavorable condition to the microorganism to grow. e.g., acidic pH of skin, gastric juice in the stomach, acidic pH of the vagina and acidic pH of the urinary tract.
8. **Ans. is 'c'** i.e., Immunologic memory (***Ref:*** *Jawetz, 27th/e, p. 143*)
   - Vaccination is based on the principle of immunogenic memory.
9. **Ans. is 'c'** i.e., IL-2 (***Ref:*** *Ananthanarayan, 8th/e, p. 139*)
   APC – IL1- TH1 cell – IL2 – enhances action of Natural killer cell?
   - IL-2 is secreted by T_H 1 cells and it induces proliferation activated NK cells, T_H cells and T_C cells and IL-12 Dendritic cells, macrophages, B cells induce production of IFN-γ, TNF-α, and IL-2 by resting and activated T and NK cells.
10. **Ans. is 'd'** i.e., IgM (***Ref:*** *Ananthanarayan, 8th/e, p. 139*)
    - Secondary exposure to an antigen results in sudden increase of IgM followed by massive production of IgG.
    - IgM is the first antibody produced in both primary as well as secondary response.
11. **Ans. is 'b'** i.e., IgG (***Ref:*** *Essential Immunology, p. 126*)
    - Anamnestic response is the secondary immune response. This response is through memory cells, which store information regarding the recognition of a pathogen based on previous interaction.
12. **Ans. is 'd'** i.e., Thymus (***Ref:*** *Ananthanarayan, 9th/e, p. 130, Fig. 14.3 and 8th/e, p. 123*)
    - Central (Primary) lymphoid organs and Peripheral (secondary) lymphoid organs.

    (See Fig. on the next page)

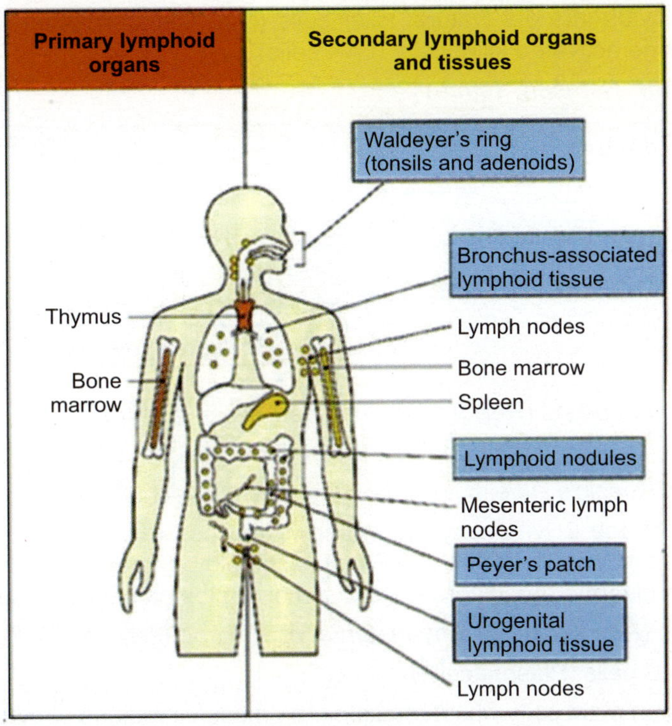

13. Ans. is 'a' i.e., Origin from same cell lineage (***Ref:*** *Ananthanarayan, 9th/e, p. 130-137 and 8th/e, p. 128-131*)

- They both originate from bone marrow but they differ in:

B cell	T cell
Has surface immunoglobulin	Has thymus specific antigen
Receptor for Fc piece of IgG present	CD3 receptor present
Forms EAC rosetteQ	Forms SRBC or E rosetteQ
CD2; measles receptor	C3 receptor; CR2; EBV receptor

- T cells undergo blast transformation (multiplication) on treatment with mitogens such as **Phytohemagglutinin, Concanavalin-A (Con A), Anti CD3.**
- B cell undergoes similar transformation with **Bacterial endotoxins, Staph aureus, EB virus, Anti Ig.**

14. Ans. is 'b' i.e., Decreased size of paracortical areas (***Ref:*** *Ananthanarayan, 9th/e, p. 130 and 8th/e, p. 127*)

- Neonatal thymectomy leads to depletion of thymus dependent areas (paracortical areas between cortical follicles and medullary cords and periarterial lymphoid collection known as malpighian corpuscles in white pulp).

15. Ans. is 'd' i.e., Paracortical layer (***Ref:*** *Baveja, 5th/e, p. 128*)

Thymus Dependent (T cell collection)

(a) **Spleen** – Periarterial lymphoid organs, Malphigian corpuscle in white pulp.

(b) **Lymph node** – Paracortical area.

Thymus Independent (B cell collection)

(a) **Spleen** – Perifollicular and Mantle layer.

(b) **Lymph nodes** – Cortical follicle, Germinal follicle and Medullary cords.

16. Ans. is 'c' i.e., NK cells (***Ref:*** *Ananthanarayan, 9th/e, p. 132 and 8th/e, p. 130*)

- Lymphocytes are classified by their surface markers into T and B cells, about 5-10% of cells are found to lack features of either type they are called null cells/Large granular lymphocytes and it is activated by IL-2. NK cells play an important role in destruction of malignant cells and virally infected host cells.

- Large granular lymphocytes include: Natural killer cells (N.K. Cells), Antibody dependent cytotoxic cells/killer cells (ADCC), Lymphokine activated killer cells (LAK cells).

17. Ans. is 'd' i.e., CD45RO (***Ref:*** *Harrison, 19th/e*)

Surface antigen	Distribution
CD 45	All leukocytes
CD45RA	Medullary T cells (Naïve T cells)
CD45RB	All leucocytes
CD45RC	Subset, T medullary thymocytes
CD45RO	Cortical thymocytes 'Memory cells'

18. Ans. are 'a, c' i.e., T cells, Fibroblasts (***Ref:*** *Ananthanarayan, 9th/e, p. 138*)

- Antigen presenting cells are – (a) Macrophages, (b) Dendritic cell, (c) B cell, (d) Langerhans cell.

19. Ans. is 'b' i.e., B cells (***Ref:*** *Robbin's 7th/e, p. 198, 199; Ananthanarayan, 9th/e, p. 136*)

- An antigen interacts with the B lymphocyte that shows the best "fit" by virtue of its immunoglobulin surface receptor. When antigen binds to this BCR, the B cell is stimulated to divide and form a clone (clonal selection). Such selected B cells proliferate and differentiate to become plasma cells that secrete antibody.

20. Ans. is 'd' i.e., Plasma cells (***Ref:*** *Ananthanarayan, 9th/e, p. 136 and 8th/e, p. 96, 130*)

- All Abs are secreted by B cells (Plasma cells).
- IgE Abs have receptors on mast cells which mediates the massive release of cytokines and responsible for Type I hypersensitivity.

21. Ans. are 'b, c' (***Ref:*** *Ananthanarayan, 9th/e, p. 136 and 8th/e, p. 100*)

- IgM and IgD present on B cell.
- All immature B cells carry IgM immunoglobulin on their surface, and most also express IgD.

22. Ans. is 'd' i.e., There is antibody induced proliferation of NK cells

(***Ref:*** *Ananthanarayan, 9th/e, p. 137 and 8th/e, p. 131; Harrison, 18th/e, p. 2658-2664 and 17th/e, p. 2025, 2028*)

- Cytotoxicity of NK cells is not antibody dependent or MHC restricted.

23. Ans. is 'a' (***Ref:*** *Ananthanarayan, 8th/e, p. 131*)

Virus infected cells are killed by:

(i) Innate immunity → by NK cells.

(ii) Adaptive immunity → by cytotoxic T cells.

24. Ans. is 'd' i.e., B cells (***Ref:*** *Ananthanarayan, 9th/e, p. 97*)

- B cells are not macrophages.

25. Ans. are 'a, c'

(***Ref:*** *Ananthanarayan, 9th/e, p. 138 and 8th/e, p. 132; Harrison, 18th/e, p. 2654-2658 and 17th/e, p. 2022, 2024*)

APCs are – Macrophages, B cells, Dendritic cells (most potent and effective activator), Langerhans cells.

26. Ans. is 'a' i.e., Mature dendritic cells (***Ref:*** *Robbins, 8th/e, p. 189*)

- Dendritic cells originate from bone marrow and are nonphagocytic in nature. They are most efficient (APCs), their function is to capture, process and present the antigenic peptide on their cell surface to the helper T cells.

27. Ans. is 'b' i.e., Phagocytosis (***Ref:*** *Ananthanarayan, 9th/e, p. 137 and 8th/e, p. 131-132*)

- Monocytes and Macrophages originate from bone marrow and their main functions are phagocytosis and Ag presentation.

28. Ans. is 'a' i.e., T cells (***Ref:*** *Ananthanarayan, 9th/e, p. 133 and 8th/e, p. 128*)

- Both T cell and B cell (T cells > B cells) form rosette with sheep erythrocytes. But best answer is T cells because T cells directly react with sheep erythrocytes, whereas B cells react with sheep erythrocytes that are coated with antibody and complement.

29. Ans. is 'a' i.e., Phytohemagglutinin (***Ref:*** *Ananthanarayan, 8th/e, p. 128*)

- Mitogens like Phytohemagglutinin (PHA), Concanavalin (Con A), and Anti CD-3 induces T cell blast transformation (multiplication).

30. Ans. is 'a' i.e., Positive Selection during Development (***Ref:*** *Lippincott's Immunology, Illustrated Review*)

- During development T cells undergo both positive selection and negative selection while B cells undergo only negative selection.

31. Ans. is 'c' i.e., CD4 (***Ref:*** *Ananthanarayan, 9th/e, p. 133 and 8th/e, p. 128*)

- Markers present on T cells are CD1, CD3, CD4, CD5 and CD8.

32. Ans. is 'c' i.e., Present antigens for recognition by T cell antigen receptors
(***Ref:*** *Robbin's 9th/e, p. 194-195 and 8th/e,p. 190-192; Ananthanarayan, 8th/e, p. 129, 133, 134*)

- Major role of MHC molecule is to bind peptide fragments of foreign proteins for presentation to antigen specific T cells.

33. Ans. is 'a' i.e., All nucleated cells (***Ref:*** *Jawetz, 27th/e, p. 139*)

- HLA class I Ag – present on the surfaces of all nucleated cells.
- HLA class II Ag – only on cells of immune system (macrophages, dendritic cells, activated T cells and B cells).

34. Ans. are 'a, b, c'
(***Ref:*** *Harrison, 17th/e, p. 2045-53; Robbins, 7th/e, p. 203; Ananthanarayan, 9th/e, p. 140 and 8th/e, p. 132-135*)

35. Ans. is 'a' i.e., T-lymphocytes (***Ref:*** *Ananthanarayan, 9th/e, p. 154 and 8th/e, p. 147*)

- Principally secreted by macrophages and monocytes; and epithelial cells and other sources are B lymphocytes, fibroblasts and endothelial cells.
- Formerly called as leucocyte activating factor (LAF) or B cell activating factor (BAF).
- Immunological functions are – Activation of T cells for the production of IL – 2, B cell proliferation and antibody synthesis, Neutrophil chemotaxis and increased PMN release from bone marrow, Increases body temperature (important endogenous pyrogen), Bone marrow cell proliferation, Induction of acute phase protein.

36. Ans. is 'a' i.e., Macrophage (***Ref:*** *Ananthanarayan, 9th/e, p. 154 and 8th/e, p. 147*)

- Principally secreted by macrophages and monocytes; and epithelial cells and other sources are B lymphocytes, fibroblasts and endothelial cells.

37. Ans. is 'a' i.e., CD4 lymphocytes (***Ref:*** *Ananthanarayan, 9th/e, p. 155 and 8th/e, p. 148; Jawetz, 23rd/e, p. 139*)

- Major source – Th1 (CD4) – induces growth and differentiation of TH1 and B cells, cytotoxicity of T and NK cells.

38. Ans. are 'a, e' (***Ref:*** *Guyton, 10th/e, p. 409; Ananthanarayan, 9th/e, p. 137 and 8th/e, p. 131; Robbin's 7th/e, p. 218*)

- Perforins are hole forming proteins and produced by: Cytotoxic T cells and N.K. Cells.

39. Ans. is 'b' i.e., Inhibits viral replication in cells (***Ref:*** *Ananthanarayan, 9th/e, p. 448-449 and 8th/e, p. 447-448*)

- Interferon by itself has no direct action on viruses but it acts on other cells of same species, rendering them refractory to viral infection.
- On exposure to interferon, cells produce a protein (translation inhibiting protein TIP) which selectively inhibits translation of mRNA.

40. Ans. is 'c' i.e., Endothelin (***Ref:*** *Ananthanarayan, 8th/e, p. 221; Greenwood, 10th/e, p. 124*)

- Endothelins are peptides (produced by vascular endothelium) that constrict blood vessels and raise blood pressure. They are normally kept in balance by other mechanisms but when they are over expressed causes hypertension and heart disease.

41. Ans. is 'c' i.e., Raised in acute inflammation (***Ref:*** *Ananthanarayan, 9th/e, p. 223*)

- C-reactive protein (CRP) is an acute phase protein. It is a beta 1 globulin which is produced in the liver (not by pneumococci).

42. Ans. are 'b, d' (***Ref:*** *Ananthanarayan, 9th/e, p. 223 and 8th/e, p. 221; Greenwood, 16th/e, p. 124*)

43. Ans. is 'c' i.e., 2 light chains, 2 heavy chains (***Ref:*** *Ananthanarayan, 9th/e, p. 94 and 8th/e, p. 96*)

- Already explained in book text.

44. Ans. is 'd' i.e., Fc fragment (***Ref:*** *Ananthanarayan, 8th/e, p. 97*)

- Fc fragment consist of parts of both H chains, composed of carboxyterminal portion of the H chains and it determines biological properties of Ig molecule such as complement fixation, placental transfer, skin fixation and catabolic rate.

45. Ans. is 'b' i.e., H-chain (***Ref:*** *Chatterjee Shinde, 4th/e, p. 92, 93; Chandrasoma Taylor, 3rd/e, p. 61, 62; Ananthanarayan, 9th/e, p. 94 Table 11.1*)

- The five classes of Igs are classified based on the amino acids sequence of the heavy chain. The basic immunoglobulin molecule is composed of two heavy (H) chains and two light (L) chains which are connected by disulfide bonds.

46. Ans. is 'b' i.e., N-Terminal (***Ref:*** *Ananthanarayan, 9th/e, p. 95 and 8th/e, p. 97*)

- Carboxy terminal (C-terminal) – Constant region (Fc region) – complement binding, NK, monocyte adherence site.
- Amino terminal (N-terminal) – Variable region (Fab region) – Ag binding site.

47. Ans. are 'd, e'

(***Ref:*** *Harrison, 18th/e, p. 2672, 2673; 17th/e, p. 2036; Ananthanarayan, 9th/e, p. 95 and 8th/e, p. 97*)

- The sites on the hypervariable regions that make actual contact with the epitopes are called "complementarity determining regions (CDRs)", "The idiotype is defined as the specific region of the Fab portion of the Ig molecule to which antigen binds".

48. Ans. is 'd' i.e., Amino end (***Ref:*** *Harrison, 18th/e, p. 2672, 2673; Ananthanarayan, 9th/e, p. 95*)

Idiotype markers are located in **hypervariable regions** of the immunoglobulin molecule and by immunization with Fab fragments anti-idiotypic abs can be produced.

49. Ans. is 'b' i.e., Constant region of heavy chain (***Ref:*** *Ananthanarayan, 9th/e, p. 99*)

- **Immunoglobulin Class Switching:** Initially, all B cells bound to an antigen carry IgM specific for that antigen and produce IgM in response to this antigen. Later, gene rearrangement generates antibodies of the same antigenic specificity but of different immunoglobulin classes. In class switching, the same assembled VH gene can sequentially associate with different CH genes, so that the immunoglobulin produced later (IgG, IgA, or IgE) has the same specificity as the original IgM but with different biologic characteristics. Class switching is dependent on cytokines released from T cells. Recently, IL-4, IL-5, IFN-γ, and transforming growth factor-beta (TGF-β) have been shown to play a role in regulating Ig class switching.

50. Ans. is 'e' i.e., IgE (***Ref:*** *Harrison, 18th/e, p. 2674 and 16th/e, p. 1922; Ananthanarayan, 9th/e, p. 98*)

- IgG has maximum serum concentration and IgE has minimum serum concentration.

51. Ans. is 'c' i.e., IgE (***Ref:*** *Harrison, 18th/e, p. 2674*)

- It is only Ig which is heat labile (inactivated at 56°C for one hour), daily production is minimum and has shortest half-life.

52. Ans. are 'b and d'

(***Ref:*** *Harrison, 18th/e, p. 2674 and 17th/e,p. 2036; Ananthanarayan, 9th/e, p. 96-99*)

- IgE has highest carbohydrate concentration, Serum half life of IgG is maximum–23 days and IgE has minimum half life–2.5 days. Remember – treatment of serum with 2-mercaptoethanol selectively destroys IgM without affecting IgG, so utilized for estimation of IgG and IgM.

53. Ans. is 'c' i.e., IgM (***Ref:*** *Ananthanarayan, 9th/e, p. 98*)

- IgM is mainly intravascular (80%), it's a pentamer and monomer, millionnaire, molecule with T1/2 is **5 days.**

54. Ans. is 'a' i.e., IgG (***Ref:*** *Jawetz, 27th/e, p. 138*)

- Once healthy babies reach six months of age, their IgG production reaches at normal level, it is major immunoglobulin (80%), max t1/2 – 23 days, passes through placenta, four subclasses IgG1, IgG2, IgG3, IgG4 have been recognized, IgG1 is maximum in amount.

55. Ans. is 'a' (***Ref:*** *Ananthanarayan, 9th/e, p. 97 and 8th/e, p. 98 (t 12.1); Harrison, 18th/e, p. 2674; 17th/e, p. 2036*)

In contrast, IgA is the predominate class of immunoglobulin found in extravascular secretions. Thus, plasma cells located in glands and mucous membranes mainly produce IgA. Therefore, IgA is found in secretions such as milk, saliva, in tears, and in other secretions of the respiratory, intestinal, and genital tracts. (*Jawetz*)

56. Ans. is 'a' i.e., IgG 1

(***Ref:*** *Harrison, 18th/e, p. 2674 and 17th/e, p. 2036; Ananthanarayan, 9th/e, p. 97 and 8th/e, p. 98*)

- IgG1- 65% > IgG2-23%> IgG3-8% > IgG4-4%.

57. Ans. is 'c' i.e., IgG2 (***Ref:*** *Harrison, 18th/e, p. 2674; Ananthanarayan, 9th/e, p. 98*)

- Already explained in book text.

58. Ans. is 'c' i.e., Differential RNA processing (***Ref:*** *Kuby Immunology, 6th/e, p. 130-131*)

- Differential RNA processing of a common primary transcript determines whether the secreted or membrane form of an immunoglobulin will be produced.
- Membrane bound or secreted form of immunoglobulin differs in the amino acid sequence of the heavy chain carboxyl terminal domains.

59. Ans. is 'c' i.e., IgM (***Ref:*** *Ananthanarayan, 9th/e, p. 98 and 8th/e, p. 98; Harrison, 18th/e, p. 2674/e, p. 2036*)

- Decreasing order of ability of Abs to fix complement is in Classical pathways: IgM > IgG1> IgG2 > IgG3 and Alternative pathway: IgA > IgD > IgG4.

60. Ans. is 'c' i.e., IgM (***Ref:*** *Harrison, 18th/e, p. 2674; Ananthanarayan, 9th/e, p. 98 and 8th/e, p. 98*)

- Both IgM and IgG acts as opsonin, however, IgM is more effective opsonin.

61. Ans. is 'a' i.e., IgA (***Ref:*** *Ananthanarayan, 9th/e, p. 97-98 and 8th/e, p. 98-99*)

- IgA (Secretory IgA) is selectively concentrated in secretions and on mucous surfaces forming an antibody paste and is believed to play, an important role in local immunity against respiratory and intestinal pathogens.

62. Ans. is 'a' i.e., Bence Jones protein (***Ref:*** *Ananthanarayan, 9th/e, p. 97 and 8th/e, p. 98*)

- Bence Jones protein is abnormal immunoglobulin found in urine.
- Coagulates at 50°C, redissolves at 70°C.
- Elevated in Multiple myeloma.

63. Ans. is 'c' i.e., IgE (***Ref:*** *Ananthanarayan, 9th/e, p. 98-99; 8th/e, p. 100*)

- The Prausnitz-Küstner test is an immunologic test formerly used by physicians to determine if a patient has an allergic reaction to a specific antigen.
- IgE is homocytotropic, i.e., species specific. Only human IgE can fix to the surface of human cells. This is the basis of Prausnitz-Küstner reaction, which was the original method of detecting atopic antibody.

64. Ans. is 'b' i.e., IgE (***Ref:*** *Ananthanarayan, 9th/e, 8th/e, p. 97, 98*)

65. Ans. is 'c' i.e., Kappa and Lambda chains (***Ref:*** *Ananthanarayan, 9th/e, p. 99 and 8th/e, p. 100*)

- A Bence Jones protein is a monoclonal globulin protein or immunoglobulin light chain found in the urine, with a molecular weight of 22-24 kDa. Detection of Bence Jones protein may be suggestive of multiple myeloma or Waldenström's macroglobulinemia.
- Bence Jones proteins are light chains of immunoglobulins so may occur as Lambda or Kappa forms, but in any other patient the chain is either Kappa or Lambda, never both.

66. Ans. is 'c' i.e., Specific antibody (***Ref:*** *Harper, 27th/e, p. 604; Ananthanarayan, 7th/e, p. 137*)

- Monoclonal antibodies are produced by Hybridoma technique which is specific Abs to a particular Ag.

  (See Figure on the Next Page)

67. Ans. is 'b' i.e., It needs carrier to induce immune response (***Ref:*** *Ananthanarayan, 9th/e, p. 87 and 8th/e, p. 91*)

- Haptens are small molecules that elicit an immune response only when attached to a large carrier such as a protein; the carrier may be one that also does not elicit an immune response by itself. (In general, only large molecules, infectious agents, or insoluble foreign matter can elicit an immune response in the body).

68. Ans. is 'b' i.e., Epitope

(***Ref:*** *Ananthanarayan, 9th/e, p. 88 and 7th/e, p. 81; Harrison, 18th/e, p. 2673 and 17th/e, p. 2036*)

- The part of the antibody or T cell receptor that interact with the epitope.

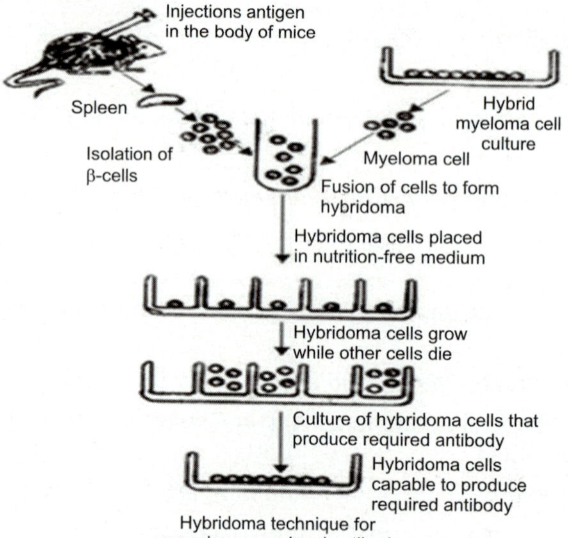

Hybridoma technique for preparing monoclonal antibody

69. Ans. is 'a' i.e., Protein coat (***Ref:*** *Ananthanarayan, 9th/e, p. 88-89 and 7th/e, p. 81-83*)

Antigenicity = protein > carbohydrates > lipid and nucleic acids.

70. Ans. is 'd' i.e., Memory response is seen (***Ref:*** *Ananthanarayan, 9th/e, p. 88-89 and 7th/e, p. 81 83*)

- These antigens directly stimulate B cells processing by antigen presenting cells and their immune response does not require activation of T cells so there is no memory response.

71. Ans. is 'a' i.e., Antigenic cross-reactivity (***Ref:*** *Ananthanarayan, 7th/e, p. 81, 82*)

- Antigenic cross reactivity – Sometimes single antigen stimulates production of variety of antibodies that more or less resemble the correct fit for the antigen. Each of these antibodies may attack different antigens that more or less resemble one another.

72. Ans. is 'a' i.e., Polyclonal activation of T cells

(***Ref:*** *Harrison, 18th/e, p. 2671, 2672; Ananthanarayan, 9th/e, p. 90 and 8th/e, p. 145*)

- Superantigens (S Ags) are a class of antigens that cause non-specific activation of T cells resulting in polyclonal T cell activation and massive cytokine release.

73. Ans. are 'a, c' (***Ref:*** *Ananthanarayan, 9th/e, p. 90; Greenwood, 16th/e, p. 92*)

Examples:

1. Staphylococcus – TSST, Exfoliative toxin, Enterotoxins.Q
2. Streptococcus – Str pyrogenic exotoxin A, B, C.Q
3. Fungus – Malassezia furfur.
4. Mycoplasma arthritidis.Q
5. Yersinia enterocolitica.Q
6. Virus – EBV, CMV, HIV, Rabies nucleocapsid.Q

74. Ans. is 'd' i.e., Covalent bond (***Ref:*** *Ananthanarayan, 9th/e, p. 103 and 8th/e, p. 102; Jawets, 23rd/e, p. 128*)

- Covalent bond is not involved in Ag-Ab reaction.

75. Ans. is 'b' i.e., Precipitation (***Ref:*** *Ananthanarayan, 9th/e, p. 105 and 8th/e, p. 104*)

Abs + soluble Ag + electrolytes = precipitation.

Abs + particulate Ag + electrolytes = agglutination.

76. Ans. is 'c' i.e., Slide flocculation (Already explained in book test)

- The Venereal Disease Research Laboratory test (VDRL) is a non-specific test for syphilis and it is a slide flocculation (precipitation) test.

77. Ans. is 'a' i.e., Widal (***Ref:*** *Ananthanarayan, 9th/e, p. 109*)

- Widal test – slide or tube agglutination test for diagnosis of Typhoid.
- Other options – precipitation tests.

78. Ans. is 'd' i.e., Schick test (***Ref:*** *Ananthanarayan, 9th/e, p. 112 and 8th/e, p. 111*)

- Schick test is a neutralization test.

79. Ans. is 'a' i.e., Neutralization reaction (***Ref:*** *Ananthanarayan, 9th/e, p. 112 and 8th/e, p. 104-111*)

- Nagler reaction is an in-vitro neutralization test.

80. Ans. is 'b' i.e., Agglutination test (***Ref:*** *Ananthanarayan, 9th/e, p. 109 and 8th/e, p. 108*)

- Coombs test (antiglobulin test or anti-Rh antibody test) is an agglutination test.
- The direct Coombs test is used to detect antibodies that are stuck to the surface of red blood cells. Many diseases and drugs can cause this. These antibodies sometimes destroy red blood cells and cause anemia. Your doctor may order this test if you have signs or symptoms of anemia or jaundice.
- The indirect Coombs test looks for free-flowing antibodies against certain red blood cells. It is most often done to determine if you may have a reaction to a blood transfusion.

81. Ans. are 'b, d' (***Ref:*** *Ananthanarayan, 9th/e, p. 105 and 8th/e, p. 104*)

- Prozone phenomenon is a false negative response resulting from high antibody titer which interferes with formation of antigen-antibody lattice, necessary to visualize a positive flocculation test. We present a case of secondary syphilis who presented to us with features of contact irritant dermatitis.

82. Ans. is 'a' i.e., Southern blot (***Ref:*** *Harrison, 18th/e, p. 521 and 17th/e, p. 390*)

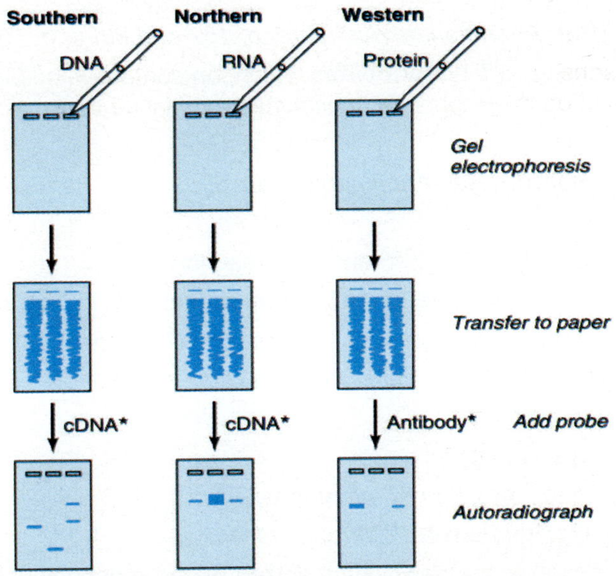

83. Ans. is 'a' i.e., RIA (***Ref:*** *Obs Dutta, 6th/e, p. 67*)

84. Ans. is 'c' i.e., C3 (***Ref:*** *Ananthanarayan, 9th/e, p. 124 and 8th/e, p. 119*) already explained in book text.

85. Ans. is 'a' i.e., C5a (***Ref:*** *Ananthanarayan, 9th/e, p. 123, 125 and 8th/e, p, 120,121*)

86. Ans. are 'b, d' (***Ref:*** *Harrison, 18th/e, p. 2683 and 17th/e, p. 2043; Integrated Medical Sciences, p. 281*)

- Complement deficiencies are said to comprise between 1 and 10% of all primary immunodeficiencies. The genetic deficiencies of early components of the classical pathway (C1q, C1r/s, C2 and C4) tend to be linked with autoimmune diseases, whereas C5 to C9 may have enhanced susceptibility to meningococcal disease. Some new clinical entities are linked with partial complement defects.

87. Ans. is 'b' i.e., C3b (***Ref:*** *Jawetz, 23rd/e, p. 121-123*)

- C3b and C4b are the major opsonins that coat the immune complexes and particulate Ags. Phagocytic cells have receptors for C3b, C4b and are able to bind to complement (C3b, C4b) coated Ags followed by phagocytosis.

88. Ans. is 'd' i.e., IgE (***Ref:*** *Ananthanarayan, 9th/e, p. 162 and 8th/e, p. 162*)

- Type I reactions (immediate hypersensitivity) – IgE (Fab) binds to Ag → mast cell degranulation – release of Histamine and other mediators.

89. Ans. is 'b' i.e., Mast cells (***Ref:*** *Ananthanarayan, 9th/e, p. 162; Robbin's 7th/e, p. 206*)

- Priming Ag→ Antigen presenting cell → T cell → Th 2 → B cell → IgE → Mast cell coated with IgE (Fc).
- Shocking dose → IgE (Fab) binds to Ag → **Mast cell degranulation.**
- Primary mediator (Histamine, Serotonin, chemotactic factor) and secondary factor (PG and cytokines) → Typical manifestations like Anaphylaxis etc.

90. Ans. is 'a' i.e., May be complement mediated (***Ref:*** *Ananthanarayan, 8th/e, p. 162*)

- Effector mechanism – ADCC and Complement mediate cytolysis.
- Complement dependent cytolysis – Transfusion reaction, erythroblastosisfetalis, Autoimmune hemolytic anemia.

91. Ans. are 'b, e' (***Ref:*** *Robbin's 7th/e, p. 210; Ananthanarayan, 8th/e, p. t741*)

- Graves' disease is type-2 hypersensitivity, and sometimes considered as type-5 hypersensitivity.

92. Ans. is 'b' i.e., Immune complex mediated (***Ref:*** *Ananthanarayan, 9th/e, p. t621*)

- Type III reactions differ from type II reactions because its antigens are not attached to the surface of the cell.
- Immune complex mediated (Ag-Ab mediated) – deposited in tissue.
- Usually complement bound to complex – so serum level falls.
- Neutrophil attracted and release enzymes.

93. Ans. is 'd' i.e., Lymphocytes (***Ref:*** *Ananthanarayan, 9th/e, p. 167 and 8th/e, p. 168*)

- Reaction is mediated by sensitized **T-lymphocytes** which, on contact with specific antigen, release lymphokines that cause biological effects on macrophages, leucocytes and tissue cells.
- Delayed type by CD4 Th1 cell.

94. Ans. is 'd' i.e., Granulomatous reaction (***Ref:*** *Ananthanarayan, 9th/e, p. 167 and 7th/e, p. 166; Robbin's 7th/e, p. 216*)

- Explained in book text.

95. Ans. is 'b' i.e., Serum sickness is a type II hypersensitivity reaction

(***Ref:*** *Ananthanarayan, 9th/e, p. 162 and 8th/e, p. 162; Chandrasoma Taylor, 3rd/e, p. 103*)

- Systemic Serum sickness is a type III hypersensitivity reaction not type II.

96. Ans. is 'c' i.e., Casoni's test (***Ref:*** *Chatterjee Parasitology, 12th/e, p. 127*)

- Casoni's test is type I hypersensitivity.
- Arthus reaction is type III hypersensitivity.
- Lepromin test and tuberculin test are type IV hypersensitivity.

97. Ans. is 'b' i.e., Prostaglandin D2 (***Ref:*** *Jawetz, 27th/e, p. 141*)

- Prostaglandins and thromboxanes are newly synthesized by the mast cell using the cyclo-oxygenase pathway. The leukotrienes B_4, C_4 and D_4 (slow reacting substance of anaphylaxis, SRS-A) are also newly synthesized by the mast cell, in this instance using the lipoxygenase pathway.

98. Ans. is 'a' i.e., Autoimmune hemolytic anemia (***Ref:*** *Ananthanarayan, 9th/e, p. 162 and 8th/e, p. 162*)

- Autoimmune hemolytic anemia is type II HSN.
- In type II Hypersensitivity reaction (Ab mediated) various mechanisms involves up: (1) Opsonization, complement and Fc receptor mediated phagocytosis (C3b acts as opsonin). (2) Complement and Fc receptor mediated inflammation (C5a acts as chemokine for neutrophil and monocyte. (3) Antibody mediated cellular dysfunction.

99. Ans. is 'b' i.e., Type II (***Ref:*** *Ananthanarayan, 9th/e, p. 162 and 8th/e, p. 162; Chandrasoma Taylor, 3rd/e, p. 103*)

- Actually Myasthenia gravis is Type V hypersensitivity subtype of type II – Abs are formed against Cell surface receptor impaired or deregulated function.

100. Ans. is 'c' i.e., Type III (***Ref:*** *Robbins, 7th/e, p. 219, 220; Chandrasoma Taylor, 3rd/e, p. 119, 120*)

- Pre-existing antibody against donor graft antigens can cause hyperacute graft rejection.

  The antigen-antibody, reaction produces an Arthus-type (type-III) immune complex injury in the vessels of the transplant.

Remember – Principal morphological manifestation of type III reaction is necrotizing vasculitis and fibrinoid necrosis.

101. Ans. is 'a' i.e., T cells (***Ref:*** *Ananthanarayan, 9th/e, p. 167 and 8th/e, p. 168*)

- Type IV HSN – T-cell, Delayed type hypersensitivity-CD4 T cells and macrophages are primarily involved characterized by Granuloma formation (Activated macrophages (Epitheloid cells) surrounded by collar of lymphocytes and giant cells.
- Th1 plays important role because the expression of delayed hypersensitivity largely depends on the cytokines secreted.
- Other examples are Tuberculin test, Lepromin test, Sarcoidosis, Tuberculosis and granulomatous inflammation.

102. Ans. is 'c' Negative selection of T cell in thymus

Negative selection is needed to prevent autoreactive T cells to come into circulation and cause autoimmunity, cryptic antigens are antigenic epitopes which are normally hidden and their exposure leads to development of immune response and in appropriate expression of MHC proteins also leads to development of self-destructive immune system.

103. Ans. is 'b' i.e., Systemic lupus erythematosus (***Ref:*** *Jawetz, 27th/e, p. 149*)

- SLE is a disease involving antibodies to non-organ specific antigens such as DNA and induces immune complexes which deposit in the vascular bed causing kidney, skin, joint and cerebral lesions.

104. Ans. is 'c' i.e., Higher incidence among males

(***Ref:*** *Ananthanarayan, 9th/e, p. 178-182 and 8th/e, p. 171-175; Harrison, 17th/e, p. 2071-74*)

- Autoimmune diseases are syndromes caused by activation of T and B cells or both. Costimulatory molecules such as B7-1 or B7-2 are involved in autoimmunity. Higher incidence is seen in females.

105. Ans. is 'd' i.e., Polyclonal B cell activation (***Ref:*** *Harrison, 18th/e, p. 1467*)

- Polyclonal activation of B cells leads to the production of antibodies to host cell and viral proteins.

106. Ans. is 'd' i.e., Isograft (***Ref:*** *Ananthanarayan, 9th/e*)

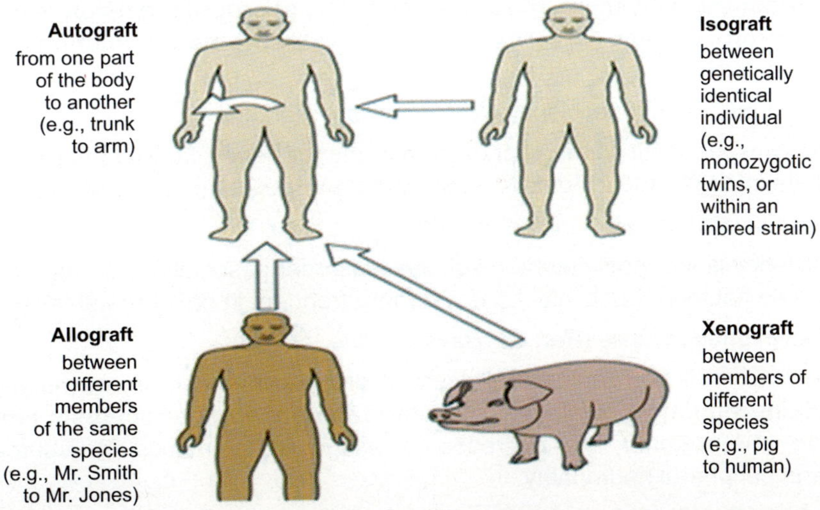

107. Ans. is 'b' i.e., Red cell agglutination by all blood group sera (***Ref:*** *Ananthanarayan, 9th/e, p. 195*)

- **Thomsen Friedreich phenomenon** – Red cell suspension contaminated with certain bacteria, e.g., Pseudomonas aeruginosa, become agglutinable by all blood group sera and even by normal human sera. It is due to unmasking of a hidden antigen normally present on all human erythrocytes, i.e., T antigen and anti T agglutinins are normally present in human sera. This panagglutinability is observed in persons suffering from systemic bacterial infections.

108. Ans. is 'b' i.e., T-lymphocytes (***Ref:*** *Ananthanarayan, 9th/e, p. 186 and 8th/e, p. 180*)

- T-lymphocytes are responsible for the Graft versus Host reaction and in this **Billingham criteria** is followed – Graft contain immunocompetent T cells, Host is immunodeficient, HLA mismatch.

109. Ans. is 'b' i.e., Severe combined immunodeficiency

(***Ref:*** *Ananthanarayan, 9th/e, p. 174 and 8th/e, p. 158; Robbin's 7th/e, p. 244*)

(1) **X-linked recessive** is most common type of SCID and is due to mutation in common chain of cytokine receptors.

(2) **Most common cause of autosomal recessive form** of severe combined immunodeficiency is due to **adenosine deaminase deficiency** and others are JAK-3 gene, RAG-1 or RAG-2 or class II MHC.

- All patients with SCID have small thymus, fail to ascend from neck, Lymph nodes, tonsils, adenoids and peyers patches are absent.
- Only available treatment is BMT (Bone marrow transplantation) and Gene therapy is found to be successful in X-linked SCID.

In AR (ADA deficiency) there is a rib cage abnormality and bone in bone effect is observed.

110. Ans. are 'b, d'

(***Ref:*** *Ananthanarayan, 9th/e, p. 175 and 8th/e, p. 159; Harrison, 18th/e, p. 478, 479 and 17th/e, p. 380, 381, 382*)

- The bacteria involved in recurrent infections are catalase positive pyogenic pathogens such as staphylococci and coliforms. Catalase negative pathogens such as streptococci and pneumococci are handled normally.
- Leucocytes from the patients of chronic granulomatous disease fail to reduce nitroblue tetrazolium NBT) during phagocytosis. This property has been used as a screening method (NBT test) for the diagnosis of chronic granulomatous disease.

111. Ans. is 'c' i.e., Determine whether polymorphonuclear leucocytes can produce superoxide

(***Ref:*** *Ananthanarayan, 9th/e, p. 175 and 8th/e, p. 59*)

- Nitro blue tetrazolium is used in a diagnostic test, particularly for chronic granulomatous disease and other diseases of phagocyte function. When there is an **NADPH oxidase defect** the phagocyte is unable to make reactive oxygen species or radicals required for bacterial killing. As a result, bacteria may thrive within the phagocyte. **The higher the blue score, the better the cell is at producing reactive oxygen species,** other test employed are **Dihydrorhodamine** (DHR) **oxidation test, cytochrome C reduction assay** and **immunoblot** for NADPH oxidase component.

112. Ans. is 'b' i.e., Isolated IgA immunodeficiency (***Ref:*** *Harrison, 18th/e, p. 2704 and 17th/e, p. 2058*)

Selective IgA deficiency is the most common primary immunodeficiency, familial (more common), naïve B cells are not able to differentiate into IgA producing cells. Along with IgA, IgG2 and IgG4 may also be reduced.

113. Ans. is 'd' i.e., IgA+IgG2 (***Ref:*** *Jawetz, 27th/e, p. 149*)

- IgG2 immunodeficiency is the most common subclass disorder associated with recurrent infections by polysaccharide encapsulated bacteria. Such infections are more frequent in patients with associated IgA deficiency.

114. Ans. is 'a' i.e., Defect in phagocytosis (***Ref:*** *CP Baveja, 5th/e, p. 150*)

- Chédiak-Higashi syndrome is a rare autosomal recessive disorder that arises from a mutation of LYST gene codes for **lysosomal trafficking regulator protein,** which leads to a **decrease in phagocytosis. Failure of phagolysosomal fusion, defective chemotaxis.** The decrease in phagocytosis results in recurrent pyogenic infections, partial albinism and peripheral neuropathy.

115. Ans. is 'a' i.e., Candida (***Ref:*** *Harrison, 16th/e, p. 697; Jawetz, 23rd/e, p. 641*)

- Cell mediated immune responses, especially CD4 cells, are important in controlling mucocutaneous candidiasis. The neutrophil is probably crucial for resistance to systemic candidiasis.

MISCELLANEOUS IMMUNOLOGY MCQs

1. As part of the innate immune response, which cells participate in phagocytosis?

(a) Macrophages and mast cells
(b) Macrophages and plasma cell
(c) NK cells and neutrophils
(d) Macrophages and neutrophils

Ans. is 'd'

2. MHC class II molecules are critically important in what immunologic process?

(a) Antigen presentation
(b) Phagocytosis
(c) Immunoglobulin class switching
(d) CD8 T cell cytotoxicity

Ans. is 'a' MHC class II relates to antigen presentation and MHC class I relates to CD8 T cell cytotoxicity.

3. The host response to the interaction of a pathogen with its specific TLR generates which of the following?

(a) IgG production
(b) Cell activation and production of cytokines and chemokines
(c) Immunoglobulin class switching
(d) Phagocytosis

Ans. is 'b'

4. The interaction of two IgG molecules binding to antigen followed by the binding of C1 to the Fc portion of the antibody results in which of the following?

(a) Initiation of antigen presentation
(b) Initiation of classic complement pathway
(c) Initiation of alternative complement pathway
(d) Initiation of the mannose-binding lectin-binding complement pathway

Ans. is 'b'

5. What is a characteristic of the adaptive immune response and not of the innate response?

(a) Physical barriers
(b) Chemical barriers
(c) Clonal expansion of effector cells
(d) Inflammatory mediators

Ans. is 'c'

6. Which genetic mechanism generates antibodies of the same specificity but different immunoglobulin classes?

(a) V gene segment recombination
(b) Class switching
(c) Somatic hypermutation
(d) Junctional variability due to imprecise V, D and J joining

Ans. is 'b'

7. A man in his twenties presents in the emergency room with shortness of breath and fatigue. He is also very pale. Two days earlier he was given penicillin for an infection. He had penicillin previously without problems and stated that he had "no allergy" to penicillin. Laboratory testing shows that antibodies to penicillin are present in the patient's serum and that he is breaking down his own red blood cells. He is diagnosed with immune hemolytic anemia. The patient has which type of hypersensitivity reaction?

(a) Type I
(b) Type II
(c) Type III
(d) Type IV (DTH)

Ans. is 'b'

8. NK cells express a killer immunoglobulin-like receptor (KIR), which recognizes:

(a) MHC class I molecules
(b) Cell adhesion molecules
(c) Glycophospholipid molecules
(d) CD40 molecules

Ans. is 'a'

9. IFN alpha and IFN gamma are produced by the virus-infected cell due to the interaction of virus nucleic acid with which of the following?

(a) C3 (third component of complement)
(b) Defensins
(c) TLR pathway
(d) IL-12

Ans. is 'c'

10. Which two cytokines play an important role in attracting neutrophils to the site of an infection?

(a) IFN Alpha and IFN-Gamma
(b) IL-8 and IL-17
(c) IL-2 and IL-4
(d) IL-6 and IL-12

Ans. is 'b'

11. Which one of the following laboratory assays is considered to be an in vitro counterpart of the type IV hypersensitivity reactions seen in the TB skin test?

(a) Immunoblot for TB antigen
(b) EIA analysis of sera from TB patient
(c) Immunofluorescence assay for TB antibody
(d) IFN-gamma production by white blood cell (WBC) treated with TB antigen

Ans. is 'd'

12. Which of the following laboratory assays can be used to detect the number and types of immune cells in the peripheral blood?

(a) Immunofixation electrophoresis
(b) EIA
(c) Flow cytometry
(d) Immunoblot

Ans. is 'c'

13. What is the minimum percentage of children which needs to be vaccinated successfully in order to achieve herd immunity to diphtheria?

(a) 100%
(b) 10%
(c) 50%
(d) 75%

Ans. is 'd'

Herd immunity can only be achieved in those diseases which depend on human transmission, such as diphtheria. Thus, in the case of tetanus, active immunization is of benefit to the individual, but not to the community, since it will not eliminate the organism which is found in the feces of domestic animals and persists in soil as highly resistant spores.

14. DNA vaccines:

(a) Are relatively poor at stimulating cytotoxic T lymphocyte responses in mice
(b) Must be administered on gold particles if they are to be effective
(c) Are only effective if followed by a protein boost
(d) May have distinct advantages when preparing subunit vaccines against viruses which frequently alter their antigens

Ans. is 'd'

15. Pattern recognition receptors (PRR) include:

(a) LPS
(b) PAMPs
(c) Lipoteichoic acid
(d) Lectin-like molecules

Ans. is 'd'

16. lysozyme:

(a) It is a cytoplasmic organelle
(b) Activates complement
(c) It is a proteolytic enzyme
(d) Splits peptidoglycan

Ans. is 'd'

17. Mutations in the gamma chain of the receptors for IL 2, 4, 7, 9 and 15 leads to:

(a) Reticular dysgenesis
(b) Bare lymphocyte syndrome
(c) Hyper IgM syndrome
(d) Severe combined immunodeficiency (SCID)

Ans. is 'd'

18. The specialized cells involved in entry of lymphocytes in lymph nodes are called:

(a) M cells
(b) Mesangial cells
(c) PALS
(d) HEV endothelial cells

Ans. is 'd'

The high-walled endothelium of the post-capillary venules (HEV) in lymph nodes express vascular addressins which are recognized by homing receptors on lymphocytes passing through the afferent lymphatics and which mediate entry of the lymphocytes into the lymph nodes.

19. On entering a germinal centre, primary B blasts grow exponentially to form which cell type in the dark zone?

(a) Secondary B blasts
(b) Centrocytes
(c) Centroblasts
(d) Memory B cells

Ans. is 'c' Centroblasts are found in the dark zone and are highly mitotic cells with no surface IgD and very little surface IgM.

20. In a lymph node, antigen pneumococcus polysaccharide leads to:

(a) Lymphocyte proliferation in the paracortex
(b) PALS development
(c) Proliferation in cortical lymphoid cells
(d) Absence of germinal centres

Ans. is 'c' Stimulation of antibody-formation by this thymus-independent antigen leads to proliferation in this location with development of germinal centers while the paracortical region remains inactive, reflecting the inability to develop cellular hypersensitivity to the polysaccharide.

21. Which of the following is seen in African children with Burkitts lymphoma?

(a) Absence of EBV
(b) T cell neoplasia
(c) Deletion of C myc gene
(d) Chromosome 8q24 to chromosome 14q32 translocation

Ans. is 'd' The *c-myc* gene (chromosome 8q24) involved in the entry of cells from resting G_0 into the cell cycle is translocated to the mu heavy chain gene (chromosome 14q32) in most cases of Burkitt's lymphoma studied.

22. The following is feature of B cell not T cell:

(a) Class I MHC
(b) CD3
(c) Measles virus receptor
(d) Surface immunoglobulin

Ans. is 'd' B cells express surface immunoglobulin of a specificity created by that cell's particular immunoglobulin gene recombinations. A totally different gene set encodes the T cell receptor for antigen.

23. T cell ligand binding B7 on a professional APC is:

(a) CD28 (b) CD2 (c) LFA-1 (d) ICAM1

Ans. is 'a' An alternative ligand for B7, present on activated T cells, is CTLA-4.

24. Skin transplant was done from sister to brother after few years, brother to sister transplant was done, but rejection occurred, what is the phenomenon called as?

(a) Schwartzman reaction

(b) Theobald Smith phenomenon

(c) Eichwald silmer effect

(d) Schultz dale phenomenon

Ans. is 'c' Unilateral sex linked histoincompatibility is known as **Eichwald silmer effect,** Grafts from female to male will succeed but male to female transplant don't succeed.

25. All of the following statements about hybridoma technology are true *except*:

(a) Specific antibody producing cells are integrated with myeloma cells

(b) Myeloma cells with mutation in salvage pathway grows well in HAT medium

(c) Aminopterin, a folate antagonist, inhibits de novo pathway

(d) HGPRTase and thymidylate synthetase are required for salvage pathway.

Ans. is 'b' Any cell that lacks HGPRT cannot grow on HAT medium.

RED ALERT POINTS

1. **Type-I** hypersensitivity is mediated by**: IgE, examples are PK reaction, Theobald Smith phenomenon, Casoni reaction, atopy, Asthma.**
2. The serum concentration of which human IgG subclass maximum: **IgG1, passes thru placenta, major antibody in secondary immune response, highest T1/2.**
3. Epsilionaminocaproic acid given prophylactically is useful if used in**: C1 esterase inhibitor deficiency, deficiency of this leads to Hereditary angioneurotic edema.**
4. Nitroblue Tetrazolium test is used for: **Phagocytes, it is negative in Chronic granulomatous disease and positive in normal individuals. These patients are suspectible for catalase positive organisms.**
5. Intermediate host for hydatid disease: **Man, Definitive host is dog, Infective form is egg, Inner layer endocyst is most active and secrete Hydatid fluid by which Casoni test (Type I hypersensitivity) is demonstrated.**
6. Most reliable investigation for diagnosis in syphilis is**: FTA-ABS (most sensitive) and TPI (most specific). Wassermann test is complement fixation test and VDRL is used to assess prognosis of the disese.**
7. **Herd immunity** is Not useful in protection against: **Tetanus.**
8. Rheumatoid factor is: **19 S globulin (IgM against IgG).**
9. Most common immunoglobulin deficiency is of: **IgA deficiency, common variable immunodeficiency is associated with Giardiasis, IgA deficiency leads to recurrent sinusitis and other infections.**
10. **Type-IV** hypersensitivity reaction is: **Mantoux test, lepromin reaction, Contact dermatitis IVY poisoning, Fries skin test.**
11. **IgM:** Activites classical complement.
12. First immunoglobulin to appear infection**: IgM (Slow, sluggish and short lived).**

    And IgG is in secondary immune response (Prompt, powerful and prolonged).
13. **Widal test** is an example of**: Agglutination test, comes positive in 2 weeks.**

    And paired test is to be done which shows 4 fold increase in titre of Abs.
14. **HLA-I (MHC-I** is involved in: Graft rejection, cell mediated cytolysis of viral infected or tumor cells. **HLA-II (MHC-II)** is involved in: Graft versus host response, Mixed leukocyte reaction. **HLA-III (MHC-III)** is involved in: Susceptibility to autoimmune disease.
15. **C-C (Beta) chemokines** are: MCP-I, Eotaxin, MIP-1a, RANTES.

    Other chemokines: C-X-C/alpha (IL-1, IL-8, TNF), **C/gamma** (lymphotactin), **CX3C** (fractalkine).
16. True about **C-reactive protein:** Beta globulin, non-specific inflammatory protein, produced in liver, raised in infections (including pneumococcal infection) and inflammatory conditions (like RA), detected by passive latex agglutination.
17. Important **acute phase proteins:** CRP, fibrinogen, hepatoglobulin, ceruloplasmin, transferrin, MBP, α-1 antitrypsin, ferritin, Serum amyloid A.
18. **Idiotype** class of antibody is determined by: N-terminal (amino end).

    Antibody isotype variation is due to: Variation in amino-acid sequence in constant region of heavy chain.
19. **Most avidly complement fixing antibody:** IgM. Antibodies activating classical complement pathway: IgM and IgG (IgM >IgG). Fc piece which fixes C1: CH2 of IgG and CH4 of IgM.
20. Precipitates at 50°C-60°C and dissolutes (disappears) on further heating upto 100°C: Light chains (Bence-Jones protein). Bence-Jones proteins are: Kappa and Lambda chains (light chains) in ratio of (2:1) of immunoglobulins.
21. **Widal test is:** Agglutination test (tube agglutination test) for typhoid. Coomb test is: Agglutination test. Rosewaaler test is: Passive haemagglutination test for RA.

    VDRL is: Precipitation test (slide precipitation test) for syphilis.

22. **C3 convertase** in classical pathway: C4b2a.C3 convertase in alternative pathway: C3bBb.
23. **Hereditary angioneurotic edema** is due to deficiency of: C1 esterase inhibitor.
24. Process of increasing the ability for phagocytosis of foreign body: Opsonization.

    Opsonization is caused by (Opsonins are): Antibodies (IgM>IgG), complement (C3b).
25. **Important type I hypersensitivities:** Eczema, hay fever, asthma, anaphylaxis, Casoni's test. **Important type II hypersensitivities:** Transfusion reaction, erythroblastosisfetalis, autoimmune hemolytic anemia, Graves' disease, myastheniagravis. **Important type III hypersensitivities:** Arthus reaction, serum sickness, Schick test, PAN, SLE, RA, Type II lepra reaction (ENL), Glomerulonephritis. **Important type IV** hypersensitivity Tuberculin test. Lepromin test, Type-1 lepra reaction. Granulomatous inflammation, contact dermatitis, sarcoidosis, TB, Graft rejection.
26. **Important features of Digeorge syndrome:** Thymic hypoplasia, hypocalcemic tetany, CHDs, facial abnormalities, Decreased T-cells, normal B-cells.

    Adenosine deaminase deficiency is seen in: Severe combined immunodeficiency (SCID).

    Job's syndrome is defect in: Phagocytosis. Nucleotidase deficiency causes: Humoral immunity deficiency. **Bloom syndrome** is characterized by: Decreased IgA and IgM with or without IgG changes.
27. **Most common fungal infection in neutropenia:** Candida. Candida infection is seen in: Myeloperoxidase deficiency.
28. **Wiskott aldrich syndrome** is: **Wasp gene mutation, RET triad is seen – recurrent infections, Eczema, thrombocytopaenia, IgE is increased, IgM decreases, IgG and IgA remains normal.**
29. **Casoni reaction is type I hypersensitivity whereas contact dermatitis is type IV.**
30. Wassermann reaction – Complement fixation test for Syphilis, Kahn flocculation test – Tube precipitation, Rosewaaler test – Passive hemagglutination test used for Rheumatoid arthritis.
31. Rosalyn yallow – developed radioimmunoassay. Stanley B prusiner – described Prion and PK reaction, Laveran – Discovery of malarial parasite.
32. TH1 helper T cell produce IL2, IFN gamma, IL12.

    TH2 helper T cell produce IL4, IL5, IL6, IL13.
33. Test for chronic brucellosis – 2 mercaptoethanol test, ELISA, CFT and Coombs test.

PRACTICE QUESTIONS

1. **Following are true of passive immunity *except*:**
   (a) Effective immediately
   (b) Applicable in immuno deficient host
   (c) Prolonged protection
   (d) Conferred by antibodies
2. **Adjuvants are used in vaccine to:**
   (a) Enhance immune response
   (b) To act as preservative
   (c) Provide correct pH
   (d) Act as media
3. **The first immunoglobulin synthesizes by the fetus is:**
   (a) IgA (b) IgD (c) IgM (d) IgD
4. **Which of the following is used in providing adoptive immunity?**
   (a) Hyper immune sera
   (b) Immunoglobulins
   (c) Live vaccines
   (d) Lymphocyte suspension
5. **Which of the following protein is not antigenic?**
   (a) Collagen
   (b) Gelatin
   (c) Myosin
   (d) Hemoglobin
6. **The different immunoglobulins are identified by different:**
   (a) L chain
   (b) H chain
   (c) Inter chain bond
   (d) Sporteins
7. **The action of papain on a molecule of IgG produces:**
   (a) Two fab + two Fc
   (b) Two fab + one Fc
   (c) One fab + two Fc
   (d) F (ab) + amino acids
8. **The only maternal immunoglobulin that is transported across the placenta is:**
   (a) IgA (b) IgD (c) IgG (d) IgE
9. **The immunoglobulin which is present in least amounts in serum is:**
   (a) IgA (b) IgG (c) IgM (d) IgE
10. **Following immunoglobulins are heat stable *except*:**
    (a) IgG (b) IgA (c) IgE (d) IgM
11. **Colostrum contains:**
    (a) IgG
    (b) IgA
    (c) All immunoglobulins
    (d) A + b
12. **Which of the following antibodies is a classical example of IgM antibodies?**
    (a) Blood group antibodies
    (b) SLE antibodies
    (c) Antibodies to typhoid 'O' antigen
    (d) All of the above
13. **Homocytotropism is a feature of:**
    (a) IgG (b) IgA (c) IgE (d) IgD
14. **Prausnitz-Kustner reaction is mediated by:**
    (a) IgA (b) IgD (c) IgE (d) IgM
15. **Bence-Jones proteins are formed of:**
    (a) Heavy chains
    (b) Light chains
    (c) J chains
    (d) T protein

16. Which of the following is most effective in precipitation reaction?

(a) IgA (b) IgG (c) IgM (d) IgE

17. Felix tubes in Widal test are used in detection of:

(a) H agglutination (b) Agglutination
(c) Both (d) None

18. Reversed passive agglutination test is used in the detection of:

(a) Antigen (b) Antibody (c) Both (d) None

19. Pfeiffer's phenomenon is due to:

(a) Antibodies (b) Complement (c) Opsonin (d) Enzymes

20. Deficiency of CI inhibitor is associated with:

(a) Angioneurotic edema (b) SLE
(c) Gram negative septicemia (d) Recurrent infections

21. Following are features of T cells *except*:

(a) E – rosette formation (b) Thymus specific antigens present
(c) Numerous cytoplasmic projections (d) Blast transformation with mitogens

22. Which of the following is seen in macrophages and not seen in lymphocytes?

(a) EAC rosette (b) Receptor for Fc
(c) Blast transformation (d) Adherence to glass surface

23. Follwoing are features of Blymphocytes *except*:

(a) Surface immunolglobulins (b) EAC rosette formation
(c) Phagocytic action (d) Blast transformation with endotoxin

24. What percentage of lymphocytes in peripheral circulation are T cells?

(a) 15-20% (b) 35-45% (c) 55-75% (d) 85-95%

25. Antibody dependent cell mediated cytotoxicity is function of:

(a) Null cells (b) T cells (c) B cells (d) Killer cells

26. Which of the following cells is specially involved in tumor immunity?

(a) T suppressor (b) Thelper (c) Plasma cell (d) NK cell

27. Follwoing are feature of plasma cells *except*:

(a) Cartwheel appearance of nucleus (b) Abundant endoplasmic reticulum
(c) Long life span of 20-30 days (d) Makes single specific type of immunoglobulin

28. Mast cells are produced in:

(a) Spleen (b) Bone marrow
(c) Liver (d) Thymus

29. Antibody mediated immunity is useful in following situations *except*:

(a) Defense against extracellular bacteria (b) Fungal infections
(c) Respiratory viral infections (d) Type I hypersensitively response

30. T cells mediated immunity is responsible for which type of hypersensitivity reaction?

(a) Type I (b) Type II (c) Type III (d) Type IV

31. Sulzberger chase phenomenon refers to antigenic tolerance based on:

(a) Size of antigen (b) Route of administration
(c) Adjuvants used (d) Host immunity

32. A person who had typhoid may produce antityphoid antibodies to a streptococcal sore throat infection is called as:

(a) Prozone phenomenon
(b) Anamnestic reaction
(c) Antigenic competition
(d) Antigenic memory

33. The drug most widely used for immunosuppression is:
(a) Cyclophosphamide
(b) Cyclosporine
(c) Methotrexate
(d) 5FU

34. Cyclophoosphamide selectively inhibits:
(a) Suppressor T lymphocytes
(b) Helper T lymphocytes
(c) B lymphocytes
(d) NK cells

35. Congenital agammaglobulinemia is inherited through:
(a) Autosomal dominant
(b) Autosomal recessive
(c) X-linked recessive
(d) Y linked

36. Which of the following disorder of vitamin metabolism is associated with immunodeficiency?
(a) Vitamin C
(b) Vitamin B12
(c) Vitamin A
(d) Vitamin #

37. Combined immunodeficiency is seen in:
(a) Nazel of syndrome
(b) Ataxia telangiectasia
(c) Wiskott Aldrich syndrome
(d) All of the above

38. Which of the following enzyme deficiency is associated with immunodeficiency?
(a) Adenosine deaminase
(b) Carbonic anhydrase
(c) DNA polymerase
(d) ATPase

39. Following are feature of jobs syndrome *except*:
(a) Mycobacterial infections
(b) Atopic eczema
(c) Elevated IgE levels
(d) Defective phagocytosis

40. Pancreatic malfunction, bony abnormalities and decreased neutrophil motility is seen in:
(a) Chediak Higashi syndrome
(b) Shwachmann's disease
(c) Job's syndrome
(d) Lazy leucocyte syndrome

41. The minimum interval between the sensitizing and shocking dose of antigen in apahylaxis should be:
(a) 24 hours
(b) 48 hours
(c) 3 days
(d) 2 weeks

42. The first autoimmune disease to be described in man is:
(a) Hashimoto's thyroditis
(b) Paroxysmal cold hemoglobinuria
(c) Myasthenia gravis
(d) SLE

43. Which of the following viral infection is known to predispose to autoimmune disease?
(a) Poliomyelitis
(b) Adeno virus infections
(c) Infections mononucleosis
(d) Hepatitis A

44. Antibodies in paroxysmal cold hemoglobinuria belong to:
(a) IgA
(b) IgG
(c) IgD
(d) IgM

45. Warm auto antibodies leading to hemolytic anemia is seen with intake of:
(a) Alpha methyldopa
(b) Phenytoin
(c) INH
(d) Digoxin

46. Which of the following antibody is found in pernicious anemia?
(a) Parietal cell antibody
(b) Intrinsic factor antibody
(c) Anti-erythrocyte antibody
(d) Both (a) and (b)

47. Anti DNA antibodies are characteristics of:

(a) Rheumatoid arthritis (b) SLE

(c) Pernicious anemia (d) Guillain-Barré syndrome

48. Which of the following drugs is known to produce a syndrome like SLE?

(a) Phenytoin (b) Isoniazid

(c) Procainamide (d) All of the above

49. Rheumatoid factor is predominantly made of:

(a) IgM (b) IgA (c) IgG (d) Collagen

50. The best method of choosing a compatible donor for organ transplantation is:

(a) Coomb's test (b) HLA typing

(c) Mixed leukocyte (d) Cross matching

ANSWERS

1.	(c)	2.	(a)	3.	(c)	4.	(d)	5.	(b)	6.	(b)	7.	(b)	8.	(c)
9.	(d)	10.	(c)	11.	(d)	12.	(c)	13.	(c)	14.	(c)	15.	(b)	16.	(b)
17.	(b)	18.	(a)	19.	(b)	20.	(a)	21.	(c)	22.	(c)	23.	(c)	24.	(c)
25.	(d)	26.	(d)	27.	(c)	28.	(d)	29.	(b)	30.	(d)	31.	(b)	32.	(b)
33.	(b)	34.	(b)	35.	(c)	36.	(b)	37.	(d)	38.	(a)	39.	(a)	40.	(b)
41.	(d)	42.	(b)	43.	(c)	44.	(d)	45.	(a)	46.	(d)	47.	(b)	48.	(d)
49.	(a)	50.	(c)												

MUST KNOW IMMUNOLOGY MCQs

1. Natural killer cells assess whether other cells are abnormal by detecting types and levels of surface associated:

(a) MHC class I molecules
(b) Non self molecules
(c) Pattern recognition receptors
(d) Pathogen associated molecular patterns

Ans. (a)

MHC class I molecules are self-identification molecules found on all nucleated host cells. Natural killer cells, after making contact with cells expressing stress signals make the decision whether to kill them or not by assessing whether they express MHC class I molecules. Although they are members of the innate immune system, natural killer cells do not recognize non-self, pattern recognition receptors or pathogen associated molecular patterns.

2. Pattern recognition receptors bind to:

(a) Pathogen associated molecular patterns
(b) B & T lymphocytes
(c) MHC class I molecules
(d) Natural killer cells

Ans. (a)

PRRs are germline-encoded host sensors, which detect molecules typical for the pathogens. They are **proteins** expressed, mainly, by cells of the **innate immune system**, such as dendritic cells, macrophages, monocytes, neutrophils and epithelial cells, to identify two classes of molecules: **Pathogen-associated molecular patterns** (PAMPs), which are associated with microbial **pathogens**, and **damage-associated molecular patterns** (DAMPs), which are associated with components of host's cells that are released during cell damage or death. They are also called primitive pattern recognition receptors because they evolved before other parts of the immune system, particularly before adaptive immunity. PRRs also mediate the initiation of antigen-specific adaptive immune response and release of inflammatory cytokines.

3. Antibody mediated recruitment of macrophages occurs through the action of:

(a) Complement receptors
(b) Fc receptors
(c) Killer activation receptors
(d) Pattern recognition receptors

Ans. (b)

Binding of an epitope causes a conformational change in the Fc portion of the antibody molecule. Fc receptors (FcRs) recognize and bind to the confirmationally altered antibody molecule, and this engagement of epitope-bound antibody molecule by FcRs stimulates phagocytosis of cells and molecules tagged by antibodies for destruction. Complement receptors bind and facilitate the phagocytosis of cells and molecules tagged by complement components or fragments. Killer activation receptors and pattern recognition receptors do not recognize antigen antibody complexes.

4. Which of the following is a correct pairing of a soluble molecule with its microcidal action in the respiratory tract?

(a) B-defensins increase microbial susceptibility to phagocytosis
(b) DNase enzymatically damages microbial membranes
(c) Fatty acids of commensal microbes degrade microbial peptidoglycan
(d) Lacrimal secretions facilitate ingestion of microbes by phagocytes

Ans. (a)

Peptidoglycan is degraded not by fatty acids or DNase but by lysozyme. Lacrimal fluid contains Lysozyme that acts on microbial peptidoglycan not on host phagocytes.

5. When an immunoglobulin molecule is subjected to cleavage by pepsin, the product:

(a) Are individual heavy and light chains
(b) Can no longer bind to antigen
(c) Consist of two separated antigen binding fragments
(d) Is a dimeric antigen binding molecule

Ans. (d)

Enzymatic cleavage of the immunoglobulin monomer by pepsin occurs distal to the variable domain and distal to heavy-heavy chain disulfide bonds, which remain intact, resulting in a molecule with two epitope binding sites.

Interchain disulfide bonds are unaffected by pepsin cleavage. The epitope binding site remains intact upon pepsin cleavage of the heavy chain. Papain cleavage of the immunoglobulin monomer occurs distal to the variable domain but proximal to the heavy–heavy chain disulfide bond, resulting in two separate epitope binding Fab fragments. Pepsin enzymatically degrades the CH2 portion of the immunoglobulin molecule resulting in fragments that rarely, if ever, form crystals.

6. A state of T lymphocyte non-responsiveness that occurs following peptide + major histocompatibility complex (pMHC) engagement is known as:

(a) Allergy (b) Apoptosis
(c) Anergy (d) Autoimmunity

Ans. (c)

Anergy is a state of non-activity that occurs when a lymphocyte receives a stimulus through its TCR or BCR in the absence of the additional appropriate signals provided by antigen presenting cells or T cells. Allergy involves the degranulation of mast cells following binding of antigen IgE molecules already affixes to the mast cell surfaces. Apoptosis is the programmed cell death of a cell through degradation of its nucleic acids. Autoimmunity is the active response of the immune system against self-epitopes.

7. The Foxp3 nuclear transcription factor is expressed within:

(a) B cells (b) CD4+CD8+(double positive) thymocytes
(c) CD8+cytotoxic cells (d) CD4+CD25+T regulatory cell

Ans. (d)

Expression of the Foxp3 nuclear transcription factor is a distinctive feature of CD4+CD25+ Treg cells. Foxp3 is not expressed by any of the other cell types indicated.

8. Which of the following cells require interaction with both pMHC and a set of costimulatory second signals from an antigen presenting cell (usually a dendritic cell) to become activated?

(a) Anergized T cell (b) B cells
(c) Mast cells (d) Naïve T cells

Ans. (d)

Dendritic cells are the usual participants in the activation of naïve cells. Anergized T cells remain refractory to subsequent engagement of pMHC and remain quiescent. B cells do not require binding of pMHC for activation. Mast cells become activated and degranulate via binding of antigen to IgE molecules already affixed to the mast cell surfaces.

9. In a patient with a Salmonella infection, which of the following mechanisms will most likely be the earliest adaptive response for clearing the infection while bacteria are present within intracellular endosomes?

(a) Antibody mediated neutralization of free bacteria
(b) Complement mediated lysis of infected host cells
(c) CTL recognition of bacterial peptides presented by MHC class II
(d) DTH responses generated by CD4+T cells

Ans. (d)

DTH responses are generally the first effective responses involved in clearance of intraendosomal microbes. Later in such infections, the microbes or their molecules may escape into the cytoplasm, making it possible for Cytotoxic T lymphocyte responses to develop. Complement does not clear active intracellular infections. Antibodies maybe effective in inhibiting reinfection but do not cleat active intracellular infections.

10. A 25-year-old man is exposed to Ascaris but does not develop clinical signs of infection. Which of the following mechanisms is likely to be responsible for his resistance to infection?

(a) Antibody mediated destruction of worm infected host cells
(b) CTL induced apoptosis of worm infected host cells
(c) Complement mediated lysis of worm attached to host tissues
(d) IgE mediated type I hypersensitivity disrupting worm attachment

Ans. (d)

Local inflammatory responses such as that induced by IgE can inhibit attachment of roundworms to the intestinal wall. Ascaris is a large worm and is not damaged by antibodies directed at it or by complement, CTLs or phagocytes.

11. **Which of the following is the predominant immunoglobulin isotype secreted in the human MALT?**
(a) IgA (b) IgD
(c) IgG (d) IgE

Ans. (d)

The vast majority of the antibody generated in the human MALT (Mucosal Associated Lymphoid Tissues) is of the IgA isotype. IgE, IgG and IgM are present, but at far lower levels, and IgD is essentially absent.

12. **Which of the following is characteristic of the mucosal immune system?**
(a) A vigorous response is made to all nonself antigens encountered
(b) Chronic inflammation makes an inhospitable environment for microbes
(c) IL-2 and IFN-γ contribute to a Th-1 like environment
(d) Tolerance to foreign antigens is the norm rather than the exception

Ans. (d)

Because the mucosal immune system is constantly exposed to so many nonself epitopes that are essentially harmless, it is tolerant of most of them. Although it can respond to microbes that pose a pathogenic threat, the mucosal system generally avoids the development of chronic inflammation because of the damage that could be inflicted on the delicate mucosal linings. The immunologic environment is generally described as more Th-2 like than Th-1 like. IgG is present at far lower levels than is IgA.

13. **Complement components are:**
(a) lipopolysaccharides (b) Glycoproteins
(c) Polysacchrides (d) Lipid

Ans. (b)

14. **A 3-year-old boy with an X linked defect in the Bruton tyrosine kinase gene is impaired in which of the following mechanisms?**
(a) Antibody mediated bacterial clearance (b) Formation of the membrane attack complex
(c) Delayed hypersensitivity responses (d) IFN-γ secretion by CD4+ T cells

Ans. (a)

Bruton's agammaglobulinemia results in a near or total absence of B cells and immunoglobulins, hence antibody-mediated responses to microbes are severely impaired. Even in the absence of antibodies and the classical pathway of complement activation, the membrane attack complex can be generated through the MBL and alternative pathways. Antibodies are not involved in the other choices.

15. **A 21-year-old woman has a history since childhood of recurrent episodes of swelling of the submucosal and subcutaneous tissue of the gastrointestinal and respiratory tracts. Her C1 inhibitor level is less than 5% of the reference value. These findings support a diagnosis of:**
(a) DiGeorge syndrome (b) Hereditary angioedema
(c) Nutritional based immune deficiency (d) Paroxysmal nocturnal hemoglobinuria

Ans. (b)

Hereditary angioedema is caused by deficient levels of C1 inhibitor. DiGeorge syndrome is caused by aberrant development of the thymus. Nutrition based immunodeficiencies are not characteristically identified by severely reduces levels of specific cell types or related molecules. Paroxysmal nocturnal hemoglobinuria is caused by the deficiency of CD59.

16. **During an infection with Streptococcus pyogenes, an individual generated sufficiently high levels of IgM and IgG antibodies against Streptococcus pyogenes antigen with structural similarities to the heart that cardiac damage was caused. In this example the microbe contributed to autoimmunity via a process known as:**
(a) Anergy (b) Central tolerance
(c) Epitope spreading (d) Molecular mimicry

Ans. (d)

Molecular mimicry contribute to autoimmunity by triggering responses with microbial molecules that are cross reactive with host molecules. Anergy and central tolerance are mechanisms for preventing autoimmunity. Epitope spreading involves the generation of responses to a series with different antigens, not to cross reactive ones.

17. **Graves disease is an example of which of the following immunologic processes?**
(a) Autoimmune disease associated with HLA gene B27

(b) Autoimmune disease associated with HLA gene DR3
(c) Immune deficiency associated with HLA gene DR2
(d) Immune deficiency associated with HLA gene DR4

Ans. (b)

Graves disease is an autoimmune disease that is associated with the **presence of the HLA DR3 gene**. It is not associated with HLA B 27, DR2, DR4 or Cw6. It does not result from immunodeficiency.

18. A 47-year-old male has a history of end stage renal failure and required a kidney transplant. Approximately four weeks after receiving his transplanted kidney he developed oliguria, fever, hypertension and pain or tenderness over his allograft. On the basis of the findings, the most likely underlying immunological process is:

(a) Autoimmunity
(b) Acute rejection
(c) Chronic rejection
(d) Hyperacute rejection

Ans. (b)

The time span is appropriate for acute rejection of the transplanted organ but not for chronic or hyperacute rejection. There is no information suggesting autoimmunity. Peripheral tolerance is a mechanism for preventing responses to self antigen.

19. A 76-year-old man is diagnosed with *E.coli* septicemia. The initial immune response to *E.coli* will incude:

(a) Binding by LPS- binding proteins and delivery to receptor on macrophages
(b) Formation of specific somatically generated receptors to bind *E.coli*
(c) Generation and secretion of specific antibodies to recognize *E.coli*
(d) Production of *E.coli* specific cytokines by lymphocytes

Ans. (a)

LPS of gram negative bacteria is recognized by LPS binding protein in the blood stream and tissue fluids. The LPS-LPS binding protein complex is then delivered to a cell membrane of a macrophage, where resident LPS receptors, composed of a complex of proteins (TLR-CD14, MD2) bind to the bacterial LPS. As a result of receptor engagement, the microbes are ingested and degraded, the macrophage is activated, and cytokine production and inflammation result. Actions of somatically generated receptors of B and T cells and of antibodies are part of the adaptive immune response as opposed to the innate response. Cytokines do not have antigen-specific activities, and killer activation receptors on NK cells recognize stress-related molecules of the surface of abnormal host cells.

20. All the following forces are involved in antigen antibody reaction except:

(a) Vander waals forces
(b) Electrostatic bond
(c) Hydrogen bond
(d) Covalent bond

Ans. (d)

Combination between antigen and antibody is firm but reversible and is effected by weak intermolecular forces such as Vander waals forces, ionic bonds and hydrogen bonding, not by the firmer Covalent bonds.

The firmness of the union is influenced by affinity and avidity.

21. Peptide binding site on Class 1 MHC molecule for presenting processed antigens to CD8 T cells is formed by:

(a) Proximal domain of alpha subunits
(b) Distal domain of alpha subunits
(c) Proximal domains of alpha and beta subunits
(d) Distal domains of alpha and beta subunits

Ans. (b)

Distal domains of alpha subunits

MHC class 1 – Antigen binding site is between alpha1 and alpha 2

MHC class 2 – Antigen binding site between alpha 1 and beta 1

22. Follicular dendritic cells, main function is:

(a) Catches antigen and presents it to T cells
(b) Catches antigen and presents it to B cells
(c) Phagocytic activity
(d) Produce immunoglobulin .

Ans. (b)

Follicular dendritic cells are located on B cells containing germinal centres of the follicles in the spleen and lymphnodes

They do not produce MHC class II

Hence they do not present antigen to helper T cells

They directly capture antigen ab complexes and presents to B cells.

23. Which is not shared between T cells and B cell?

(a) Positive selection during development (b) Class 1 MHC expression

(c) Antigen specific receptors (d) All of the above

Ans. (a)

During development – immature cells develop into mature cells.

In this process T cells first acquire Double negative cells–then double positive–single positive cells which is acquired by process called positive selection followed by negative selection (remember **TPN – Tcell have positive selection and negative selection).**

B cells have only **negative selection.**

24. Thymus dependent area in spleen:

(a) Mantle layer (b) Perifollicular cells

(c) Malphigian corpuscle (d) All of the above

Ans. (c)

T cell dependent (Thymus) areas in spleen are periarterial lymphoid collections, malphigian corpuscles in white pulp whereas in Mantle layer and perifollicular follicle area it is B cell.

In lymph nodes T cell dependent area is paracortical area, whereas B cell area is cortical follicle.

25. Molecular mass of IgG is:

(a) 150 (b) 400

(c) 1000 (d) 1500

Ans. (a)

Ig A–160 (monomer), 400 (dimer)

IgG–150, IgM–1000, IgE–190, IgD–175

26. Variable portion of antibody is:

(a) C terminal (b) N terminal

(c) CHO moiety (d) None

Ans. (b)

Aminoterminal (N)–variable unit

Carboxy terminal (C)–constant unit

27. Prozone phenomenon is seen in:

(a) Tularaemia (b) Legionnares disease

(c) Plague (d) Secondary syphilis

Ans. (d)

Antibodies starts to raise during secondary stage of syphilis

Leads to high titre sera – false negative

Serial dilutions done to avoid prozone phenomenon.

28. Polysaccharide antigens are:

(a) T cell independent antigens (b) T cell dependent antigens

(c) MHC I dependent antigens (d) MHC II dependent antigens

Ans. (a)

For proteins and erythrocytes – T cell dependent antigens.

For polysaccharides – T cell independent antigens.

Protein antigens eliminated in days to weeks whereas polysaccharide antigens persist for months to years e.g., pneumococcal polysaccharide may persist upto 20 years in humans following a single injection.

29. Distinct amino acid sequence at the antigen combining site is called:
(a) Idiotype (b) Allotype (c) Epitope (d) Paratope

Ans. (a)

Idiotype is based on antigenic difference in the hypervariable region.
Allotype is based on alleleic difference in immunoglobulins e.g., Gm type.
Isotype is antigenic differences in constant regions of heavy chain decide isotypes.

30. Who got nobel prize for discovery of split genes?
(a) Burnet (b) Susumu Tonegawa
(c) Neils K jerne (d) Paul Ehrlich

Ans. (b)

One gene – one protein concept in past.
But it was overcome by discovery of split genes for immunoglobulins.
Discovered by Susumu Tonegawa and awarded nobel prize for it.

31. Mechanism similar to Schwartzman reaction occurs in:
(a) Fitz Hugh Curtis syndrome (b) Waterhouse Friderichsen syndrome
(c) Eichwald slimser effect (d) Anaphylactoid reaction

Ans. (b)

Factors affecting intravascular coagulation is affected.
Not actually immune mediated reaction.
Smilar reactions happens in Waterhouse Friderichsen syndrome.

32. Passive cutaneous anaphylaxis detect:
(a) Heterocytotropic ab (b) Wheal and flare reaction
(c) Atopy (d) Cutaneous anaphylaxis

Ans. (a)

Passive cutaneous anaphylaxis–in vivo method for detection of antibodies.
Antigen injection intradermally then same antigen with a dye injected IV – after 4 to 24 hours – wheal flare reaction occurs in intradermal site.
Helps to detect IgG ab which is heterocytotropic, not for IgM which is homocytotropic.

33. Reaction due to lysis of bacterial cell wall and necrotic cell product is:
(a) Arthus reaction (b) Serum sickness
(c) Jarish Herxheimer reaction (d) Infectious mononucleosis ampicillin reaction

Ans. (c)

Cell wall antibiotics e.g., penicillin causes rapid cell wall lysis.
Release of proinflammatory cytokines or toxic bacterial products and occurs in treatment of primary and secondary syphilis.

34. The defect in reticular dysgenesis of de vaal is:
(a) Multipotent Haemotopoietic stem cells (b) Lymphoid stem cells
(c) Myeloid stem cells (d) Erythroid stem cells

Ans. (a)

SCID – three forms.
Swiss type agammaglobulinaemia.
Reticular dysgenesis.
Adenosine deaminase (ADA deficiency).
Reticular dysgenesis of devaal is defect at multipotent haematopoietic stem cell.

35. Ataxia telangiectasia patients have a deficiency of:
(a) IgM (b) IgA
(c) IgD (d) IgG

Ans. (b)

Ataxia telangiectasia – combined deficiency, Autosomal recessive, Ataxia telangiectasia, ovarian dysgenesis, chromosomal abnormalities, Death due to sinopulmonary infection, Serum and secretory IgA absent, IgE deficiency seen.

Chapter 10

RECENT NEET PATTERN ALL INDIA, AIIMS AND PGI QUESTIONS

NEET PATTERN ALL INDIA 2018

1. Cutaneous larva migrans caused by:

(a) Nector Americanus
(b) Ankylostoma duodenale
(c) Ankylostoma brazilensis
(d) Ankylostoma caninum

Ans. (c) Ankylostoma brazilensis

Non-human ankylostoma species cause cutaneous larvae migrans.

LARVA MIGRANS

Infection with helminth larvae not adapted to humans.

Cutaneous larva migrans (creeping eruption)

- **Ancylostoma braziliense (Most common)**
- A. caninum
- Uncineria stenocephala
- Gnathostoma spinigerum
- Bunostomum phlebotomum

Visceral larva migrans

- **Toxocara canis (Most common)**
- T. catis
- Angiostrongylus cantonensis
- A. costaricensis
- Anisakine spp.

2. Adult form of Echinococcus granulosus has definite host as:

(a) Dog
(b) Cat
(c) Cattle
(d) Pig

Ans. (a) Dog

Definitive host: Dog, jackal, fox; adult worm resides in the small intestine and discharges eggs in the feces. **Intermediate host:** Sheep, pig, goat, cattle, **man** (**Dead end host**).

3. Slide of peripheral blood smear of a patient suffering with fever and chills is shown. Vector for the disease shown in the image is:

(a) Hard tick
(b) Anopheles
(c) Culex
(d) Tse Tse fly

Ans. (a) Hard tick

Ticks transmit the human strain of babesiosis, Babesia species are in the phylum Apicomplexa, which also has the protozoan parasites that cause malaria, toxoplasmosis, and cryptosporidiosis. Babesia parasites reproduce in red blood cells, where they can be seen as cross-shaped inclusions (four *merozoites* asexually budding, but attached together forming a structure looking like a *"Maltese cross"*) and cause hemolytic anemia, quite similar to malaria.

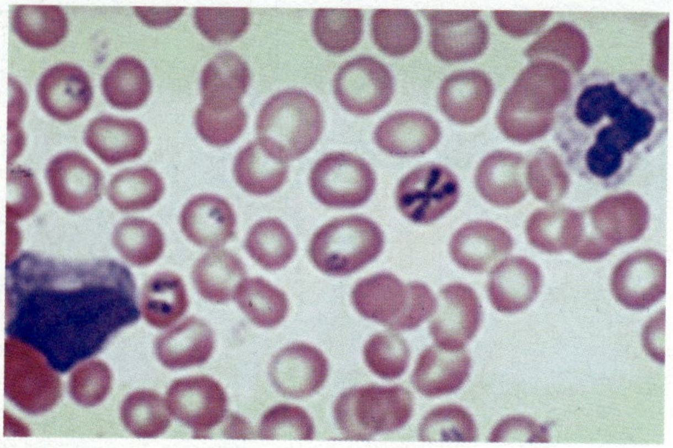

"Maltese cross formations" on the blood film are diagnostic (pathognomonic) of babesiosis, since they are not seen in malaria, the primary differential diagnosis. Careful examination of multiple smears may be necessary, since *Babesia* may infect less than 1% of circulating red blood cells, thus be easily overlooked.

Serologic testing for antibodies against *Babesia* (both IgG and IgM) can detect low-level infection in cases with a high clinical suspicion, but negative blood film examinations. Serology is also useful for differentiating babesiosis from malaria in cases where people are at risk for both infections. Since detectable antibody responses require about a week after infection to develop, serologic testing may be falsely negative early in the disease course.

A polymerase chain reaction (PCR) test has been developed for the detection of *Babesia* from the peripheral blood. PCR may be at least as sensitive and specific as blood-film examination in diagnosing babesiosis, though it is also significantly more expensive. Most often, PCR testing is used in conjunction with blood film examination and possibly serologic testing.

4. Which can grow in acidic medium?

(a) Lactobacillus
(b) Peptostreptococcus
(c) Staphylococcus
(d) Streptococcus

Ans. (a) Lactobacillus

Lactobacillus is a genus of Gram-positive, facultative anaerobic or microaerophilic, rod-shaped, non-spore-forming bacteria. They are a major part of the lactic acid bacteria group (i.e., they convert sugars to lactic acid). *Lactobacillus* species are normally a major part of the vaginal microbiota.

5. What is Dane's particle?

(a) HBV DNA
(b) Hbs Ag
(c) HCV
(d) Hbe Ag

Ans. (b) Hbs Ag

The Hepatitis B virion is a double-walled, spherical structure and measures 42 nm in diameter. It was first demonstrated by Dane in 1970 and so is known as Dane particle. By electron microscopy three types of particles can be seen in the serum from patients with hepatitis B. These are (i) spherical particles measuring 22 nm in diameter, (ii) filamentous or tubular particles with a diameter of 22 nm and of varying length, and (iii) double-walled, spherical structures measuring 42 nm in diameter. The former two particles are antigenically identical and are known as hepatitis B surface antigen, or HBsAg. The latter particle is the complete hepatitis viral particle known as Dane particle.

6. Burkholderia cepacia is intrinsically resistant to:

(a) Ceftazidime
(b) Trimethoprim-sulfamethoxazole
(c) Temocillin
(d) Carbapenems

Ans. (c) Temocillin

Temocillin is a β-lactamase-resistant penicillin and it is used primarily for the treatment of multiple drug-resistant, Gram-negative bacteria. It is a carboxypenicillin.

B. cepacia complex strains are intrinsically resistant to a wide range of antimicrobial agents, including aminoglycosides, polymyxin, first and second-generation cephalosporins, and carboxypenicillins. Antimicrobial agents that are effective against B. cepacia complex in vitro include trimethoprim-sulfamethoxazole, ceftazidime, carbapenems, ureidopenicillins, fluoroquinolones, minocyline and chloramphenicol.

7. Acute Hemorrhagic conjunctivitis is caused by which enterovirus?

(a) Enterovirus 70
(b) Enterovirus 71
(c) Adenovirus
(d) Enterovirus 69

Ans. (a) Enterovirus 70

Enterovirus 70 is a member of the genus of viruses called Enterovirus and family of the viruses *Picornaviridae*. Usually very small (about 30 nm in diameter), it is non-enveloped (meaning it only has a *nucleic acid* core and protein *capsid*) and has a single-stranded *positive-sense RNA genome*; the protein capsid the virus itself is surrounded by is *icosahedral*. It is known as one of the more new enteroviruses within this category. It spreads easily from one person's eyes to another's through contact with infected objects, like fingers, or through the eye secretion itself. Enterovirus 70 infrequently causes polio-like permanent paralysis.

Coxsakievirus A24 variant

The Coxsakievirus is another member of the genus of viruses called Enterovirus and family of the viruses Picornaviridae. Its isolation host is human. It is an *antigenic* variant of the Coxsakievirus A24. It was studied independently for the first time in Singapore in 1970.

Adenovirus 11

Adenoviruses are a medium-sized variant that are *nonenveloped*, like Enterovirus 70. They have a double-stranded linear *DNA genome*. There are 57 variants of this virus, that each cause 5-10% of *upper respiratory infections* in humans. These viruses are some of the largest nonenveloped viruses in existence, and because of this, they can pass through the *endosome* without any necessary envelope fusion.

8. Transduction is mediated by:

(a) Bacteriophage
(b) Plasmid
(c) Metaphage
(d) Cosmids

Ans. (a) Bacteriophage

Transduction is the process by which foreign DNA is introduced into a cell by a virus or viral vector. An example is the viral transfer of DNA from one bacterium to another. Transduction does not require physical contact between the cell donating the DNA and the cell receiving the DNA (which occurs in conjugation), and it is *DNase* resistant (*transformation* is susceptible to DNase).

9. Scromboid fish poisoning is due to which of the following gram negative bacteria?

(a) E. coli
(b) Salmonella
(c) Enterococcus
(d) Shigella

Ans. (a) E. coli

Scombroid food poisoning is a foodborne illness that results from eating spoiled (decayed) fish. Along with ciguatera, it is listed as a common type of seafood poisoning. The toxin believed to be responsible is histamine, formed as the flesh of the fish begins to decay. As histamine is also the natural agent involved in allergic reactions, scombroid food poisoning often gets misidentified as a food allergy. Histidine is an amino acid that exists naturally in many types of food (including fish) and at temperatures above 16°C it is converted to the biogenic amine histamine via the enzyme histidine decarboxylase produced by these bacteria (primarily Morganella morganii but also other bacteria such as Escherichia, Proteus, Salmonella and Shigella species) degrade histidine present in the musculature of the fish to heat-stable histamine and a histamine-like substance termed saurine (this is one reason why fish should be stored in the freezer).

10. Mycoplasma is inherently resistant to:

(a) Doxycycline
(b) Azithromycin
(c) Ceftriaxone
(d) Ciprofloxacin

Ans. (c) Ceftriaxone

Mycoplasma is a genus of bacteria that lack a cell wall around their cell membrane. Without a cell wall, they are unaffected by many common antibiotics such as penicillin or other betalactam antibiotics that target cell wall synthesis. DOC - Oral Azithromycin.

11. Sabin Feldman dye test is done for:

(a) Toxoplasmosis
(b) Echinococcosis
(c) Chaga's disease
(d) Sleeping sickness

Ans. (a) Toxoplasmosis

A **Sabin–Feldman dye test** is a serologic test to diagnose for toxoplasmosis. The test is based on the presence of certain antibodies that prevent methylene blue dye from entering the cytoplasm of *Toxoplasma* organisms. Patient serum is treated with Toxoplasma trophozoites and complements as activator, and then incubated. After incubation, methylene blue is added. If anti-Toxo antibodies are present in the serum, because these antibodies are activated by complements and lyse the parasite membrane, Toxoplasma trophozoites are not stained (positive result); if there are no antibodies, trophozoites with intact membrane are stained and appear blue under microscope (negative result).

AIIMS AND PGI 2017

1. Beta 1,3 glucan assay is used for diagnosis of:

(a) Invasive candidiasis
(b) Cryptococcosis
(c) Rhinocerebral zygomycosis
(d) Mycetoma

2. Lipoarabinomannan assay in urine is used for screening infection of:

(a) M. tuberculosis
(b) Cryptococcosis
(c) Zygomycosis
(d) Aspergillosis

3. Identify the image:

(a) Vibrio
(b) Leptospira
(c) Helicobacter
(d) Campylobacter

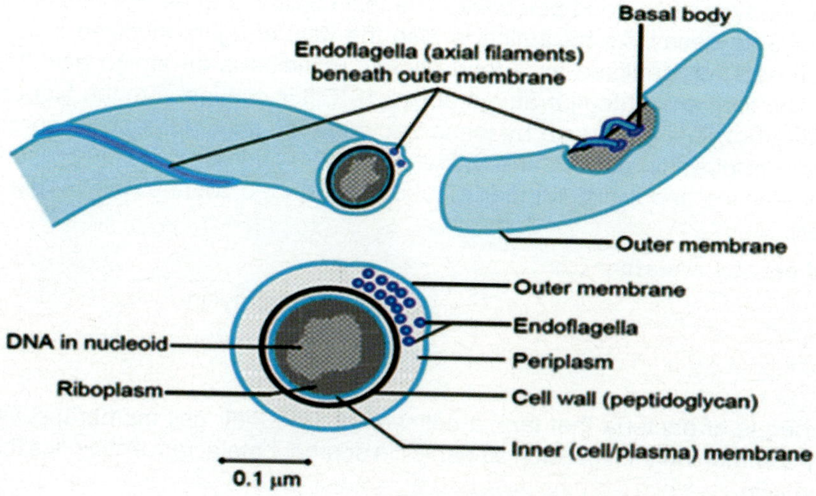

4. Identify the image:

(a) Coxsackie virus
(b) Pox virus
(c) Varicella zoster
(d) Herpes simplex

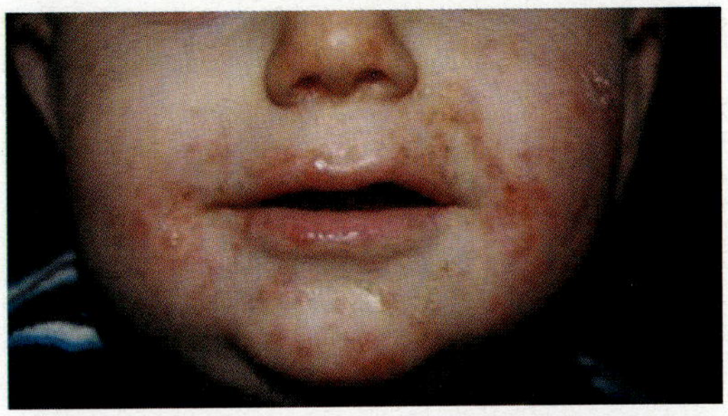

5. Identify the image:

(a) Mycetoma
(b) Sporotrichosis
(c) Chromomycosis
(d) Tinea nigra

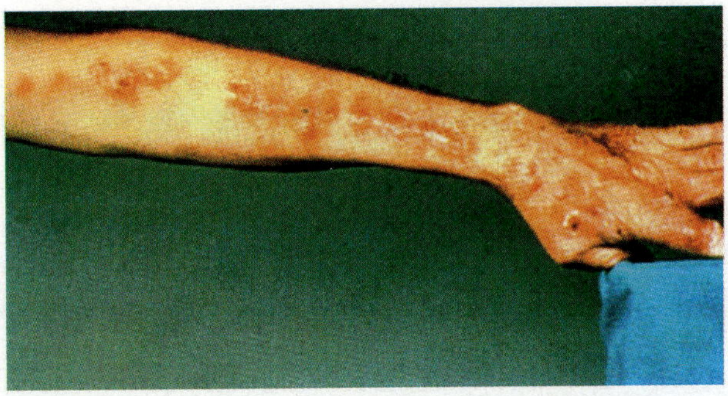

6. Identify the image:

(a) HIV
(b) HBV
(c) EBV
(d) Polio

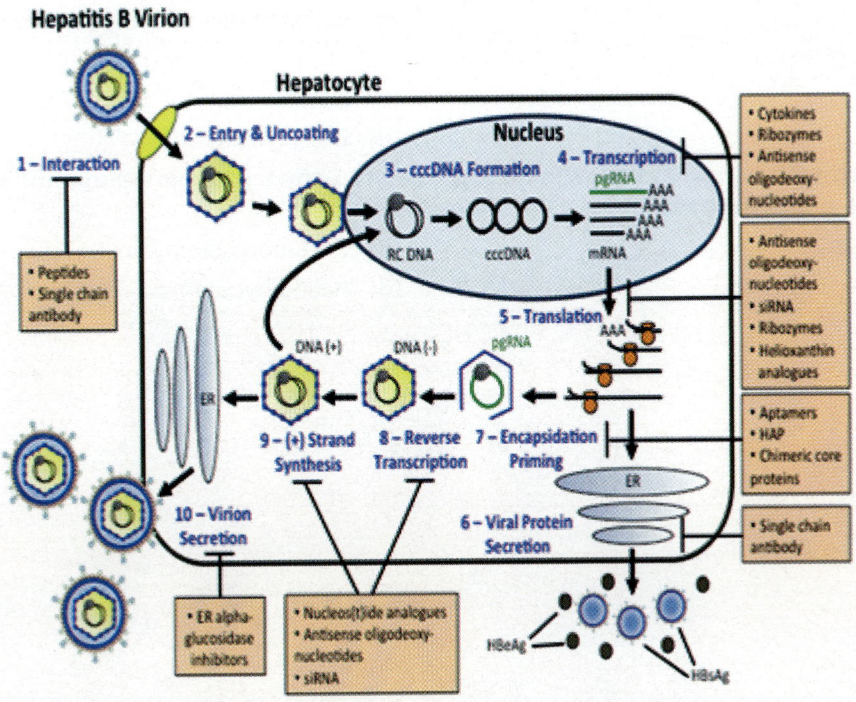

7. Lung biopsy of a neutropenic patient shows these structures on staining. What could be the diagnosis?

(a) Pneumocystis pneumonia
(b) Histoplasmosis
(c) Aspergillosis
(d) Mucormycosis

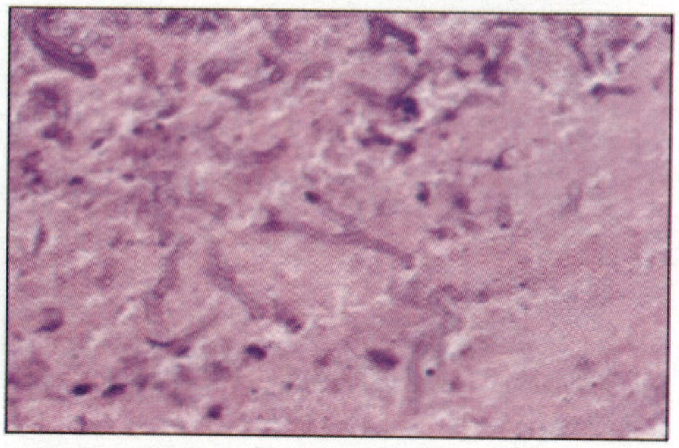

8. Most important mechanism of antibiotic resistance in biofilms is:

(a) Increased adhesion
(b) Increased effect of antibiotics
(c) Low mitotic rate
(d) Mechanical barrier

9. Viral haemorrhagic fever reported in India is:

(a) Crimean congo
(b) Yellow fever
(c) Marburg
(d) Ebola

10. Dimorphic fungi include all *except*:

(a) Pneumocystis carnii
(b) Penicillium marneffi
(c) Blastomyces dermatidis
(d) Histoplasma capsulatum

11. Treatment for gonococcal and nongonococcal urethritis:

(a) Ceftriaxone 250 mg single parenteral dose
(b) Azithromycin single dose PO
(c) Cefixime 400 mg single dose PO
(d) Ciprofloxacin 1 gm single dose PO

12. Disinfectant used for disinfection of hospital floors:

(a) Phenol
(b) Quartenary ammonium compound
(c) Alcohol
(d) Chlorine based compounds

13. DOC in scrub typhus:

(a) Ampicillin
(b) Ceftriaxone
(c) Gentamicin
(d) Doxycycline

14. A lady presented with verrucous growth on leg, Biopsy shows granulomatous inflammation with giant cell containing large pigmented muriform cells, diagnosis is:

(a) Sporotrichosis
(b) Chromoblastomycosis
(c) Eumycetoma
(d) Actinomycetoma

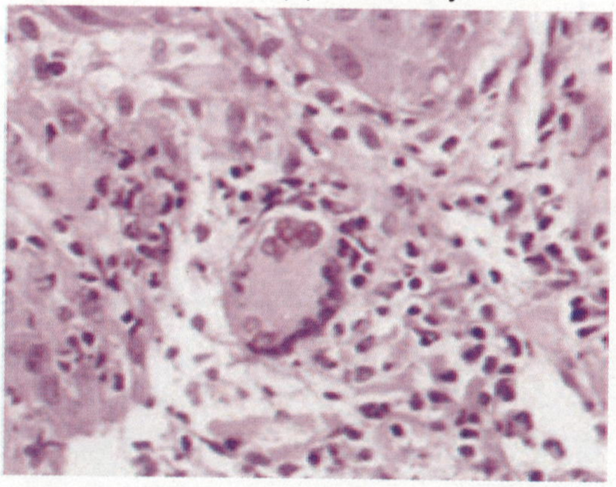

15. Gardasil 9 vaccine provides protection against to which of the papilloma viruses:

(a) 6,11,16,18
(b) 16, 18
(c) 16, 18,31,33,45
(d) 6, 11, 16, 18, 31, 33, 45, 52, 58

16. Best sample to detect CMV in congenital infections:

(a) Blood
(b) CSF
(c) Saliva
(d) Liver biopsy

17. A HIV infected patient was suspected to have diarrhoea by Cyclospora, was treated for it and it got worse, and shifted to ICU and bone marrow aspirate collected, diagnosis of fungal infection was made. All true about fungal image all *except*:

(a) Doesn't grow on SDA
(b) Spore is infectious form
(c) Cause disseminated disease
(d) It is an intracellular pathogen

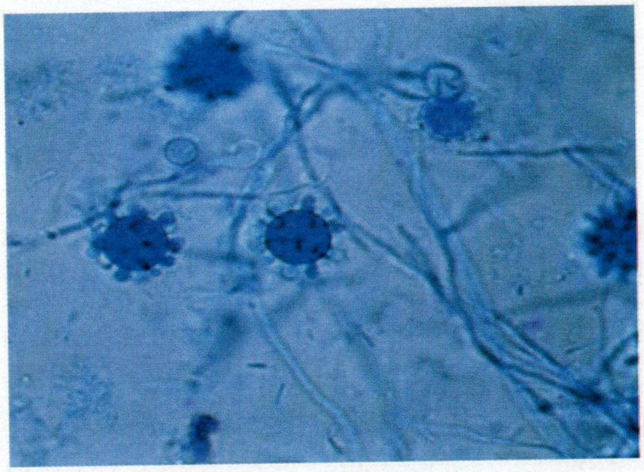

18. PEP is indicated in:

(a) Hepatitis A
(b) Hepatitis B
(c) Rabies
(d) Hepatitis C
(e) Varicella

19. Immunotherapy for leprosy can be done with:

(a) BCG vaccine
(b) M. indicus pranii
(c) ICRC bacillus
(d) Mycobacterium leprae Hsp65
(e) M. vaccae

20. Sporotrichoid pattern of skin lesions are seen in:

(a) Sporotrichosis
(b) Nocardiosis
(c) Fish tank granuloma
(d) Mycetoma
(e) Cutaneous leishmaniasis

21. Ebola virus:

(a) Belongs to family filoviridae
(b) Incubation period is 2-21 days
(c) BSL4 is used
(d) IOC is real time PCR
(e) Spread by contact with secretion of patient

22. True about Adenovirus:

(a) Satellite shape
(b) Used as gene vectors
(c) Oncolytic virus
(d) 6 groups (A-F), 51 serotypes
(e) DNA virus

ANSWERS AND EXPLANATIONS

1. **Ans. is 'a'** i.e., Invasive candidiasis

(1, 3)-β-D-glucan medical application:

An assay to detect the presence of (1, 3)-β-D-glucan in blood is marketed as a means of identifying invasive or disseminated fungal infections. This test should be interpreted within the broader clinical context, however, as a positive test does not render a diagnosis, and a negative test does not rule out infection. False positives may occur because of fungal contaminants in the antibiotics *amoxicillin-clavulanate*, and *piperacillin/tazobactam*. False positives can also occur with contamination of clinical specimens with the bacteria *Streptococcus pneumoniae*, *Pseudomonas aeruginosa*, and *Alcaligenes faecalis*, which also produce (1→3) β-D-glucan. This test can aid in the detection of *Aspergillus*, Candida, and *Pneumocystis jirovecii*. This test cannot be used to detect Mucor or Rhizopus, the fungi responsible for *mucormycosis*, as they do not produce (1, 3)-beta-D-glucan.

2. **Ans. is 'a'** i.e., M. tuberculosis

Determine™ TB LAM Ag test (LF-LAM) is an urine test for the detection of LAM antigen, a lipopolysaccharide present in mycobacterial cell walls, which is released from metabolically active or degenerating bacterial cells. LAM appears to be present predominately in people with active TB disease.

3. **Ans. is 'b'** i.e., Leptospira

These are found in the corkscrew shaped spirochetes. Although these bacteria are gram negative (with a double membrane envelope structure), they possess only 2 to 4 rings (the S, M and presumably the C rings and sometimes an extra pair) in the basal complex – they lack the P and L rings. The result is that the basal complex does not cross the outer membrane and the filaments lie between the peptidoglycan and outer membrane (in the periplasm) wrapped around the cell (giving it a spiral appearance) as shown above. Otherwise, these flagella possess the usual basal body (discs), hook and filament. These internal flagella form a bundle or axial filament. The filaments contain a core of flagellin (FlaB) and in some species also contain a sheath of a second type of flagellin (FlaA). The sheathed filaments are thicker (about 25 nanometres in diameter). These non-emergent flagella, or endoflagella (endo- meaning 'internal').

4. **Ans. is 'a'** i.e., Coxsackievirus

Hand, foot and mouth disease (**HFMD**) is a common infection caused by a group of viruses. It typically begins with a fever and feeling generally unwell. This is followed a day or two later by flat discolored spots or bumps that may blister, on the hands, feet and mouth, and occasionally buttocks and groin. Signs and symptoms normally appear 3–6 days after exposure to the virus. The rash generally goes away on its own in about a week. Fingernail and toenail loss may occur a few weeks later, but will regrow with time.

The viruses that cause HFMD are spread through close personal contact, through the air from coughing, and the feces of an infected person. Contaminated objects can also spread the disease. *Coxsackievirus* A16 is the most common cause and Enterovirus 71 is the second-most common cause. Other strains of coxsackievirus and enterovirus can also be responsible. Some people may carry and pass on the virus despite having no symptoms of disease. Other animals are not involved. Diagnosis can often be made based on symptoms. Occasionally a throat or stool sample may be tested for the virus. Handwashing may prevent spread and those infected should not go to work, daycare, or school.

5. **Ans. is 'b'** i.e., Sporotrichosis

Sporotrichosis (also known as "**rose gardener's disease**") is a disease caused by the infection of the *fungus Sporothrix schenckii*. This fungal disease usually affects the *skin*, although other rare forms can affect the *lungs, joints, bones*, and even the *brain*. Because *roses* can spread the disease, it is one of a few diseases referred to as *rose-thorn* or *rose-gardeners' disease*.

- *Cutaneous or skin sporotrichosis, pulmonary sporotrichosis and disseminated sporotrichosis.*

6. **Ans. is 'b'** i.e., HBV

The life cycle of hepatitis B virus is complex. Hepatitis B is one of a few known *non-retroviral* viruses which use *reverse transcription* as a part of its replication process.

Attachment

The virus gains entry into the cell by binding to receptors on the surface of the cell and entering it by *endocytosis* mediated by either *clathrin* or *caveolin-1*. HBV initially binds to *heparin sulfate proteoglycan*. The pre-S1 segment of the HBV L protein then binds tightly to the cell surface receptor *sodium taurocolate cotransporting polypeptide* (NTCP). NTCP is mostly found in the *sinusoidal membrane* of *liver cells*. The presence of NTCP in liver cells correlates with the tissue specificity of HBV infection.

Penetration

Following endocytosis, the virus membrane fuses with the host cell's membrane, releasing the nucleocapsid into the cytoplasm.

Uncoating

Because the virus multiplies via RNA made by a host enzyme, the viral genomic DNA has to be transferred to the cell nucleus. It is thought the capsid is transported on the *microtubules* to the *nuclear pore*. The core proteins dissociate from the partially double stranded viral DNA, which is then made fully double stranded (by host DNA polymerases) and transformed into covalently closed circular DNA (*cccDNA*) that serves as a template for transcription of four viral *mRNAs*.

Replication

The largest mRNA, (which is longer than the viral genome), is used to make the new copies of the genome and to make the *capsid* core protein and the **viral RNA-dependent-***DNA-polymerase*.

Assembly

These four viral transcripts undergo additional processing and go on to form progeny virions which are released from the cell or returned to the nucleus and re-cycled to produce even more copies.

Release

The long mRNA is then transported back to the cytoplasm where the virion P protein synthesizes DNA via its reverse transcriptase activity.

7. **Ans. is 'c'** i.e., Aspergillosis

   Image is showing a 45 degree branching septate hyphae, suggestive of Aspergillus species.

8. **Ans. is 'd'** i.e., Mechanical barrier

   The protective mechanisms at work in biofilms appear to be distinct from those that are responsible for conventional antibiotic resistance. In biofilms, poor antibiotic penetration, nutrient limitation and slow growth, adaptive stress responses, and formation of persister cells are hypothesized to constitute a multi-layered defence.

9. **Ans. is 'a'** i.e., Crimean congo

   Crimean Congo haemorrhagic fever (CCHF) is one of the deadly haemorrhagic fevers that are endemic in Africa, Asia, Eastern Europe and the Middle East. It is a tick-borne zoonotic viral disease caused by CCHF virus of genus *Nairovirus* (family Bunyaviridae). CCHF not only forms an important public health threat but has a significant effect on the health care personnel, especially in resource-poor countries. India was always a potentially endemic area until an outbreak hit parts of Gujarat, taking four lives including the treating medical team.

10. **Ans. is 'a'** i.e., Pneumocystis carnii

    Dimorphic fungi are Fungi that can exist as mold/hyphal/filamentous form or as yeast. An example is *Penicillium marneffei*, a human pathogen that grows as a mold at room temperature, and as a yeast at human body temperature.

    Several species of dimorphic fungi are important pathogens of humans and other animals, including Coccidioides immitis, Paracoccidioides brasiliensis, Blastomyces dermatitidis, Histoplasma capsulatum, Sporothrix schenckii.

    Mold in the **Cold** (25°C), **Yeast** in the **Heat** (37°C).

11. **Ans. is 'a'** i.e., Ceftriaxone 250 mg single parenteral dose

12. **Ans. is 'a'** i.e., Phenol

    Cresol, xylenol, Lysol and ortho-phenylphenol are the common phenolics used in laboratories and hospitals as disinfectants.

13. Ans. is 'd' i.e., **Doxycycline**

The drug most commonly used is *doxycycline* or *tetracycline*, but *chloramphenicol* is an alternative. Strains that are resistant to doxycycline and chloramphenicol have been reported. *Rifampicin* and *azithromycin* are alternatives. **Azithromycin is an alternative in children and pregnant women with scrub typhus, and when doxycycline resistance is suspected.**

Zoonotic tetrad: Rich in scrub jungles, provide the perfect ecological niche for the existence of the essential **"zoonotic tetrad"** (chiggers, rodents, scrub forest and mites) which helps sustaining a sylvatic cycle among the chiggers and rodents. Man trespassing these so called "mite islands" for collection of woods, is bitten by the chiggers.

14. Ans. is 'b' i.e., Chromoblastomycosis

Medlar bodies, also known as **sclerotic** or **muriform cells**, are thick walled cells (5-12 microns) with multiple internal transverse septa or chambers that resemble copper *pennies*. When present in skin or subcutaneous tissue, the cells are indicative of *chromoblastomycosis*.

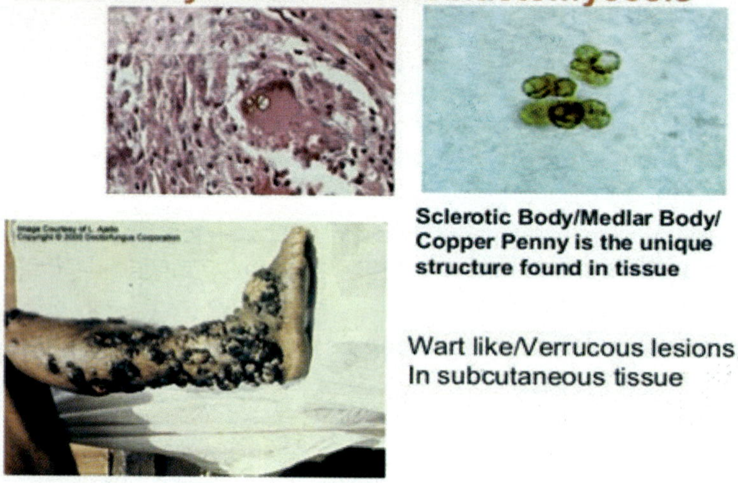

15. Ans. is 'd' i.e., 6, 11, 16, 18, 31, 33, 45, 52, 58

Gardasil 9 is a vaccine indicated in females 9 through 26 years of age for the prevention of cervical, vulvar, vaginal, and anal cancers caused by human papillomavirus (HPV) Types 16, 18, 31, 33, 45, 52 and 58; precancerous or dysplastic lesions caused by HPV Types 6, 11, 16, 18, 31, 33, 45, 52 and 58; and genital warts caused by HPV Types 6 and 11.

Note: Gardasil 9 is indicated in males 9 through 26 years of age for the prevention of anal cancer caused by HPV Types 16, 18, 31, 33, 45, 52 and 58; precancerous or dysplastic lesions caused by HPV Types 6, 11, 16, 18, 31, 33, 45, 52 and 58; and genital warts caused by HPV Types 6 and 11.

16. Ans. is 'c' i.e., Saliva

Diagnosis of acute maternal CMV infection by the presence of IgM and low IgG avidity requires confirmation of fetal infection which is typically performed by CMV PCR of the amniotic fluid.

Viral culture of the urine and saliva obtained within the first two weeks of life continue to be the gold standard for diagnosis of congenitally infected infants.

In the immunocompromised host, newer rapid diagnostic assays such as pp65 antigenemia and real-time CMV PCR of blood or plasma.

17. Ans. is 'a' i.e., Doesn't grow on SDA

Histoplasma capsulatum appears to be strongly associated with the droppings of certain bird species as well as bats. A mixture of these droppings and certain soil types is particularly conducive to proliferation. The patient may feel fever, chest pains, a general ill feeling, and a dry cough. Nutrient that is important for the growth of *Histoplasma capsulatum is* ***Iron****. Iron is essential in redox reaction related to its existence in reduced Fe2+ and oxidized Fe3+ states.*

Narrow based budding yeast cells at 37°C and tuberculate macroconidia are seen at 25°C on SDA or BHI agar.

18. Ans. are 'a, b, c, e'

Hepatitis A – Human normal immunoglobulin can be combined with Hepatitis A vaccine, it is used as PEP for all nonimmune household contacts of a diagnosed case of Hepatitis A.

Hepatitis B – In a newborn born to Hepatitis B positive mother – Hepatitis B vaccine with immunoglobulins is indicated, if a person exposed is already immunized booster dose is indicated.

Rabies – Category II bites need post exposure prophylaxis with Rabies vaccine, category III bites – Rabies immunoglobulin along with Rabies vaccine is given.

Varicella – PEP is indicated for unvaccinated healthy aged > 12 months and without other evidence of illness. Vaccine is to be given within 5 days of exposure.

Hepatitis C – Currently no PEP is indicated.

Note – In Tetanus and HIV PEP is indicated.

19. Ans. are 'a, b, c, e'

Addition of immunotherapy to chemotherapy aims at efficient killing of viable bacilli.

(a) Antigenically related mycobacteria – BCG, Mycobacterium w, ICRC bacillus and Mycobacterium vaccae have been found to be safe adjuncts to chemotherapy. It helps in reducing duration of treatment and also incidence of reactions.

(b) Drugs–Oflox, Rifampicin, Clarithromycin.

(c) Other immunomodulators.

Mycobacterium indicus pranii vaccine – Indigenous leprosy vaccine.

20. Ans. are 'a, b, c, e'

Sporotrichoid lymphocutaneous infection is a syndrome characterised by superficial cutaneous lesions that progress along dermal and subcutaneous lymphatics.

This pattern is known as sporotrichoid after the infection of:

- Dimorphic fungus – Sporothrix schenkii.
- Nocardia brasilensis.
- Mycobacterium marinum.
- Leishmania brasilensis.

21. Ans. are 'a, b, c, d, e'

Ebola virus is the single member of the *species Zaire ebolavirus*, which is the *type species* for the *genus Ebolavirus, family Filoviridae, order Mononegavirales*.

The natural reservoir of Ebola virus is believed to be *bats*, particularly *fruit bats*, and it is primarily transmitted between humans and from animals to humans through *body fluids*.

EBOV carries a *negative-sense* RNA genome in virions that are cylindrical / tubular, and contain *viral envelope*, matrix, and nucleocapsid components.

Ngoy mushula described ebola as –The illness is characterized with a high temperature of about 39°C, *hematemesis*, diarrhoea with blood, retrosternal abdominal pain, prostration with "heavy" articulations, and rapid evolution death after a mean of three days.

22. Ans. are 'a, b, c, d, e'

Adenoviruses (members of the family Adenoviridae) are medium-sized (90–100 nm), nonenveloped (without an outer lipid bilayer) viruses with an icosahedral nucleocapsid containing a double stranded DNA genome. Their name derives from their initial isolation from human adenoids in 1953.

Adenoviruses have long been a popular *viral vector* for *gene therapy* due to their ability to affect both replicating and non-replicating cells, accommodate large *transgenes*, and code for proteins without integrating into the host cell genome. More specifically, they are used as a vehicle to administer *targeted therapy*, in the form of *recombinant DNA* or protein. This therapy has been found especially useful in treating cystic fibrosis.

Strange but true – In China, *oncolytic adenovirus* is an approved cancer treatment.

AIIMS MAY 2017

Recent Exam Points

1. **Trichomonas vaginalis**
   - Trichomonas vaginalis exists only as a trophozoite (no cyst stage).
   - **Incubation period** is 5 to 28 days.
   - Infection is more common in women than in men.
   - **Clinical complications** in females: Vaginal discharge, foul smelling frothy, **itching (strawberry appearance);** males: Urethritis, balanoposthitis.
   - **Lab diagnosis** is based on demonstration of trophozoites in clinical specimen. **DOC – Metronidazole and Tinidazole.**
2. **Sputum microscopy negative tuberculosis diagnosis**
   - Many TB patients have negative AFB smears with a subsequent positive culture. Negative smears do not exclude TB disease.
   - **The CB NAAT (Cartridge Based Nucleic Acid Amplification Test)** is known as the **GeneXpert** in most countries other than India. This is the preferred first diagnostic test in smear negative tuberculosis, children and people with TB and HIV coinfection.
   - This test is a molecular test which detects the DNA in TB bacteria. It uses a sputum sample and can give a result in less than 2 hours. It can also detect the genetic mutations associated with resistance to the drug Rifampicin. The Genexpert MTB/RIF cannot be used for treatment monitoring, as it detects DNA of both live and dead bacteria.
3. **Liver fluke cycle**
   - **Fascioliasis is caused by Fasciola hepatica** and less often by F. gigantica, which are flat worms classified as liver flukes (trematodes).
   - **Mode of infection: Ingestion of aquatic vegetation contaminated with encysted metacercaria. Definitive host:** Sheep, goat, cattle and Intermediate host: snail.
4. **IgG Fragments**
   - IgG is the major class of immunoglobulin present in the serum. IgG is the only immunoglobulin class to cross the placenta and therefore is the most abundant immunoglobulin in newborns. Isotype-specific transport of IgG across the placenta occurs with preference for IgG1 and IgG3 subclasses. IgG also mediates opsonization of antigen through binding of antigen-antibody complexes to Fc receptors on macrophages and other cells.

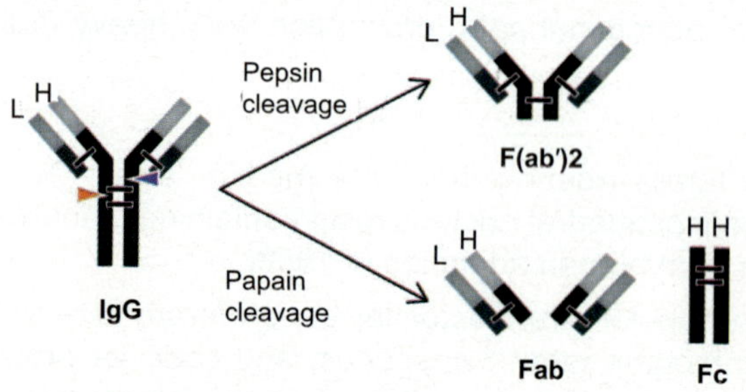

5. **Zika virus**
   - **Zika virus disease** is caused by a virus transmitted primarily by **Aedes mosquitoes.** People with Zika virus disease can have symptoms including mild fever, conjunctivitis, muscle and joint pain, malaise or headache. These symptoms normally last for 2-7 days.

- **There is scientific consensus that Zika virus is a cause of microcephaly and Guillain-Barré syndrome.** Links to other neurological complications are also being investigated. Infection with **Zika virus may be suspected based on symptoms and recent history of travel (e.g., residence in or travel to an area with active Zika virus transmission).** A diagnosis of Zika virus infection can only be confirmed through laboratory tests on blood or other body fluids, such as urine, saliva or semen.

6. **Red bag** (Red coloured non-chlorinated plastic bags or containers)
   - **Contaminated Waste (Recyclable):** Wastes generated from disposable items such as tubing, bottles, intravenous tubes and sets, catheters, urine bags, syringes (without needles and fixed needle syringes) and vaccutainers with their needles cut) and gloves.
   - **Treatment and Disposal Options:** Autoclaving or microwaving/hydroclaving followed by shredding or mutilation or combination of sterilization and shredding. Treated waste to be sent to registered or authorized recyclers or for energy recovery or plastics to diesel or fuel oil or for road making, whichever is possible. Plastic waste should not be sent to landfill sites.
7. **Aspergillosis treatment**
   - **Invasive aspergillosis** needs to be treated with prescription antifungal medication, usually voriconazole. Other antifungal medications used to treat aspergillosis include lipid amphotericin formulations, posaconazole, isavuconazole, itraconazole, caspofungin and micafungin.
   - **For allergic forms of aspergillosis such as allergic bronchopulmonary aspergillosis (ABPA) or allergic Aspergillus sinusitis, the recommended treatment is itraconazole, a prescription antifungal medication.** Corticosteroids may also be helpful.
8. **Treatment of Burkholderia mallei**
   - **B. mallei, earlier known as Pseudomonas mallei, was first isolated by Loeffler and Scotch in 1882 from a horse suffering from glanders.** The bacterium is known to cause glanders, which is a serious disease of equine animals, but capable of transmission to other animals (goats, dogs and cats) and humans.
   - **B. mallei is usually sensitive to Trimethoprim-sulfamethoxazole (TMP-SMX), ciprofloxacin, streptomycin, novobiocin, gentamicin, imipenem and sulfonamides.**
   - **Burkholderia cepacia:** Opportunistic respiratory infections in patients with cystic fibrosis or chronic granulomatous disease and urinary tract infections in patients with indwelling catheters.
   - **Burkholderia mallei:** Acute or chronic infection with infection localized to the skin, subcutaneous tissue, or respiratory tract.
   - **Burkholderia pseudomallei** – Melioidosis.Q
9. **Treatment of pneumocystis**
   - **Pneumocystis pneumonia (PCP) is a serious infection caused by the fungus Pneumocystis jirovecii.**
   - P. jiroveci pneumonia (PJP) does not respond to anti-fungal treatment. **The treatment of choice is TMP-SMX,** with second-line agents including pentamidine, dapsone (often in combination with pyrimethamine), or atovaquone.
10. **Klebsiella pneumoniae**
    - **Klebsiella is Gram-negative bacteria** that can cause different types of health care-associated infections, including pneumonia, bloodstream infections, wound or surgical site infections and meningitis.
    - Increasingly, Klebsiella bacteria have developed anti-microbial resistance (KPC), most recently to the class of antibiotics known as carbapenems. Klebsiella bacteria are normally found in the human intestines (where they do not cause disease). They are also found in human stool (feces).
11. **Nocardia**
    - Nocardia are Gram-positive bacilli showing a branching, beaded, and filamentous form. They stain poorly with Gram stain and appear to be Gram-negative with intracellular Gram-positive granules. Nocardia organisms like that of mycobacteria contain mycolic acid in their cell wall. **They are usually weakly acid fast. Acid fastness (1% H_2SO_4) is a property of Nocardia by which it can be differentiated from other similar bacteria, such as actinomycetes.**

12. Eggs of Enterobius vermicularis

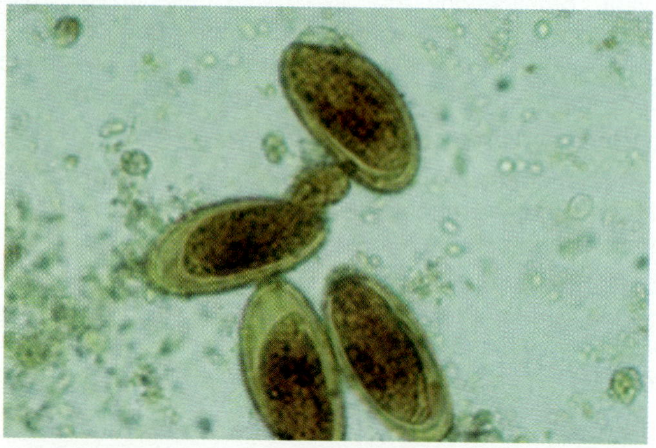

Eggs of Ascaris

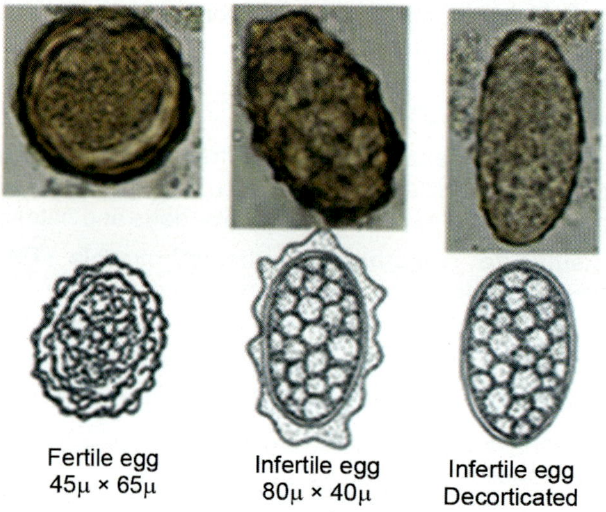

13. Milky white discharge with fishy odor

- **Bacterial vaginosis:** The most common symptom is an abnormal vaginal discharge that varies depending upon the cause of infection.
- **Bacterial vaginosis:** Thin, watery discharge, heavier than usual, grayish white or yellow, often with a strong fishy odor, mild burning or irritation of the vulva and vagina, often without redness or itching.
- **Whiff test:** Vaginal discharge smells fishy when mixed with 10% potassium hydroxide.

14. Microbial contamination of disinfectants

- Pseudomonas species is the most common bacteria which can survive in presence of disinfectant like Cetrimide. Cetrimide Agar is used for the selective isolation and presumptive identification of Pseudomonas aeruginosa.

15. Mechanism of action of MRSA

- There are three known mechanisms for which staphylococcus aureus become resistant to methicillin:
  (i) Presence of an acquired penicillin binding protein (PBP2a) – most cases.
  (ii) Modification of normal (Intrinsic) penicillin binding proteins.
  (iii) Hyperproduction of β-lactamase → Rare.

16. Plasmodium falciparum vaccine

- **Status of vaccine development:** Despite many decades of intense research and development effort, there is no commercially available malaria vaccine at the presenttime. **RTS, S/AS01 is the most advanced vaccine candidate against the most deadly form of human malaria.**
- **RTS, S/AS01 is a pre-erythrocytic stage hybrid recombinant protein vaccine, based on the RTS, S recombinant antigen.**

  It comprises the hybrid polypeptide RTS in which regions of the P. falciparum circumsporozoite protein known to induce humoral (R region) and cellular immune (T region) responses are covalently bound to the hepatitis B surface antigen (S). This recombinant fusion protein (RTS) is expressed in Saccharomyces cerevisiae together with free hepatitis B surface antigen (S), to form RTS, S virus-like particles.

17. Swollen belly syndrome

- **S. fuelleborni** kellyi is also the **aetiological agent of swollen baby (or belly) syndrome in New Guinea,** in which neonatal infants acquire overwhelming intestinal infections which can also disseminate (Ashford and Barnish, 1989). This is also fatal in the absence of anti-Strongyloides therapy.

MICROBIOLOGY PGI QUESTIONS (2016)

1. Bacteriorhodopsin is associated with:

(a) Helicobacter
(b) Halobacteria
(c) Hafnia
(d) Antibacterial protein
(e) Act as proton pump

Ans. (b), (e)

(a)	False	Helicobacter has no correlation with this protein.
(b)	True	**Bacteriorhodopsin protein is associated with Halobacteria.**
(c)	False	Hafnia has no correlation with this protein.
(d)	False	**Bacteriorhodopsin donot have antibacterial properties.**
(e)	True	**Bacteriorhodopsin protein acts as proton pump.**

Khorana HG. Two light-transducing membrane proteins: Bacteriorhodopsin and the mammalian rhodopsin. *Proceedings of the National Academy of Sciences of the United States of America* 1993;90(4):1166-1171.

2. Bacteria used in Griffith experiment is:

(a) Streptococcus pyogenes
(b) Capsulated Streptococcus pneumoniae
(c) Staphylococcus aureus
(d) MRSA
(e) Non capsulated Streptococcus pneumoniae

Ans. (b), (e)

(a)	False	Streptococcus pyogenes was not used in **Griffith experiment.**
(b)	True	Capsulated Streptococcus pneumoniae (Pathogenic and Smooth colonies on solid media) strain was used in **Griffith experiment.**
(c)	False	Staphylococcus aureus strain was not used in **Griffith experiment.**
(d)	False	Methicillin resistant Staphylococcus aureus strain is resistant to all beta lactum groups of drugs and has no association with **Griffith experiment.**
(e)	True	Non capsulated Streptococcus pneumoniae (Nonpathogenic and Rough colonies on solid media) was used in **Griffith experiment.**

Keyser, Medical Microbiology, 2005, Pg. 174

3. Which fungus gives germ tube test positive?

(a) Cryptococcus
(b) Aspergillus
(c) Candida albicans
(d) Candida dubliniensis
(e) All Candida species

Ans. (c), (d)

(a)	False	Cryptococcus is capsulated Yeast and identified by India ink preparation.
(b)	False	Aspergillus – Mould and identified by culture on SDA.
(c)	True	**Germ tube test helps in speciation of Candida species and** Candida albicans, Candida dubliniensis are +ve.
(d)	True	–do–
(e)	False	Only Candida albicans and Candida dubliniensis are +ve for germ tube test.

Root, Clinical Infectious Diseases, Pg. 178

4. NNN Media used for isolation of:

(a) Leishmania donovani
(b) Giardia
(c) E. histolytica
(d) Trichomonas vaginalis
(e) Trypanosoma cruzi

Ans. (a), (e)

(a)	True	Novy-Mac Neal-Nicolle (NNN) medium, RPMI 1640 and Evans and Schneider medium are used for cultivation of Trypanosoma cruzi and Leishmania donovani.
(b)	False	Diamond's media is used for isolation of E. histolytica and Giardia.
(c)	False	Diamond's media is used for isolation of E. histolytica and Giardia.
(d)	False	Various culture media (gold standard) are used for isolation of Trichomonas vaginalis like Lash's cysteine hydrolysate serum media, Diamond's trypticase yeast maltose media and McCoy cell line.
(e)	True	Novy-Mac Neal-Nicolle (NNN) medium, RPMI 1640 and Evans and Schneider medium are used for cultivation of Trypanosoma cruzi and Leishmania donovani.

Ref: *Hunter's Tropical Medicine, 9th edition, Pg. 1083*

5. Human papilloma virus (HPV) causes cancer of all *except*:

(a) Bladder cancer
(b) Oropharyngeal carcinoma
(c) Squamous cell carcinoma
(d) Cervical cancer
(e) Testicular cancer

Ans. (a), (e)

(a)	True	HPV has no association with bladder cancer.
(b)	False	Oropharyngeal carcinoma can cause by HPV.
(c)	False	Squamous cell carcinoma can cause by HPV.
(d)	False	99% Cervical cancer–caused by HPV.
(e)	True	HPV has no association with testicular cancer.

Jawetz, Medical Microbiology, 23rd edition, Pg, 633, 646

Lange Review of Medical Microbiology and Immunology, 13th edition, Pg. 674

6. Gel diffusion tests used for detection of Ag or Ab.

Which one is the example of gel precipitation test?

(a) Immunoelectrophoresis
(b) VDRL
(c) WIDAL
(d) Coombs test
(e) Elek's test

Ans. (a), (e)

(a)	True	Immunoelectrophoresis is a type of gel diffusion.
(b)	False	VDRL – Slide flocculation test.
(c)	False	WIDAL – Slide or Tube agglutination test.
(d)	False	Coombs test – Direct Hemagglutination test.
(e)	True	Elek's test also known as the immunodiffusion technique, is an in vitro virulence test performed upon Corynebacterium diphtheriae.

Ananthnarayan and Paniker Textbook of Microbiology, 7th edition, Pg. 96

(Lange), Pg. 1176

(Jawetz), Pg. 781

7. Specific test for identification of infectious diseases agent is/are?

(a) Microscopy
(b) Culture method
(c) PCR
(d) NAAT
(e) MGIT system

Ans. (c), (d)

(a)	False	Microscopy has less specificity compared to other diagnostic tests.
(b)	False	Some infectious agents cannot be cultured.
(c)	True	PCR detects the nucleic acid of causative microorganism and is very specific test.
(d)	True	NAAT are very specific tests like PCR, RFLP, Ligase chain reaction, etc.
(e)	False	MGIT system – only used for isolation of Mycobacterium species.

8. Methods of bacteria acquiring drug resistance:

(a) Conjugation
(b) Transduction
(c) Transformation
(d) Satellitism
(e) Swarming

Ans. (a), (b), (c)

(a)	True	Bacteria can acquire drug resistance by conjugation, transduction and transformation.
(b)	True	–do–
(c)	True	–do–
(d)	False	Satellitism phenomenon is shown by haemophilus influenzae.
(e)	False	Swarming phenomenon is type of motility on blood agar.

Ref: *1. (Lange), 35, 57* *2. (Jawetz), 107*

9. Microbiological organisms used in sterilization control.

Sterilization accuracy is assessed by using:

(a) Clostridium perfringenes
(b) Geobacillus stereothermophilus
(c) Staphylococcus aureus
(d) Clostridium botulinum
(e) Bacillus subtilis subsp. niger

Ans. (b), (e)

(a)	False	Spores of Clostridium perfringenes are not used in sterilization control.
(b)	True	Spores of Geobacillus stereothermophilus are used in sterilization control of Autoclaving and Plasma sterilization.
(c)	False	Staphylococcus aureus is used in sterilization control.
(d)	False	Spores of Clostridium botulinum are not used in sterilization control.
(e)	True	Spores of Bacillus subtilis subsp. niger are used in sterilization control of Hot air oven.

10. Which is not member of Enterobacteriaceae family?

(a) E. coli
(b) Salmonella
(c) Citrobacter
(d) Vibrio
(e) Pseudomonas

Ans. (d), (e)

(a)	False	E. coli is member of Enterobacteriaceae family.
(b)	False	Salmonella is member of Enterobacteriaceae family.
(c)	False	Citrobacter is member of Enterobacteriaceae family.
(d)	True	Vibrio belongs to family Vibrionaceae.
(e)	True	Pseudomonas belongs to family Pseudomonadaceae.

Enterobacteriaceae:

(Lange) 339

(Jawetz) 229

11. Which one cannot act as definitive host of Clonorchis sinensis?

(a) Dogs (b) Pigs (c) Cats (d) Cows (e) Goats

Ans. (d), (e)

(a)	False	Dogs, pigs and cats serve as definitive host of Clonorchis sinensis.
(b)	False	–do–
(c)	False	–do–
(d)	True	Cow as definitive host in Dicrocoelium dendriticum infection. Cow as intermediate host in ***Taenia saginata*** infection.
(e)	True	Goat – Serve as an intermediate host in ***Echinococcus granulosus*** infection.

Ref: *(Jawetz) 745*

(Lange) 1008

12. Effective drugs for Fasciola hepatica:

(a) Bithionol
(b) Praziquantel
(c) Triclabendazole
(d) Metronidazole
(e) Niclofolan

Ans. (a), (b), (c)

(a)	True	Bithionol, Praziquantel and Triclabendazole are recommended and effective drugs in Fasciola hepatica infection.
(b)	True	–do–
(c)	True	–do–
(d)	False	Metronidazole is DOC for Amoebiasis, Trichomoniasis and Giardiasis.
(e)	False	Niclofolan is no longer recommended for Fasciola hepatica infection due to toxicity.

Ref: *(Lange) 1010*

13. Stain for M.Tb (Staining techniques for Mycobacterium tuberculosis):

(a) Auramine
(b) ZN
(c) Gram stain
(d) Giemsa stain
(e) Albert stain

Ans. (a), (b)

(a)	True	Auramine – Fluorescent stain for Mycobacterium.
(b)	True	ZN staining – used for stain acid fast structures like Mycobacterium.
(c)	False	Gram staining is not useful in case of Mycobacterium.
(d)	False	Giemsa stain is not used for staining of Mycobacterium.
(e)	False	Albert Stain is used for identification Corynebacterium diphtheria.

14. Which is immune complex mediated disease?

(a) SLE
(b) Bronchial asthma
(c) RA
(d) Goodpasture
(e) Tuberculin skin test

Ans. (a), (c)

(a)	True	SLE – Type III reactions (i.e., immune complex reactions)
(b)	False	Bronchial asthma – Type I reactions (i.e., immediate hypersensitivity reactions)
(c)	True	RA – Type III reactions (i.e., immune complex reactions)
(d)	False	Goodpasture – Type II reactions (i.e., cytotoxic hypersensitivity reactions)
(e)	False	Tuberculin skin test – Type IV reactions (i.e., delayed hypersensitivity reactions, cell-mediated immunity)

15. Giardia, true is:

(a) Mostly invade into small intestine
(b) Present with bloody diarrhea
(c) Mostly in hyperglobulinemia patient
(d) Nitroimidazole is effective
(e) Trophozoites passed in stool but non infectious

Ans. (a), (e)

(a)	True	Commonly found in Duodenum and upper jejunum.
(b)	False	Causes Non-invasive infection.
(c)	False	Not associated with hyperglobulinemia patients.
(d)	False	DOC – Metronidazole.
(e)	True	Cysts are infective forms.

Ref: *(Jawetz) 719*
(Lange) 926

16. Characteristic morphological form associated with Pl. falciparum is/are:

(a) RBC enlarged
(b) Ring shaped gametocytes
(c) Crescent shape gametocytes
(d) Multiple rings trophozoite
(e) Developmental stages are not seen in peripheral smears

Ans. (c), (d)

(a)	False	RBC size will be normal in P. falciparum infection, RBC enlarged = P. vivax and P. ovale.
(b)	False	P. falciparum have crescent or banana shaped Gametocytes.
(c)	True	–do–
(d)	True	Multiple rings only present in trophozoite of P. falciparum.
(e)	False	Developmental stages are seen in peripheral smears.

1. *http://www.cdc.gov/dpdx/malaria/dx.html*
2. *(Lange) 938*
3. *(Jawetz) 728*

17. True about diagnosing babesiosis:

(a) Culture
(b) PCR
(c) RFLP
(d) Peripheral smear examination is gold standard investigation
(e) Malaria and babesia ring forms can be difficult to distinguish one from the other

Ans. (b), (d), (e)

(a)	False	Culture method is not useful in diagnosis of Babesiosis.
(b)	True	PCR can be used in diagnosis of Babesiosis when microscopy fails.
(c)	False	RFLP is not used in diagnosis of Babesiosis.
(d)	True	Peripheral smear examination–gold standard investigation.
(e)	True	Malaria and babesia ring forms can be difficult to distinguish as they look similar.

(*Lange*) *975*

18. Common causative agent of hand-foot-and-mouth disease is:

(a) Enterovirus
(b) Coxsackie B4
(c) Coxsackievirus A16
(d) HPV
(e) HAV

Ans. (a), (c)

(a)	True	Enterovirus also causes hand-foot-and-mouth disease.
(b)	False	Coxsackie B4 – can cause a varying range of symptoms like gastrointestinal distress myocarditis.
(c)	True	Coxsackievirus A16–most common cause of hand-foot-and-mouth disease.
(d)	False	HPV don't cause hand-foot-and-mouth disease.
(e)	False	HAV don't cause hand-foot-and-mouth disease.

19. IP < 4 weeks is for:

(a) Gonorrhea
(b) Hep B
(c) Babesiosis
(d) Tertiary syphilis
(e) Filariasis

Ans. (a), (c)

(a)	True	IP for Gonorrhea = 2-15 days
(b)	False	IP for HBV = average 4 months
(c)	True	IP for Babesiosis = between 1-6 weeks
(d)	False	IP for Tertiary syphilis = 10-30 years
(e)	False	IP for Filariasis = 8 to 16 months

20. Category C Bioterrorism Agents is/are:

(a) Hanta virus
(b) Ebola virus
(c) Crimean congo virus
(d) Tuberculosis
(e) HIV

Ans. (a), (d)

(a)	True	Hanta virus – Category C
(b)	False	Ebola virus – Category A
(c)	False	Crimean congo virus – Category A
(d)	True	MDR Tuberculosis – Category C
(e)	False	HIV – Not categorized as Bioterrorism Agents

PGI 2017

1. Dimorphic fungi

- Dimorphic fungi are those fungi that can exist in two different morphological forms under two different environmental conditions. These fungi exist as moulds in their natural habitat and in vitro at room temperature and as yeasts in vivo or in vitro at 37°C. Most of the dimorphic fungi are responsible for systemic or deep mycoses. For definitive identification of the fungus, yeast to mould conversion should be demonstrated. All dimorphic Isolates known to cause systemic mycoses must be handled with caution in a biological safety cabinet.
- The dimorphic fungi are Histoplasma capsulatum, Blastomyces dermatitidis, Coccidioides immitis, Paracoccidiodes brasiliensis, Penicillium marneffi and Sporothrix schenkii.

2. Actinomycetes

- Actinomycetes are Gram-positive, catalase-positive, nonmotile bacilli. They are considered to be transitional forms between bacteria and fungi.

Human infections caused by Actinomycetes

Bacteria	Diseases
Actinomyces species	Cervicofacial actinomycosis, thoracic actinomycosis, and actinomycosis of the abdomen and pelvis
Nocardia species	Primary cutaneous nocardiosis, bronchopulmonary infection, and secondary central nervous system infection
Rhodococcus species	Pulmonary infections and opportunistic infections (traumatic endophthalmitis, peritonitis in patients undergoing dialysis, and post-traumatic skin infection)

3. Measles infectivity period

- **Incubation period:** 10 to 14 days. Patients are contagious during the prodromal phase (2–4 days) and the first 2–5 days of rash, when virus is present in tears, nasal and throat secretions, urine and blood. The characteristic maculopapular rash appears about day 14 just as circulating antibodies become detectable, the viremia disappears, and the fever falls. The rash develops as a result of interaction of immune T cells with virus-infected cells in the small blood vessels and lasts about 1 week. (In patients with defective cell-mediated immunity, no rash develops).

4. Barrel shaped eggs

- The nematode (roundworm) Trichuris trichiura, also called the human whipworm. Whipworm is a soil-transmitted helminth (STH) and is the third most common roundworm of humans. Whipworm causes an infection called trichuriasis and often occurs in areas where human feces is used as fertilizer or where defecation onto soil happens. The worms are spread from person to person by fecal-oral transmission or through feces-contaminated food.
- The standard method for diagnosing the presence of whipworm is by microscopically identifying whipworm eggs (Barrel shaped with mucous plugs at poles) in a stool sample. Because eggs may be difficult to find in light infections, a concentration procedure is recommended.

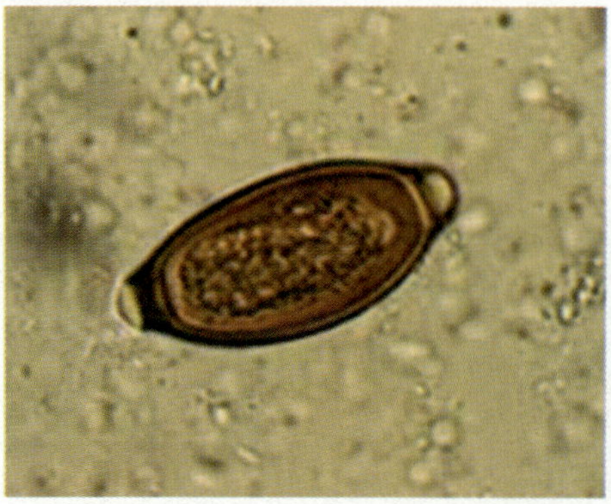

5. Tick borne diseases

- **Anaplasmosis** is transmitted to humans by tick bites primarily from the blacklegged tick (*Ixodes scapularis*) in the northeastern and upper midwestern U.S. and the western blacklegged tick (*Ixodes pacificus*) along the Pacific coast.

  Babesiosis is caused by microscopic parasites that infect red blood cells. Most human cases of babesiosis in the U.S. are caused by *Babesia microti*. *Babesia microti* is transmitted by the blacklegged tick (*Ixodes scapularis*).
- ***Borrelia mayonii*** infection has recently been described as a cause of illness in the upper midwestern United States. It has been found in blacklegged ticks (*Ixodesscapularis*) in Minnesota and Wisconsin. *Borrelia mayonii* is a new species and is the only species besides *B. burgdorferi* known to cause *Lyme disease* in North America.
- **Borrelia miyamotoi** infection has recently been described as a cause of illness in the U.S. It is transmitted by the blacklegged tick (*Ixodes scapularis*) and has a range similar to that of Lyme disease.
- **Colorado tick fever** is caused by a virus transmitted by the Rocky Mountain wood tick (Dermacentor andersoni). It occurs in the the Rocky Mountain states at elevations of 4,000 to 10,500 feet.
- **Ehrlichiosis** is transmitted to humans by the lone star tick (*Ambylomma americanum*), found primarily in the southcentral and eastern U.S.
- **Lyme disease** is transmitted by the blacklegged tick (*Ixodes scapularis*) in the northeastern U.S. and upper mid-western U.S. and the western blacklegged tick (*Ixodes pacificus*) along the Pacific coast.
- **Powassan disease** is transmitted by the blacklegged tick (*Ixodes scapularis*) and the groundhog tick (*Ixodes cookei*). Cases have been reported primarily from northeastern states and the Great Lakes region.
- **Rickettsia parkeri rickettsiosis** is transmitted to humans by the Gulf Coast tick (*Amblyomma maculatum*).
- **Rocky Mountain spotted fever (RMSF)** is transmitted by the American dog tick (*Dermacentor variabilis*), Rocky Mountain wood tick (*Dermacentor andersoni*), and the brown dog tick (*Rhipicephalus sangunineus*) in the U.S. The brown dog tick and other tick species are associated with RMSF in Central and South America.
- **Tickborne relapsing fever (TBRF)** is transmitted to humans through the bite of infected soft ticks. *Tularemia* is transmitted to humans by the dog tick (*Dermacentor variabilis*), the wood tick (*Dermacentor andersoni*), and the lone star tick (*Amblyomma americanum*). Tularemia occurs throughout the U.S.

6. Infection in Cystis fibrosis

- Biofilms are important in human infections that are persistent and difficult to treat. A few examples include *Staphylococcus epidermidis* and *S aureus* infections of central venous catheters, eye infections/ such as what occur with contact lenses and intraocular lenses, in dental plaque, and in prosthetic joint infections. Perhaps the most profound example of a biofilm in human infection is in *P aeruginosa* airway infections in cystic fibrosis patients.
- P aeruginosa in a culture can produce multiple colony types. P aeruginosa from different colony types may also have different biochemical and enzymatic activities and different antimicrobial susceptibility patterns. Sometimes, it is not clear if the colony types represent different strains of P aeruginosa or are variants of the same strain. Cultures from patients with cystic fibrosis (CF) often yield P aeruginosa organisms that form mucoid colonies as a result of overproduction of alginate, an exopolysaccharide. In CF patients, the exopolysaccharide appears to provide the matrix for the organisms to live in a biofilm.

7. Cancer causing virus

Association of Viruses with Human Cancers

S. No.	Virus	Human Cancer
1.	Human papillomaviruses	Genital tumors Squamous cell carcinoma Oropharyngeal carcinoma
2.	Epstein-Barr virus	Nasopharyngeal carcinoma Burkitt lymphoma Hodgkin disease B-cell lymphoma
	Human herpesvirus 8	Kaposi sarcoma

Contd.

Contd.

3.	Hepatitis B virus	Hepatocellular carcinoma
4.	Merkel cell virus	Merkel cell carcinoma
5.	Human T-lymphotropic virus Human immunodeficiency virus	Adult T-cell leukemia AIDS-related malignancies
6.	Hepatitis C virus	Hepatocellular carcinoma

8. Donovanosis

- **Granuloma Inguinale (Donovanosis):** Granuloma inguinale is a genital ulcerative disease caused by the intracellulargram-negativebacteriumKlebsiellagranulomatis(formerlyknownasCalymatobacteriumgranulomatis). It is endemic in some tropical and developing areas, including India; Papua, New Guinea; the Caribbean; central Australia; and southern Africa. Clinically, the disease is commonly characterized as painless, slowly progressive ulcerative lesions on the genitals or perineum without regional lymphadenopathy; subcutaneous granu-lomas (pseudobuboes) also might occur. The lesions are highly vascular (i.e., beefy red appearance) and bleed. Extragenital infection can occur with extension of infection to the pelvis, or it can disseminate to intra-abdominal organs, bones, or the mouth. The lesions also can develop secondary bacterial infection and can coexist with other sexually transmitted pathogens.
- The causative organism of granuloma inguinale is difficult to culture, and diagnosis requires visualization of dark-staining Donovan bodies on tissue crush preparation or biopsy. DOC – Azithromycin 1 g orally once per week or 500 mg daily for at least 3 weeks a nd until all lesions have completely healed.

9. Antigen presenting cells

- Antigen presenting cells (APCs) are a heterogeneous group of immune cells that mediate the cellular immune response by processing and presenting antigens for recognition by certain lymphocytes such as T cells. Classical APCs include dendritic cells, macrophages, Langerhans cells and B cells.

10. Both T and B lymphocyte involved in diseases.

- **Combined immunodeficiencies (B and T cells defects)**
  - (a) Cellular immunodeficiency with abnormal immunoglobulin synthesis (Nezelof syndrome).
  - (b) Ataxia telangiectasia.
  - (c) Wiskott-Aldrich syndrome.
  - (d) SCID.

Chapter 11

IMAGE BASED QUESTIONS

Courtesy: CDC Image Library

GENERAL MICROBIOLOGY

1.

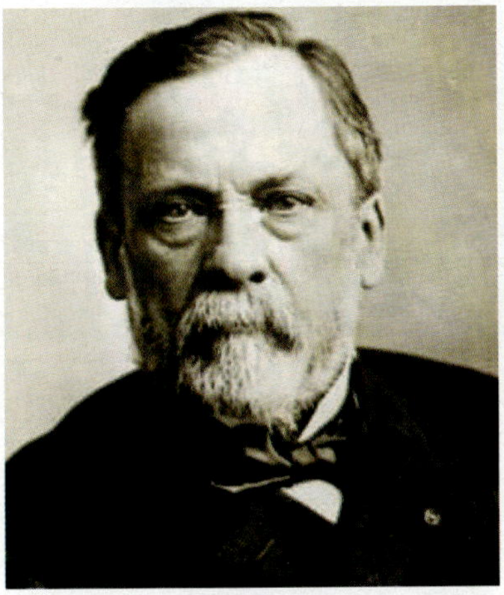

Louis Pasteur

2.

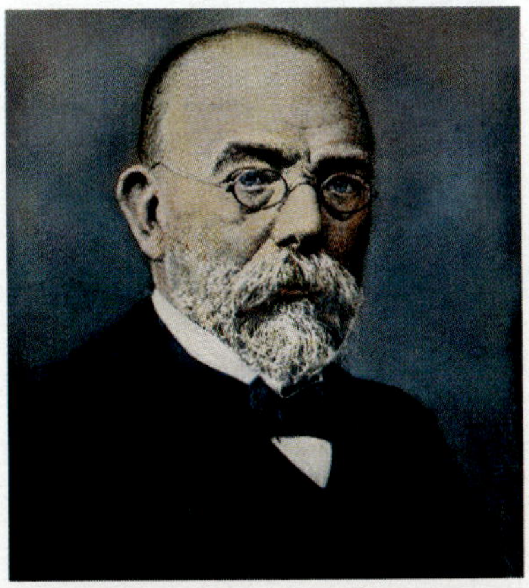

Robert Koch

3.

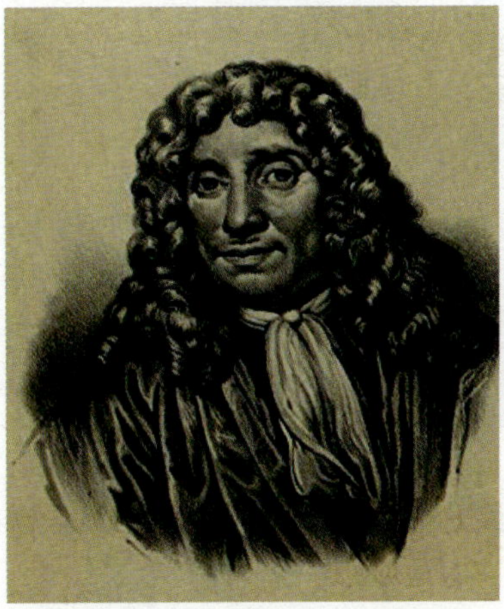

Antony van Leeuwenhoek

4.

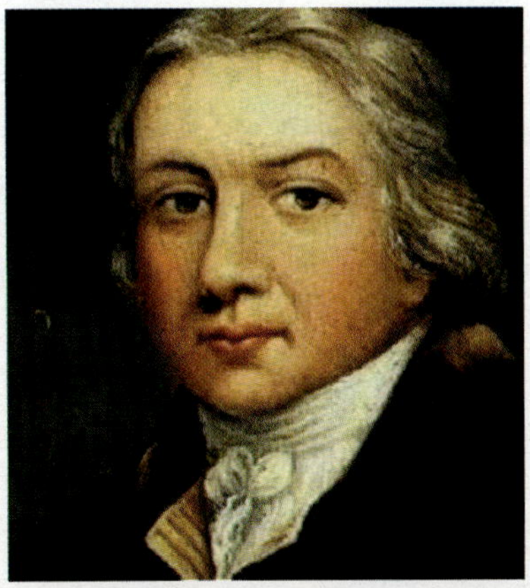

Edward Jenner

5. **Autoclave (121°C, 15 min, 15 lbs).**

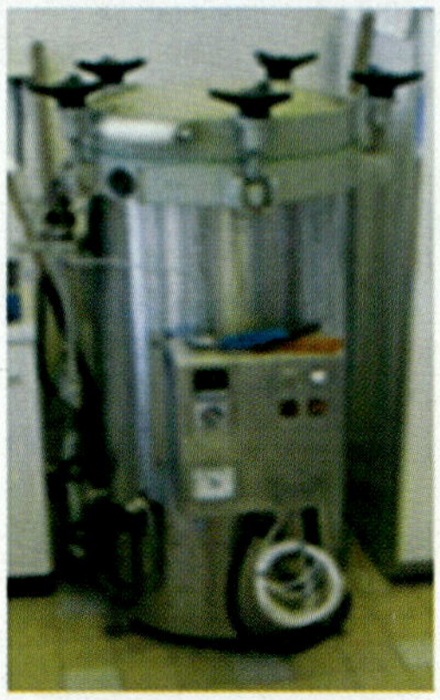

6. **Hot Air Oven (160°C for 2 hours).**

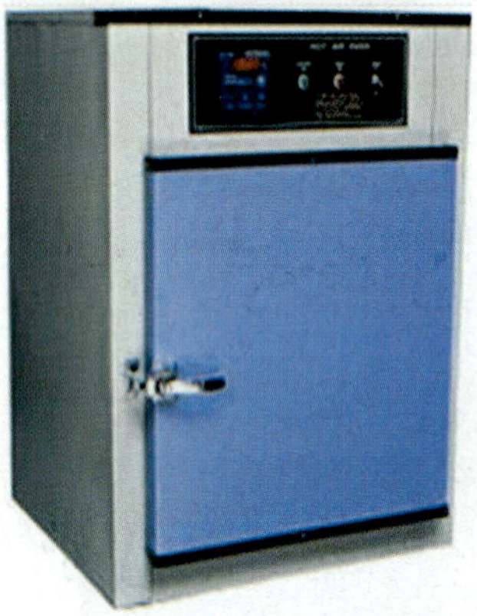

7. **Inspissator (80 to 85°C – 30 min = 3 days).**

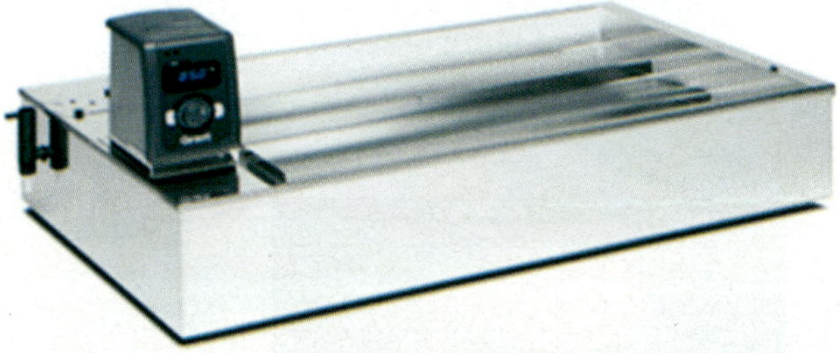

8. **Antibiotic sensitivity testing by disk diffusion (Kirby Bauer) method on MHA. See zone of inhibition around the disk.**

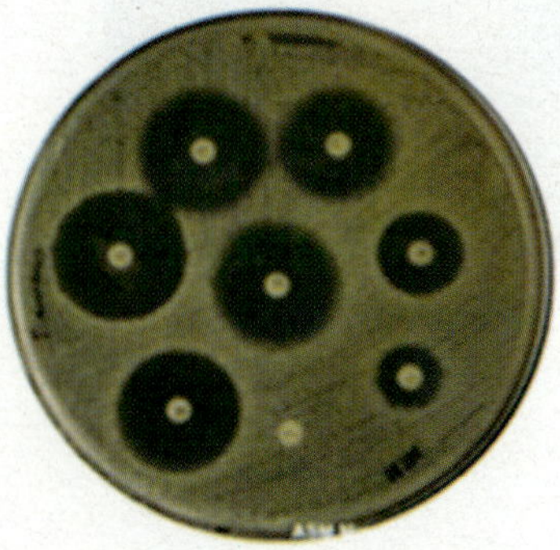

9. **McIntosh Filde's Jar (for Anaerobic culture).**

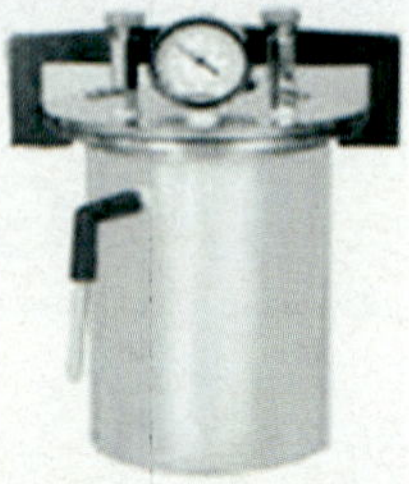

10. **Gas Pak System (for Anaerobic culture).**

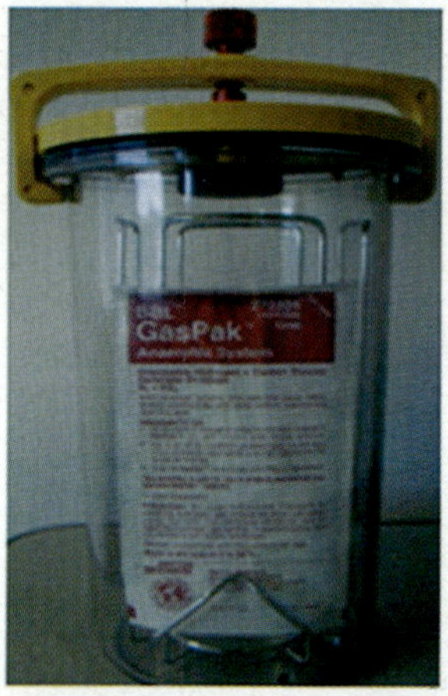

11. **Candle Jar (For culture of Capnophilic bacteria) – Pneumococcus and Meningococci.**

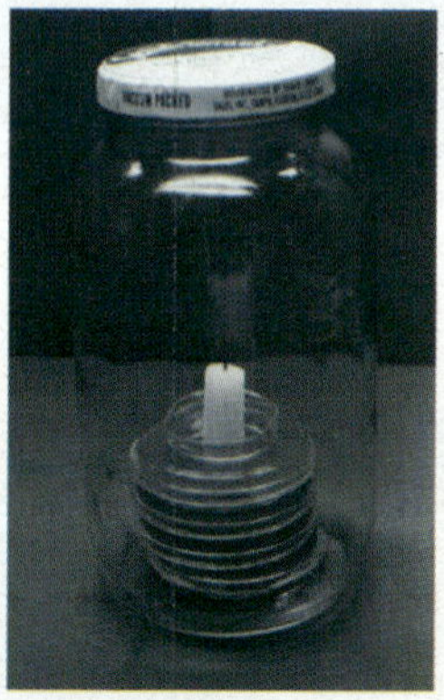

12. **Nutrient Agar (Simple or Basal Media).**

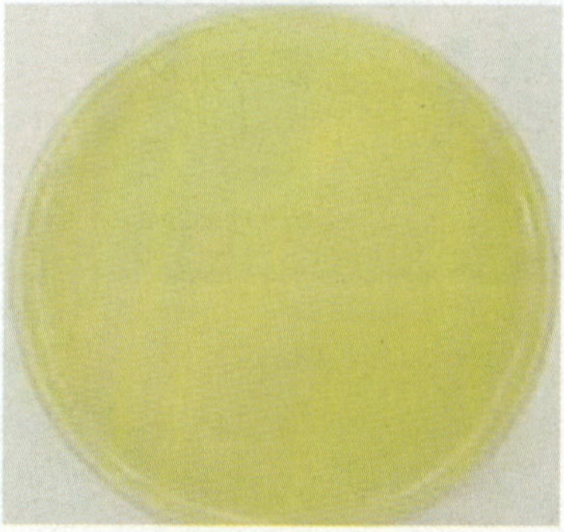

13. **Blood Agar (Enriched media).**

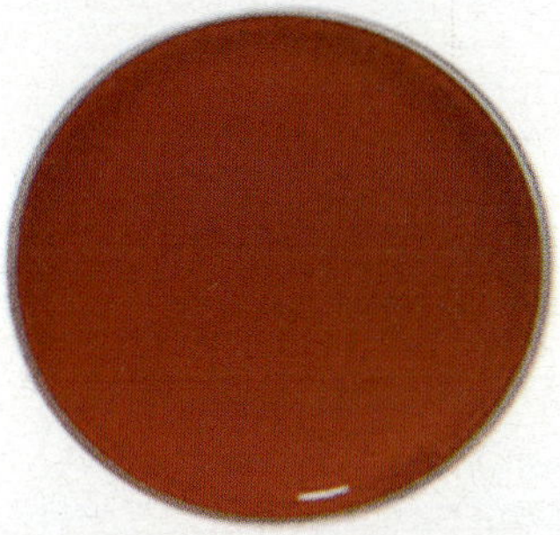

14. **Chocolate Agar (Enriched media).**

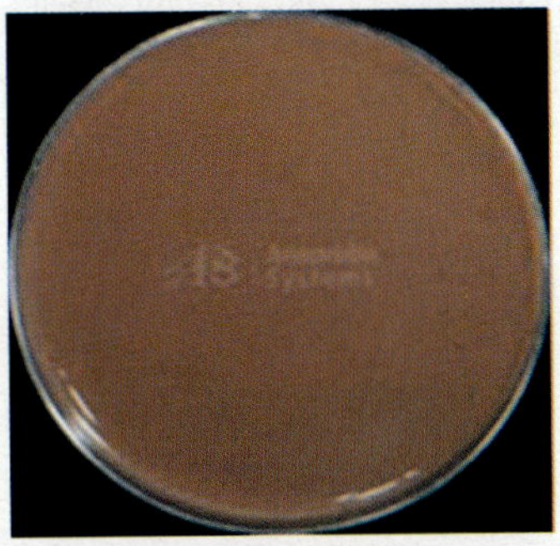

15. **MacConkey Agar (Differential or Indicator media).**

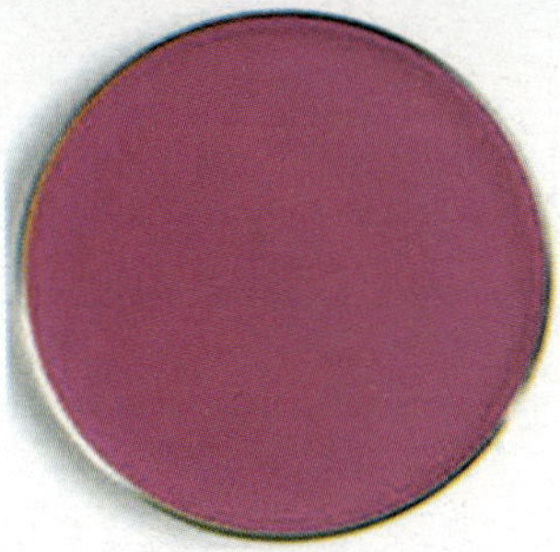

16. **Castaneda Biphasic Medium for Blood Culture.**

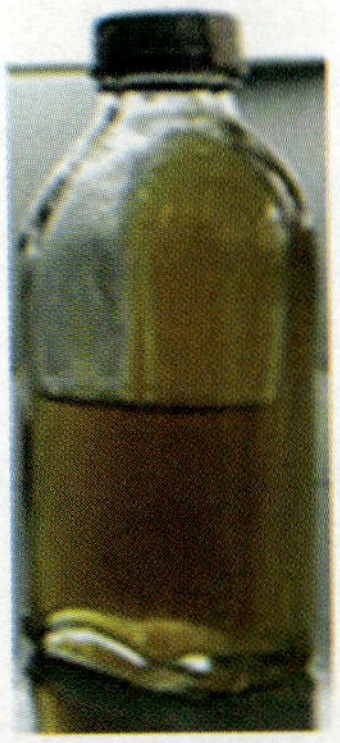

17. **Nichrome Wire Loop**

Microbiologists use inoculating loops to transfer microorganisms to growth media. It is also used for streak method for bacterial isolation from various clinical specimens. It is easy to sterilize and reuse because nichrome wire resists deterioration with repeated heat/cooling cycles. Flame sterilization is a very simple method of killing microorganisms on an inoculating loop.

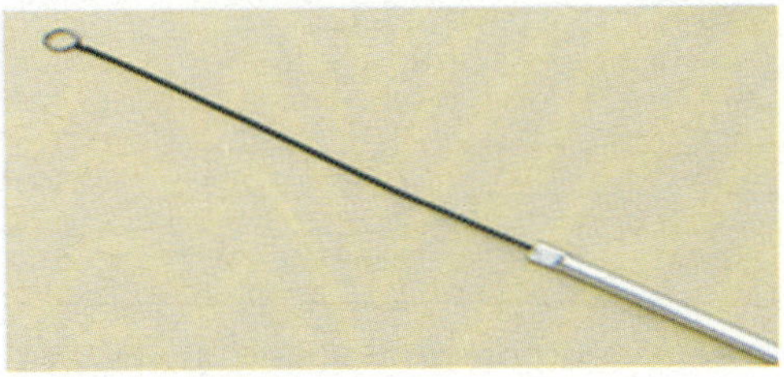

18. **Nichrome Straight Wire**

It is used for different purposes like stab culture (Motility detection), stab followed by stroke (TSI inoculation), Stroke culture on SDA slant for fungus isolation, pick up the isolated colonies from mixed bacterial colonies on solid media etc.

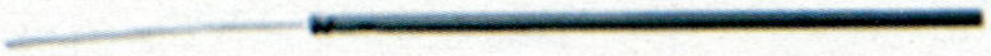

19. **Microtitre Plate**

It is used in ELISA for detection of Antibodies or Antigens from various clinical specimens.

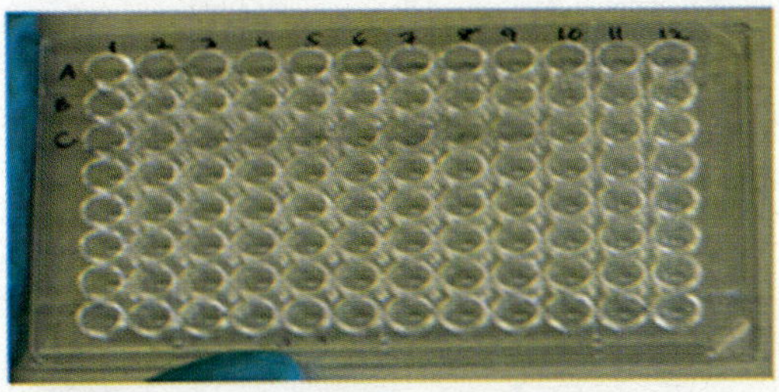

20. **Purified protein derivative (PPD) test/Mantoux test is done with the help of Tuberculin syringe.**

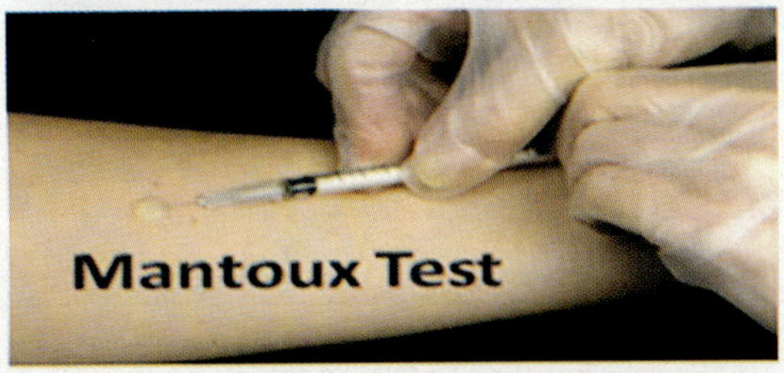

IMMUNOLOGY

1. HLA class I and class II molecules (PBR = peptide-binding region).

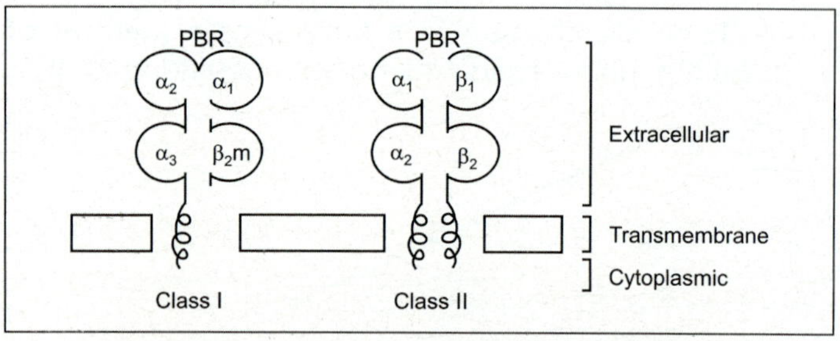

2. Different antigen-processing pathways for the MHC class I and class II molecules.

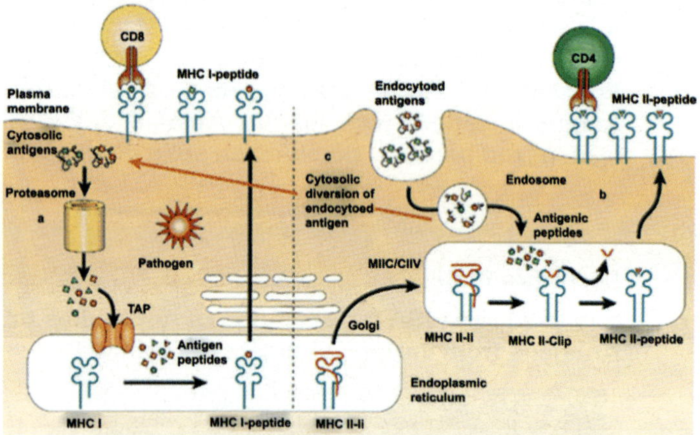

3. DiGeorge Syndrome (Genetic Thymic Hypoplasia).

Cleft palate   Skeletal differences

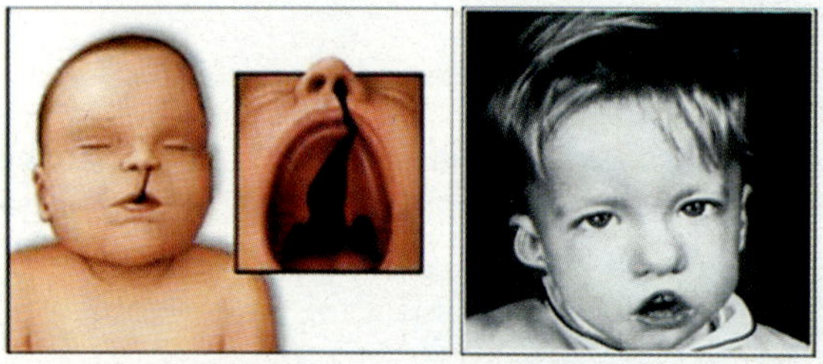

4. Classes of Antibodies.

Name	Properties	Structure
IgA	Found in mucous, saliva, tears and breast milk. Protects against pathogens.	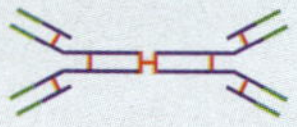
IgD	Part of the B cell receptor. Activates basophils and mast cells.	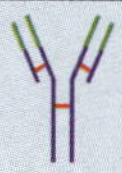

Contd.

Contd.

IgE	Protects against parasitic worms. Responsible for allergic reactions.	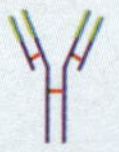
IgG	Secreted by plasma cells in the blood. Able to cross the placenta into the fetus.	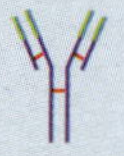
IgM	May be attached to the surface of a B cell or secreted into the blood. Responsible for early stages of immunity.	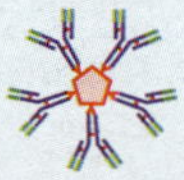

5. Antigen-Antibodies Reactions.

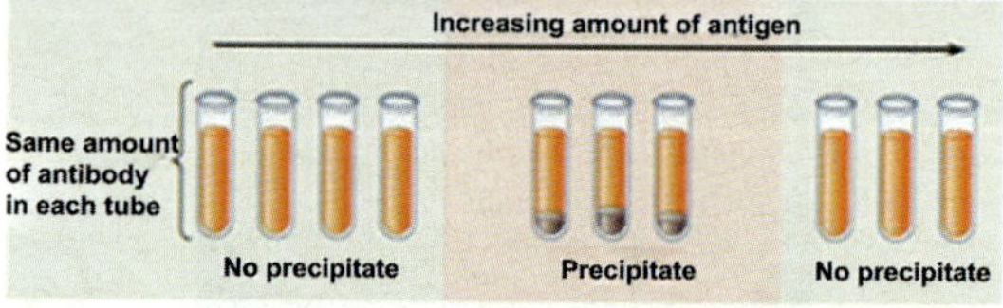

(a)

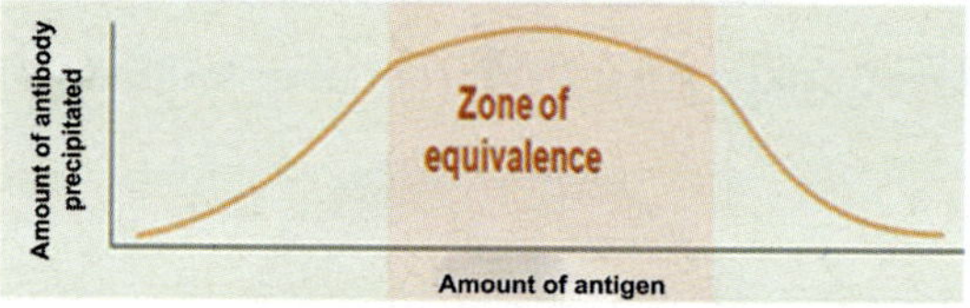

(b)

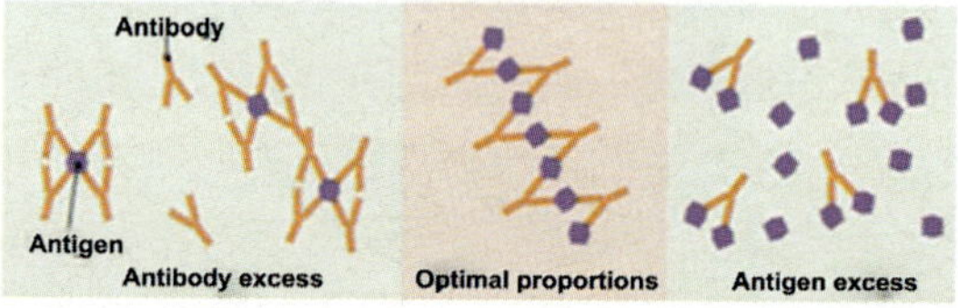

6. Analysis of Antigens and Antibodies by Immunoprecipitation.

The precipitation of protein occurs at the equivalence point, at which multivalent antibody forms large complexes with antigen.

A. **Ouchterlony immunodouble diffusion:** Antigen and antibody diffuse from wells, meet and form a precipitin line.

B. **Countercurrent Electrophoresis:** This technique is similar to the Ouchterlony method, but antigen movement is facilitated by electrophoresis.

C. **Single Radial Immunodiffusion:** This technique involves the diffusion of antigen into an antibody containing gel. Precipitin rings indicate an immune reaction, and the area of the ring is proportional to the concentration of the antigen.

D. **Rocket Electrophoresis:** Antigens are separated by electrophoresis into an agar gel that contains antibody. The length of the "rocket" indicates concentration of antigen E, immunoelectrophoresis. Antigen is placed in a well and separated by electrophoresis. Antibody is then placed in the trough, and precipitin lines form as antigen and antibody diffuse toward each other.

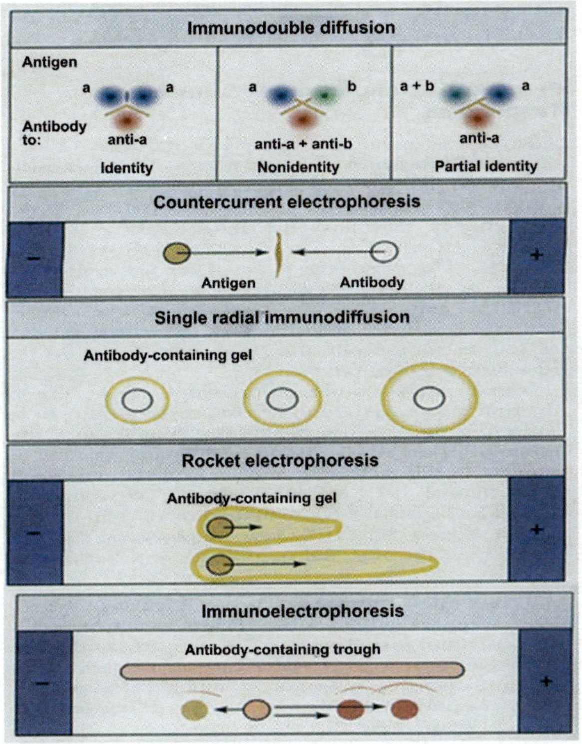

7. **Single and double diffusion in one dimension.**

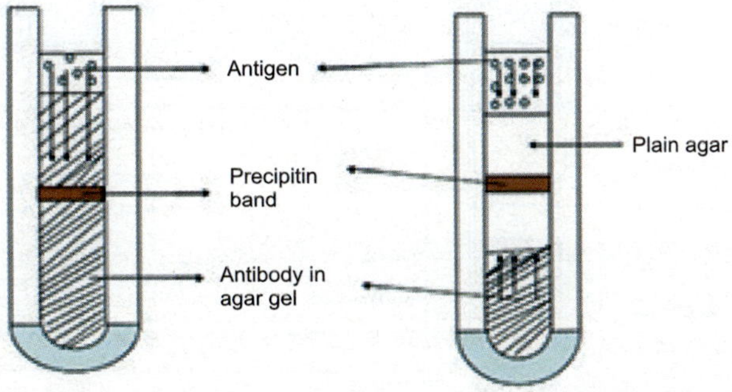

Single diffusion (Oudin procedure) Double diffusion (Okley - Fulthrope procedure)

8. **Countercurrent immunoelectrophoresis.**

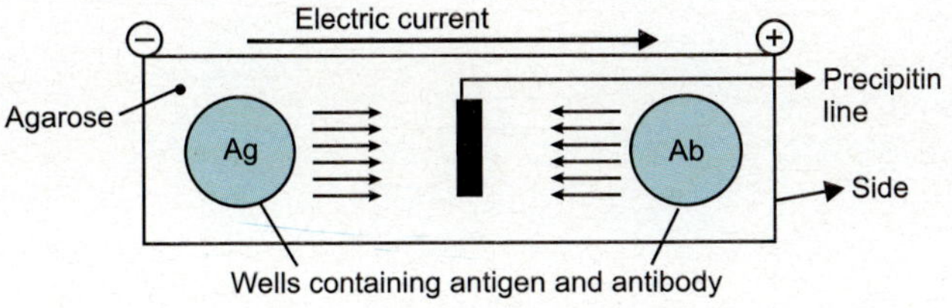

9. **96 well Microtiter plate–It is a flat plate with multiple "wells" used as small test tubes. The microplate has become a standard tool in analytical research and clinical diagnostic testing laboratories. A very common usage is in the enzyme-linked immunosorbent assay (ELISA), the basis of most modern medical diagnostic testing in humans and animals.**

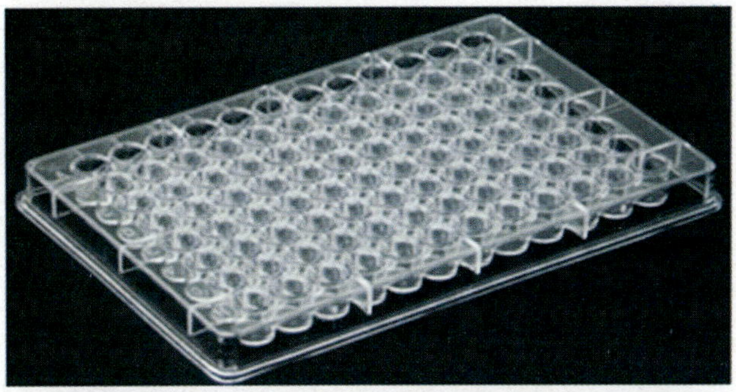

10. **Bleb formation in Mantoux tuberculin skin test.**

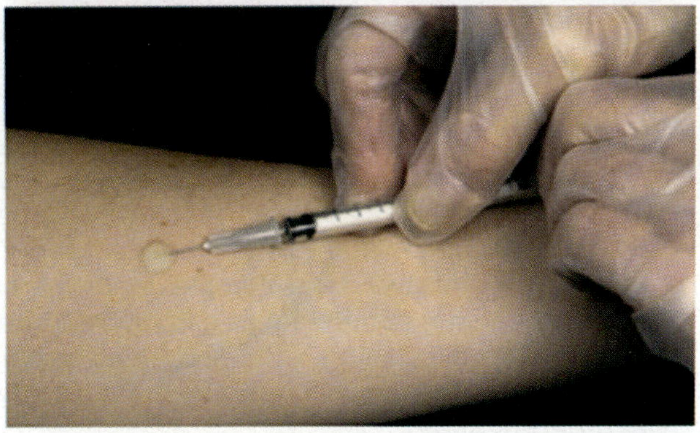

11. **Strongly positive Mantoux test.**

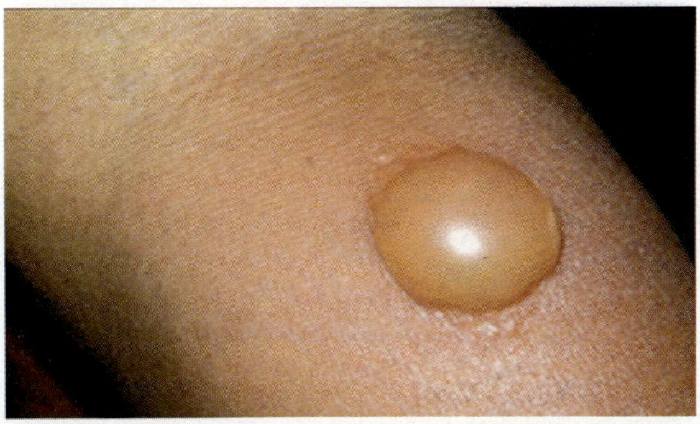

12. **An epitope, also known as antigenic determinant, is the part of an antigen that is recognized by the immune system, specifically by antibodies, B cells, or T cells. For example, the epitope is the specific piece of the antigen to which an antibody binds.**

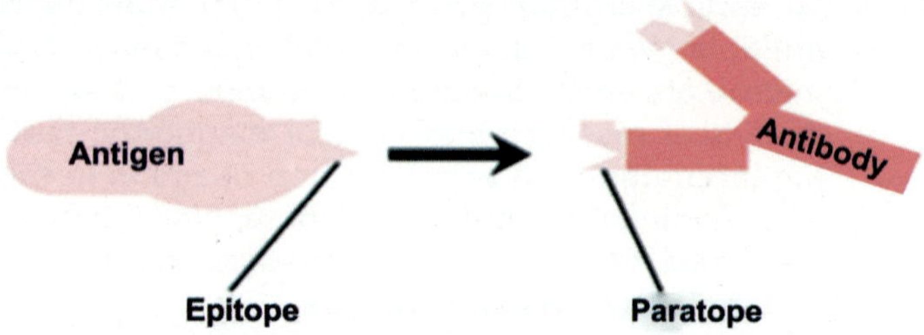

13. **Serum sickness – "It is a type of hypersensitivity, specifically immune complex (type 3) hypersensitivity. Serum sickness typically develops up to ten days after exposure to the antiserum, and symptoms are similar to an allergic reaction."**

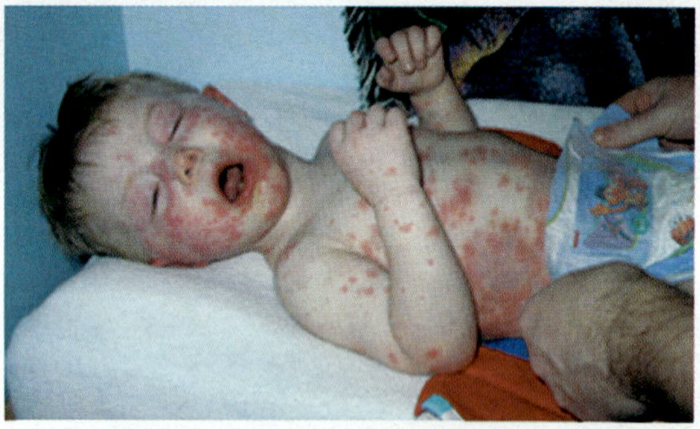

14. **Arthus reaction – Sub-acute antibody mediated hypersensitivity type III reaction – Caused by intradermal injection of antigen that induces antibodies that then form complexes in the skin causing edema, necrosis and activation of complement. Red swelling with undefined edge in 5-12 hours. (Reason why booster shots are given at different sites).**

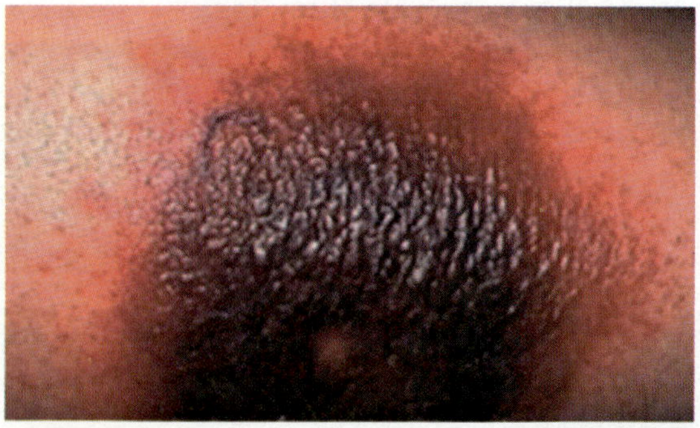

15. **Graves' Disease.**

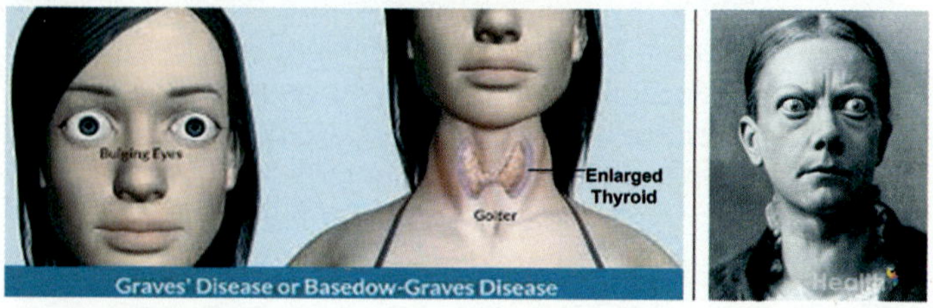

16. **Erythroblastosis Fetalis.**

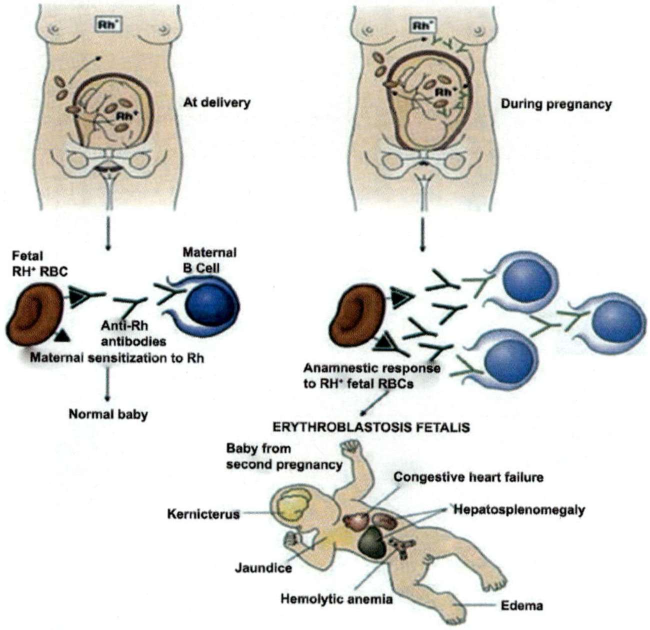

17. **ABO Blood Types.**

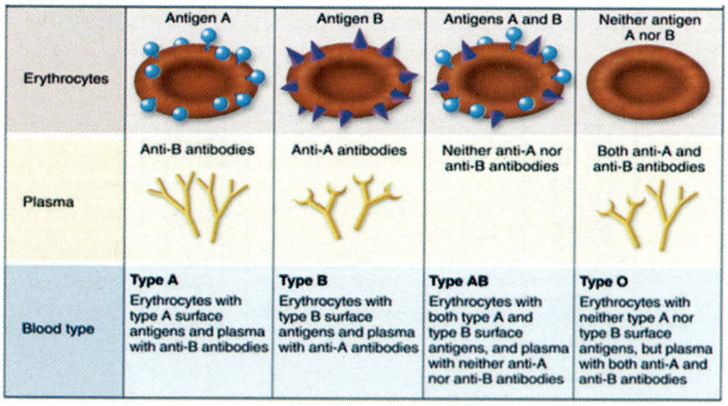

Direct Coombs test / Direct antiglobulin test

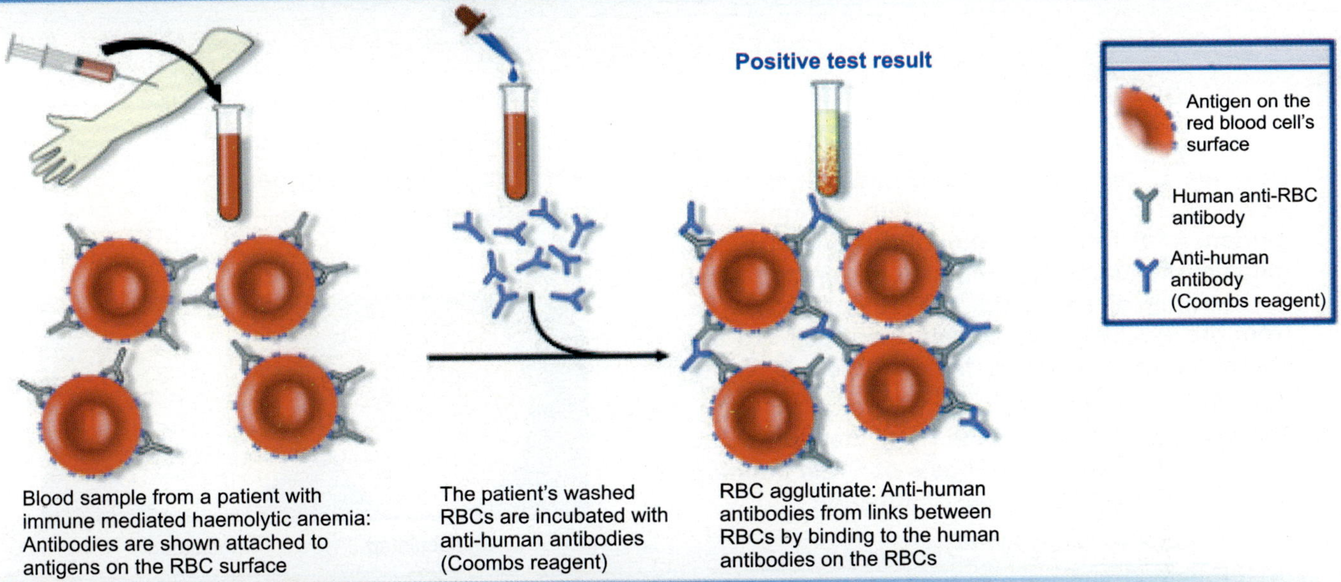

Indirect Coombs test / Indirect antiglobulin test

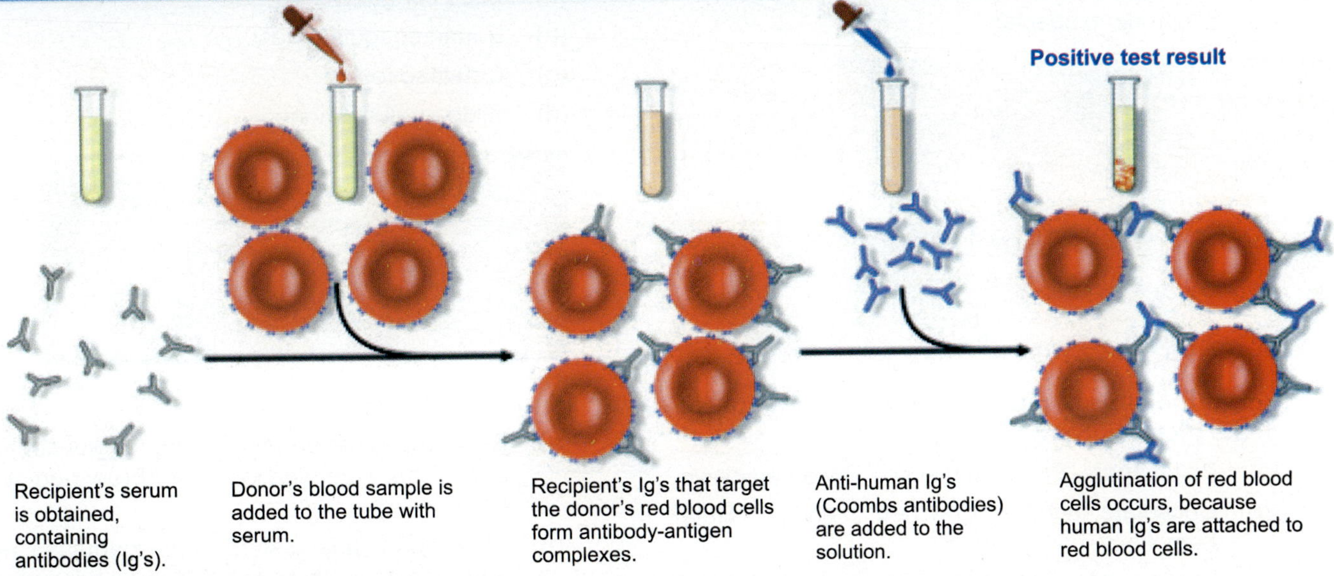

BACTERIOLOGY

GRAM-POSITIVE COCCI

1. **A 35 years old man came to the OPD with swelling of the hand. Patient had a history of skin abrasion on the hand while working in a garden. After four days, he noticed swelling and inflammation over the area of abrasion, followed by swelling of the hand. A purulent discharge from the swelling was collected and sent to the Microbiology laboratory for the Gram staining and culture sensitivity.**

   The given picture shows the Gram staining of the sample collected. On the basis of Gram staining what is the probable cause of infection?

   (a) Streptococcus pyogenes
   (b) Enterococcus
   (c) Staphylococcus aureus
   (d) Clostridium species

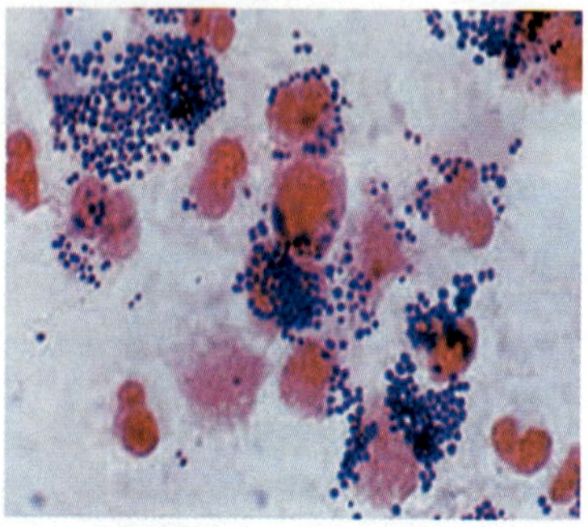

2. **Select the appropriate combination on the basis of the picture given:**

   (a) Blood agar – Enriched media – Alpha hemolysis
   (b) Chocolate agar – Enriched media – Beta hemolysis
   (c) Blood agar – Enrichment media – Beta hemolysis
   (d) Blood agar – Enriched media – Beta hemolysis

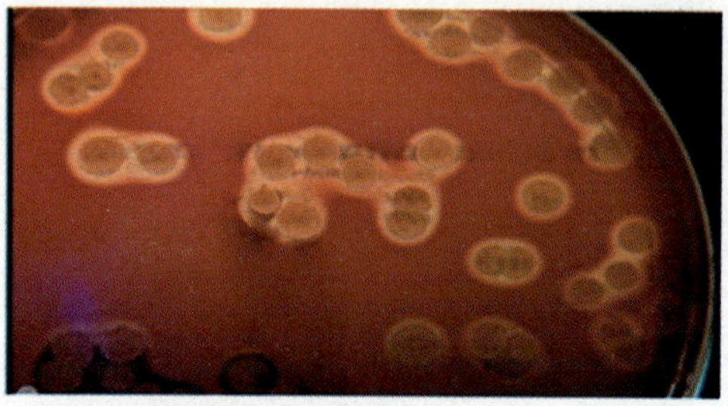

3. **A Gram positive bacteria grows on this selective media. Identify the bacteria:**

   (a) Staphyloccocus saprophyticus
   (b) Staphylococcus aureus
   (c) Staphylococcus epidermidis
   (d) Streptococcus pyogenes

Mannitol salt agar

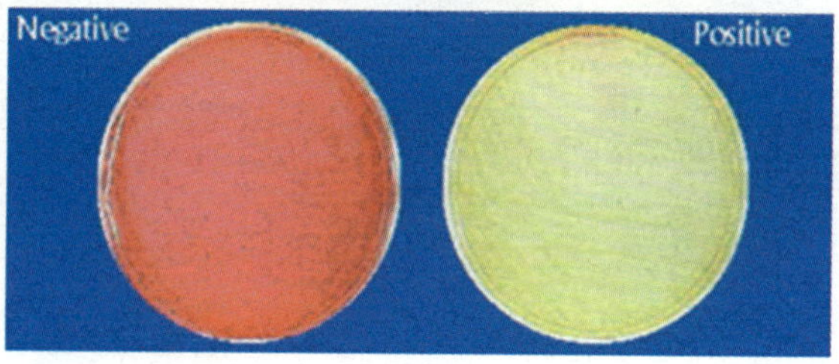

Uninoculated Inoculated

4. **Identify the test:**

   (a) Slide coagulase test
   (b) Bound coagulase test
   (c) Catalase test
   (d) Slide agglutination

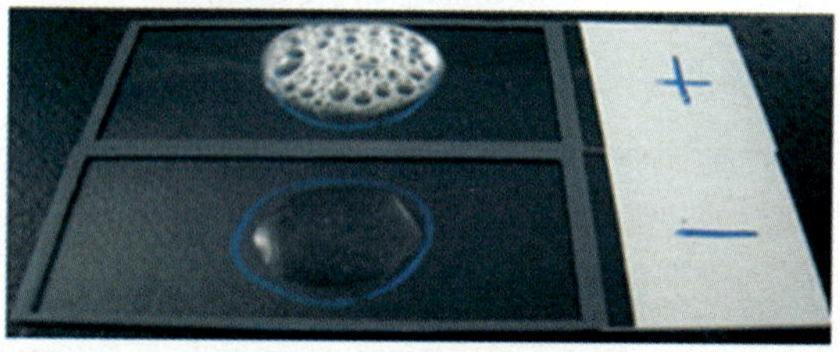

5. **Identify the test:**

   (a) Slide agglutination test (Bound agglutinin test) and Tube agglutination test (Free agglutinin test)
   (b) Slide coagulase test (Bound coagulase test) and tube coagulase test (Free coagulase test)
   (c) Slide coagulase test (Free coagulase test) and tube coagulase test (Bound coagulase test)
   (d) Slide agglutination test (Free agglutinin test) and Tube agglutination test (Bound agglutinin test)

Slide test

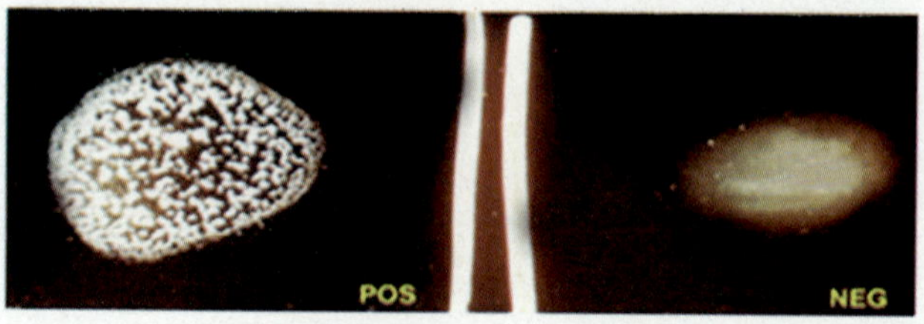

Tube test

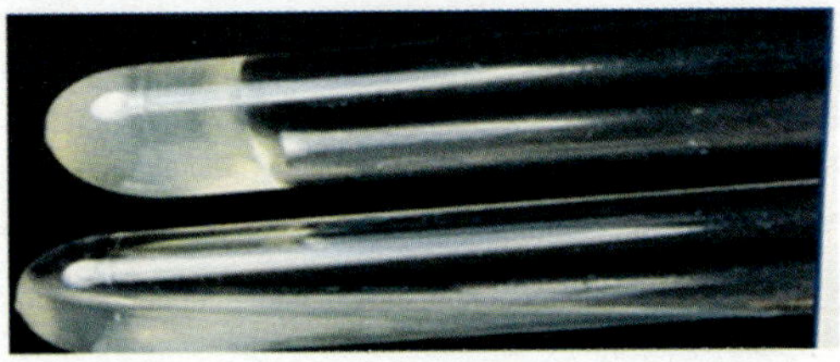

6. **Which bacteria give this type of colony morphology as shown in the given picture?**
   (a) Staph. saprophyticus
   (b) Staph. aureus
   (c) Strept. pyogenes
   (d) Staph. epidermidis

Golden yellow colonies on Nutrient agar

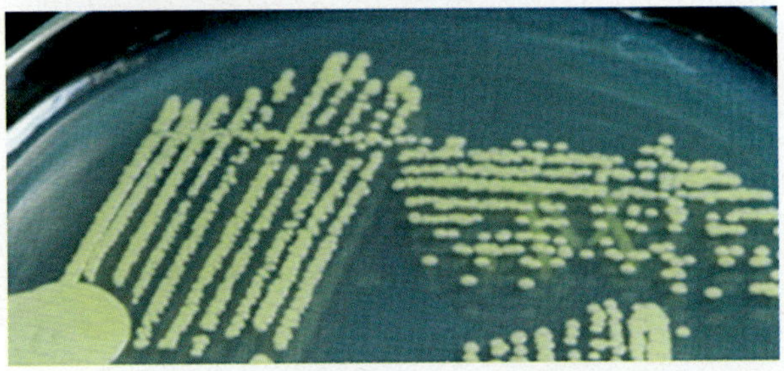

7. **On the basis of Novobiocin sensitivity testing, identify the Bacteria B.**
   Bacteria A- Sensitive **Bacteria B- Resistant**
   (a) Staph. aureus
   (b) Staph. hemolyticus
   (c) Staph. saprophyticus
   (d) Staphylococcus epidermidis

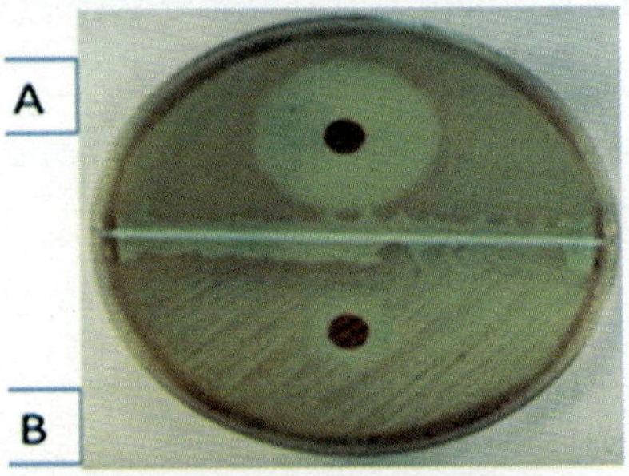

Novobiocin sensitivity testing

8. **Bacteria is cultured on blood agar and it is showing beta hemolysis followed by sensitivity to Bacitracin, identify the organism:**
   (a) Streptococcus pneumoniae
   (b) Staphylococcus aureus
   (c) Streptococcus agalactiae
   (d) Streptococcus pyogenes

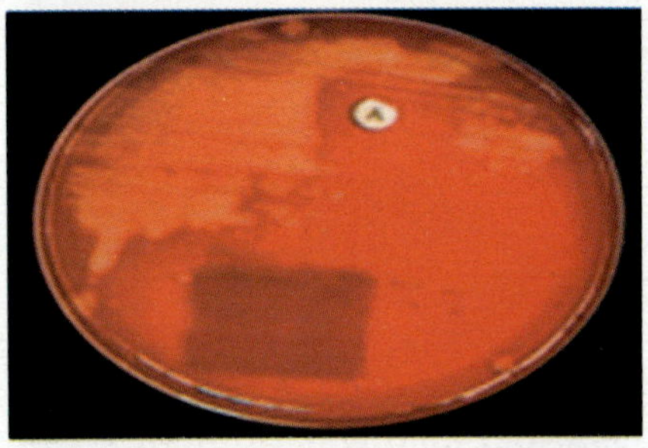

Disc A (Bacitracin) - Sensitive

9. **A seven-year-old girl presented with severe sore throat and fever up to 39 degree C for the previous three days. She denied coryza or earache. On examination she was found to have bilateral tender submandibular lymphadenopathy, enlarged tonsils pharyngeal exudates. A throat swab was taken for Gram staining and culture. The given picture shows the Gram staining of the sample collected. On the basis of Gram staining what is the probable cause of infection?**
   (a) Streptococcus pneumoniae
   (b) Staphylococcus aureus
   (c) C. diphtheriae
   (d) Streptococcus pyogenes

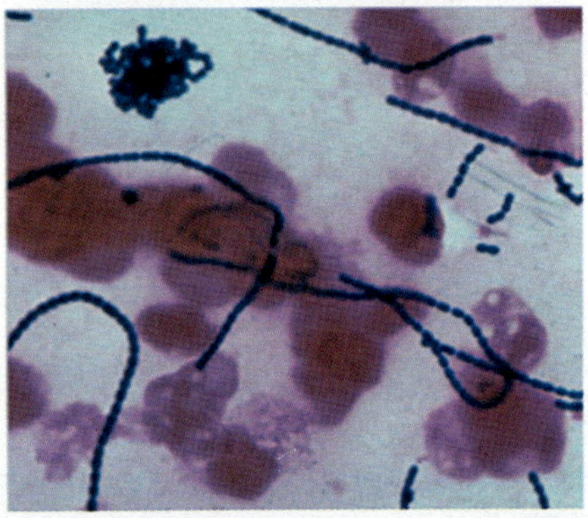

10. **Identify the test:**
    A = S. agalactiae (Arrow shaped), B = S. pyogenes
    Perpendicular streak line = S. aureus.
    (a) CAMP test
    (b) Reverse CAMP test
    (c) In vitro pathogenicity test for S. pyogenes
    (d) Demonstration of hemolytic property of S. pyogenes

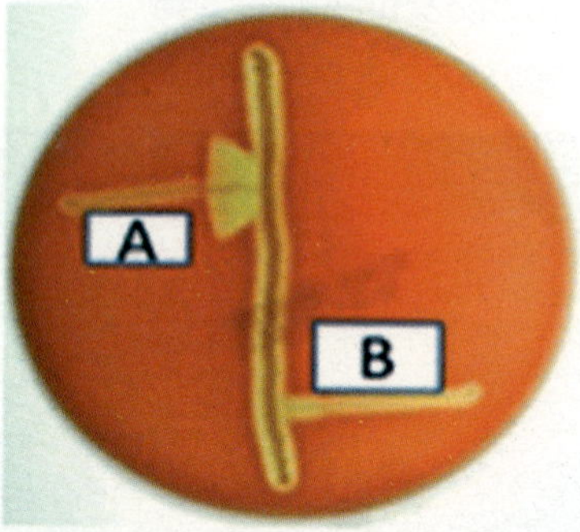

11. **A 60-year-old man was brought in with a history of high grade fever with chills and rigors for the previous two days. He also had a mild chest pain and productive cough. The sputum was submitted for investigation. X-ray chest showed consolidation in the right lower lobe. The direct smear from sputum showing this picture. On the basis of Gram staining what is the probable cause of infection?**

(a) Streptococcus pyogenes

(b) Streptococcus pneumoniae

(c) N. meningitidis

(d) Kleb. pneumoniae

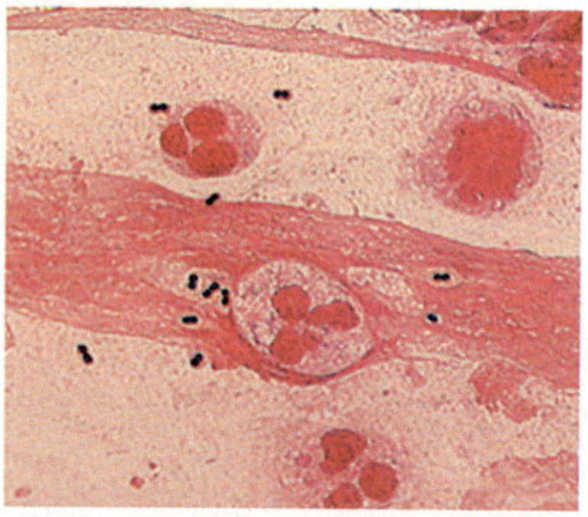

12. **Image description => Media – Blood agar, Disk – Optochin.**

Identify the bacteria on the basic of image information:

(a) Viridans streptococci (b) Enterococci

(c) Group B streptococci (d) Pneumococci

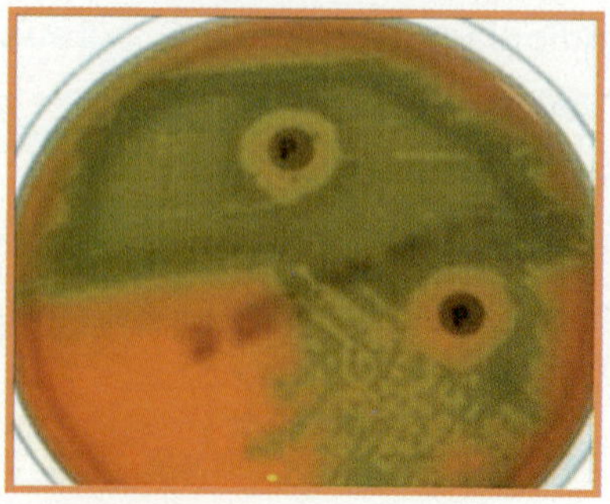

GRAM-NEGATIVE COCCI

13. **A seven-year-old boy presented to the emergency department with high-grade fever on the previous day. He complained of headache, was disoriented and had projectile vomiting. On examination, the neck rigidity was seen and kernig's sign was positive. A lumbar puncture was carried out for Gram staining, Culture, complete blood counts and serum biochemistry. Gram staining of CSF showing gram negative cocci, what would be the possible cause of infection?**

(a) E. coli

(b) Meningococcus

(c) Hemophilus

(d) Pneumococcus

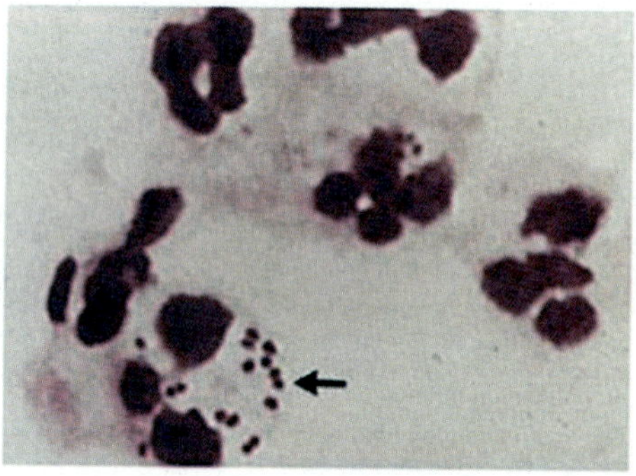

14. **A 25-year-old heterosexual male from Chandigarh came with history of dysuria and noted some pus like drainage in his underwear and at the top of his penis. He gave a history of being sexually active with five or six partners in the past 6 months. His physical examination showed yellow urethral discharge and tenderness at the tip of the penis. Gram staining of discharge showing Gram negative cocci. On the basis of Gram staining what is the probable cause of infection?**

(a) Mycoplasma hominis

(b) Ureaplasma urealyticum

(c) Gonococci

(d) Chlamydia trachomatis

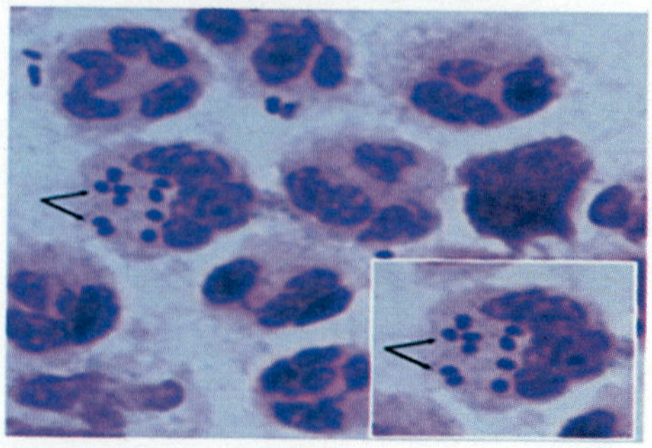

GRAM-POSITIVE BACILLI

15. **A five-year-old child presented to the pediatrics outpatient department with a history of pain in the throat and difficulty in swallowing. He had high grade fever for the previous two days. On examination, he was found to have cervical lymphadenopathy, and the tonsillar pillars were covered by a white discharge. The mother was informed that her child immunization was not complete. A throat swab was collected and submitted for microscopy and culture. Identify the staining method based on microscopic picture.**

(a) Gram staining
(b) Albert's staining
(c) Modified ZN staining
(d) McFadyean's reaction

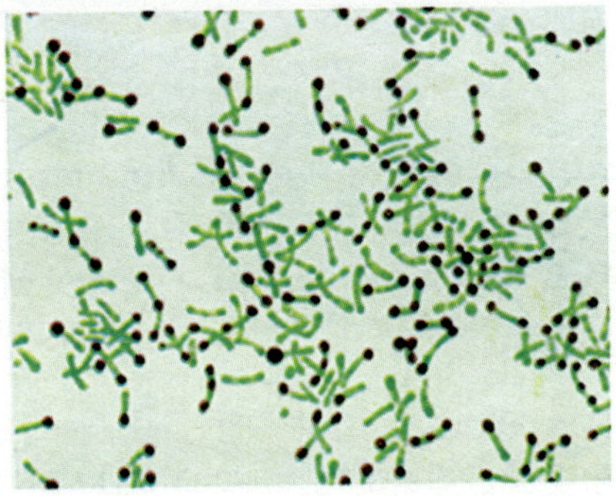

16. **Identify the test:**

(a) Cytotoxicity testing of C. diphtheriae toxin
(b) ICT for C. diphtheriae toxin
(c) Biotyping of C. diphtheriae
(d) Elek's test

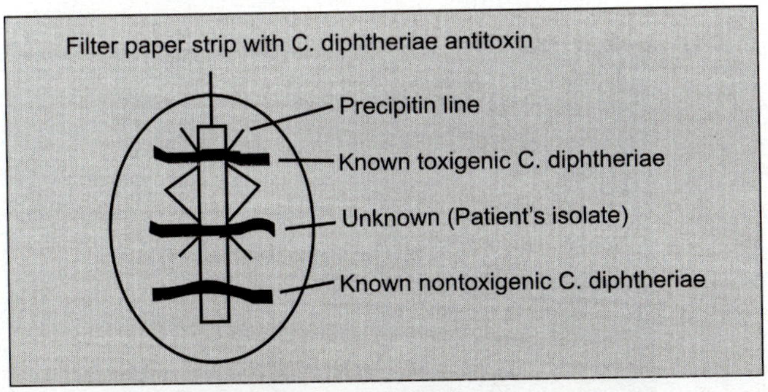

17. **Select the right combination on the basis of image:**

(a) Wilson Blair's agar – Selective media
(b) Potassium tellurite agar – Selective media
(c) XLD agar – Selective media
(d) Chocolate agar – Selective media

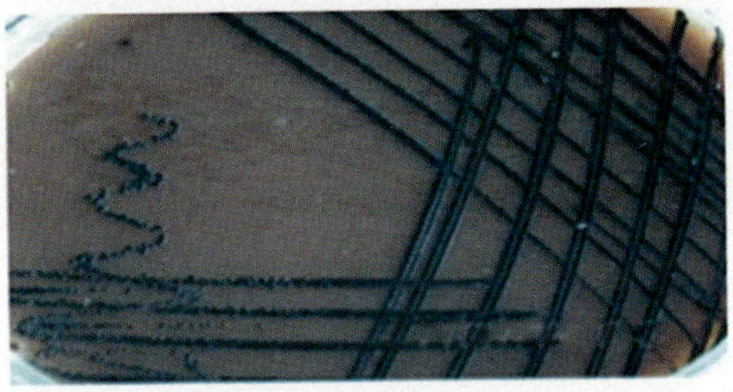

18. **Image – Loeffler's serum slope**
Select the right combination:

(a) Selective media – C. diphtheriae appears in 6-8 hours
(b) Basal media – C. diphtheriae appears in 16-18 hours
(c) Differential media – C. diphtheriae appears in 16-18 hours
(d) Enriched media – C. diphtheriae appears in 6-8 hours

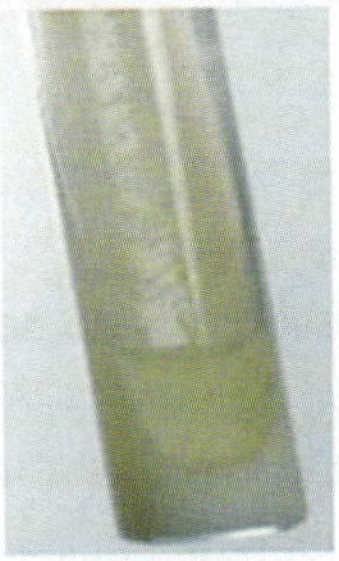

19. **A 45-year-old veterinary surgeon presented with a black eschar on the left hand. There was extensive swelling around the ulcer but it was not painful. There were few vesicular lesions surrounding the ulcer. He presented a history of injury to the hand while handling animals. What would be the presumptive diagnosis on the basis of history and culture smear of fluid from the vesicles?**

(a) Actinomycetoma
(b) Clostridium infection
(c) Cutaneous anthrax
(d) Extrapulmonary nocardiosis

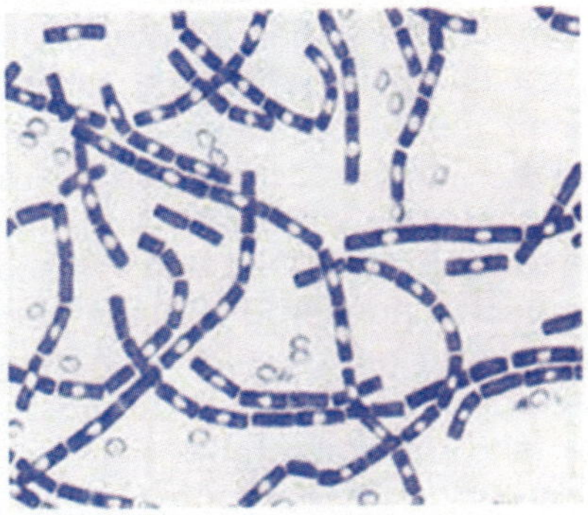

20. Identify the type of bacterial colonies on blood agar:

(a) Medusa head appearance of B. anthracis

(b) Medusa head appearance of B. cereus

(c) Greyish white frosted glass appearance of B. anthracis

(d) Greyish white frosted glass appearance of B. cereus

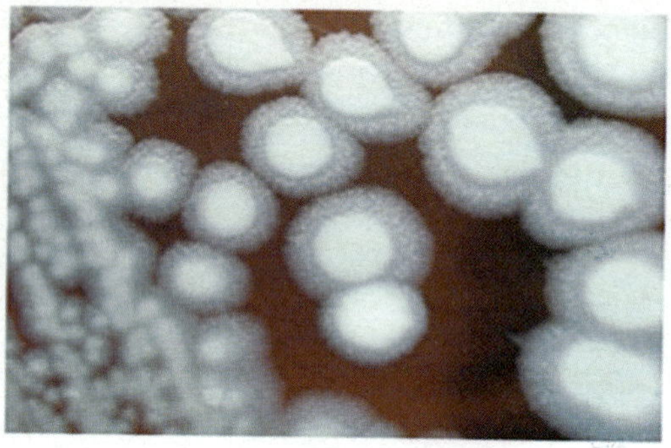

21. Identify the test:

(a) Demonstration of motility in semisolid nutrient agar

(b) Demonstration of stab culture method

(c) Gelatin liquefaction showing inverted fir tree like appearance by B. anthracis

(d) Demonstration of motility in Gelatin stab agar for B. anthracis

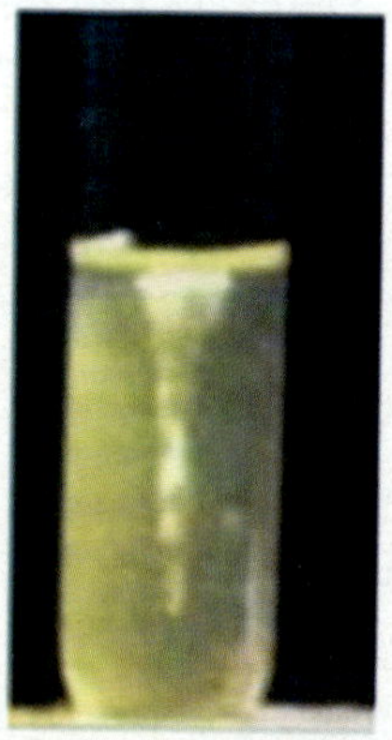

22. A 50-year-old man had a road traffic accident while travelling in a remote village area. He sustained multiple fractures with open wound in the left leg. On reaching the nearest hospital two days later, he was found to be in shock. The wound was contaminated with soil and blood; the local muscles appeared to have been crushed. He was stared on supportive therapy and antibiotics, but after two days, the edema and pain at the site increase and serious discharge developed. When the area around the wound was plated, crepitation was left. Gram staining of the wound discharge showed the presence of thick brick-shaped, Gram positive Bacilli, on the basis of microscopy what would be possible cause of infection?

(a) Clostridium histolyticum

(b) Clostridium septicum

(c) Clostridium perfringens

(d) Clostridium novyi

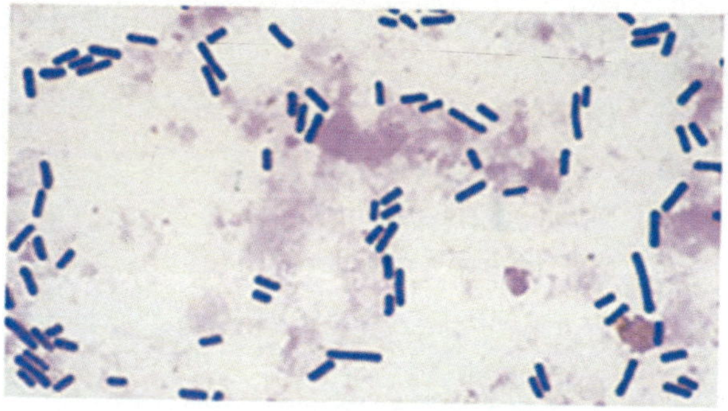

23. Choose the appropriate combination based on image description:

(a) **B** is showing Proteolytic property of Cl. perfringens and **C** is showing Saccharolytic property of Cl. tetani

(b) **B** is showing Proteolytic property of Cl. tetani and **C** is showing Saccharolytic property of Cl. perfringens

(c) **B** is showing Saccharolytic property of Cl. perfringens and **C** is showing Proteolytic property of Cl. tertium

(d) **B** is showing Saccharolytic property of Cl. perfringens and **C** is showing Proteolytic property of Cl. tetani

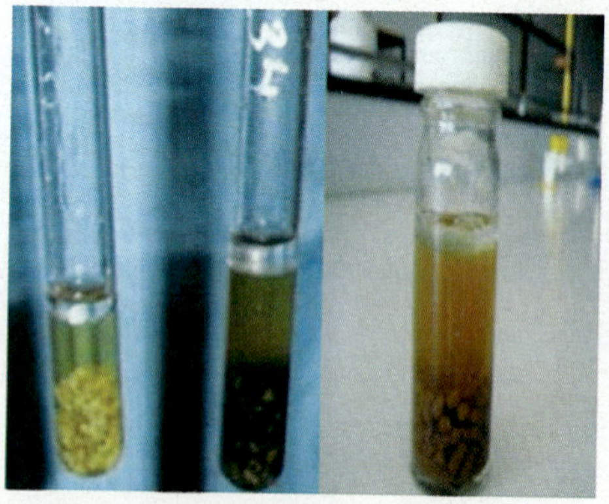

A B C

A – Uninoculated Robertson cooked meat broth
B – RCM broth turns into black color
C – RCM broth turns into pink color

24. Identify the type hemolysis and the bacteria producing it:

(a) Double zone hemolysis by Cl. tetani
(b) Target hemolysis Cl. perfringens
(c) Beta hemolysis by Cl. botulinum
(d) Incomplete hemolysis by Cl. difficile

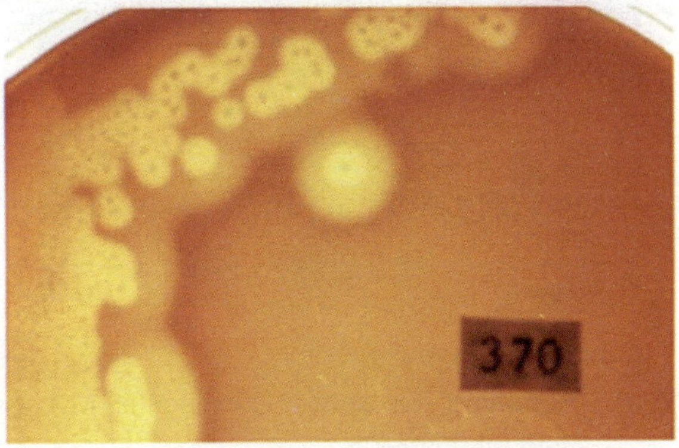

25. Identify the identification test:

(a) Litmus milk test positive for Cl. tetani
(b) Heat tolerance test for Cl. tetani
(c) Stormy clot reaction by Cl. perfringens
(d) RCM broth turns into pink color due to Saccharolytic property of Cl. perfringens

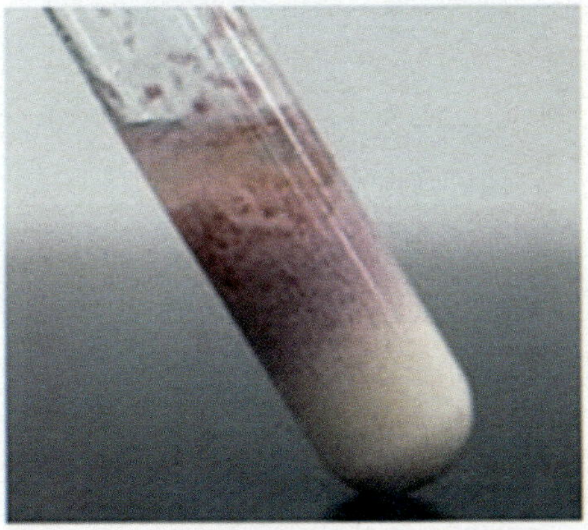

26. A = Bow tie shaped enhanced hemolysis by Cl. perfringens, B = Negative for Cl. septicum, C = Group B Streptococci (S. agalactiae).

On the basis of A, B, C – Identify the test.

(a) Reverse CAMP test
(b) CAMP test
(c) Nagler's reaction
(d) Enhanced Target hemolysis by Cl. perfringens

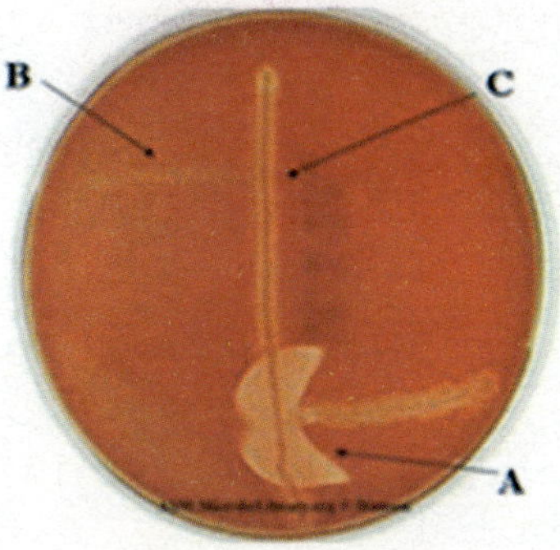

27. Identify the bacteria on the basis of gram stain:

(a) Cl. tertium having terminal spherical spores
(b) Cl. tertium having terminal oval spores
(c) Cl. tetani having terminal oval spores
(d) Cl. tetani having terminal spherical spores

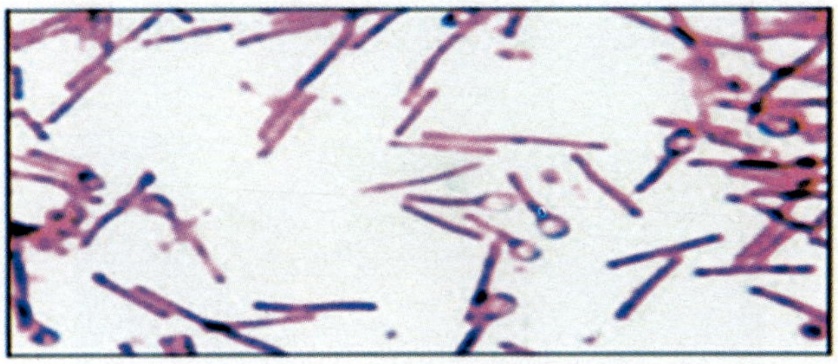

28. Three months ago, a 53-year-old woman had surgery and chemotherapy for breast cancer. Four weeks ago, she developed a cough occasionally productive of purulent sputum. About 2 weeks ago, she noted a slight but progressive weakness of her left arm and leg. On chest examination, rales were heard over the left upper back when the patient breathed deeply. Neurologic examination confirmed weakness of the left arm and leg. Chest radiography showed a left upper lobe infiltrate. Contrast enhanced computed tomography showed two lesions in the right hemisphere. Gram stain of a purulent sputum specimen showed branching Gram positive rods that were partially acid fast. Which of the following organisms is the cause of this patient's current illness?

(a) Actinomyces israelii
(b) Corynebacterium pseudodiphtheriticum
(c) Aspergillus fumigatus
(d) Nocardia
(e) Erysipelothrix rhusiopathiae

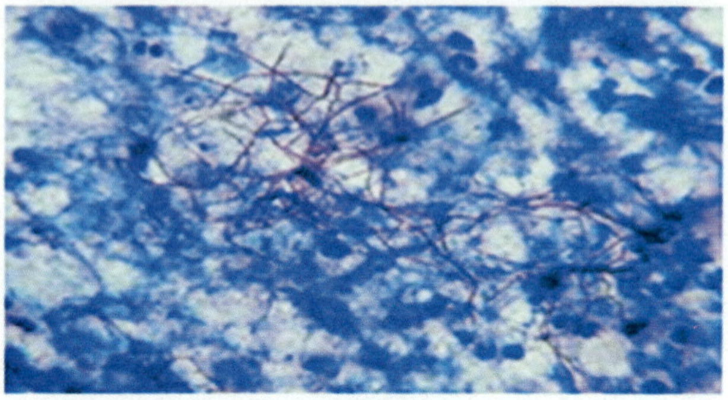

29. Identify the clinical condition:

(a) Could be Eumycetoma
(b) Could be Actinomycetoma
(c) Botryomycosis
(d) Could be one of the above

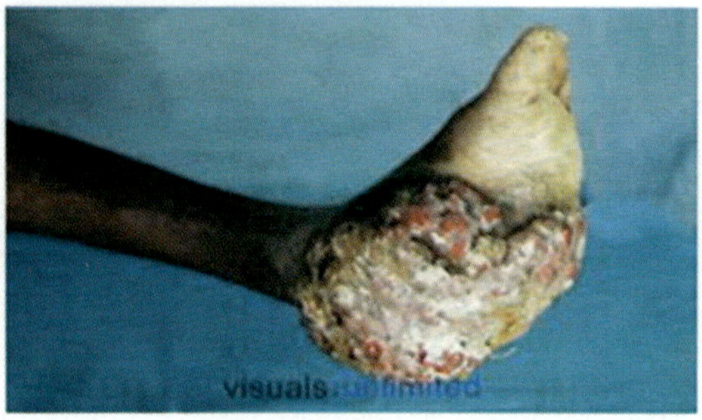

30. Image description:

Gram stain of the Gram positive bacillus Listeria monocytogenes in a blood culture. Original magnification × 1000. Red blood cells are present in the background. Listeria organisms isolated from clinical specimens frequently show variation in length and often in shape as well. Gram staining picture of Listeria resembles the Diphethroids. L. mon cytogens has a tumbling end-over-end motility at 22–28°C but not at 37°C; the motility test rapidly differentiates Listeria from diphtheroids that are members of the normal microbiota of the skin.

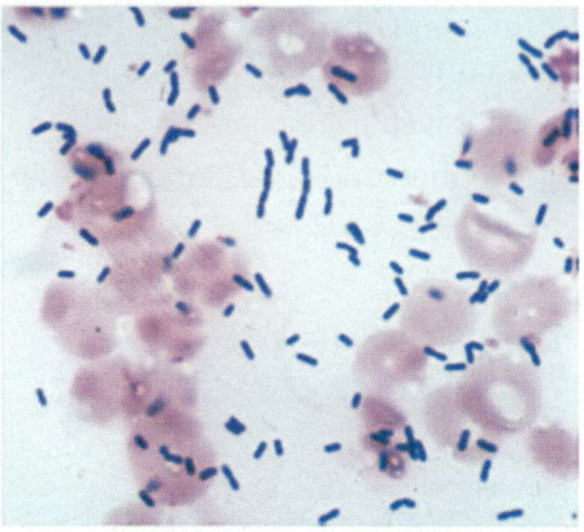

31. Choose the right combination:

(a) Gram staining – Gram negative bacilli
(b) Gram staining – Mycobacterium tuberculosis
(c) Z N staining – Mycobacterium tuberculosis
(d) Z N staining – Gram negative bacilli

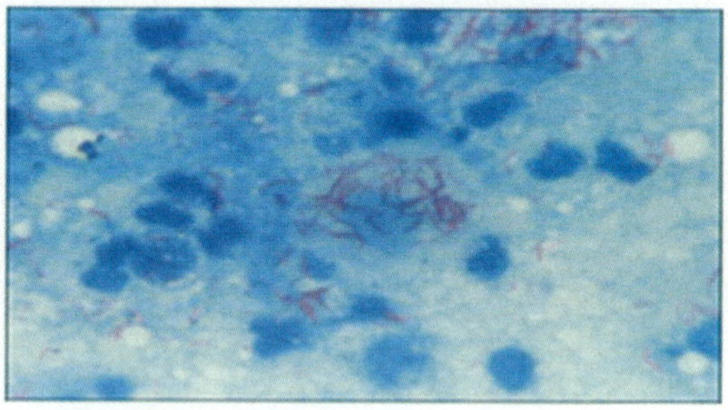

32. Identify the staining:

(a) Auramine fluorescent staining for Mycobacterium tuberculosis
(b) Modified Z. N. staining for Mycobacterium tuberculosis
(c) Cold Z. N. staining for Mycobacterium tuberculosis
(d) Auramine fluorescent staining for T. pallidum

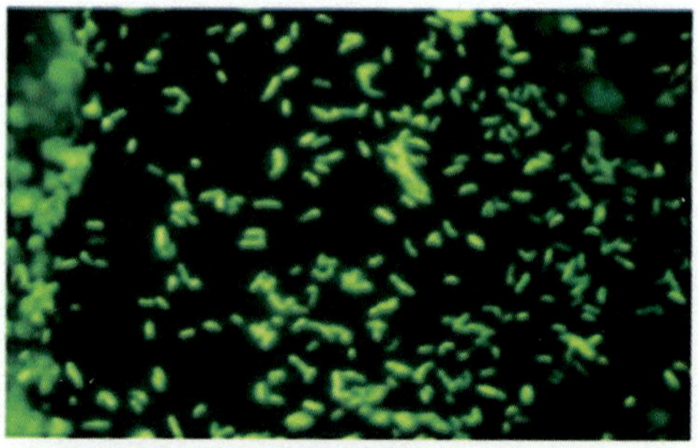

33. Identify the medium:

(a) Loeffler serum slope medium
(b) Lowenstein-Jensen medium
(c) Dorset egg slope medium
(d) Petragnami slope medium

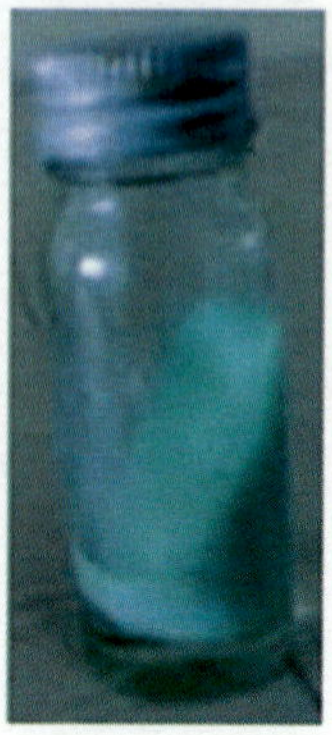

34. Identify the staining and interpret the result:

(a) Z.N. staining showing M. leprae arranged in groups in Histocytes

(b) Z.N. staining showing M. tuberculosis arranged in groups in Histocytes

(c) Modified Z.N. staining showing intracellular Nocardia

(d) Gram staining showing intracellular Klebsiella pneumoniae

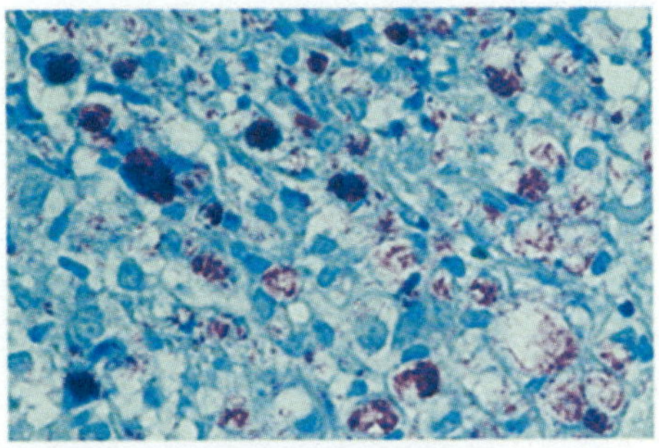

35. Identify the animal:

(a) Albino mice (b) Guinea pig

(c) Hamster (d) Nine banded armadillo

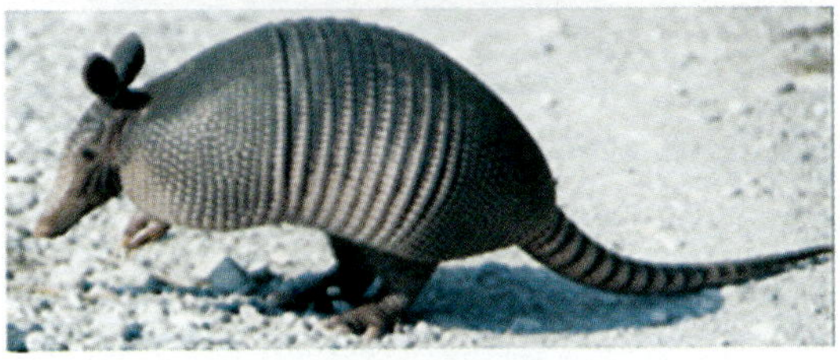

GRAM–NEGATIVE BACILLI

36. Choose the correct answer on the basis of image:

(a) Gram staining showing Gram negative cocci – Neisseria

(b) Gram staining showing Gram positive bacilli – Clostridium

(c) Negative staining for Gram negative bacilli – E. coli

(d) Gram staining of Gram negative bacilli – E. coli

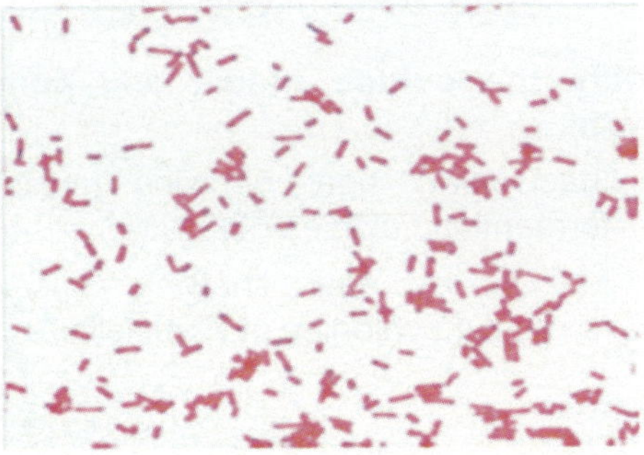

37. A 25-year-old woman consulted her family physician, complaining of frequency of urination and dysuria. Her physician advised to drink plenty of water but there was no relief. In the absence of such relief of symptoms for two days and development of fever with chills, she consulted a specialist in a hospital. Urine samples were taken and cultured on MacConkey agar after 18 hours of incubation Lactose fermenting colonies grown. Identify the causative organism.

(a) Klebsiella (b) E. coli

(c) Pseudomonas (d) Salmonella

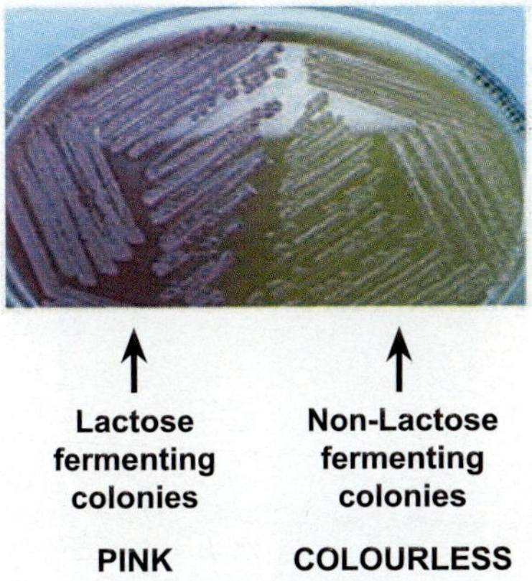

38. Which statement is not true about Indole test?

(a) Indole positive organism are E. coli, Klebsiella oxytoca, Vibrio cholerae and Proteus vulgaris

(b) Helps in identification of Gram positive bacilli

(c) Part of IMViC tests

(d) Demonstrates the presence of tryptophanase enzyme

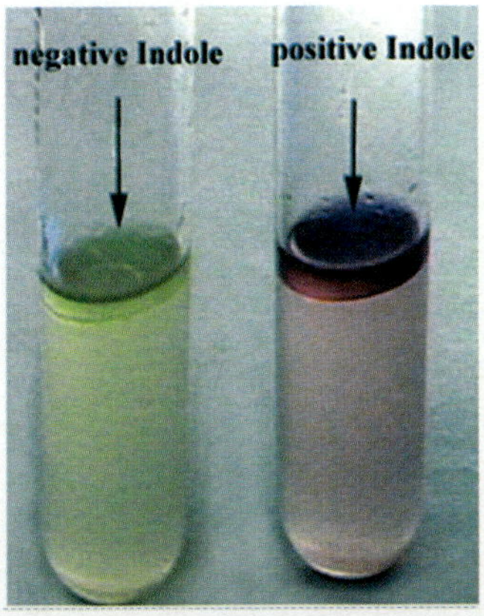

39. Identify the incorrect combination:

(a) Methyl red positive – E. coli

(b) Methyl red negative – Klebsiella

(c) Methyl red positive – Enterobacter aerogenes

(d) Methyl red negative – Hafnia

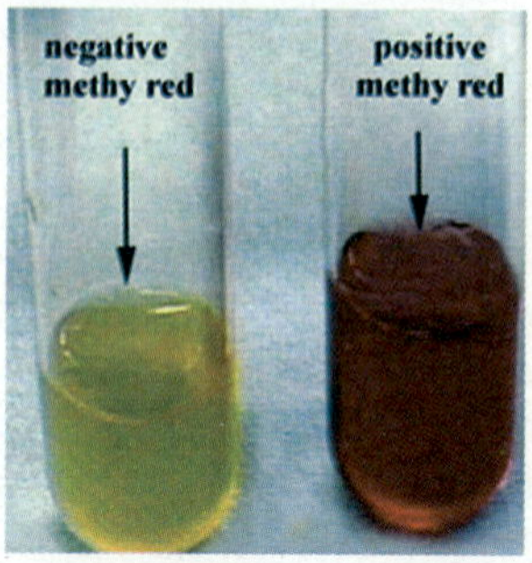

40. Which one is not true about Cystine lactose electrolyte deficient (CLED) Agar?

(a) Use for urine culture
(b) A-NLF colonies, B-LF colonies
(c) Inhibits the proteus swarming
(d) It is a selective media

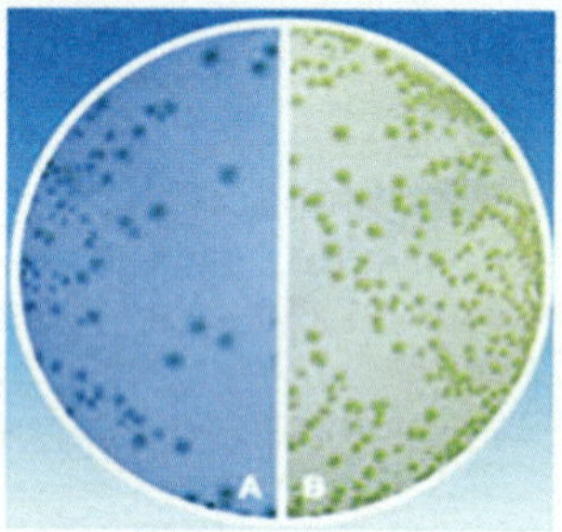

41. Identify the biochemical test and which culture method is used for it?

(a) Urea hydrolysis test by stab culture method
(b) Urea hydrolysis test by stroke culture method
(c) Citrate utilization test by stab culture method
(d) Citrate utilization test by stroke culture method

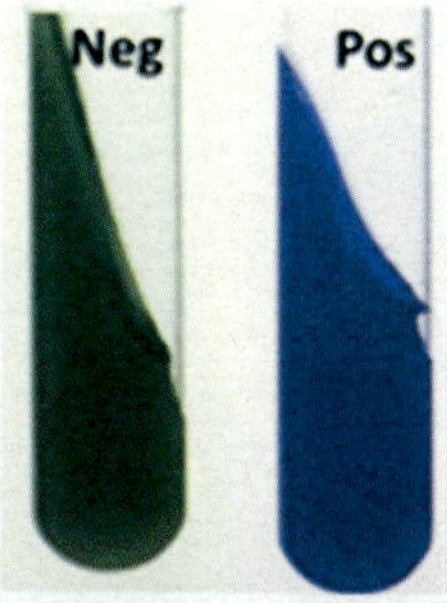

42. Identify the biochemical test and which culture method is used for it?

(a) Urea hydrolysis test by stab culture method
(b) Urea hydrolysis test by stroke culture method
(c) Citrate utilization test by stab culture method
(d) Citrate utilization test by stroke culture method

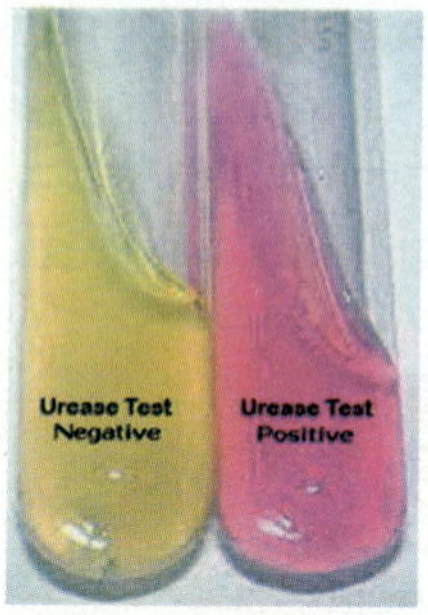

43. Identify the biochemical test:

(a) Methyl red test
(b) VP test
(c) Indole test
(d) Nitrate reduction test

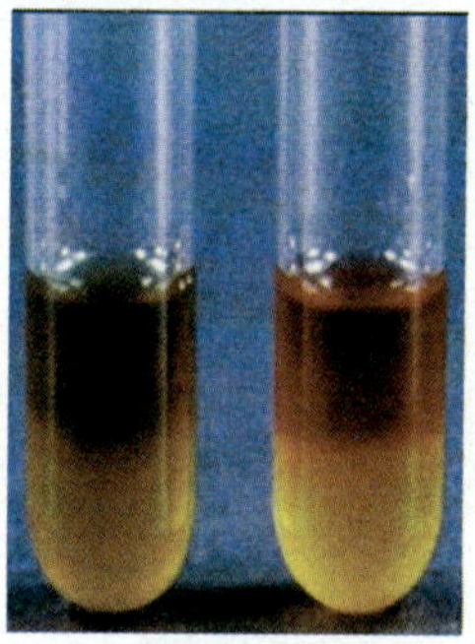

44. Identify the biochemical test:

(a) Urea hydrolysis test for different bacteria
(b) Citrate utilization test for different bacteria
(c) PPA test
(d) Triple sugar iron agar test with different reactions of bacteria

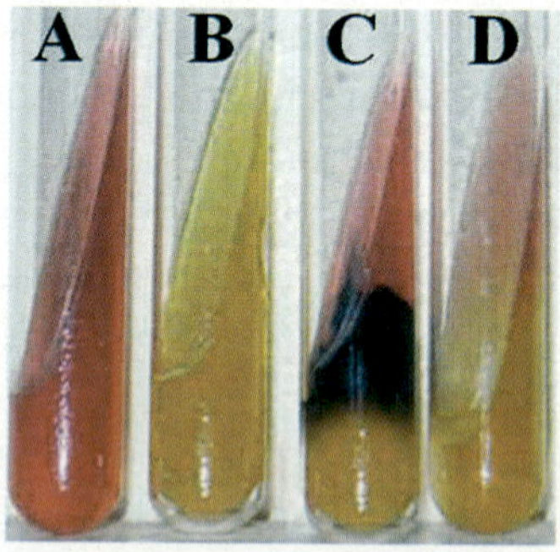

45. Identify the culture media and comment on growth:

(a) MacConkey agar showing mucoid lactose fermenting colonies of E. coli
(b) MacConkey agar showing mucoid lactose fermenting colonies of Klebsiella

(c) MacConkey agar showing non-lactose fermenting colonies of Klebsiella

(d) MacConkey agar showing non-lactose fermenting colonies of E. coli

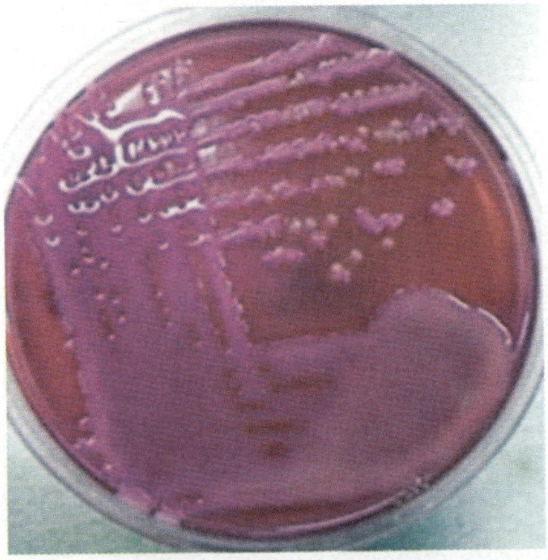

46. Identify the culture media and phenomenon:

(a) Blood agar showing Actinomycetes colonies in circular fashion

(b) Chocolate agar showing wrinkled colonies of Hemophilus influnezae

(c) Blood agar showing swarming

(d) Blood agar showing alpha hemolysis

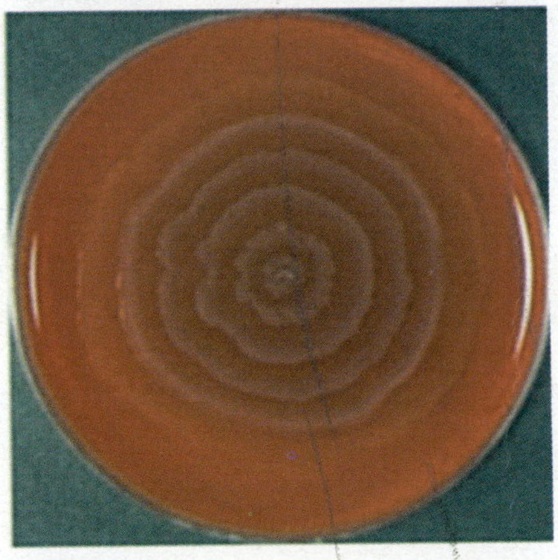

47. Choose the right statement on the basis of given media and colony characteristics:

(a) Shigella on DCA showing non lactose fermenting red colonies

(b) Shigella on XLD agar showing non lactose fermenting red colonies

(c) S. typhi on XLD agar showing red colonies with black center

(d) S. paratyphi A on XLD agar showing red colonies with black center

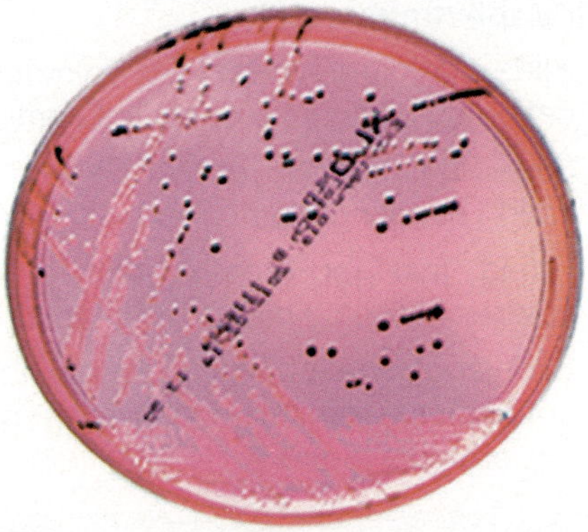

48. Choose the right statement on the basis of given media and colony characteristics:

(a) Jet black colored colonies of S. typhi on Wilson Blair's agar

(b) Jet black colored colonies of S. typhi on Deoxycholate citrate agar (DCA)

(c) Brown black colored colonies of S. typhi on Wilson Blair's agar

(d) Brown black colored colonies of S. paratyphi A on Wilson Blair's agar

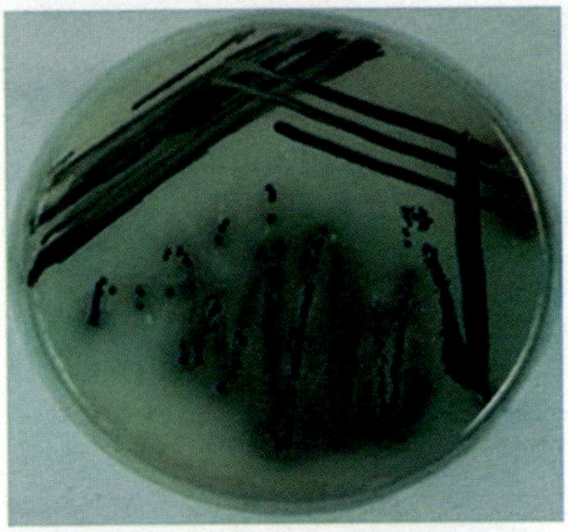

49. Identify the skin rash in typhoid:

(a) Nagayama spots (b) Koplik spots

(c) Forchheimer spots (d) Rose spots

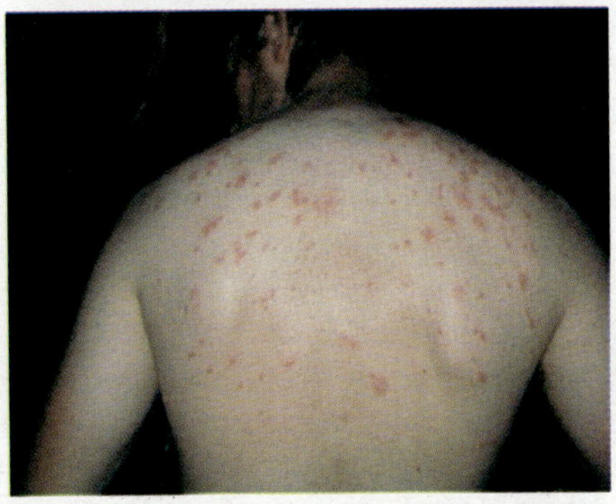

50. Identify the rapid test:

(a) Slide agglutination test for Salmonella identification by using type specific O antisera

(b) Slide agglutination test for Salmonella identification by using type specific H antisera

(c) Rapid test for identification of Salmonella species by using monoclonal antibodies

(d) Slide agglutination test for detection of H and O antibodies against H and O antigen of S. typhi, S. paratyphi A and B

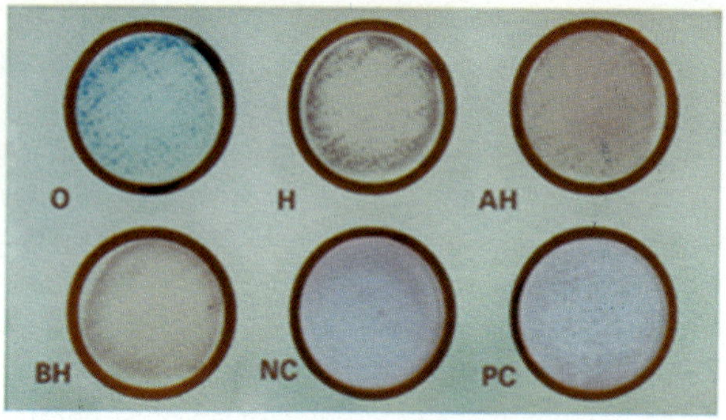

51. Identify the media and growth on it:

(a) XLD showing growth of Salmonella

(b) TCBS showing growth of Vibrio

(c) DCA showing growth of Shigella

(d) CLED showing growth of proteus

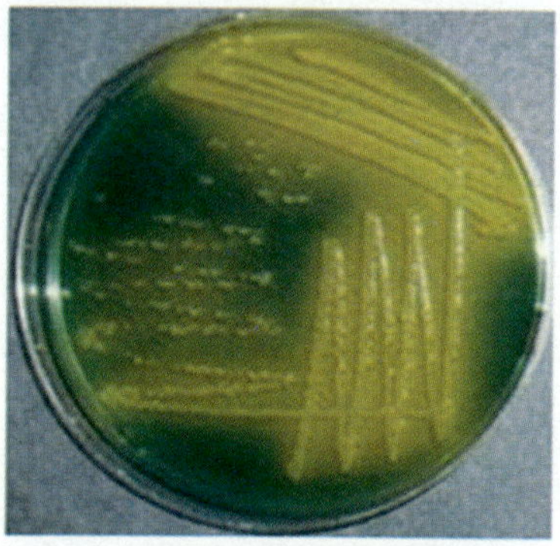

52. A10-year-old child from a suburban slum presented to the pediatric emergency departmnet during the monsoons complaining of profuse diarrhea–frequency of 10-15 times for the previous two days and vomiting 2-3 times the previous day there was no history of fever, abdominal pain and passage of blood in stools. The child complained of decreased of urine output, intense thirst and leg cramp. On examination, he was found to be moderately dehydrated. On further questioning, the family mentioned that some of the other residents of the slum were also suffering from a similar condition. The given image is stool sample of patient. What will be possible cause of infection on the basis of history and sample macroscopy?

(a) E. coli

(b) Shigella dysenteriae

(c) Vibrio cholerae

(d) Campylobacter

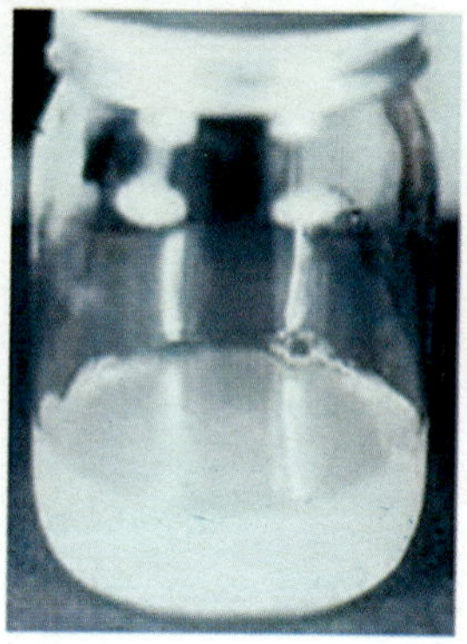

53. Identify the identification test:

(a) String test

(b) Slide coagulase test

(c) Slide catalase test

(d) Slide oxidase test

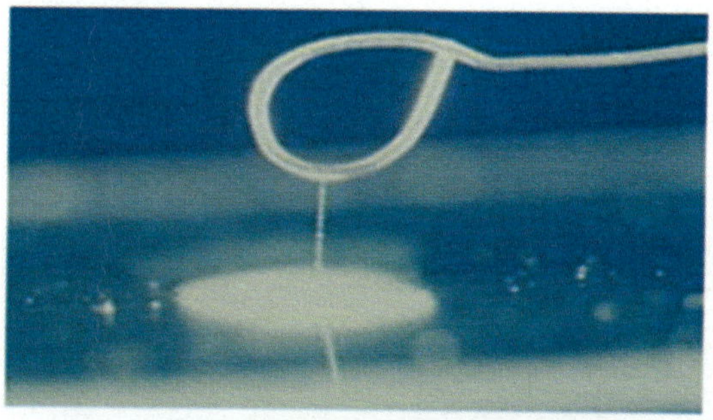

54. Identify the bacterial infection on the basis of image:

(a) Pseudomonas aeruginosa

(b) E. coli

(c) Staph aureus

(d) Strept pyogenes

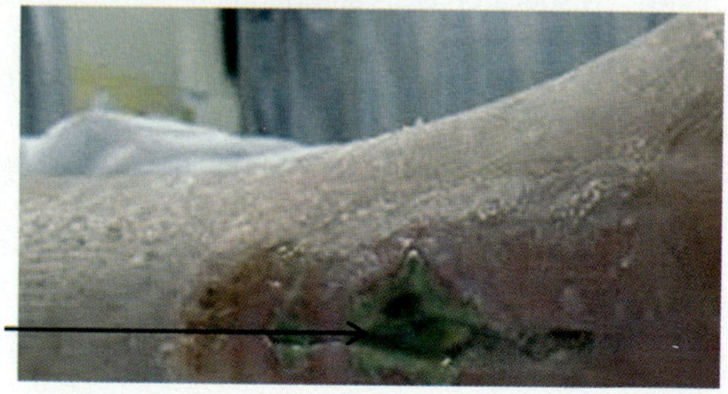

55. Pus sample came to microbiology lab to culture and sensitivity. On MHA bacteria showing pigmentation. What will be possible clinical isolate?

(a) Acinetobacter
(b) Pseudomonas
(c) Burkholderia pseudomallei
(d) Burkholderia mallei

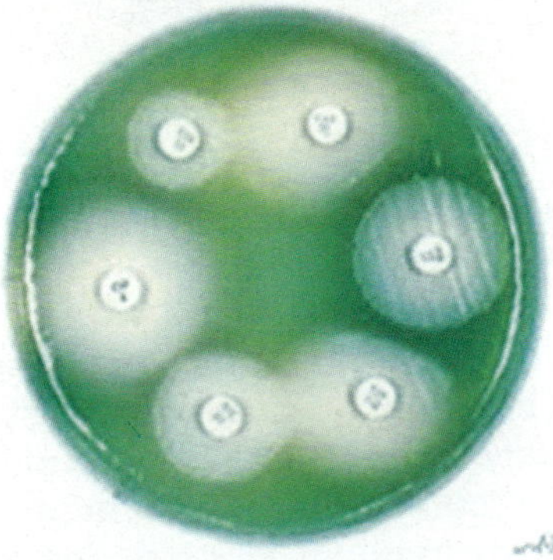

56. Oxidase test helps in identification of each bacterium except one:

(a) Brucella
(b) Vibrio
(c) Neisseria
(d) E. coli

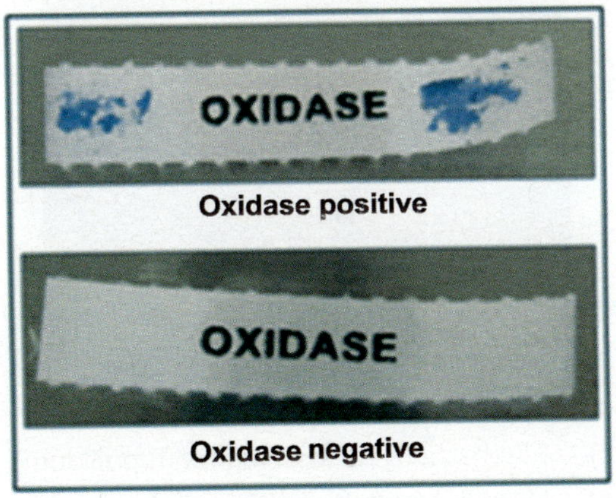

57. Identify the bacteria and staining method:

(a) Gram staining of blood showing gram positive bacilli
(b) Gram staining of blood showing gram negative bacilli
(c) Wright-Giemsa staining of blood showing blue colored bacilli stained like bipolar
(d) Gram staining of blood showing gram positive spore bearing bacilli

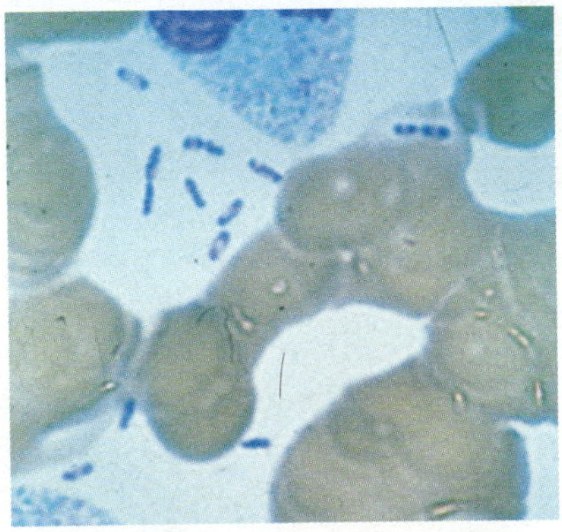

58. Identify the test:

(a) CAMP test
(b) Satellitism test
(c) Reverse CAMP test
(d) Demonstration of beta hemolysis on blood agar by Staph aureus

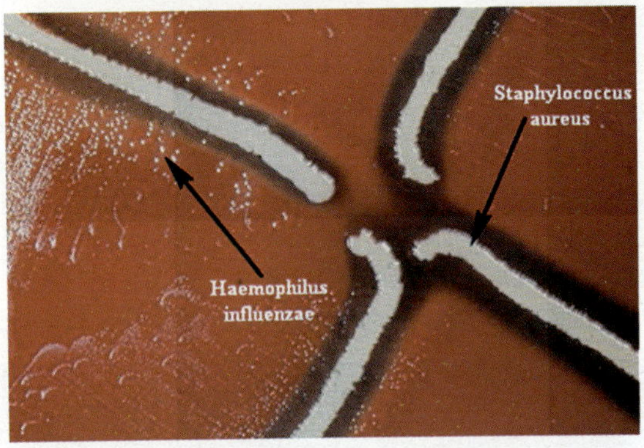

59. The lesion is painful and bleeds easily while taking the swab for gram staining. What will be the probable cause of infection?

(a) Haemophilus ducreyi
(b) Triponema pallidum
(c) HPV
(d) HSV 2

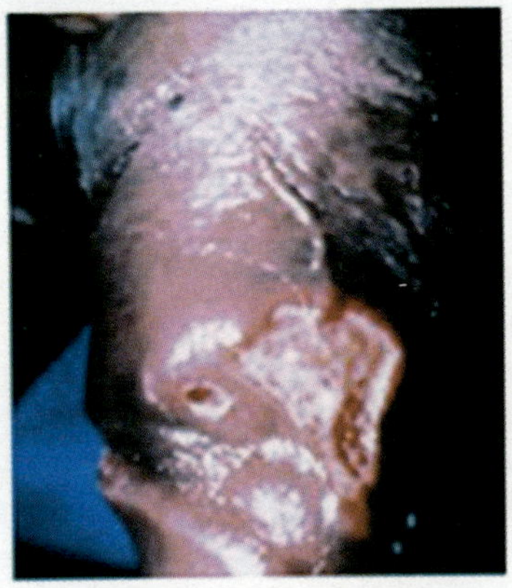

60. **Image description:**

Gram stain of Haemophilus influenzae in sputum.

The organisms are very small (0.3 × 1 μm), Gram negative coccobacilli (small arrows). The large, irregularly shaped objects (large arrow) are the nuclei of polymorphonuclear cells. Mucus is faintly stained pink in the background.

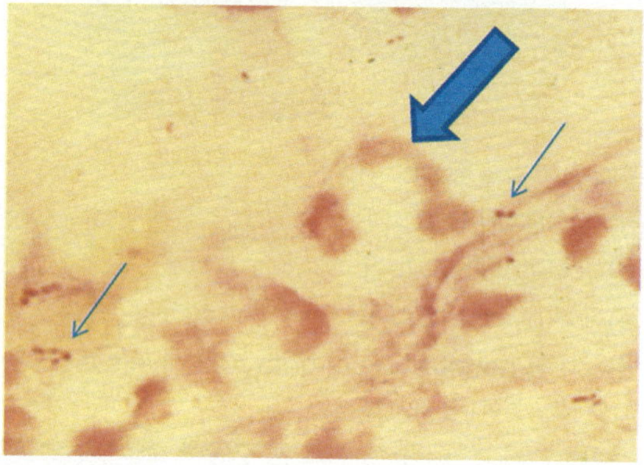

61. **Image description:**

Regan-Lowe Agar is a selective medium recommended for the isolation and cultivation of *Bordetella* spp. Mercury drop like appearance of B. pertussis on Regan-Lowe Agar.

Other selective media for B. pertussis is Bordet-Gengou medium (potato-blood-glycerol agar).

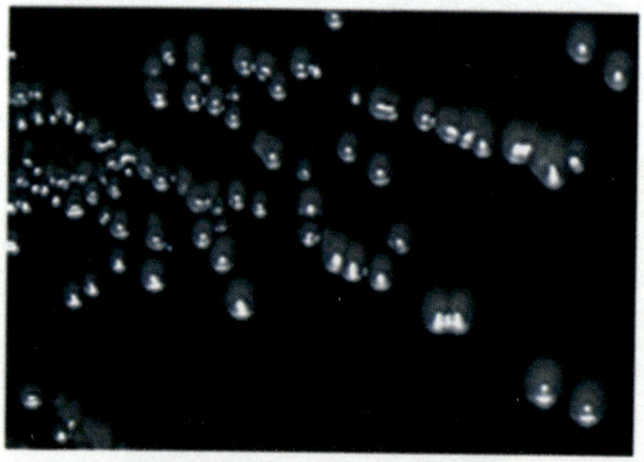

62. **Image description:**

Buffered charcoal yeast extract – Legionellae are highly fastidious and grow on complex media like BCYE with α-ketoglutarate, L-cysteine, and iron (BCYE) at a pH of 6.9, temperature of 35°C, and 90% humidity. Antibiotics can be added to make the medium selective for Legionella species. The charcoal acts as a detoxifying agent. Colonies are round with an entire edge, glistering, convex, green or pink iridescent and have speckled opalescence resembling ground glass.

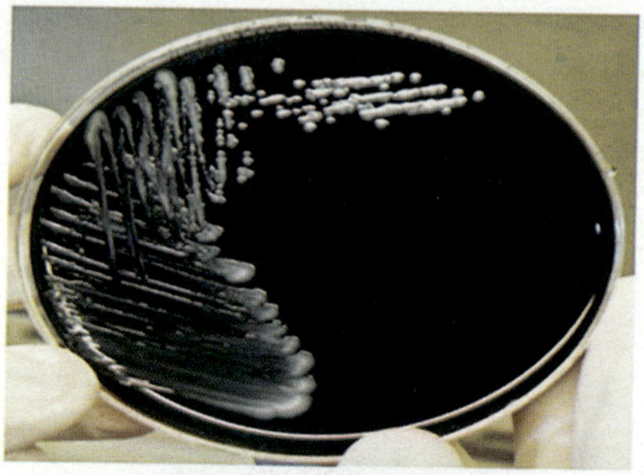

OTHER GROUPS OF BACTERIA

63. **A 20-year-old male who works as a truck driver presented to the skin and venereal disease OPD with a genital ulcer, which was painless for the last 10 days. He had unprotected sexual contact with a commercial sex worker about 2 weeks previously. On examination the ulcer was found to be circumscribed, indurated and partially healed. The inguinal lymph nodes were enlarged. What would be probable cause of infection on the basis of history and genital lesion?**

(a) HIV (b) HPV
(c) Treponema pallidum (d) HSV-2

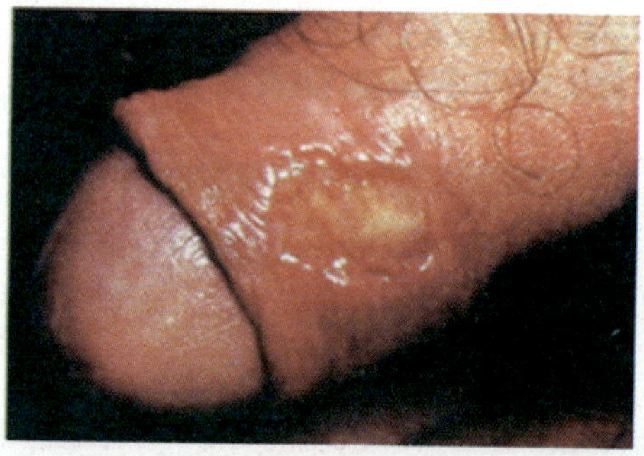

64. **Identify the bacteria with its microscopy:**

(a) Dark-field Microscopy for T. pallidum
(b) Negative staining for Borrelia
(c) Fluorescent Ab staining for T. pallidum
(d) Negative staining for T. pallidum

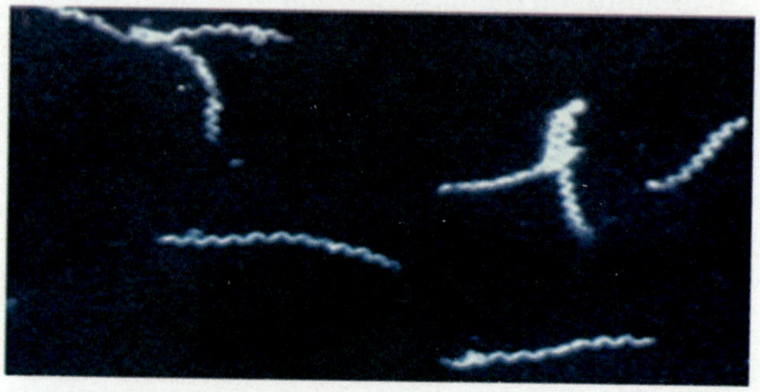

65. **Identify the staining method and microorganism:**

(a) Fluorescent staining for Mycobacterium tuberculosis

(b) Fluorescent Ab staining for T. pallidum

(c) Dark-field Microscopy for T. pallidum

(d) Dark-field Microscopy for Laptospira

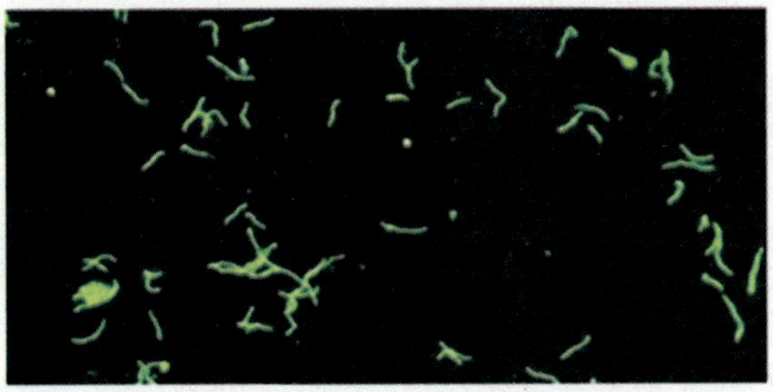

66. **Identify the staining method and microorganism:**

(a) Gram staining of T. pallidum

(b) Fluorescent Ab staining for T. pallidum

(c) Fontana (silver impregnation method) staining for T. pallidum

(d) Dark-field Microscopy for T. pallidum

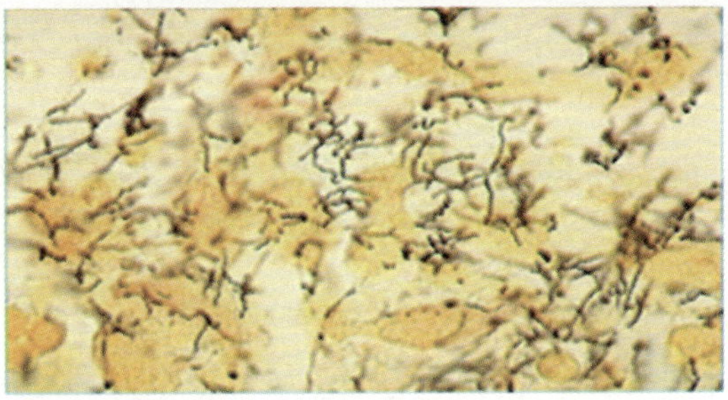

67. **Image description:**

Microscopic agglutination test (MAT) of Leptospira by using Dark-Field Microscope – Leptospirosis diagnosis is mainly based on serological tests, with the microscopic agglutination test (MAT) considered as gold standard

Principle: Antibodies in the test serum react with antigens on the surface of the bacteria and agglutinate them

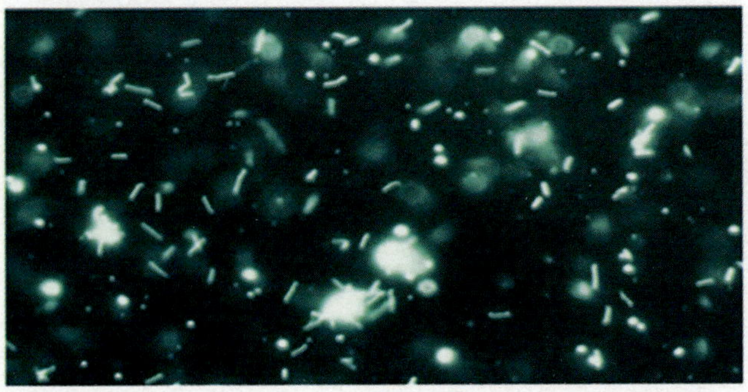

68. **Image description:**

Borreliae stain readily with bacteriologic dyes as well as with blood stains such as Giemsa stain or Wright stain. Borrelia (arrow) in a peripheral blood smear of a patient with relapsing fever. Original magnification × 1000.

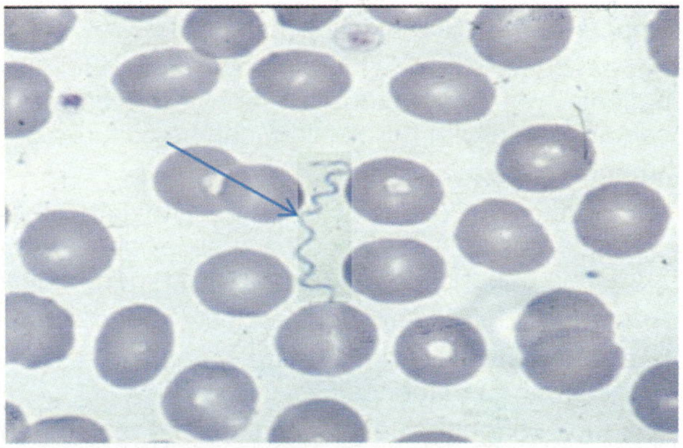

69. **Image description:**

M. bovis growing (fried egg appearance) on Mycoplasma Agar.

Other solid medium are SP-4 medium, A8 media containing urea and standard so lid medium for Mycoplasma.

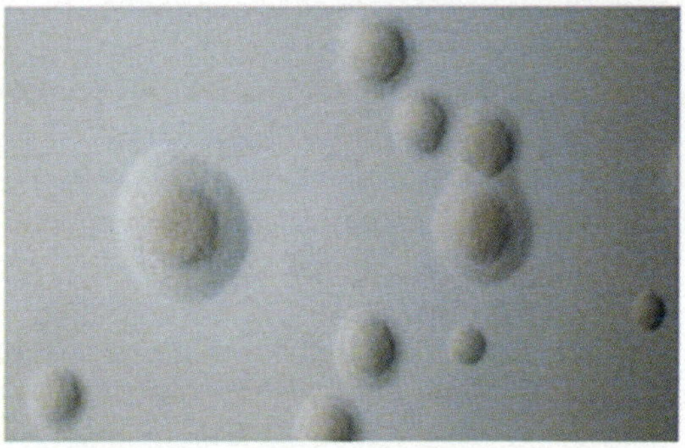

70. **Image description:**

A8 Agar containing urea. Growth of Mycoplasma is signaled by a color change indicating hydrolysis of urea.

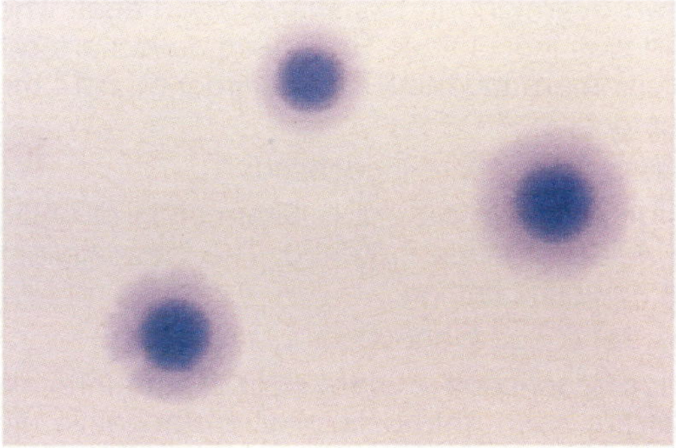

ANSWERS AND EXPLANATIONS

1. **Ans. is 'c'** i.e., Staphylococcus aureus

   Image description – Gram staining of Pus or discharge showing Gram positive cocci in clusters with numerous pus cells, suggestive of Staphylococcus aureus infection.

2. **Ans. is 'c'** i.e., Blood agar – Enrichment media – Beta hemolysis

   Image description – Blood agar showing beta hemolytic colonies of Staphylococcus aureus.

3. **Ans. is 'b'** i.e., Staphylococcus aureus

   Image description – Mannitol salt agar (Selective media) is used to screen for nasal carriers of S. aureus and patients with cystic fibrosis. Staphylococcus aureus but not other Staphylococci ferment mannitol and specimens contaminated with normal flora can be cultured on it, salt inhibits the normal flora.

4. **Ans. is 'c'** i.e., Catalase test

   Image description – This test is used to detect the presence of cytochrome oxidase enzymes. A drop of 3% hydrogen peroxide solution is placed on a slide, and a small amount of the bacterial growth is placed in the solution. The formation of bubbles (the release of oxygen) indicates a positive test result.

5. **Ans. is 'b'** i.e., Slide coagulase test (Bound coagulase test) and tube coagulase test (Free coagulase test)

   Image description – The Slide coagulase test detects bound coagulase is much simpler and usually gives results parallel with the tube test.

   The tube coagulase test detects free coagulase. When there is divergence, the tube test will be the deciding factor.

6. **Ans. is 'b'** i.e., Staph. aureus

   Image description – Staph. aureus showing golden yellow pigmented colonies on Nutrient agar. Nutrient agar is the best media to demostrate the pigment production. The pigment is believed to be a lipoprotein allied to carotene. Pigment production is enhanced by adding 1% glycerol monoacetate or milk in the media.

7. **Ans. is 'c'** i.e., Staph. saprophyticus

   Image description – Novobiocin sensitivity testing is used to identify the Staph. saprophyticus out of other Coagulase negative staphylococcus species. It causes UTI in young women.

8. **Ans. is 'd'** i.e., Streptococcus pyogenes

   Image description – Bacitracin sensitivity testing – It is an identification test of S. pyogenes. Any zone of inhibition around the disk is considered as positive, while most of the other beta hemolytic streptococci are resistant.

9. **Ans. is 'd'** i.e., Streptococcus pyogenes

   Image description – Gram staining of throat swab showing gram positive cocci (Violet color) arranged in chains with numerous pus cells suggestive of S. pyogenes according to the case.

10. **Ans. is 'a'** i.e., CAMP test

    Image description – CAMP (Christie, Atkins, Munch-Peterson) test is an identification test of group B streptococci (S. agalactiae). S. agalactiae produces phospholipase and act synergistically with beta hemolysin of S. aureus to causes an enhanced arrow shaped hemolysis at their junction on blood agar.

11. **Ans. is 'b'** i.e., Streptococcus pneumoniae

    Image description – Streptococcus pneumoniae in sputum are seen as lancet-shaped Gram positive diplococcic surrounded by clear halo (Capsule). Degenerating nuclei of polymorphonuclear cells are the large darker irregular red shapes. Mucus and amorphous debris are present in the background.

12. **Ans. is 'd'** i.e., Pneumococci

    Image description – Optochin sensitivity testing is an identification test of S. pneumoniae. The S pneumoniae were grown overnight on 5% sheep blood agar. The optochin (ethyl hydrocupreine HCl) or P disk was placed when the plate was inoculated. The pneumococci are α-hemolytic with greening of the agar around the colonies. The zone of inhibition around the P disk is larger than 14 mm, indicating that the organisms are pneumococci rather than viridans streptococci.

13. **Ans. is 'b'** i.e., Meningococcus

    Image description – It is Gram stain of CSF showing Gram negative oval cocci, arranged typically in pairs, with the adjacent sides flattened. The intracellular presence of Meningococci inside the polymorphs in CSF sample is characteristic finding.

14. **Ans. is 'c'** i.e., Gonococci

    Image description – Gram stain of a urethral exudate of a patient with gonorrhea. Nuclei of many polymorphonuclear cells are seen. Intracellular Gram negative diplococci (Neisseria gonorrhoeae) in one polymorphonuclear cell are marked by the arrow.

15. **Ans. is 'b'** i.e., Albert's staining

Image description – Albert's staining showed the presence of rod-shaped bacteria typically arranged in Chinese letter or Cuneiform (V-L shaped), green in color, along with bluish-black granules.

16. **Ans. is 'd'** i.e., Elek's test

Image description – Elek's gel precipitation test – It is a gel immunodiffusion test for demonstration of C. diphtheriae toxin in vitro. If strain produces toxin, the toxin diffuses into the agar medium and meet with the appropriate amount to antitoxin, this leads to arrow shaped precipitation band.

17. **Ans. is 'b'** i.e., Potassium tellurite agar – Selective media

Image description – Potassium Tellurite Blood Agar is a selective medium used for isolation and cultivation of Corynebacterium species. It is selective due to the presence of inhibitor and differential by means of ability of organism to reduce potassium tellurite. Potassium tellurite acts as a selective agent and has inhibitory activity against most Gram positive and Gram negative bacteria except Corynebacterium species. C.diphtheriae reduces potassium tellurite to tellurium and thereby produce gray-black coloured colonies.

18. **Ans. is 'd'** i.e., Enriched media - C. diphtheriae appears in 6-8 hours

Image description – Growth of C. diphtheriae can be detected within 6-8 hours. It also restores virulence and other identifying properties (microscopic, metachromatic granules and colonial) after they have been lost due to prolonged incubation or repeated subculturing. It is also used for demonstration of pigmentation and ascospores.

19. **Ans. is 'c'** i.e., Cutaneous Anthrax

Image description – Gram stain of culture smear of B. anthracis showing gram +ve bacilli (Bamboo stick appearance).

20. **Ans. is 'a'** i.e., Medusa head appearance of B. anthracis

Image description – Madusa head colonies of B. anthracis on Blood agar (dry wrinkled, non-hemolytic colonies).

21. **Ans. is 'c'** i.e., Gelatin liquefaction showing inverted fir tree like appearance by B. anthracis

Image description – Gelatin stab agar – B. anthracis grows as inverted fir tree appearance.

22. **Ans. is 'c'** i.e., Clostridium perfringens

Image description – Gram positive bacilli with characteristic feature of boxcar shaped, thick and stubby. Clostridium perfringens typically does not form spores when grown on laboratory media.

23. **Ans. is 'b'** i.e., **B** is showing Proteolytic property of Cl. tetani and **C** is showing Saccharolytic property of Cl. perfringens

Image description – A is uninoculated RCM broth (Anaerobic media). **B** is showing Proteolytic property (RCM turns to Black) of Cl. tetani and **C** is showing Saccharolytic property (RCM turns to pink) of Cl. perfringens.

Other clostridium species having Proteolytic and Saccharolytic property:

Proteolytic Clostridia – C. botulinum A, B and F.

Saccharolytic Clostridia – C. difficile, C. botulinum C, D and F.

24. **Ans. is 'b'** i.e., Target hemolysis Cl. perfringens

Image description – Target hemolysis (double zone hemolysis) is specifically produced by Cl. perfringens on blood agar. Inner zone (complete hemolysis) is produced by θ toxin and outer zone (incomplete hemolysis) is produced by α toxin.

25. **Ans. is 'c'** i.e., Stormy clot reaction by Cl. perfringens

Image description – It's an identification test for Cl. perfringens. In litmus milk test, lactose fermentation leads to the formation of acid which lowers the pH followed by color change of litmus milk from blue to red. The acid coagulates the casein and clotted milk is disrupted due to vigorous gas production.

26. **Ans. is 'a'** i.e., Reverse CAMP test

Image description – The Reverse CAMP test is used to identify C. perfringens, in this test C. perfringens is streaked over the centre of the plate. Strept. agalactiae is streaked at right angle to it. A positive test shows the presence of an arrow shaped zone of enhanced hemolysis towards C. perfringens.

27. **Ans. is 'd'** i.e., Cl. tetani having terminal spherical spores

Image description – Spores of C. tetani are spherical, terminal, bulging and drumstick appearance.

28. **Ans. is 'd'** i.e., Nocardia

Hint one is involvement of right hemisphere as we know, in extrapulmonary nocardiosis most common infection is **Brain abscess.**

Hint two is branching Gram positive rods with acid fastness is suggestive of Nocardia infection.

Image description – Modified acid-fast (0.5-1% H_2SO_4) staining of sample showing branching filamentous red colored acid fast bacilli.

29. Ans. is 'd' i.e., Could be one of above

On the basis of image information you cannot differentiate between all these three as clinically Mycetoma and Botryomycosis resembles to each other closely.

Image description – Mycetoma of foot

31. Ans. is 'c' i.e., Z.N. staining – Mycobacterium tuberculosis

Image description – Z.N. staining of smear showing long slender, beaded, red colored acid fast bacilli with numerous pus cells against blue background.

32. Ans. is 'a' i.e., Auramine fluorescent staining for Mycobacterium tuberculosis

Image description – Auramine fluorescent staining of sputum showing bright brilliant green Mycobacterium tuberculosis against dark black background.

33. Ans. is 'b' i.e., Lowenstein-Jensen medium

Image description – Lowenstein-Jensen medium is a selective medium (consists Malachite green as selective agent) and used for isolation of Mycobacterium species. M. tuberculosis produces rough, tough and buff colored colonies whereas M. bovis produces smooth, moist and white colored colonies on LJ medium.

34. Ans. is 'a' i.e., Z.N. staining showing M. leprae arranged in groups in Histocytes

Image description – Z.N. staining (5% H_2SO_4) – Slit skin smear – AFB arranged in groups (cigar like bundles) to from globi (AFB in Histocytes). The globi are present inside the foamy macrophages called Virchow's lepra cells or Foamy cells.

35. Ans. is 'd' i.e., Nine banded armadillo

Image description – M. leprae cannot be culture either on artificial media or in tissue culture. It can be culture in nine banded armadillo and foot pad of mice.

36. Ans. is 'd' i.e., Gram staining of Gram negative bacilli – E. coli

Image description – Gram staining of E. coli from pure culture.

37. Ans. is 'b' i.e., E. coli

Image description – MacConkey agar showing lactose fermenting pink colored non mucoid colonies and non-lactose fermenting pale colored colonies.

Hint one – Non mucoid, lactose fermenting pink colored colonies.

Hint two – Most common cause of UTI is E. coli.

38. Ans. is 'b' i.e., Helps in identification of Gram positive bacilli

Image description – Indole test is used to determine the ability of an organism to split amino acid tryptophan to form the compound indole. Tryptophan is hydrolysed by **tryptophanase** to produce three possible end products – one of which is indole. Indole production is detected by Kovac's or Ehrlich's reagent which contains **4 (p)-dimethylamino benzaldehyde**, this reacts with indole to produce a red coloured compound. Indole Test Reaction Indole test is a commonly used biochemical test (e.g., in IMVIC test, SIM test etc). Indole test helps to differentiate members of **Enterobacteriaceae** and other genera.

39. Ans. is 'c' i.e., Methyl red positive – Enterobacter Aerogenes

Image description – The Methyl Red test involves adding the pH indicator methyl red to an inoculated tube of MR-VP broth. If the organism uses the mixed acid fermentation pathway and produces stable acidic end-products, the acids will overcome the buffers in the medium and produce an acidic environment in the medium. When methyl red is added, if acidic end products are present, the methyl red will stay red.

Methyl red positive Bacteria – Except Hafnia, Enterobacter, Serratia and Klebsiella all member of family **Enterobacteriaceae** are positive for MR test.

Methyl red negative bacteria – Hafnia, Enterobacter, Serratia and Klebsiella.

40. Ans. is 'd' i.e., It is a selective media

Image description – CLED Agar is a differential medium and used for urine culture. It also inhibits the proteus swarming and L-cystine supports the growth of cysteine dependent dwarf coliform colonies of coliforms.

41. Ans. is 'd' i.e., Citrate utilization test by stroke culture method

Image description – The Citrate Utilization test is used to identify bacteria which utilize as one of their starting products of metabolism a compound called citrate (ionized form of citric acid). As citrate is utilized from the media by the bacteria, the pH of the medium changes. As the pH becomes more alkaline, the media changes from green to blue (alkaline). The blue color change is the result: blue is positive, green is negative.

Citrate positive – Citrobacter, Klebsiella, Enterobacter, Proteus etc.

Citrate negative – E. coli, Shigella, Morgenella etc.

42. Ans. is 'b' i.e., Urea hydrolysis test by stroke culture method

Image description – Urea is a diamide of carbonic acid. It is hydrolyzed with the release of ammonia and carbon dioxide. Many organisms especially those that infect the urinary tract, have a urease enzyme which is able to split urea in the presence of water to release ammonia and carbon dioxide. The ammonia combines with carbon dioxide and water to form ammonium carbonate which turns the medium alkaline, turning the indicator phenol red from its original orange yellow color to bright pink.

Urease positive – Helicobacter pylori, **P**roteus spp, **U**reaplasma, **C**ryptococcus spp, **C**orynebacterium spp, Yersinia spp, **N**ocardia, Brucella spp etc.

Mneomonics to remember urease positive organisms**: PUNCH.**

43. Ans. is 'b' i.e., VP test

Image description – Voges-Proskauer Test – The Voges-Proskauer (VP) test is used to determine if an organism produces acetylmethyl carbinol from glucose fermentation. If present, acetylmethyl carbinol is converted to diacetyl in the presence of α-naphthol, strong alkali (40% KOH), and atmospheric oxygen. The α-naphthol was not part of the original procedure but was found to act as a color intensifier by Barritt and must be added first. The diacetyl and quanidine-containing compounds found in the peptones of the broth then condense to form a pinkish red polymer.

VP positive – Hafnia, Serratia, Enterobacter, Klebsiella (HESK).

VP negative – Except HECK all memner of Enterobacteriaceae family.

44. Ans. is 'd' i.e., Triple sugar iron agar test with different reactions of bacteria

Image description – Triple sugar iron agar (TSI) is a differential medium that contains lactose, sucrose, a small amount of glucose (dextrose), ferrous sulfate, and the pH indicator phenol red. It is used to differentiate enterics based on the ability to reduce sulfur and ferment carbohydrates.

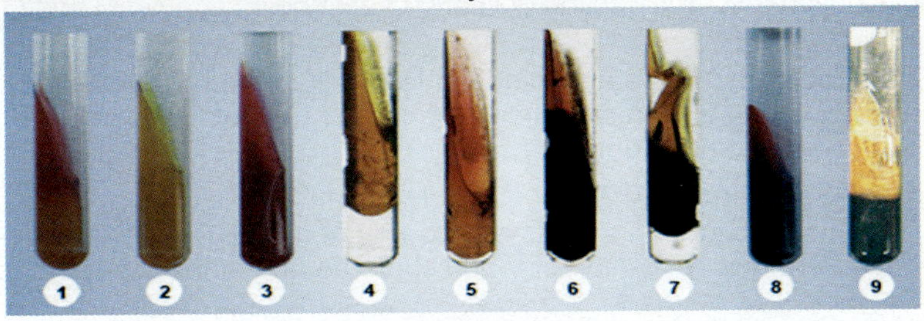

Result (slant/butt)	Symbol	Interpretation
1. Red/Yellow	K/A	Glucose fermentation only, peptone catabolized.
2. Yellow/Yellow	A/A	Glucose and lactose and/or sucrose fermentation.
3. Red/Red	K/K	No fermentation, Peptone catabolized.
4. Yellow/Yellow with bubbles	A/A,G	Glucose and lactose and/or sucrose fermentation, Gas produced.
5. Red/Yellow with bubbles	K/A,G	Glucose fermentation only, Gas produced.
6. Red/Yellow with bubbles and black precipitate	K/A,G,H_2S	Glucose fermentation only, Gas produced, H_2S produced.
7. Yellow/Yellow with bubbles and black precipitate	A/A,G, H_2S	Glucose and lactose and/or sucrose fermentation, Gas produced, H_2S produced.
8. Red/Yellow with black precipitate	K/A, H_2S	Glucose fermentation only, H_2S produced.
9. Yellow/Yellow with black precipitate	A/A, H_2S	Glucose and lactose and/or sucrose fermentation, H_2S produced.

45. Ans. is 'b' i.e., MacConkey agar showing mucoid lactose fermenting colonies of Klebsiella

Image description – MacConkey agar with LF mucoid colonies of K. pneumoniae. Klebsiella possess capsule because of which it produces mucoid colonies.

Type – Differential/Indicator media.

Sterilization – Autocalving.

Use – Diffentiate lactose fermentating colonies from non-lactose lactose fermentating colonies.

46. Ans. is 'c' i.e., Blood agar showing swarming

Image description – Blood agar with swarming of proteus.

Swarming – Growth of the bacteria in concentric circles beyond the line of inoculation.

It is the one of the type of motility which is shown by Proteus, Cl. tetani.

47. Ans. is 'c' i.e., S. typhi on XLD agar showing red colonies with black center

Image description – Xylose Lysine Deoxycholate (XLD) Agar is a selective medium for the isolation of Salmonella and Shigella spp from clinical specimens and food samples. Non lactose fermenting colonies appears pale (Shigella species) and lactose fermenting colonies appears pink in color. It also has H_2S indicator system, consisting of sodium thiosulphate and ferric ammonium citrate, is included for the visualization of hydrogen sulphide produced, resulting in the formation of colonies with black centers. H_2S producing Salmonella (S. typhi and paratyphi B) will appear like pale colored colonies with black center.

48. Ans. is 'a' i.e., Jet black colored colonies of S. typhi on Wilson Blair's agar

Image description – Wilson Blair's agar is a selective medium. It is particularly valuable for the isolation of S. Typhi from heavily contaminated specimens. The medium is highly selective for Salmonella, being inhibitory to coliforms, Proteus and Shigella; occasional strains of coliforms grow to form dull green or brown colonies, but without a surrounding metallic sheen. Ferrous sulphate is reduced by Salmonella species in presence of bismuth sulphite and dextrose to form iron sulphide, indicated by jet black coloured colonies with a metallic sheen.

49. Ans. is 'd' i.e., Rose spots

Image description – At approximately the end of the first week of Typhoid illness, the fever plateaus at 103-104°F (39-40°C). The patient develops rose spots, which are salmon-colored, blanching, truncal, maculopapules usually 1-4 cm wide and fewer than 5 in number; these generally resolve within 2-5 days. These are bacterial emboli to the dermis and occasionally develop in persons with shigellosis or non-typhoidal salmonellosis. Rose spots, usually on the skin of the abdomen or chest, are seen briefly in rare cases.

50. Ans. is 'd' i.e., Slide agglutination test for detection of H and O antibodies against H and O antigen of S. typhi, S. paratyphi A and B

Image description – Slide Widal test (Slide agglutination test) – It is a qualitative slide Widal test, showing agglutination in O and H antigen of S. typhi. Serum sample will be further test for quantitative slide Widal test for estimation of antibodies titre against S. typhi O and H antigens.

51. Ans. is 'b' i.e., TCBS showing growth of Vibrio

Image description – Thiosulfate-citrate-bile salts-sucrose agar (TCBS) – It is a selective media and recommended for the selective isolation and cultivation of Vibrio cholerae and other enteropathogenic Vibrio's causing food poisoning.

Sucrose fermenting Vibrio (V. cholerae) produces yellow colored colonies whereas sucrose non-fermenting Vibrio (V. mimicus, V. parahemolyticus) produce green colored colonies on TCBS.

52. Ans. is 'c' i.e., Vibrio cholerae

Image description – Rice watery stool

Diarrhea – Cholera-related diarrhea comes on suddenly and may quickly cause dangerous fluid loss – as much as a quart (about 1 liter) an hour. Diarrhea due to cholera often has a pale, milky appearance that resembles water in which rice has been rinsed (rice-water stool).

Complained of decreased of urine output, intense thirst and leg cramp are the classic presentation of cholera.

53. Ans. is 'a' i.e., String test

Image description – String test for the identification of Vibrio cholerae – If the result is positive, the bacterial cells will be lysed by the sodium deoxycholate or sodium taurocholate, the suspension will lose turbidity, and DNA will be released from the lysed cells causing the mixture to become viscous. A mucoid "string" is formed when an inoculating loop is drawn slowly away from the suspension.

String test is used to differentiate Vibrio cholerae (string test positive) from other Vibrio spp. (string test negative).

54. Ans. is 'a' i.e., Pseudomonas aeruginosa

Image description – Bluish green pus discharge due to pigment (Pyocyanin) production in Pseudomonas infection.

55. Ans. is 'b' i.e., Pseudomonas

Image description – Pseudomonas isolate produced pigment on MHA.

56. Ans. is 'd' i.e., E. coli

Image description – The oxidase test is used to identify bacteria that produce cytochrome C oxidase, an enzyme of the bacterial electron transport chain. When present, the cytochrome C oxidase oxidizes the reagent (tetramethyl-p-phenylenediamine) to (indophenols) purple color end product. When the enzyme is not present, the reagent remains reduced and is colorless.

Oxidase positive bacteria – Mnemonics for Oxidase Positive Organisms – PVNCH (It's just an acronyms inspired by the famous mnemonic for Urease Positive organisms–PUNCH) – **P:** Pseudomonas spp, **V:** Vibrio cholerae, **N:** Neisseria spp, **C:** Campylobacter spp, **H:** Helicobacter spp/Haemophilus spp, Aeromonas spp and Alcaligens.

57. Ans. is 'c' i.e., Wright-Giemsa staining of blood showing blue colored bacilli stained like bipolar

Image description – Polychromatic differential stains such as Wayson and Wright-Giemsa provide contrast staining so that bacteria, tissue, and blood cell components are easily seen. Basic fuchsin and methylene blue in the Wayson stain bind to the bacterial cells which, upon staining, **appear as pink-blue cells with granules at end of the cell, thus making the cell look like a closed safety pin** (hairpin-like appearance). Wright-Giemsa stain, typically used in clinical laboratories for differentiating blood cell types, binds to Y. pestis cells in much the same way as methylene blue, yielding bipolar-staining Y. pestis cells. This differential polychromatic appearance can be seen with different types of organisms; therefore, Wayson stain alone is not diagnostic for Y. pestis.

Gram staining of blood showing Gram negative, bipolar-staining bacilli →

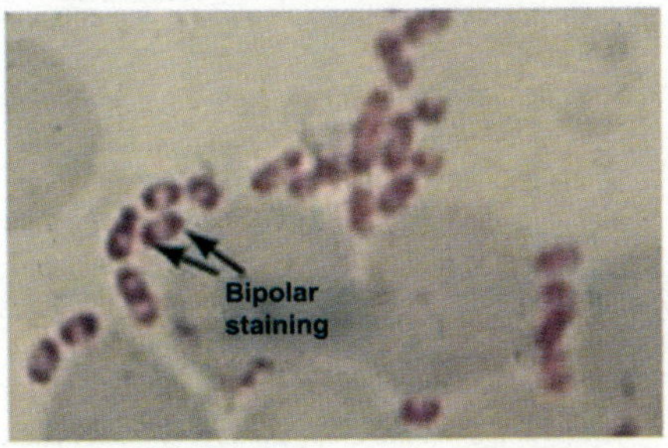

58. Ans. is 'b' i.e., Satellitism test

Image description – Satellitism test – Most strains of Haemophilus spp does not grow on 5% Sheep Blood Agar, which contains hemin (factor X) but lacks NAD (factor V). Staphylococcus aureus produce NAD as a metabolic byproduct when grow on Blood agar. Therefore, Haemophilus spp may grow on sheep blood agar very close to the colonies of Staphylococcus aureus (as it produces NAD-factor V); this phenomenon is known as satelliting.

59. Ans. is 'a' i.e., Haemophilus ducreyi

Image description – Chancroid (also known as soft chancre and ulcus molle) is a bacterial sexually transmitted infection characterized by painful ulceration on the genitalia that bleeds easily on if it is scrapped.

60. Ans. Image description on Page 467.

61. Ans. Image description on Page 467.

62. Ans. Image description on Page 467.

63. Ans. is 'c' i.e., Treponema pallidum

Image description – Chancre – A primary sore or ulcer at the site of entry of T. pallidum and it begins as a painless papule that rapidly becomes ulcerated, hard and indurated and it is very rich in T. pallidum.

64. Ans. is 'a' i.e., Dark-field Microscopy for T. pallidum

Image description – A drop of tissue fluid or exudate is placed on a slide, and a coverslip is pressed over it to make a thin layer. The preparation is then examined under oil immersion within 20 minutes of collection with darkfield illumination for typical motile spirochetes. Dark-field microscopy should not be performed on lesions within the oral cavity because it is not possible to differentiate pathogenic from commensal spirochetes. Treponemes disappear from lesions within a few hours after the beginning of antibiotic treatment.

65. Ans. is 'b' i.e., Fluorescent Ab staining for T. pallidum

Image description – Tissue fluid or exudate is spread on a glass slide, air dried, and sent to the laboratory. It is fixed, stained with a fluorescein labeled anti-treponeme antibody which are targeted against T. pallidum surface antigen and examined by means of immunofluorescence microscopy for typical fluorescent spirochetes.

66. Ans. is 'c' i.e., Fontana (silver impregnation method) staining for T. pallidum

Image description – T pallidum cannot be seen under the light microscope. Its morphology and motility can be seen under the dark ground or phase contrast microscope. It cannot be stained by ordinary bacterial stains, but can be stained by silver impregnation methods. Fontana's method is used for staining films and Levaditi's method for tissue sections. On prolonged Giemsa staining they stain pale pink.

67. Ans. Image description on Page 468.

68. Ans. Image description on Page 468.

69. Ans. Image description on Page 468.

70. Ans. Image description on Page 468.

VIROLOGY

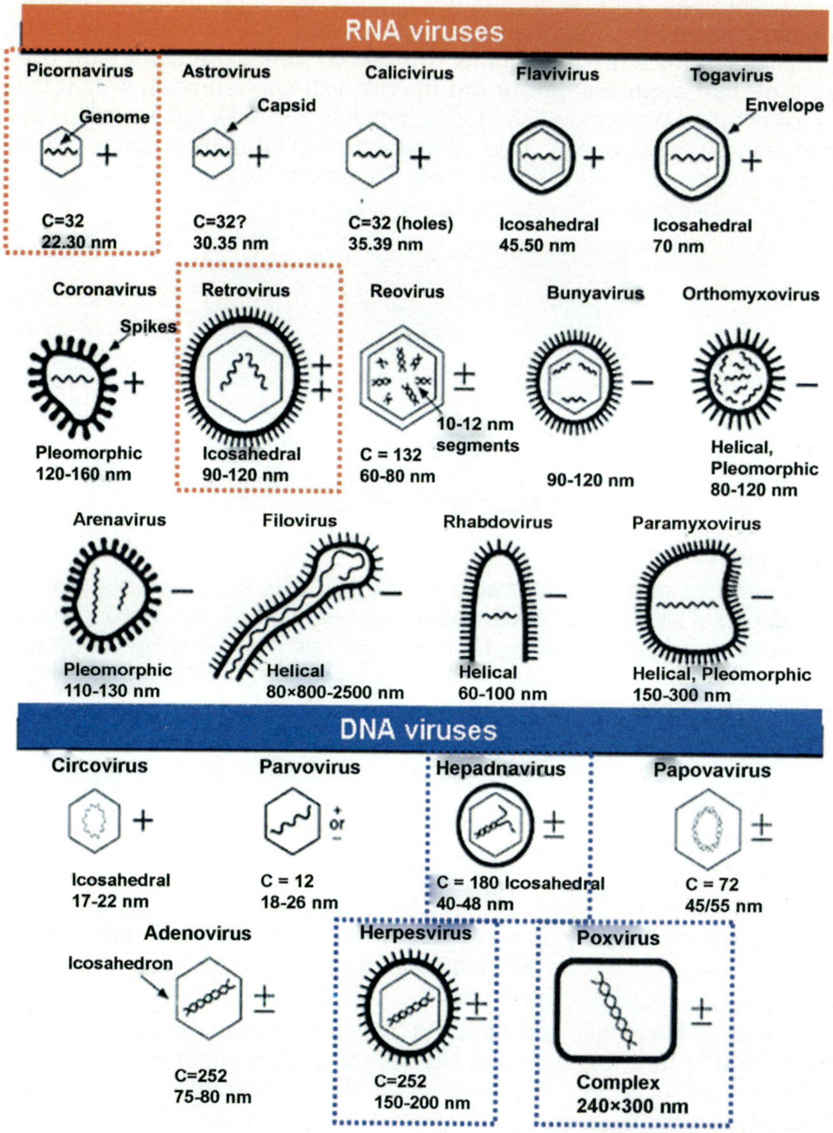

1. Routes of embryonated egg inoculation.

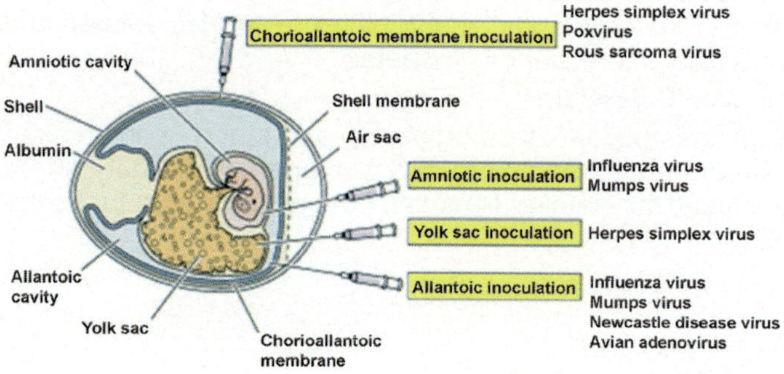

2. Tissue culture flask with cell lines.

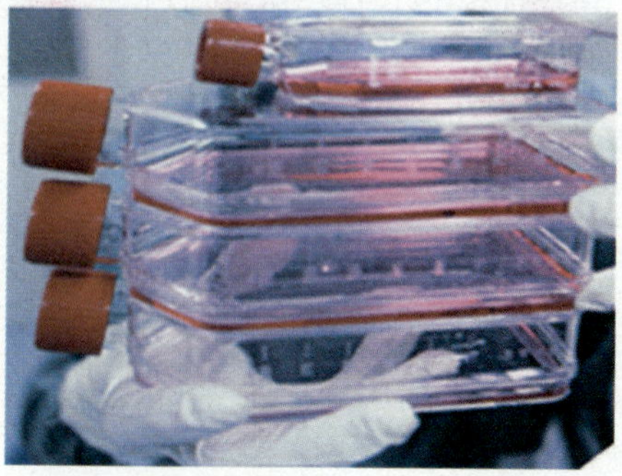

3. **Herpes simplex virus (ds linear DNA).**

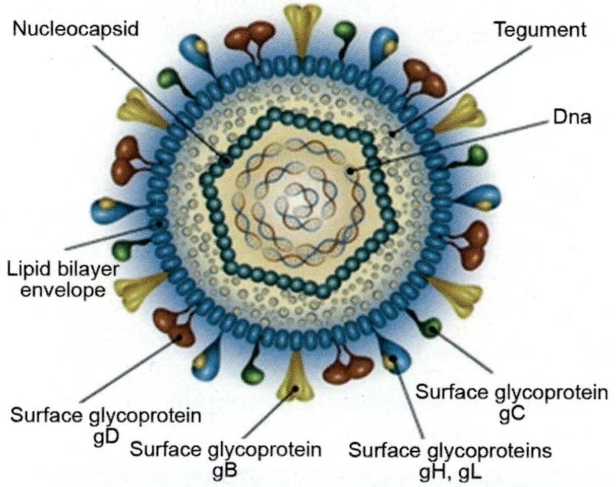

4. **Cytopathic effects induced by herpesviruses. A: Herpes simplex virus in HEp-2 cells (hematoxylin and eosin stain, 57×), with early focus of swollen, rounded cells. B: Varicella-zoster virus in human kidney cells (hematoxylin and eosin stain, 228×), with multnucleated giant cell containing acidophilic intranuclear inclusions (arrow). C: Cytomegalovirus in human fibroblasts (unstained, 35×) with two foci of slowly developing cytopathic effect. D: Cytomegalovirus in human fibroblasts (hematoxylin and eosin stain, 228×), showing giant cells with acidophilic inclusions in the nuclei (small arrow) and cytoplasm (large arrow), the latter being characteristically large and round.**

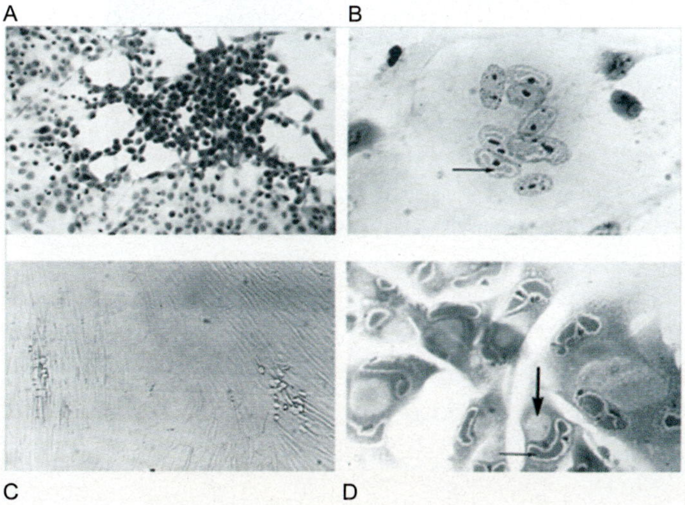

5. **Herpes labialis.**

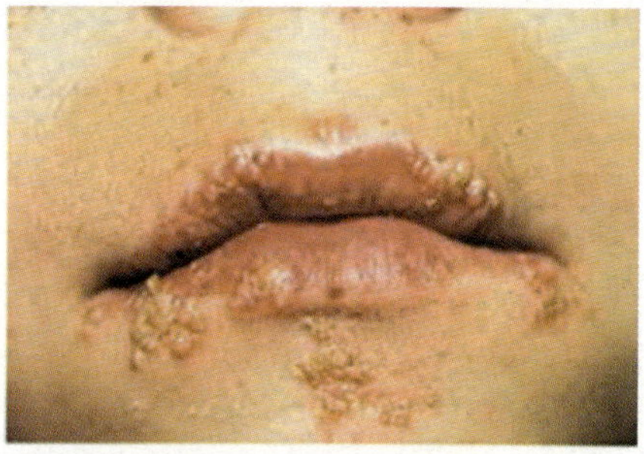

6. ***Dendritic ulcers* are the most common presentation of HSV keratitis.**

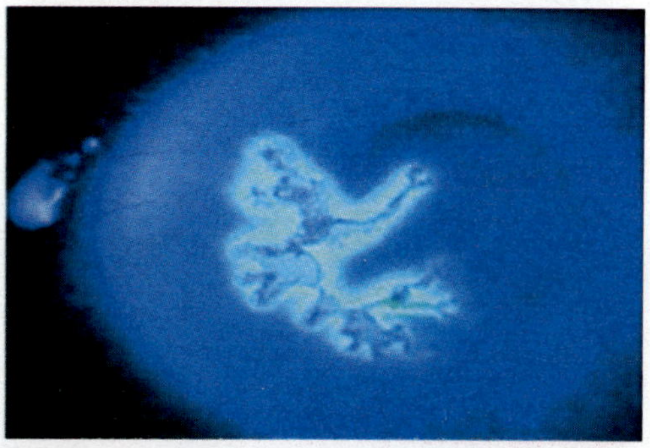

7. **Eczema herpeticum caused by HSV 1 or 2.**

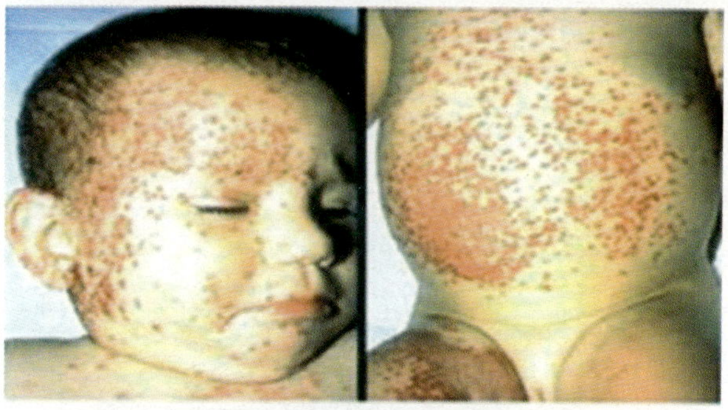

8. **Zoster ophthalmicus.**

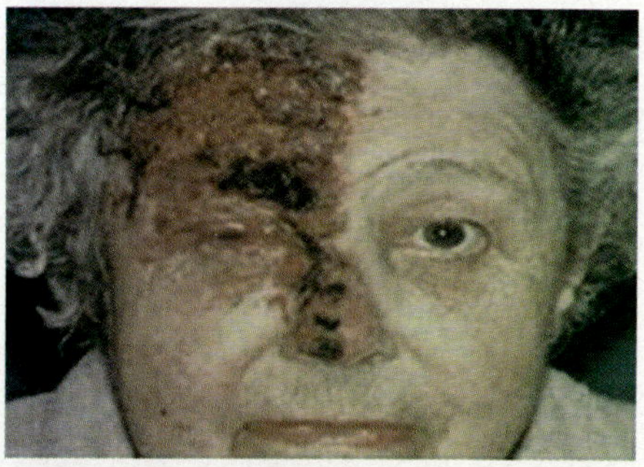

9. **Smallpox (Centrifugal) and Chickenpox (Centripetal).**

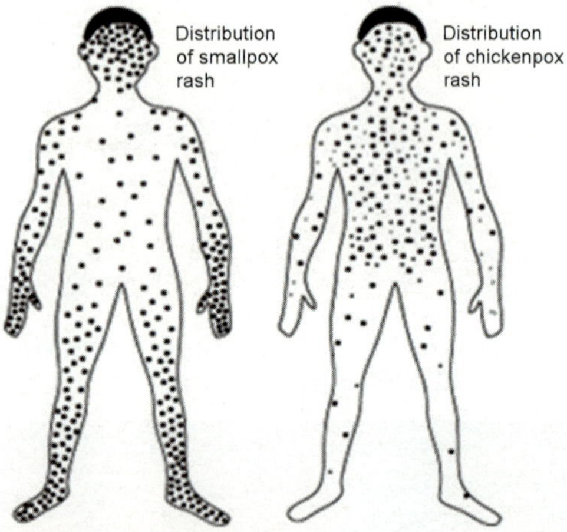

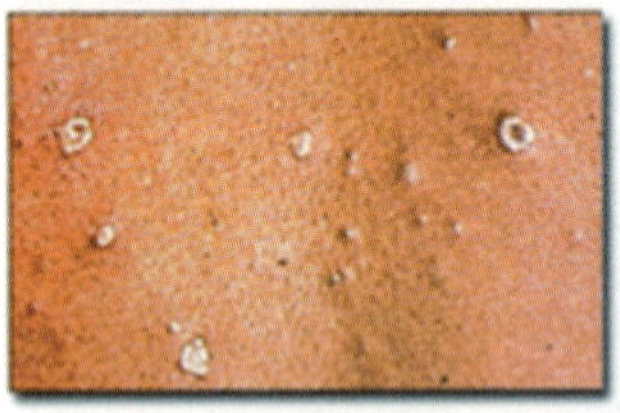

Chickenpox rash

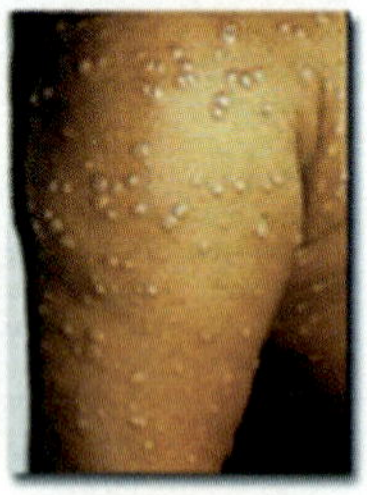

Smallpox rash

10. **Multinucleated giant cell in Tzanck smear of a tissue scraping.**

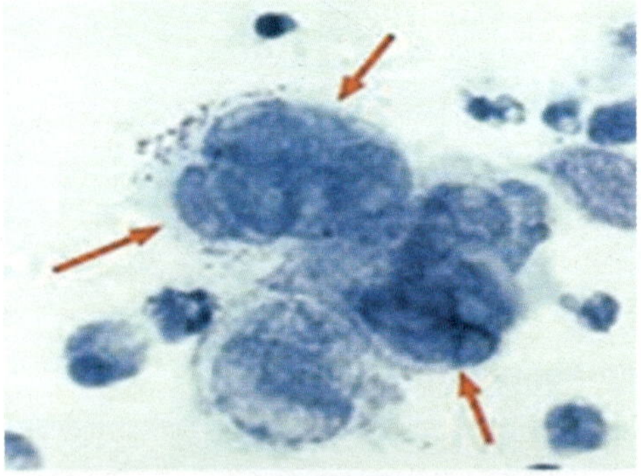

11. **Owl's eye inclusion body of CMV.**

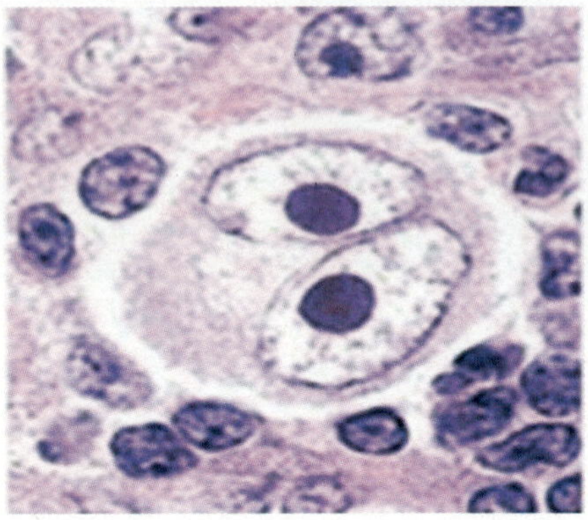

12. **Infectious mononucleosis tonsillitis (white or grayish film over enlarged tonsils).**

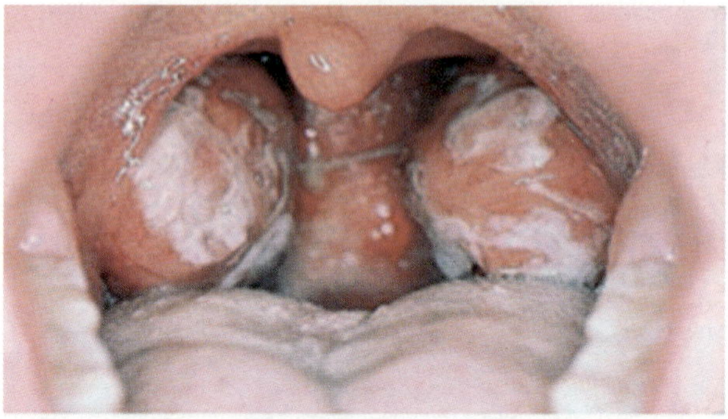

13. **Oral hairy leukoplakia of tongue (EBV infection in AIDS patients).**

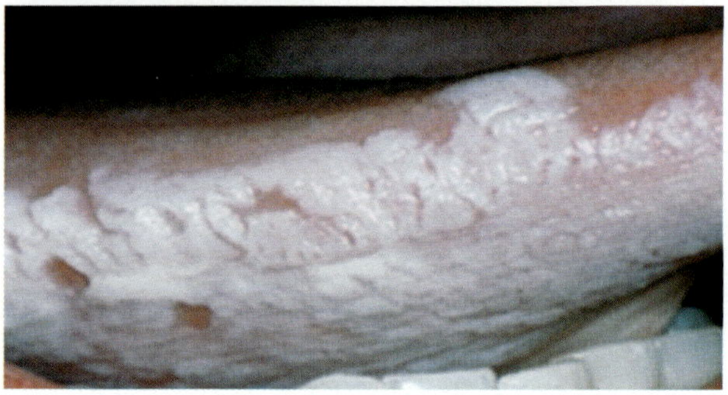

14. **Burkitt's lymphoma (Tumor of Jaw) – EBV infection in Africans (90%).**

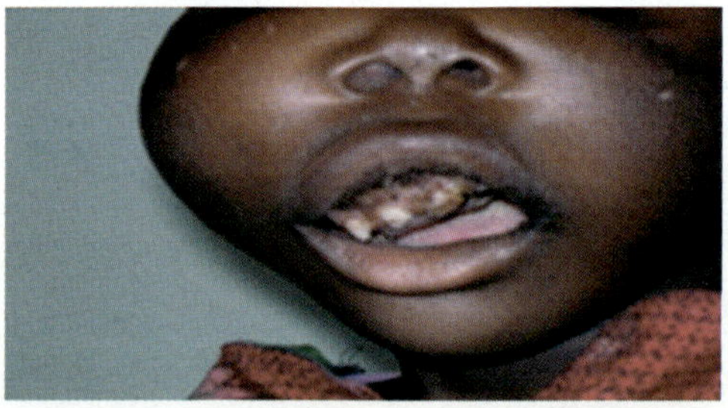

15. **Infectious mononucleosis peripheral blood smear showing Atypical lymphocyte.**

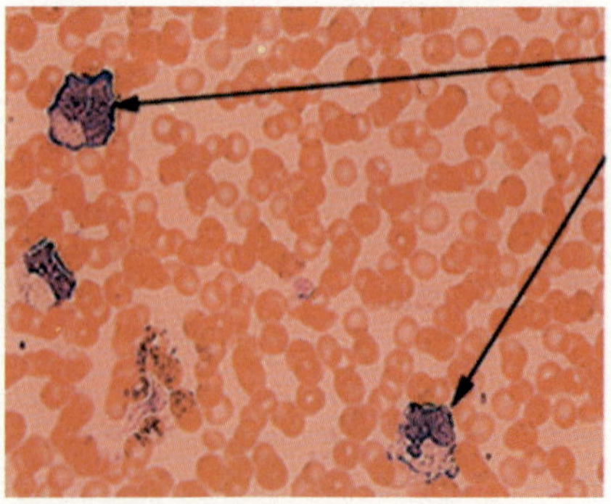

16. **Paul Bunnel test for diagnosis of infectious mononucleosis.**

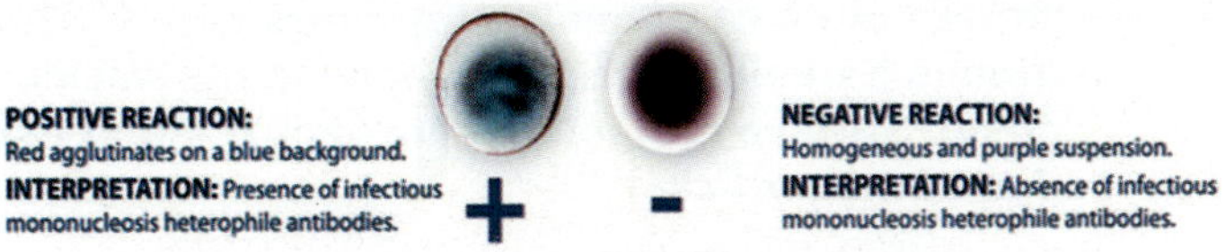

17. Roseola infantum caused by HHV-6 and HHV-7 (rarely).

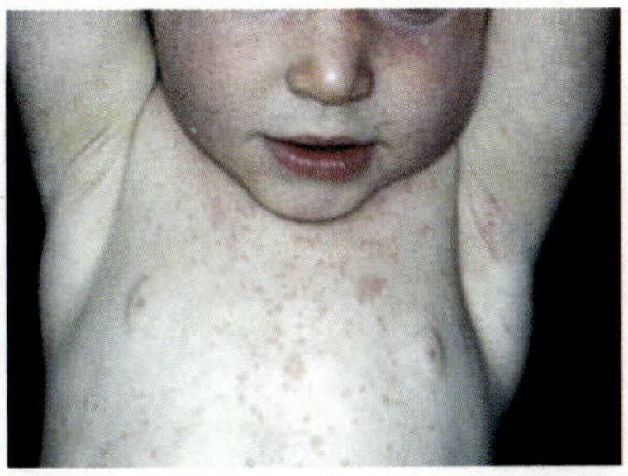

18. Kaposi's sarcoma caused by HHV 8.

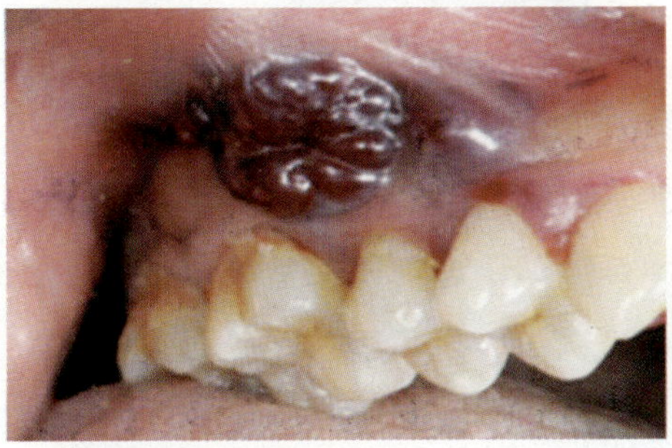

19. Slapped chick appearance in Fifth disease or Erythema infectiosum (Parvovirus B 19 infection).

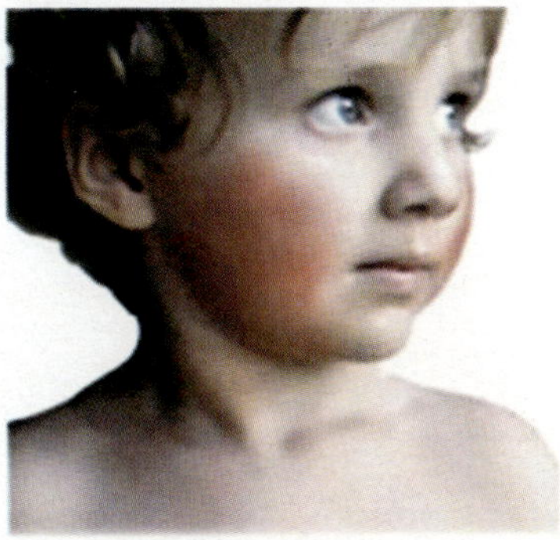

20. Perianal Condyloma acuminatum (STD) caused by Human papilloma virus (HPV).

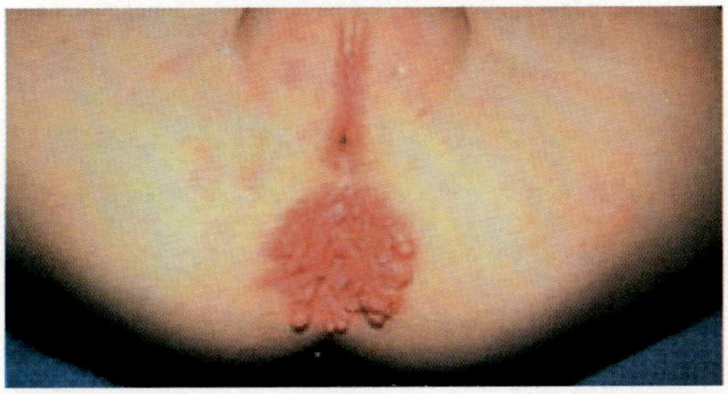

21. Penile Condyloma acuminata (STD) caused by Human papilloma virus (HPV).

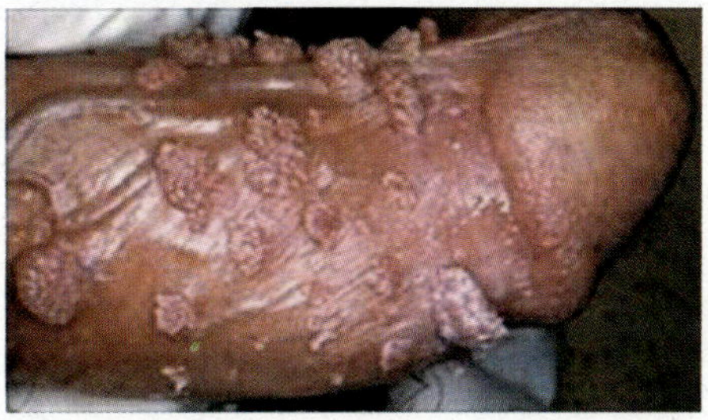

22. Adenovirus.

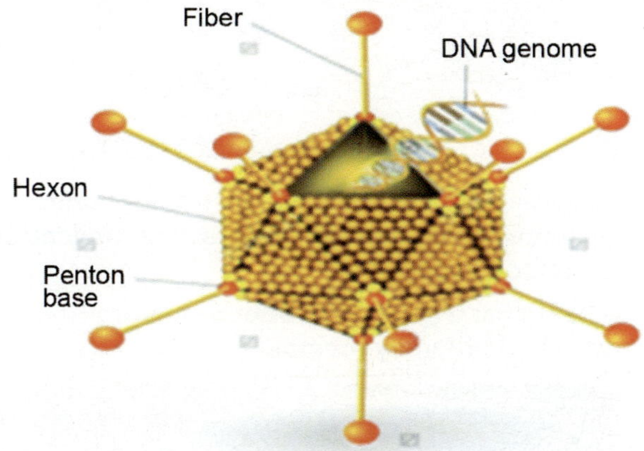

23. Adenovirus.

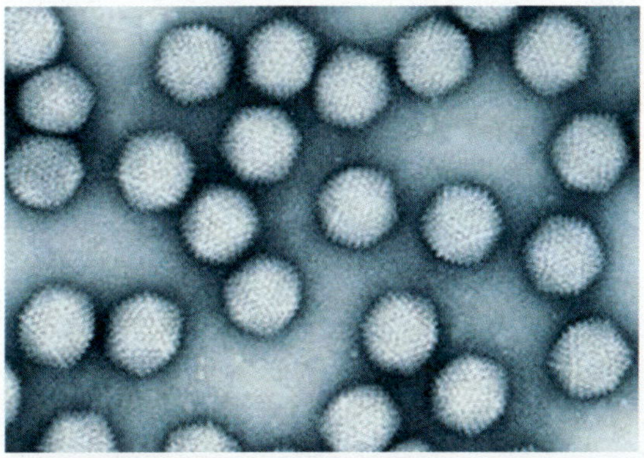

24. The chorioallantoic membrane of a developing chick covered with Smallpox virus pocks.

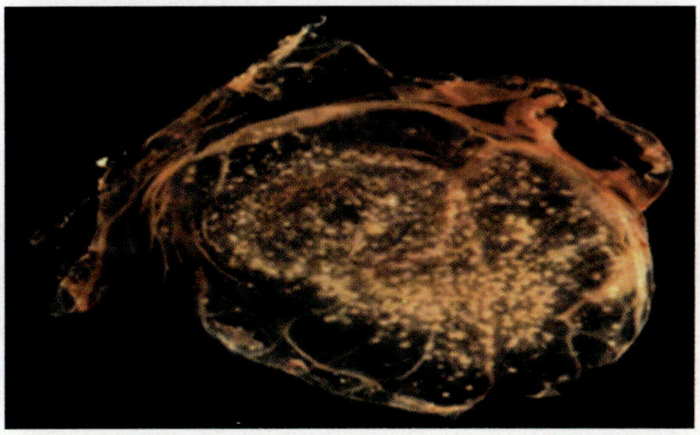

25. **Smallpox rash. A "Smallpox Recognition Card" from the World Health Organization illustrates the distribution and nature of the typical rash of smallpox in an unvaccinated child.**

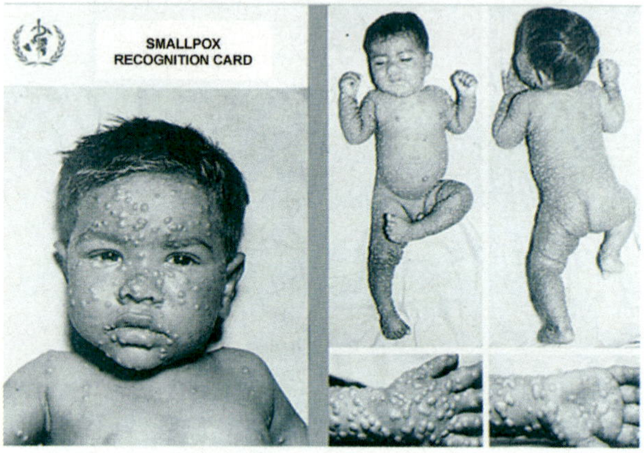

26. **Eczema vaccinatum in a young child with eczema/atopic dermatitis. It is a complication of smallpox vaccination.**

The disease developed after exposure to a newly vaccinated family member.

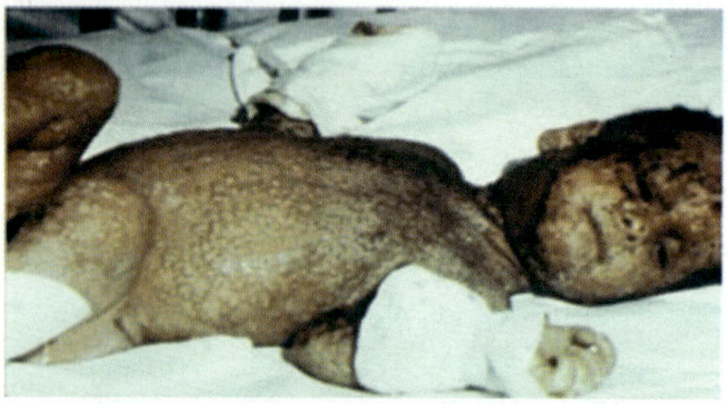

27. **Antigenic drift and Antigenic shift.**

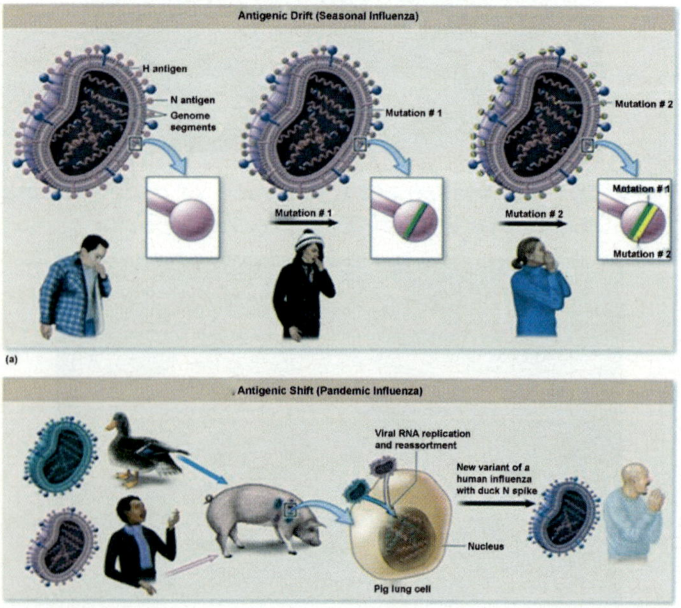

28. **Ultrastructure of parainfluenza virus type 1. The virion is partially disrupted, showing the nucleocapsid. Surface projections are visible along the edge of the particle.**

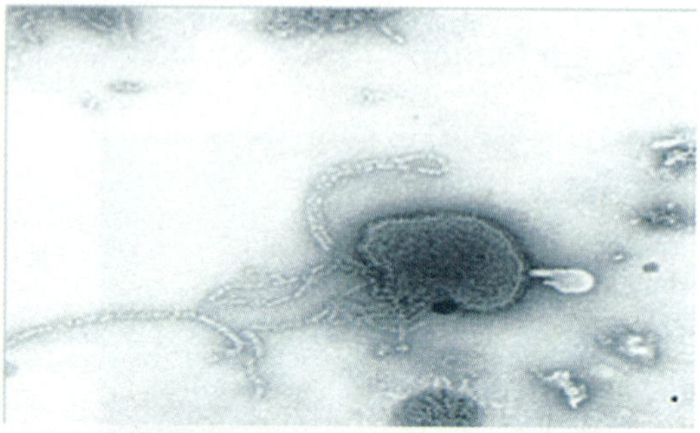

29. **Bacteriophage (Virus which infect the bacteria).**

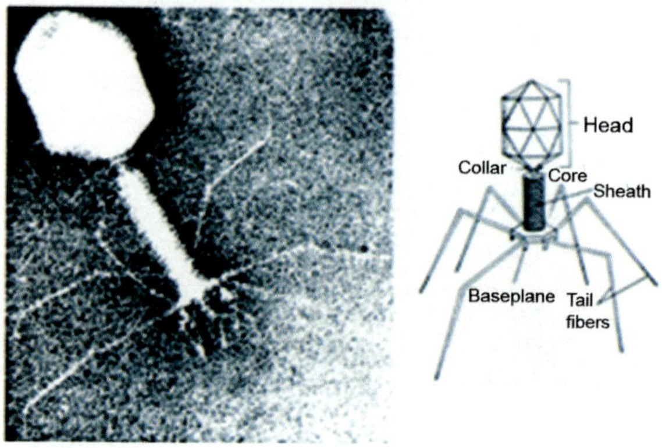

30. **Molluscum Contagiosum (Umbilicated lesions with dimple at center).**

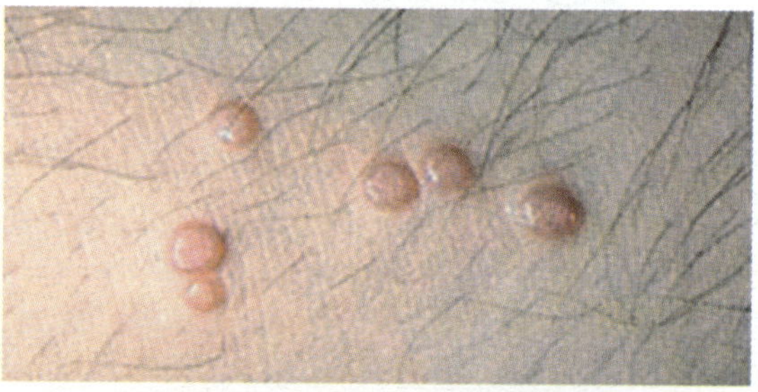

31. **Pink cytoplasmic viral inclusions "Molluscum bodies" in Molluscum Contagiosum.**

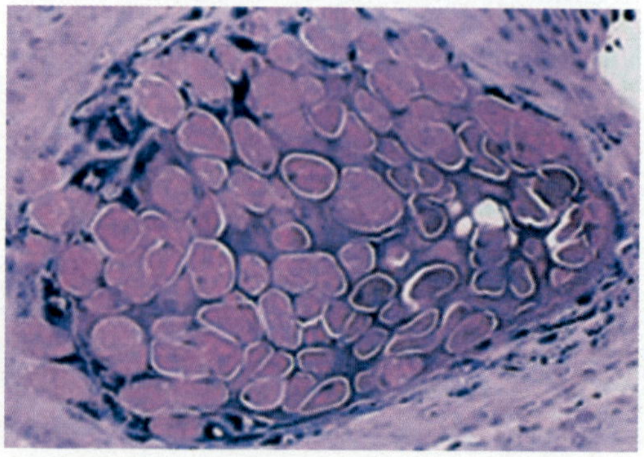

32. Child with mumps: Classic submandibular and preauricular enlargement of the parotid gland.

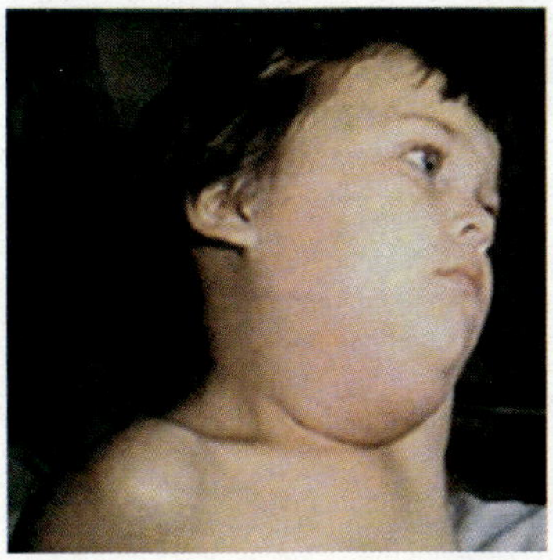

33. Koplik's spot in buccal mucosa (Measles).

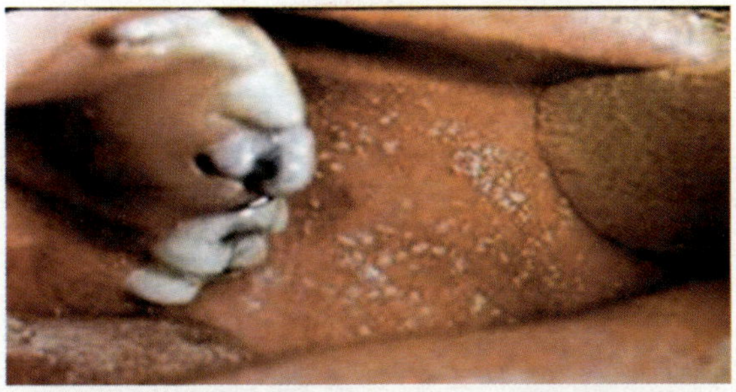

34. Cataracts due to Congenital Rubella Syndrome (CRS).

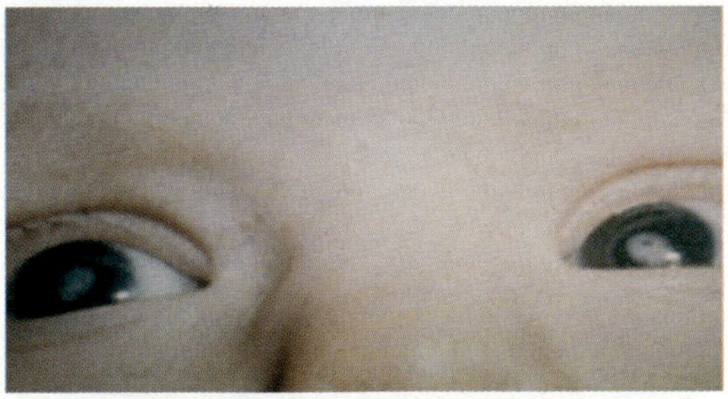

35. Forchheimer spots in Rubella.

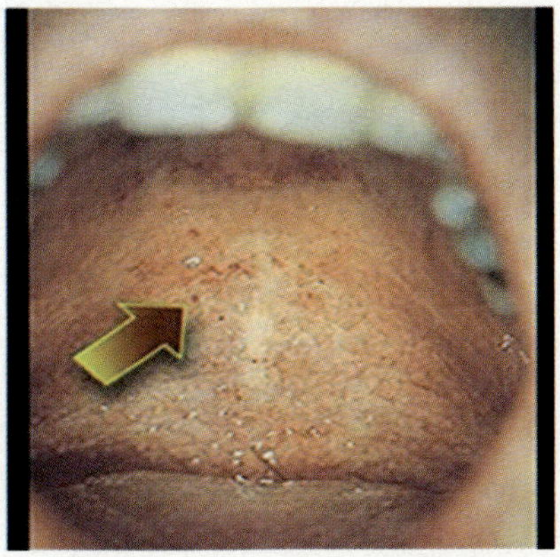

36. Rabies virus.

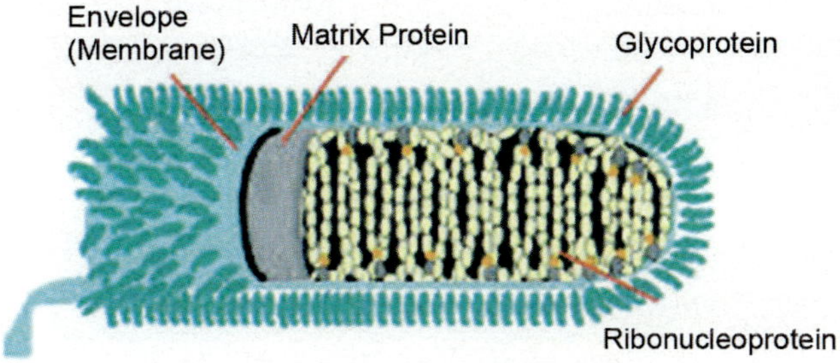

37. Inclusion bodies in Rabies infection.

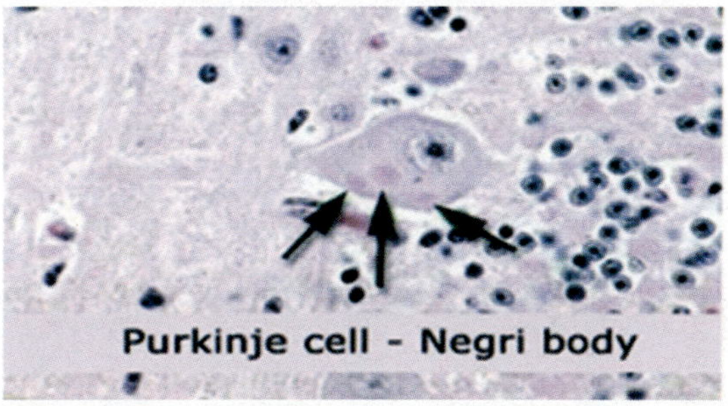

38. Contextual determinants and transmission of Japanese encephalitis.

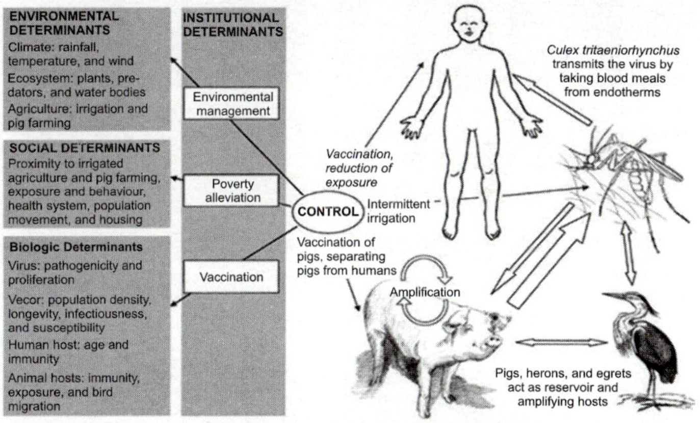

39. HIV virus.

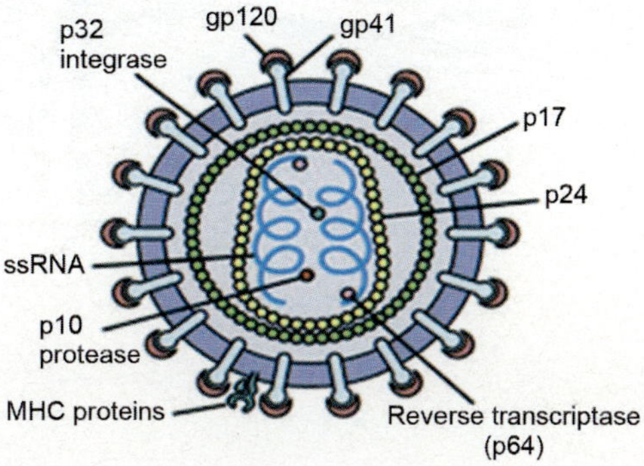

40. HIV tridot test (Rapid ICT).

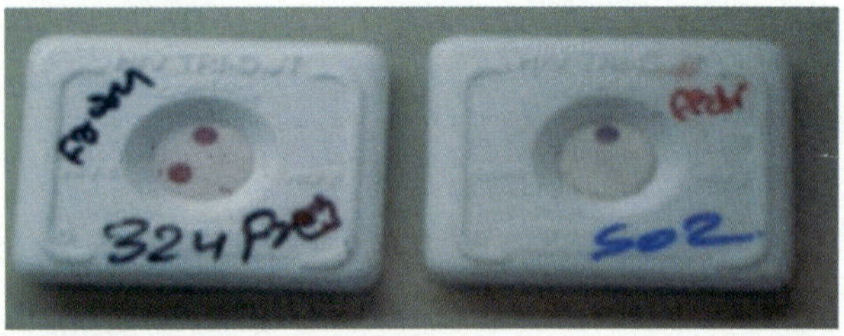

41. Western blot test for HIV (confirmation test).

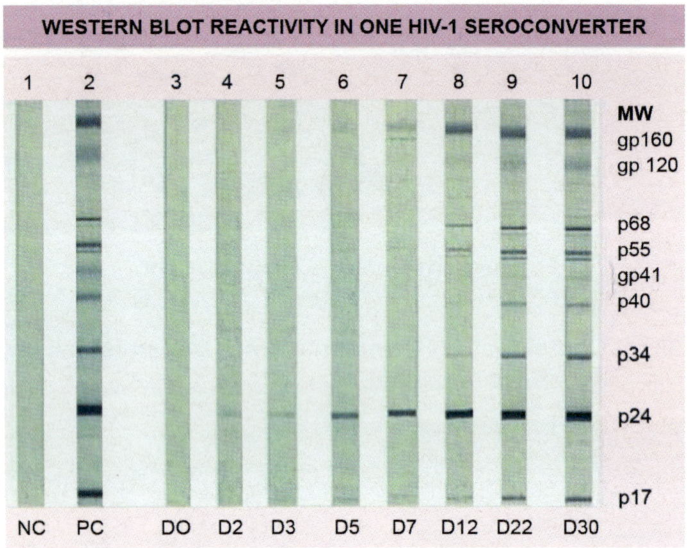

NC – Negative control

PC – Positive control

D – Patients samples

42. Ebola virus – Electron Microscopy shows filamentous appearance.

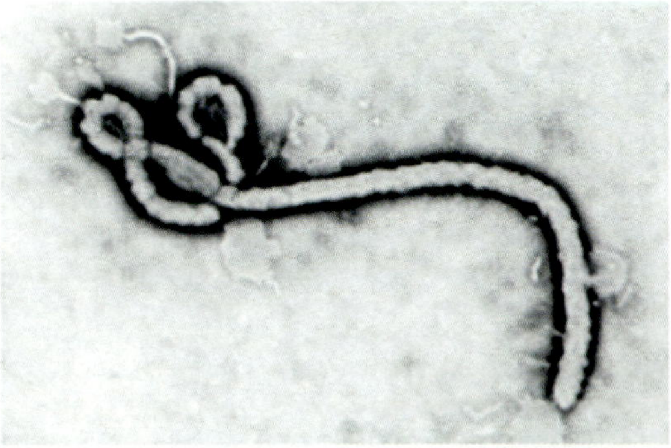

43. Hepatitis B virus – Three morphological forms (spherical, tubular and dane particle).

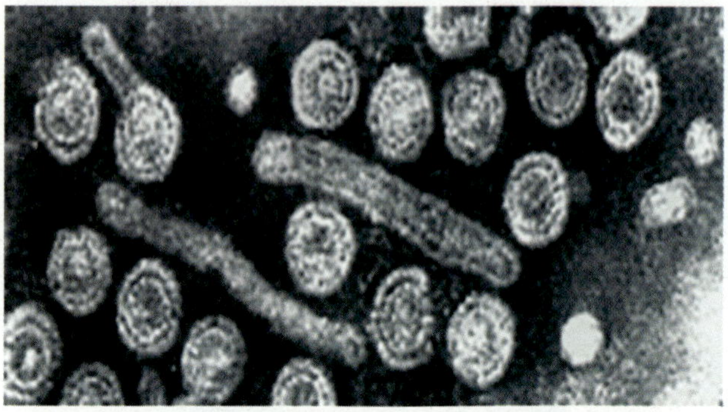

44. HBV structure.

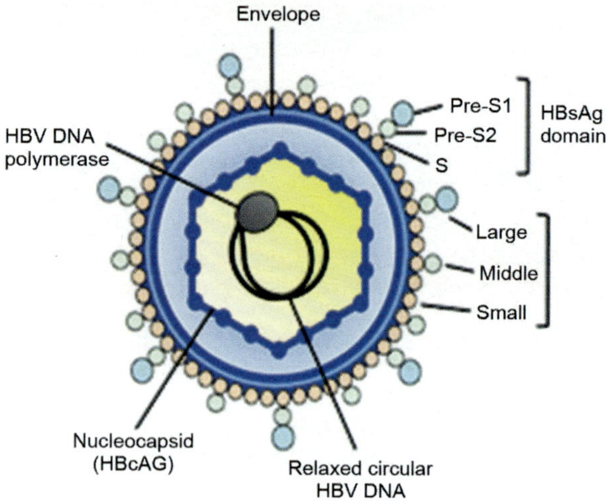

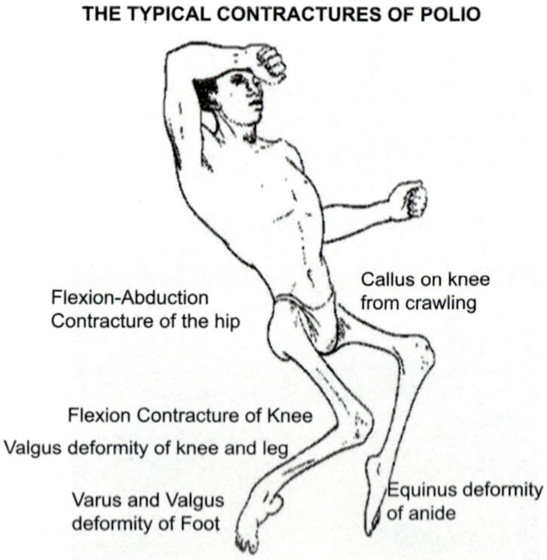

MYCOLOGY

1. Arthroconidia (arthrospores): Conidia that result from the fragmentation of hyphal cells.

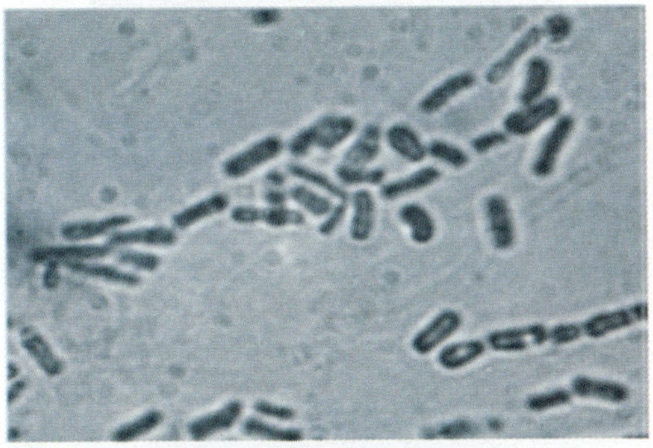

2. Tenia capitis caused by Trichophyton tonsurans and Trichophyton violaceum.

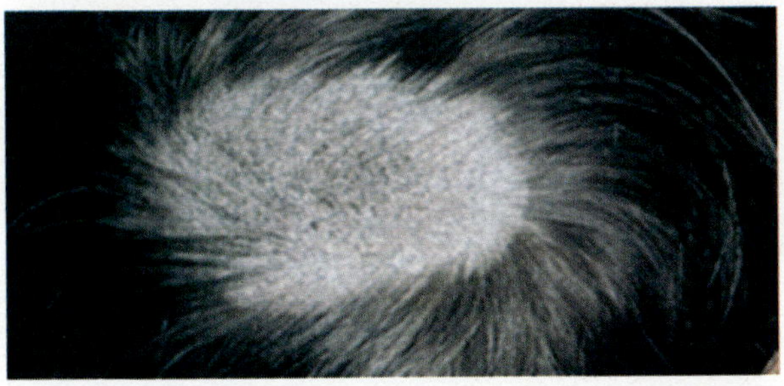

3. Kerion caused by Zoophilic Dermatophytes like Trichophyton mentagrophytes and Trichophyton verrucosum.

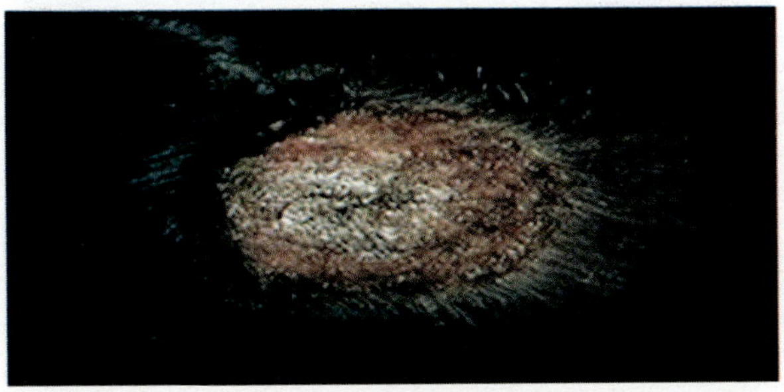

4. Tinea cruris (Jock itch) caused by Epidermophyton floccosum and T. rubrum.

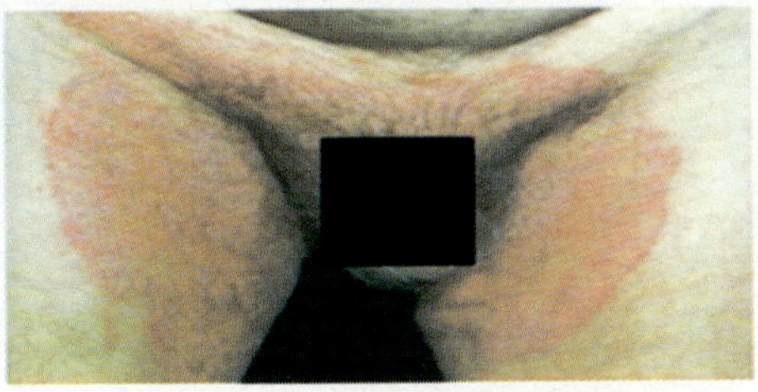

5. Tinea pedis (Athlete foot) caused by T. rubrum and Epidermophyton floccosum.

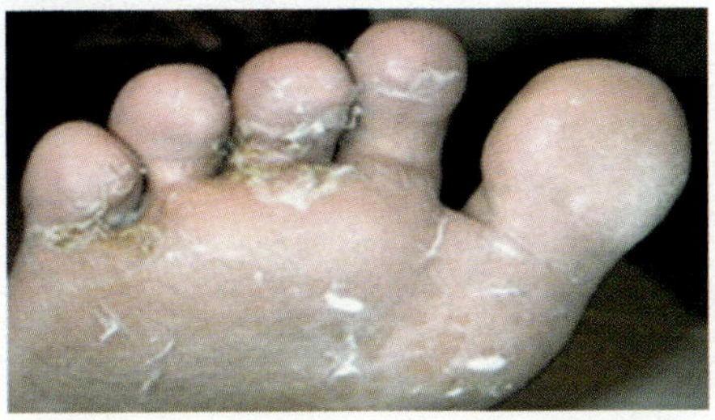

6. Favus caused by T. schoenleinii, T. violaceum, T. gypsum.

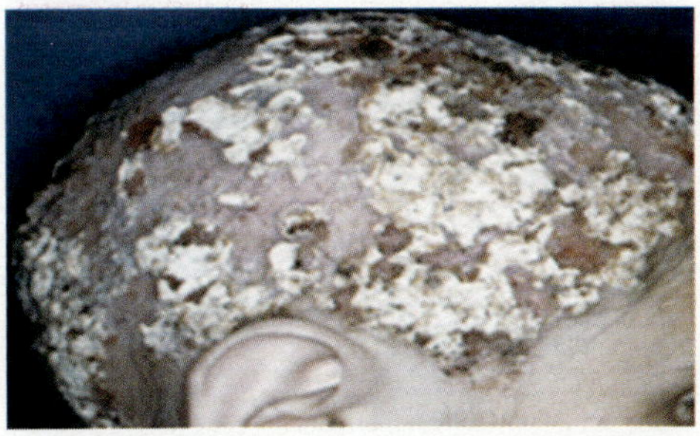

7. Black dot ringworm caused by Trichophyton.

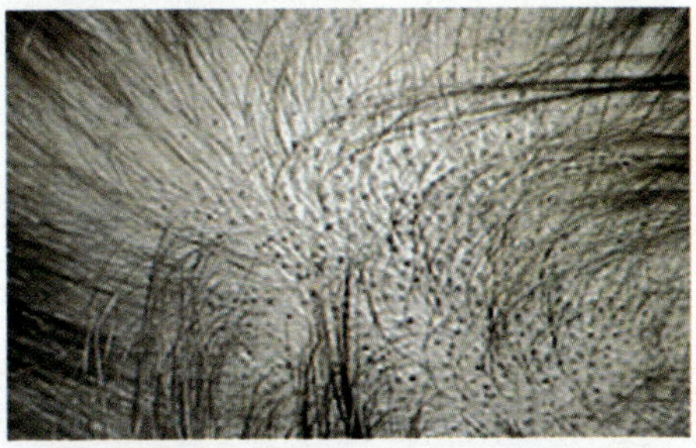

8. Piedra: White piedra hair with nodule due to growth of Trichosporon.

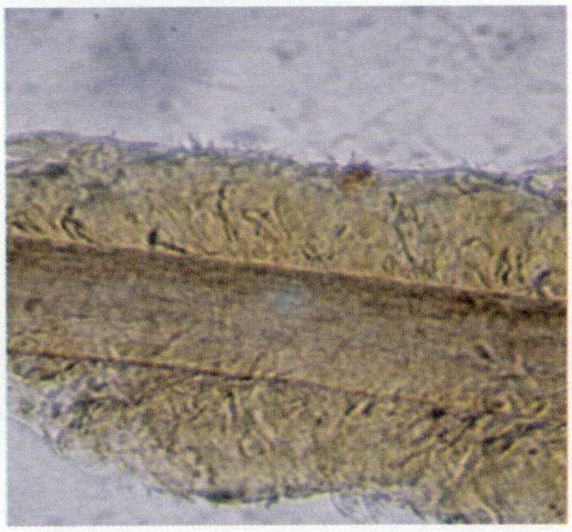

9. Black piedra hair with a hard, black nodule, caused by growth of the dematiaceous mold, Piedraia hortae.

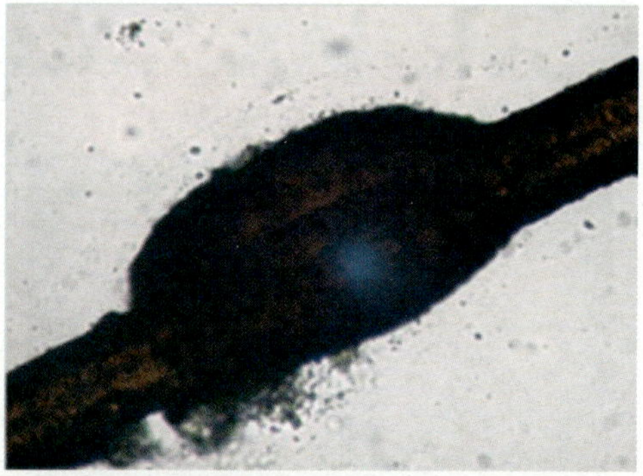

10. Pityriasis versicolor caused by M. furfur.

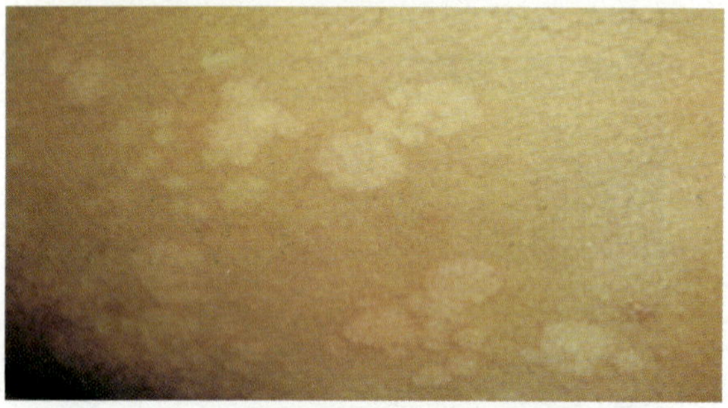

11. LPCB mount of Trichophyton showing microconidia on hyphae. This arrangement of microconidia has been described as "birds on a wire".

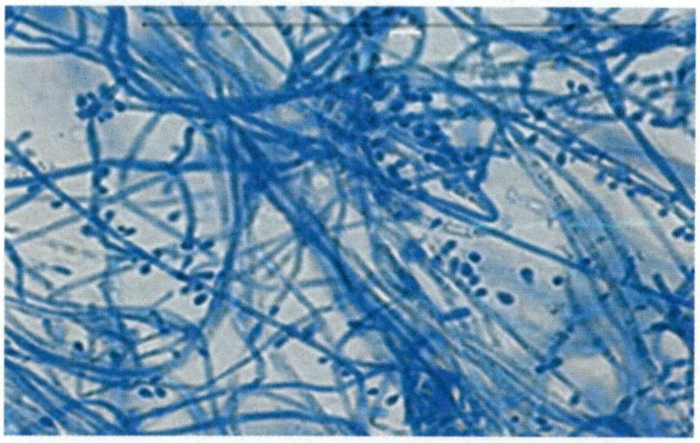

12. LPCB mount of Trichophyton showing Cylindrical Macroconidia.

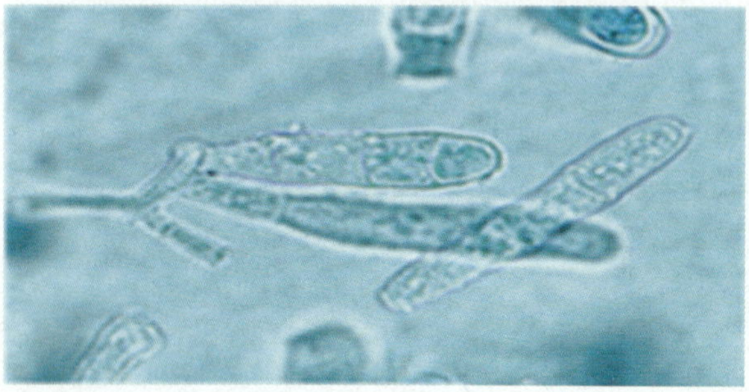

13. Conidia of Trichophyton.

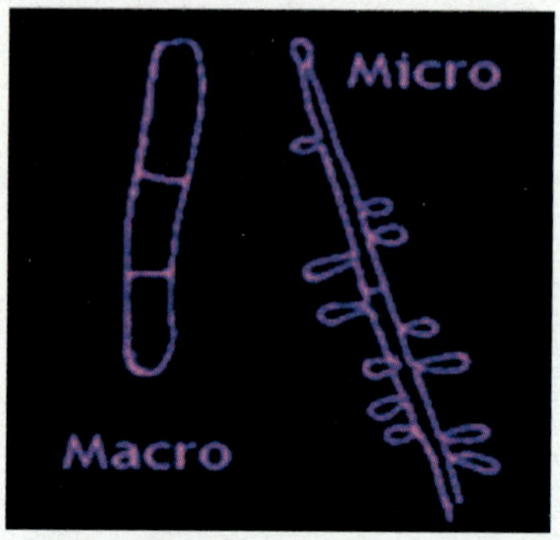

14. LPCB mount of Epidermatophyton showing Club shaped or pear shaped multicellular macroconidia.

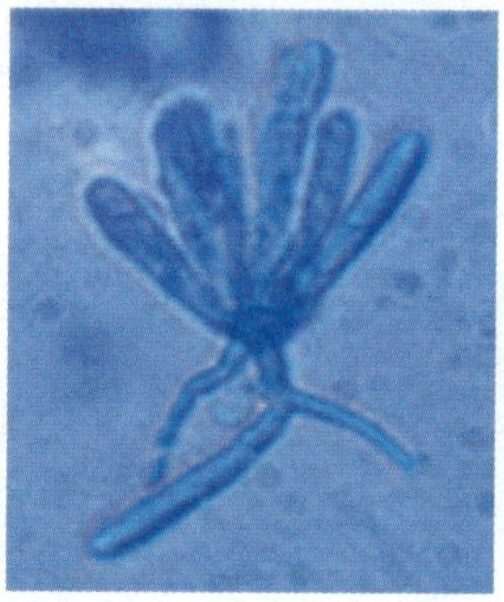

15. LPCB mount of Microsporum showing multicellular spindle or fusiform shaped Macroconidia.

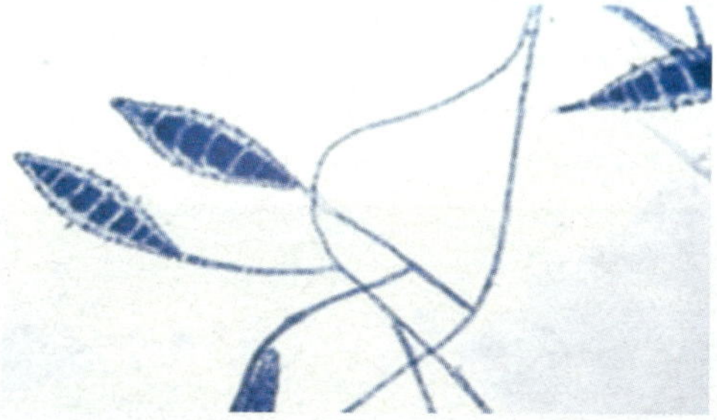

16. Dermatophytosis–KOH preparation of scrapings from a ringworm lesion. The epidermal cells are lysed by KOH to reveal hyaline branching septate hyphae.

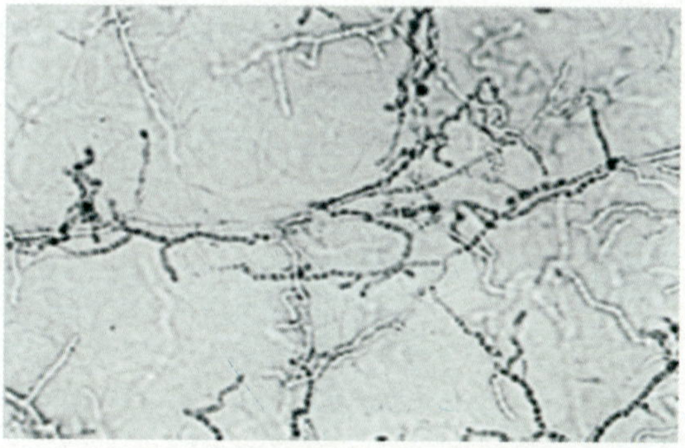

17. Ectothrix **Endothrix**

(Arthrospore form seath around the hair) **(Spores inside the hair shaft)**

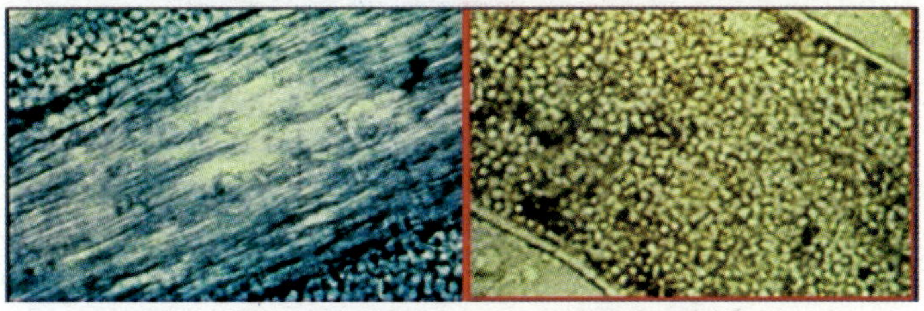

Ectothrix hair infection – Microsporum species and Endothrix hair infection – Trichophyton species

18. Sabouraud Dextrose Agar (SDA) – Selective media for isolation for Fungus.

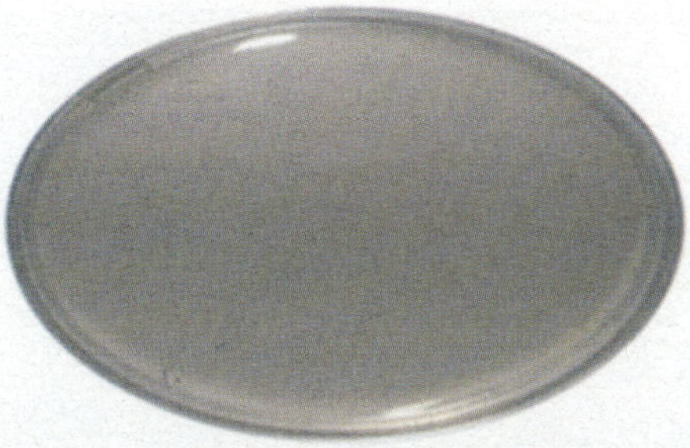

19. Sporotrichosis – Cutaneous tissue revealing the small spherical and elongated budding yeast cells (3–5 µm) of Sporothrix schenckii, which are stained black by the Gomori methenamine silver (GMS) stain.

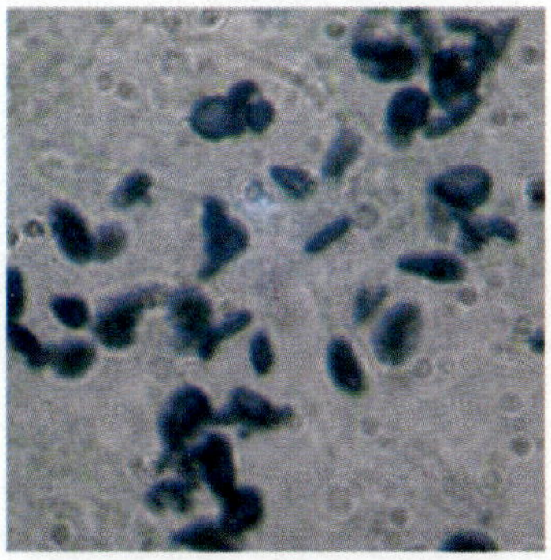

20. Chromomycosis – The diagnostic brownish, melanized sclerotic cells (4–12 µm diameter) are evident in this H and E stained cutaneous biopsy.

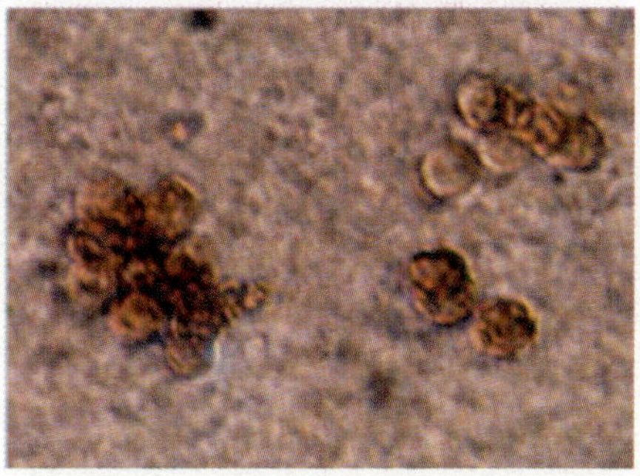

21. In culture at ambient temperatures, Coccidioides posadasii produces hyaline, septate hyphae and arthroconidia.

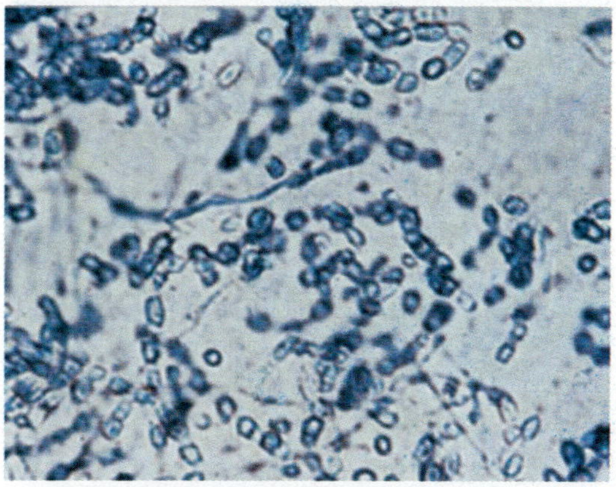

22. Coccidioidomycosis – Large spherules containing endospores can be seen in this section of lung tissue – H and E staining.

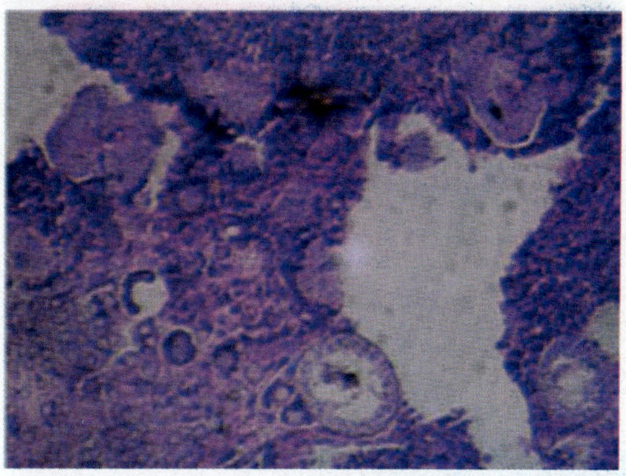

23. Blastomycosis and Blastomyces dermatitidis. Note the large, spherical thick-walled yeast cells (8–15 µm in diameter) in this section of a cutaneous abscess – H and E Staining.

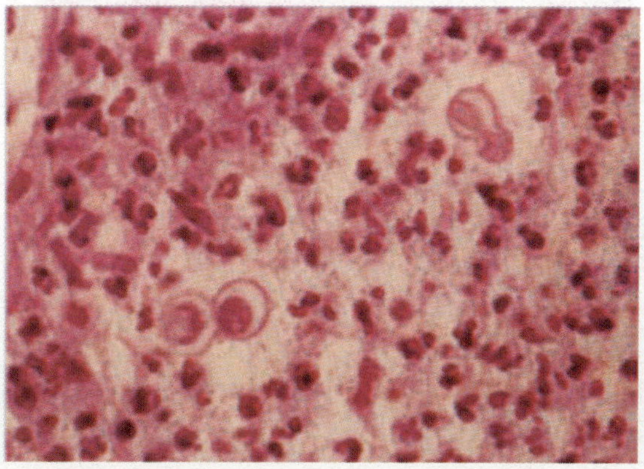

24. Paracoccidioidomycosis – Large, multiply budding yeast cells (15–30 µm) are observed in cutaneous lesion – KOH mount.

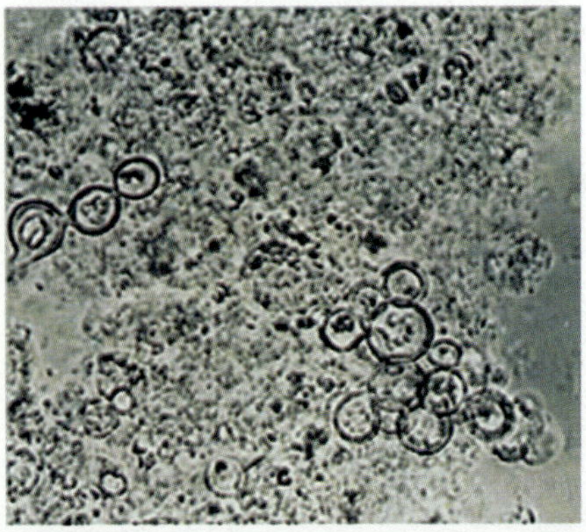

25. Oral thrush caused by Candida albicans.

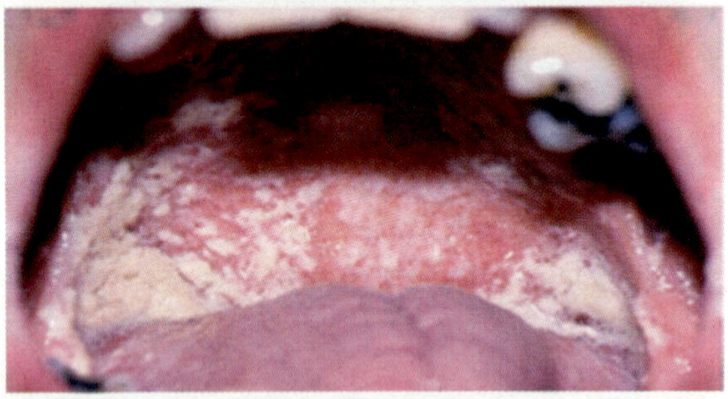

26. Germ tube test for identification of Candida albicans (+ve).

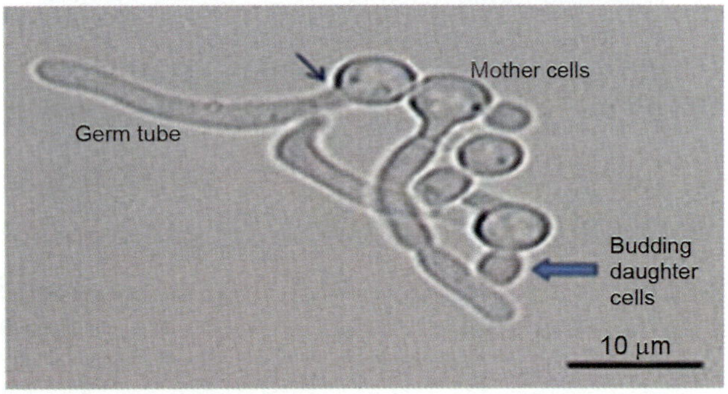

27. Chlamydospore formation on corn meal agar at 20°C.

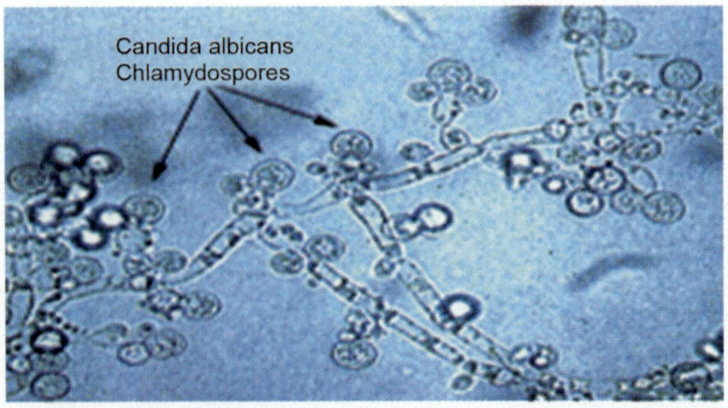

28. Gram staining of candida showing GPOBYC (Gram positive oval budding yeast cells) with pseudohyphae.

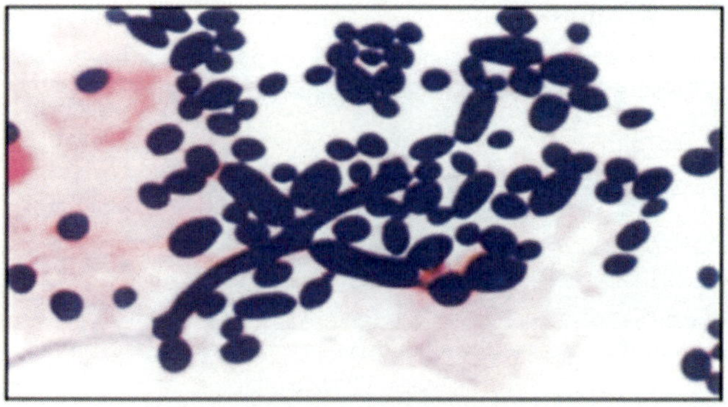

29. Candida colonies (white to cream colored, smooth, glabrous) on SDA.

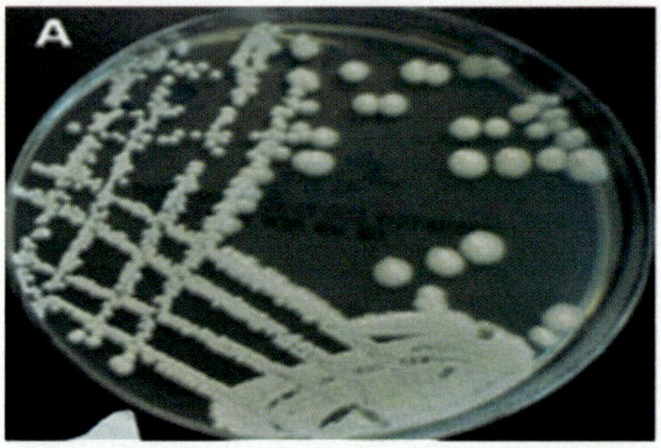

30. CHROM Agar showing different colored colonies produced by candida species which helps in identification.

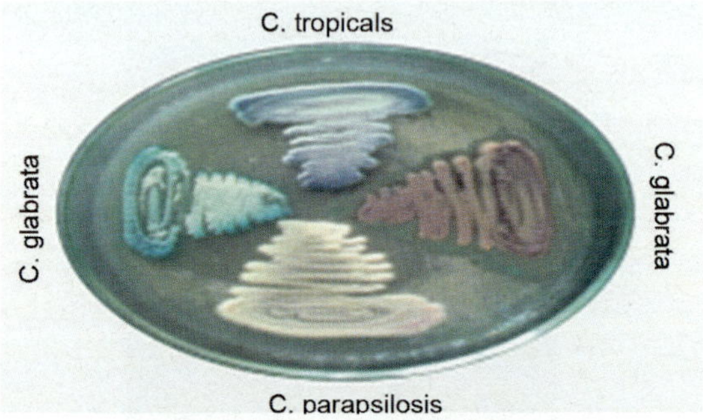

31. Candidiasis – Yeasts and pseudohyphae in tissue, stained with periodic acid-Schiff.

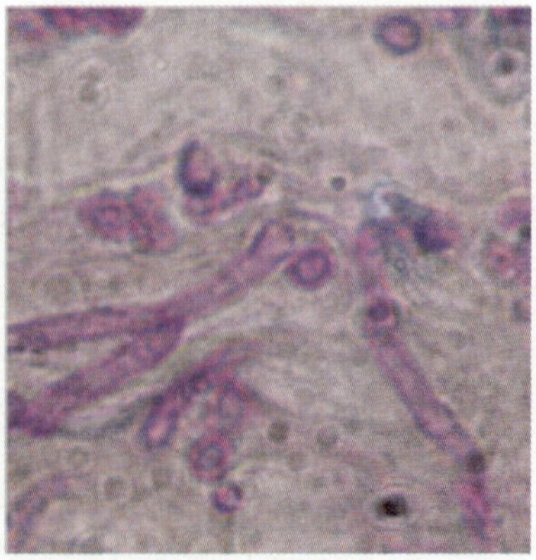

32. India ink preparation of CSF showing Cryptococcus with retractile capsule.

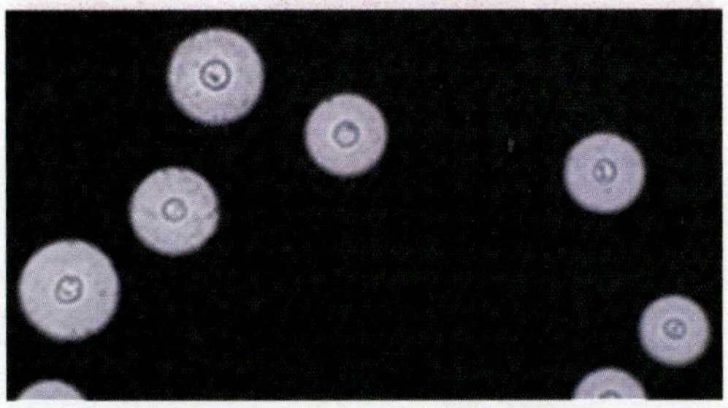

33. Cryptococcus neoformans colonies (Mucoid) on SDA.

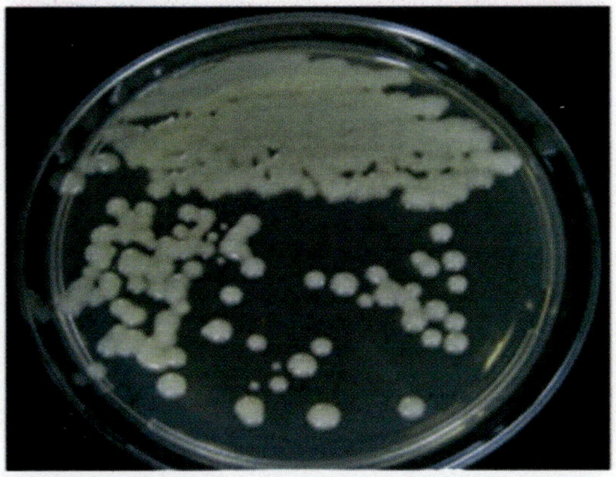

34. Gram staining of Cryptococcus neoformans showing GPRBYC (Gram positive round budding yeast cells).

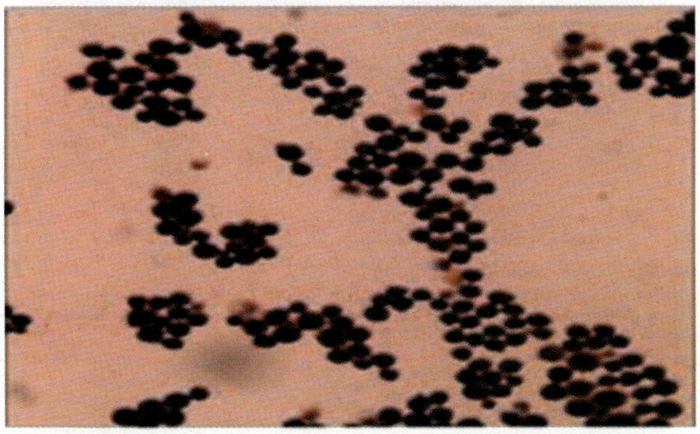

35. Urea hydrolysis test positive for Cryptococcus.

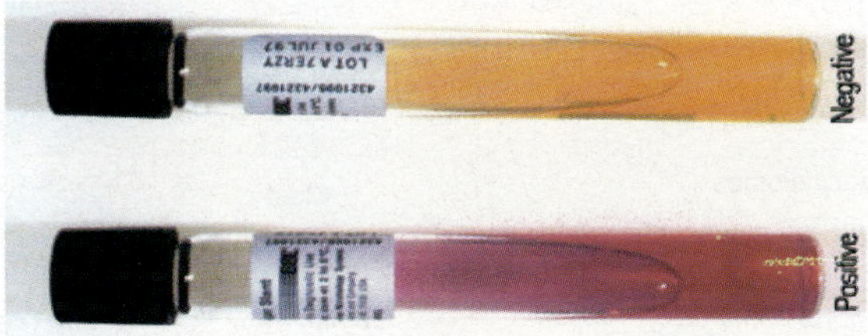

36. Latex agglutination test for detection of capsular Ag in cryptococcal meningitis.

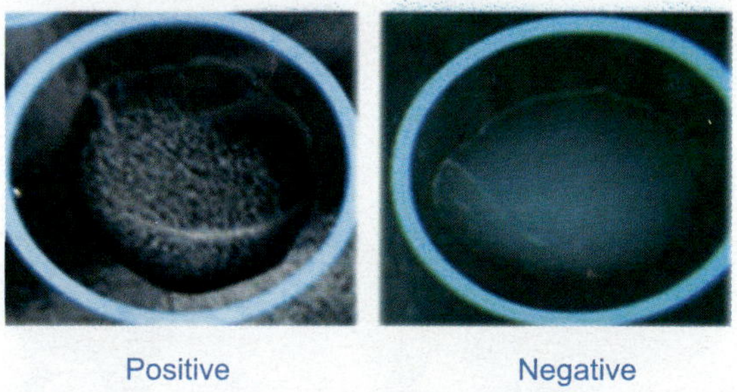

37. Maltese crosses shaped cast seen in polarized microscopy in nephrotic syndrome associated with C. neoformans infection.

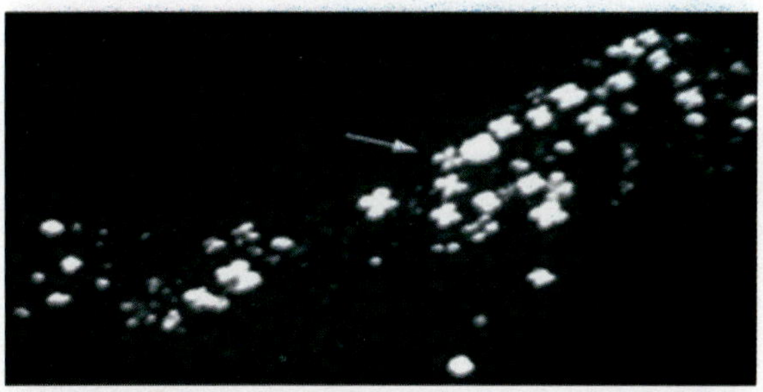

38. The spore cases (cysts) of pneumocystis stained with the Gomori methenamine silver (GMS) stain.

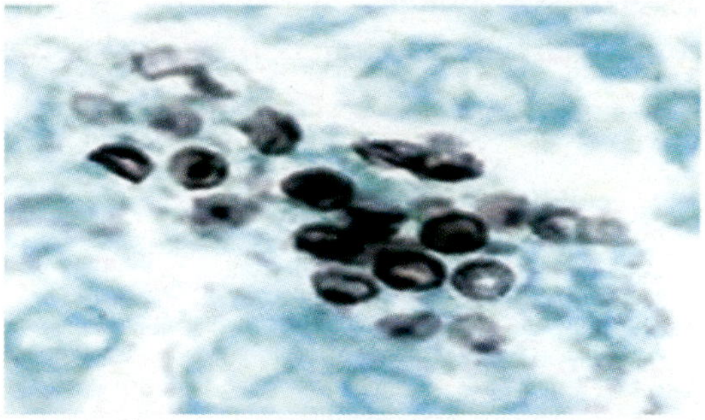

39. A smear of induced sputum stained with the Diff-Quik (Giemsa) method showing trophozoites and cysts of *Pneumocystis carinii.*

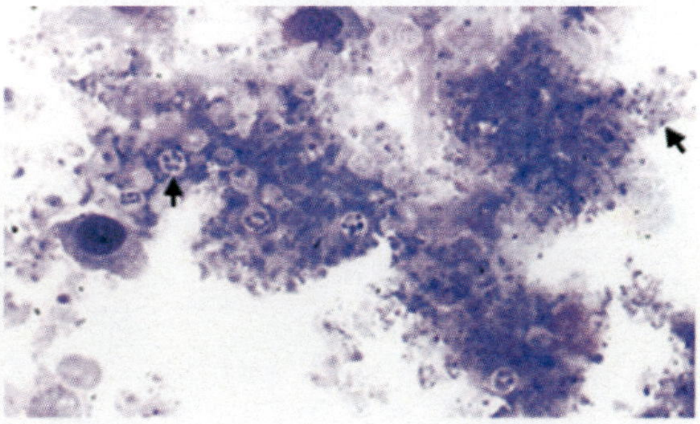

40. **LPCB mount of Aspergillus showing septate hyaline hyphae with dichotomous branching at 45°.**

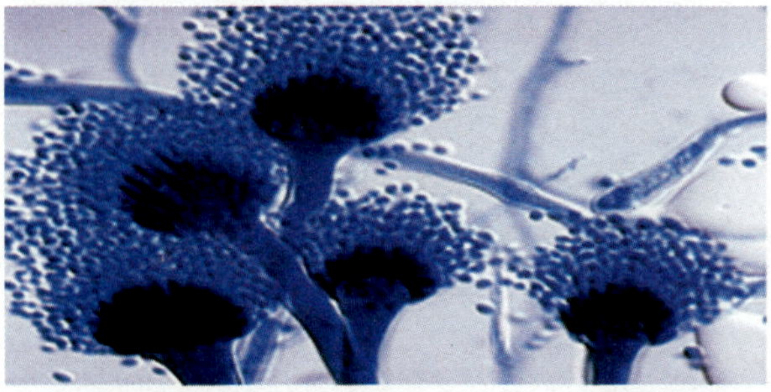

41. **Histopathological presentations of sporotrichosis showing presence of radiating star-like Asteroid body.**

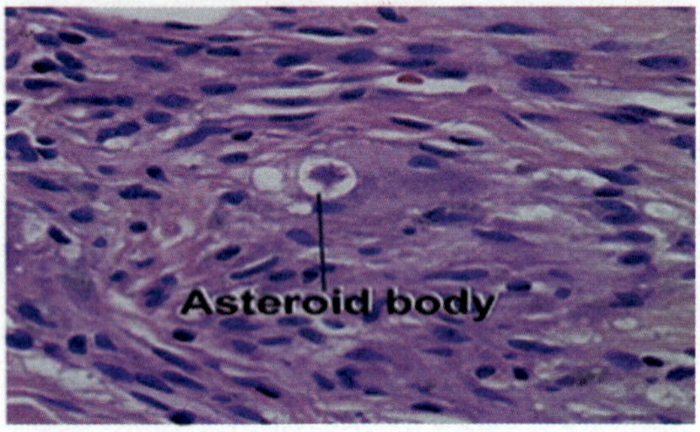

42. **Cigar- and oval-like yeast form of Sporothrix schenckii typically found in Tissue section.**

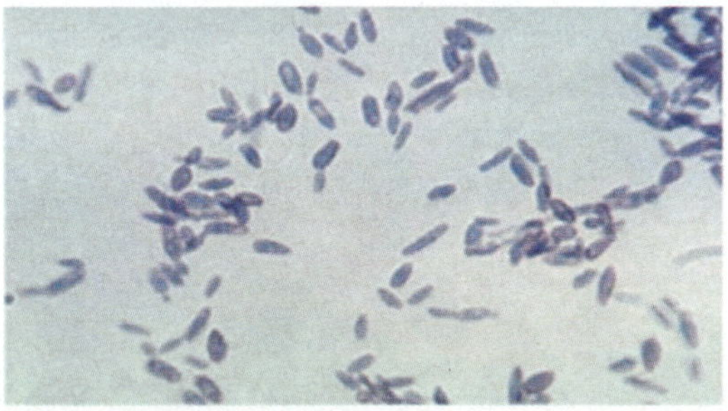

43. **Mucormycosis – Broad, ribbon-like sparsely septate hyphae (10–15 μm in width) of Rhizopus oryzae in histopathologic specimen, stained with Gomori methenamine silver.**

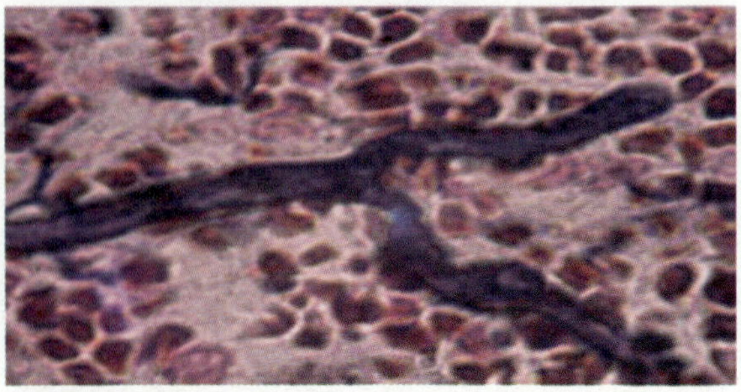

44. **Rhizopus – The sporangium of this mold has released its sporangiospores but remains attached to the supporting sporangiophore, and rhizoids are apparent at the base of the sporangiophore.**

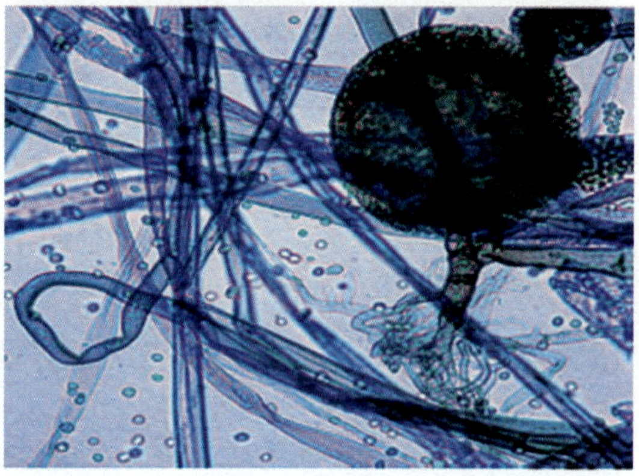

45. **Bipolaris – Dematiaceous mold that produces characteristic thick-walled macroconidia.**

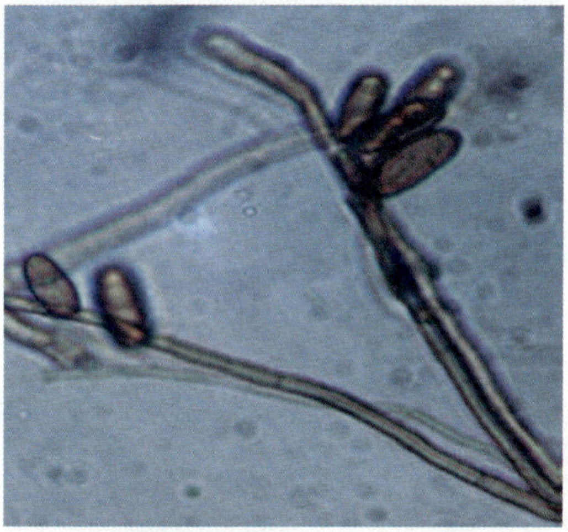

46. **Dimorphic fungi.**

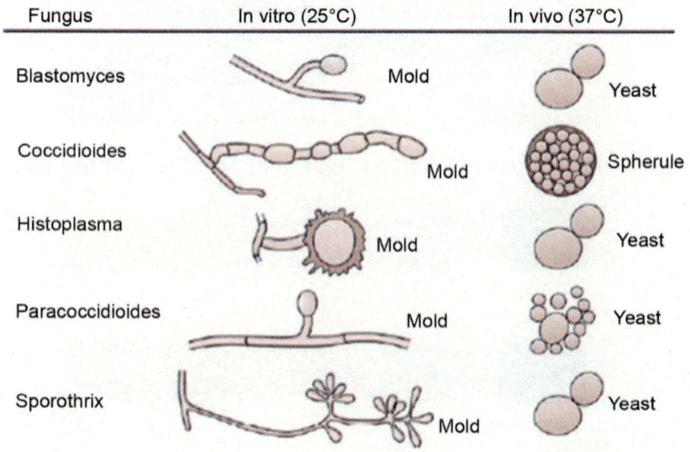

PARASITOLOGY

1. **Trichrome stain of Entamoeba histolytica trophozoites in amebiasis.**

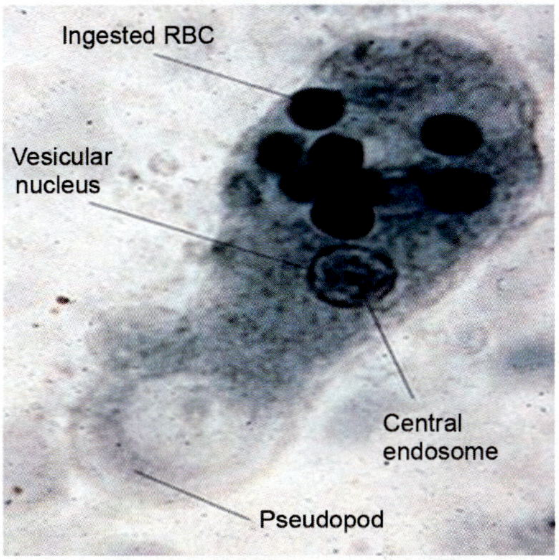

2. **Mature Cyst of Entamoeba coli in an unstained wet mount preparation with saline.**

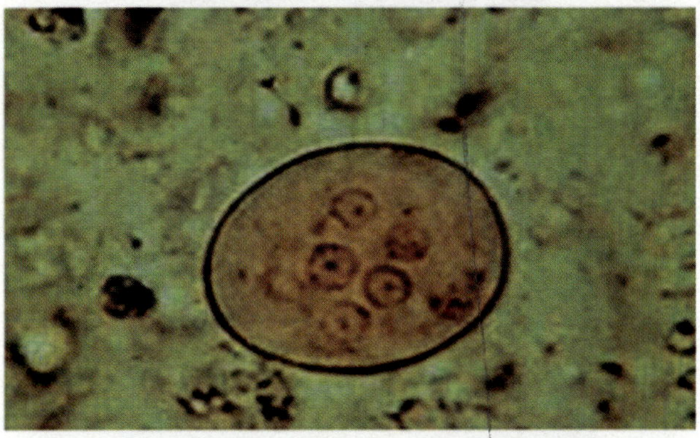

3. **Histopathology of a typical flask-shaped ulcer of intestinal amoebiasis.**

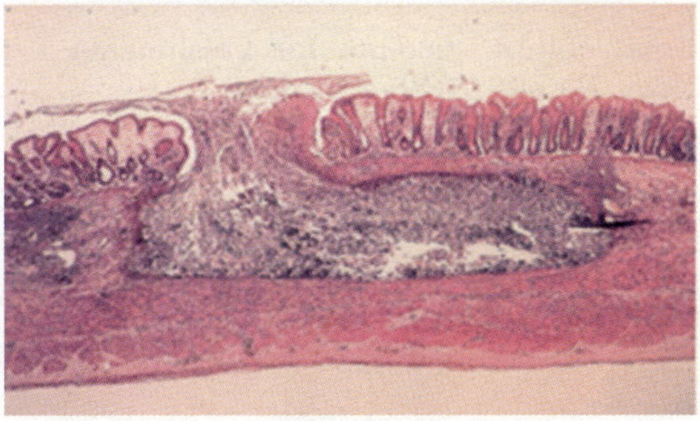

4. **Charcot-Leyden crystals – fecal smear (Trichrome stain).**

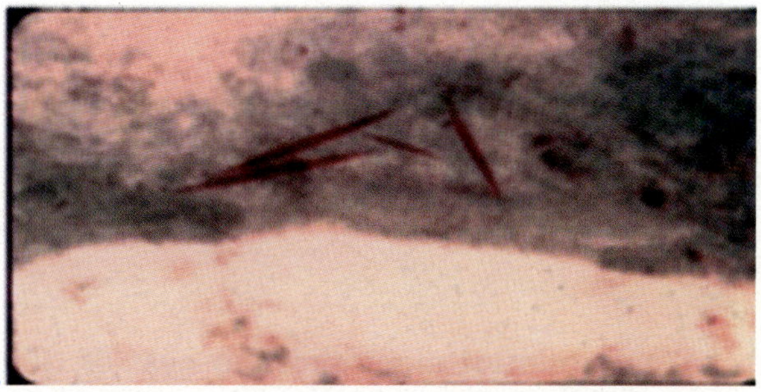

5. **Acanthamoeba: Trophozoit with thorn like pseudopodia in CSF saline mount.**

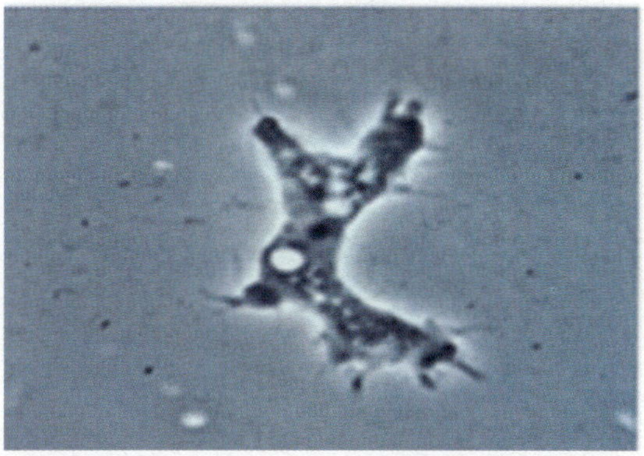

6. **Naegleria fowleri: Amoeboid trophozoite and flagellated trophozoite in saline mount.**

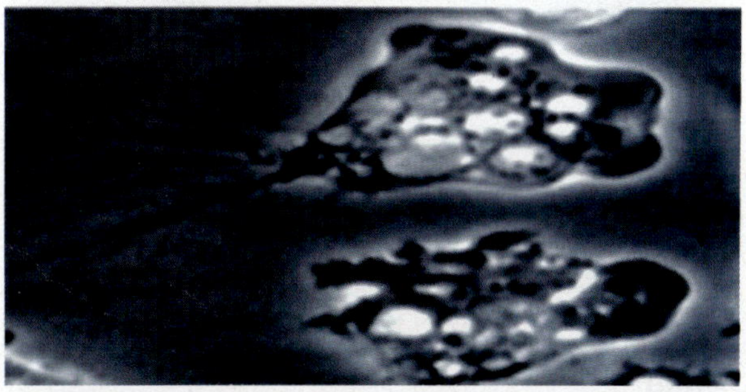

7. **Balamuthia mandrillaris: Trophozoite and Cyst in saline mount.**

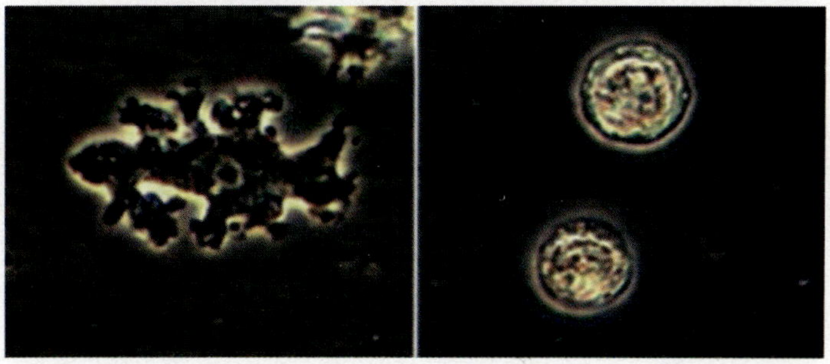

8. Giemsa staining of Giardia lamblia trophozoite in stool sample.

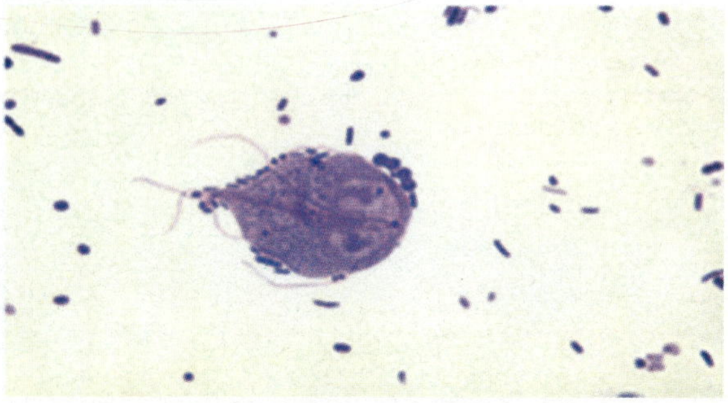

9. Saline mount of stool showing cyst of Giardia lamblia.

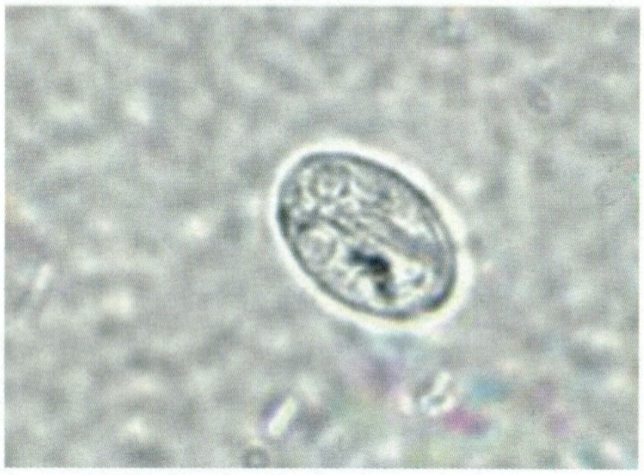

10. Trichomonas vaginalis trophozoites.

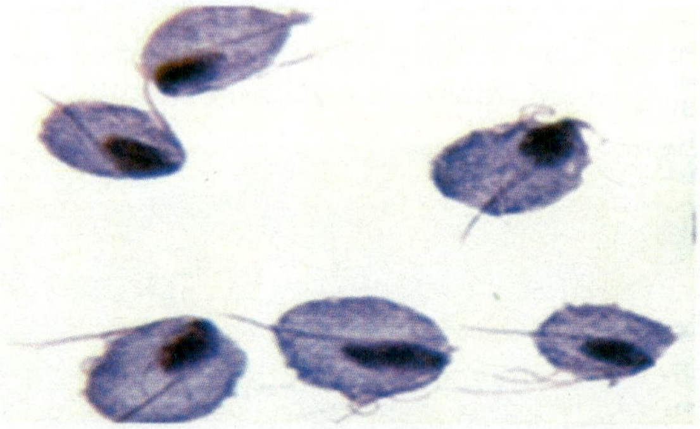

11. Leishmania donovani Promastigotes in culture fluid.

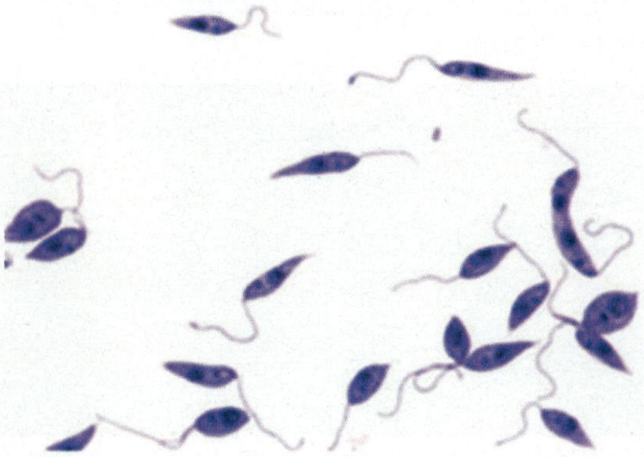

12. Leishmania donovani (LD) bodies – Amastigote form in bone marrow.

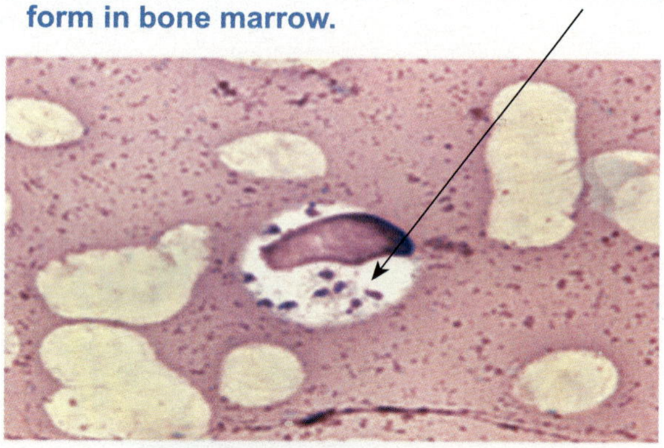

13. Visceral leishmaniasis – splenomegaly.

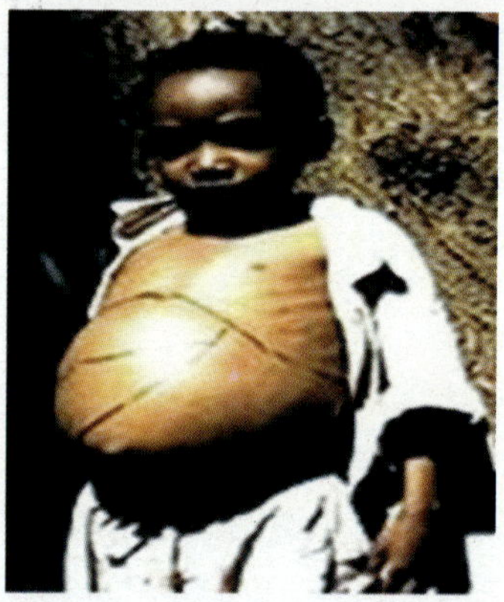

14. Post kala azar dermal leishmaniasis (PKDL).

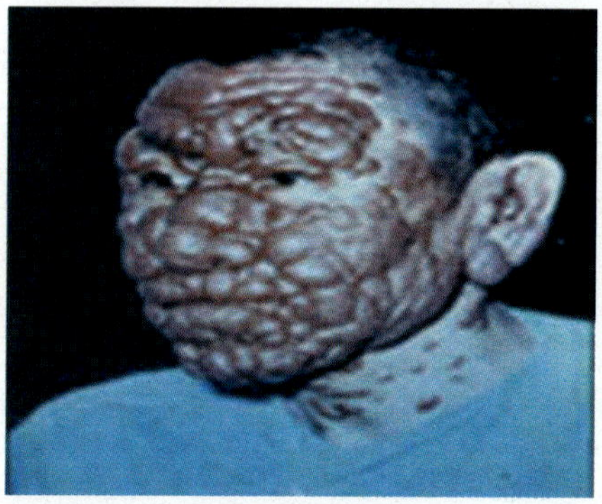

15. Solid culture medium for Leishmania – Neal, Novy, Nicolle (NNN) medium.

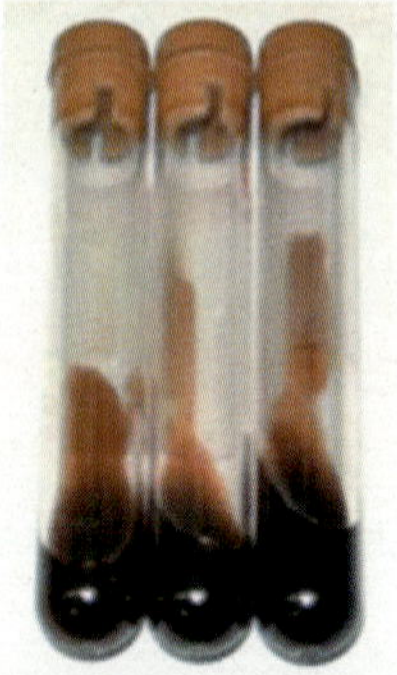

16. **Cutaneous leishmaniasis ulcerated lesion.**

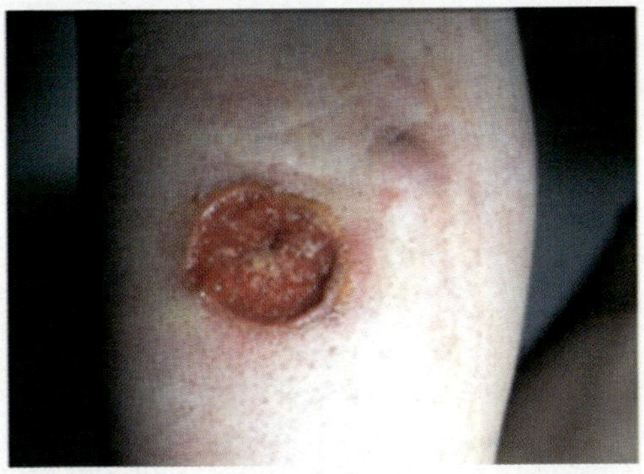

17. **Female Sand fly (Phlebotomus argentipes) – Vector for Leishmaniasis.**

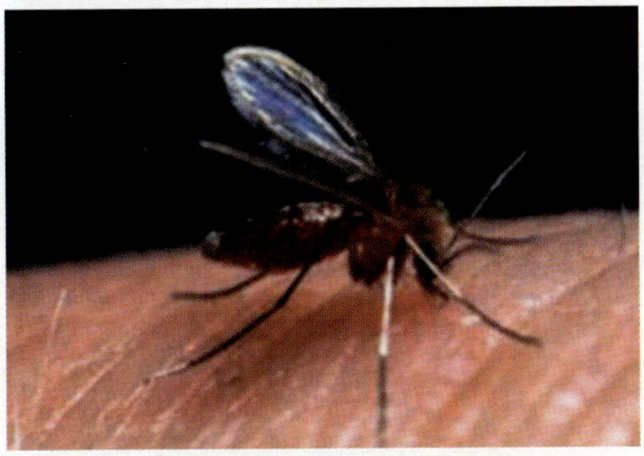

18. **A patient with espundia caused by Leishmania braziliensis.**

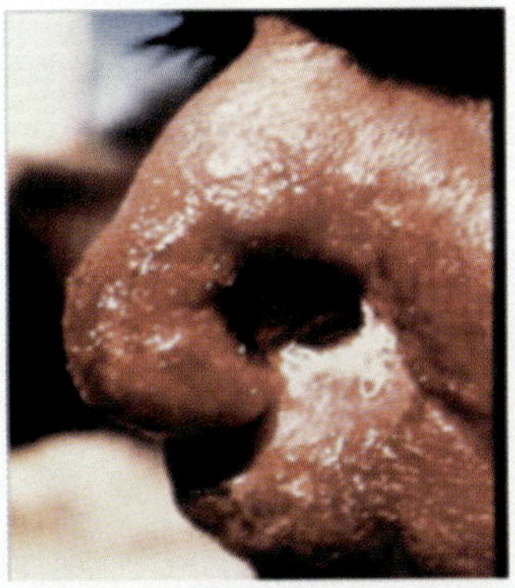

19. **Reduviid bug – Vector of Trypanosoma cruzi (Chaga's disease).**

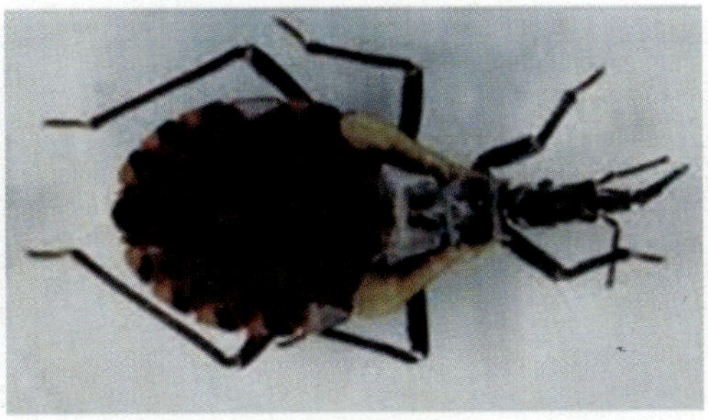

20. **Trypomastigote form of T. cruzi in thin blood smears stained with Giemsa.**

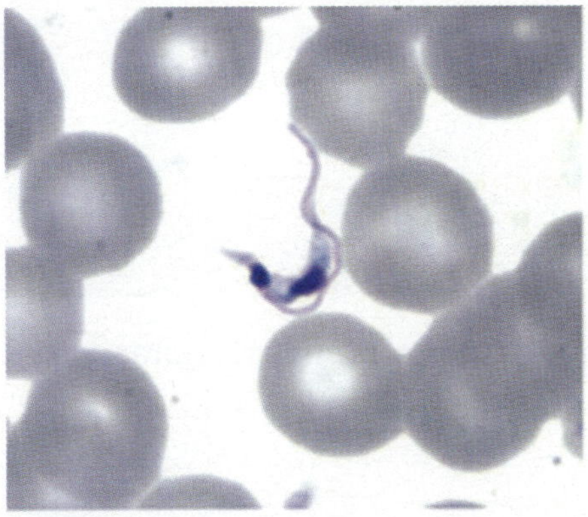

21. **Female Anopheles (Anopheline) – vector of Malaria.**

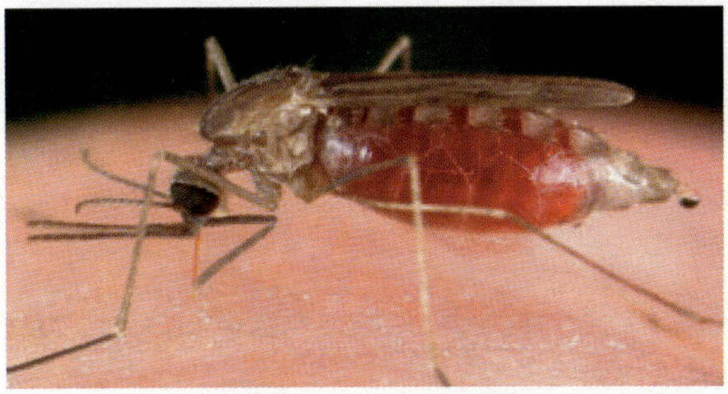

22. **QBC gametocytes of plasmodium falciparum.**

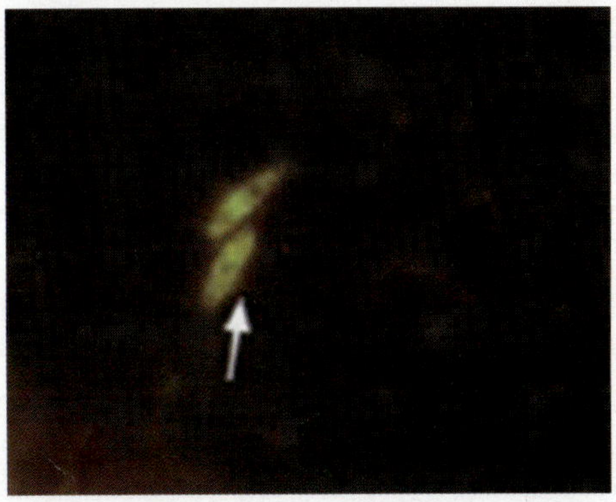

23. **Black water fever (hemoglobinuria and dark colored urine).**

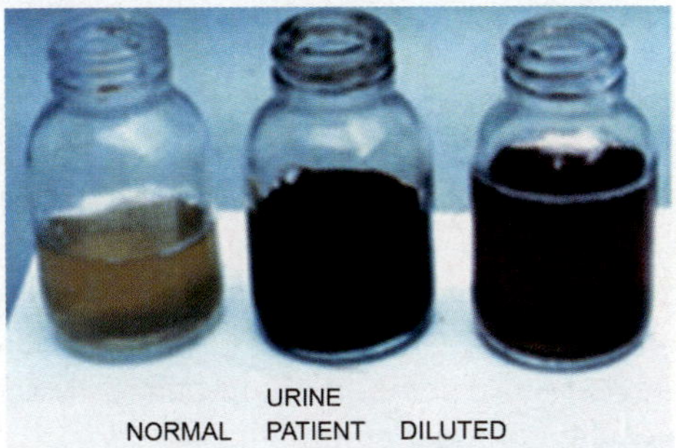

24. Rapid Malaria antigen detection test. p.v – p. vivex, p.f – p. falciparum Ag.

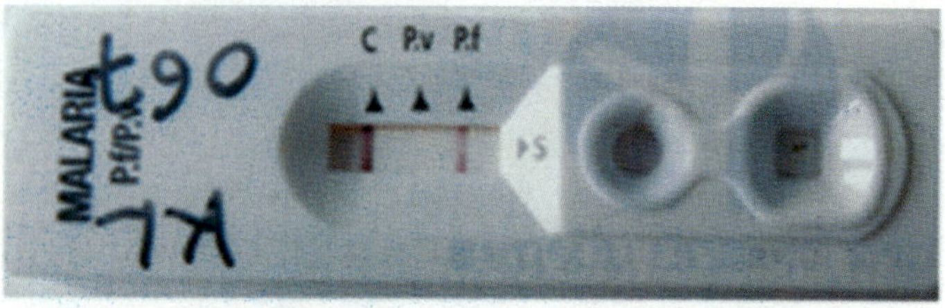

25. The morphology of malaria parasites.

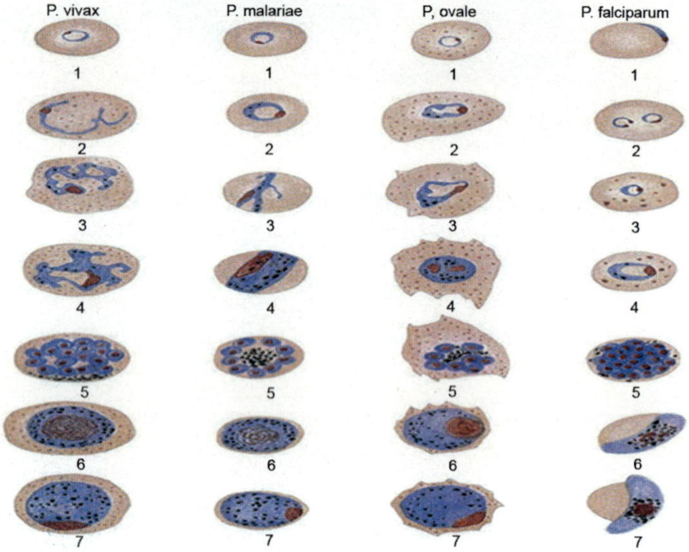

Plasmodium vivax: 1. Early trophozoite (ring form). 2. Late trophozoite with **Schüffner's dots (note enlarged red blood cell).** 3. Late trophozoite with ameboid cytoplasm (very typical of P. vivax). 4. Late trophozoite with ameboid cytoplasm. 5. Mature schizont with merozoites and clumped pigment. 6. Microgametocyte with dispersed chromatin. 7. Macrogametocyte with compact chromatin.

Plasmodium malariae: 1. Early trophozoite (ring form). 2. Early trophozoite with thick cytoplasm. 3. Early trophozoite **(band form).** 4. Late trophozoite **(band form)** with heavy pigment. 5. Mature schizont with merozoites (9) arranged in rosette. 6. Microgametocyte with dispersed chromatin. 7. Macrogametocyte with compact chromatin.

Plasmodium ovale: 1. Early trophozoite (ring form) **with James dots**. 2. Early trophozoite (note enlarged red blood cell). 3. Late trophozoite in red blood cell with fimbriated edges. 4. Developing schizont with irregularly shaped red blood cell. 5. Mature schizont with merozoites (8) arranged irregularly. 6. Microgametocyte with dispersed chromatin. 7. Macrogametocyte with compact chromatin.

Plasmodium falciparum: 1. Early trophozoite **(accolé or appliqué form).** 2. Early trophozoite (one ring is in headphone configuration/double chromatin dots). 3. Early trophozoite with **Maurer's dots.** 4. Late trophozoite with larger ring and Maurer's dots. 5. Mature schizont with merozoites. 6. Microgametocyte with dispersed chromatin. 7. Macrogametocyte with compact chromatin.

Note: Without the appliqué form, Schüffner's dots, multiple rings/cell, and other developing stages, differentiation among the species can be difficult. It is obvious that the early rings of all four species can mimic one another very easily. Remember: One set of negative blood films cannot rule out a malarial infection.

26. Toxoplasma gondii: Tachyzoites (comma-shaped) from the peritoneal exudates of infected mice stained with Giemsa.

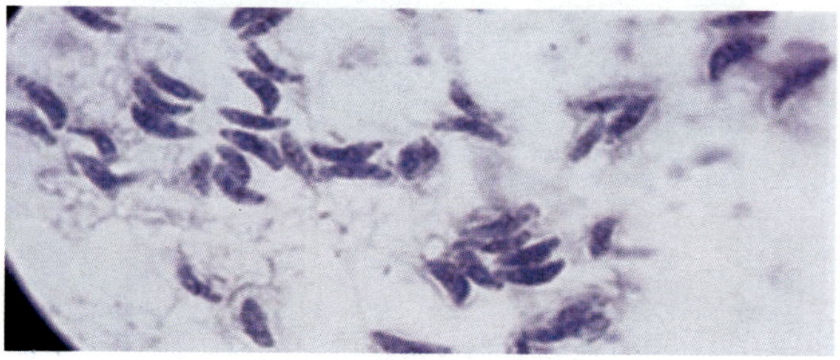

27. Toxoplasma gondii: Tissue cyst (containing bradyzoites) in organ biopsy.

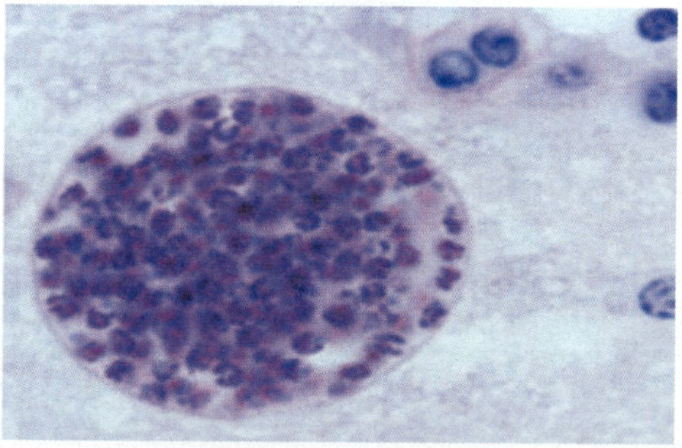

28. Toxoplasma gondii tachyzoites – detected by fluorescent antibody test.

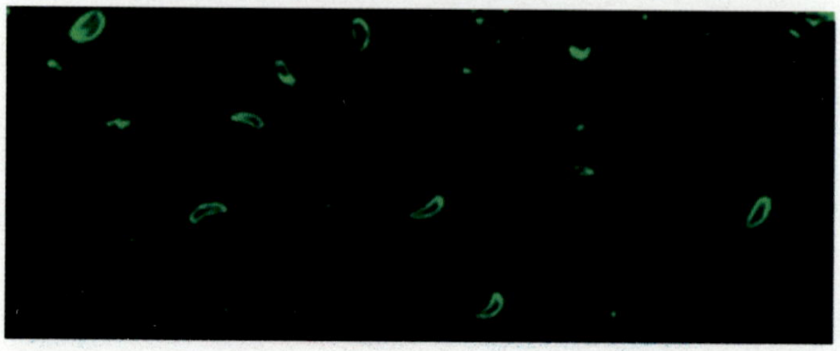

29. **Cryptosporidium parvum: 4-6 µm in size, round, acid fast (1% H_2SO_4) containing sporozoites.**

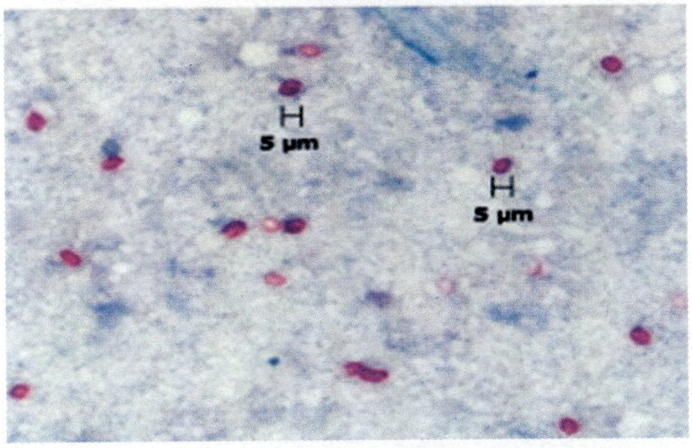

30. **Cyclospora cayetenensis: 8-12 µm in size, round, variably acid fast (1% H_2SO_4), contains two sporocyst each bearing sporozoites.**

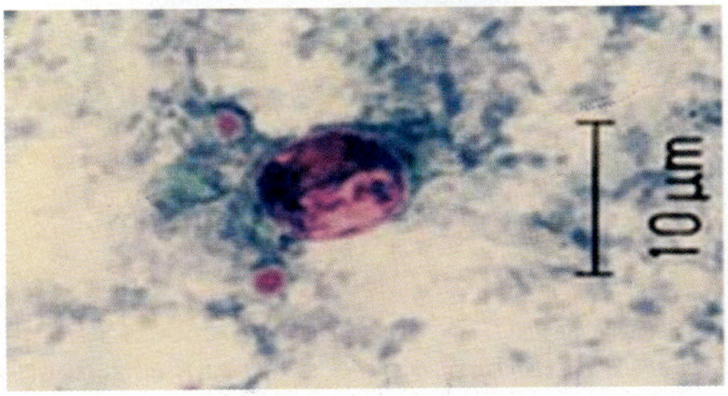

31. **Isospora belli: 23-36 µm in size, oval, uniformly acid fast (1% H_2SO_4), contains two sporocyst each bearing four sporozoites.**

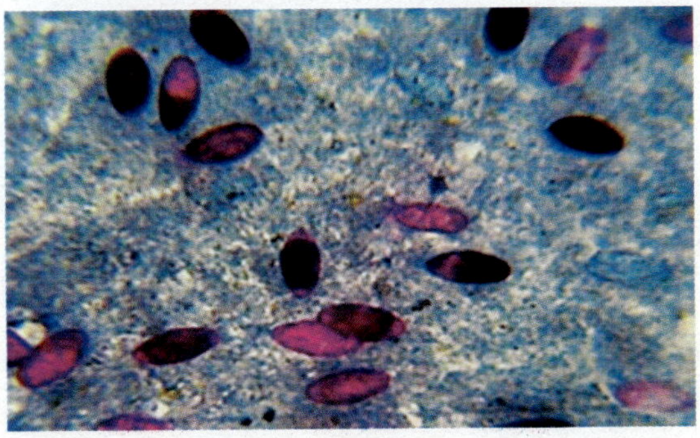

32. **Isospora belli wet mount stool smear.**

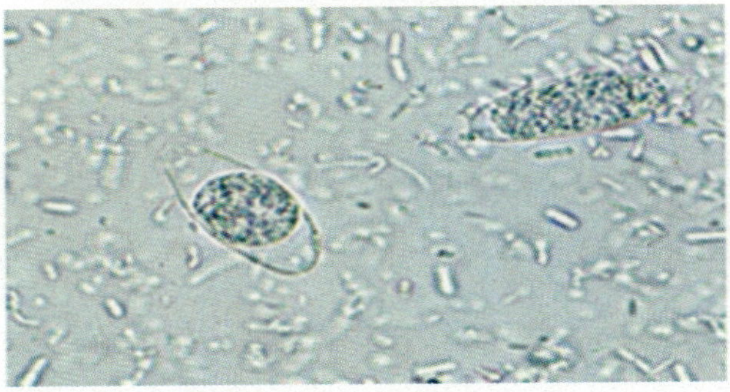

33. **Morphology of cestode.**

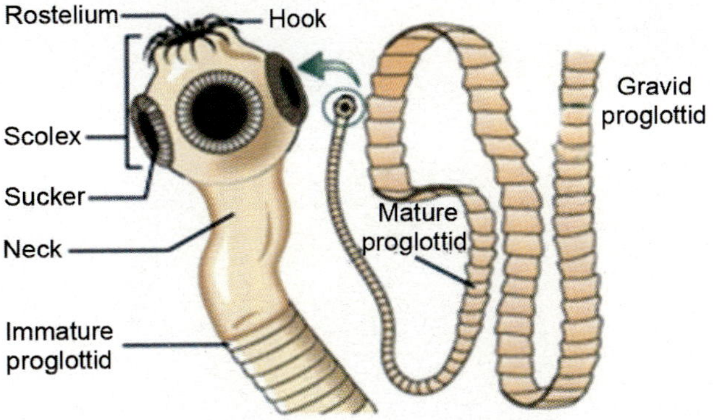

34. **Operculated eggs of Diphyllobothrium latum in stool wet mount.**

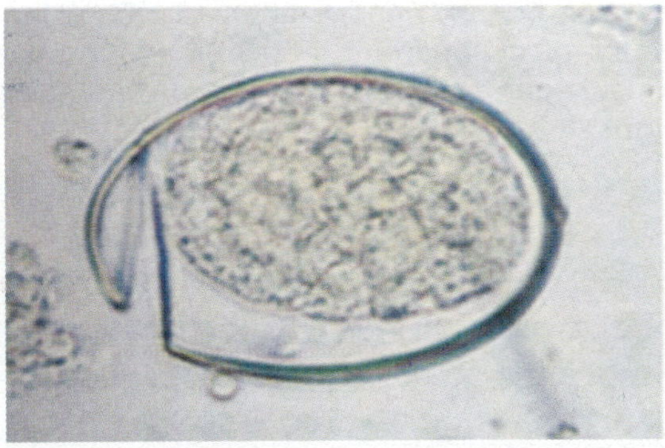

35. **Mature proglottid of T. saginata, stained with carmine.**

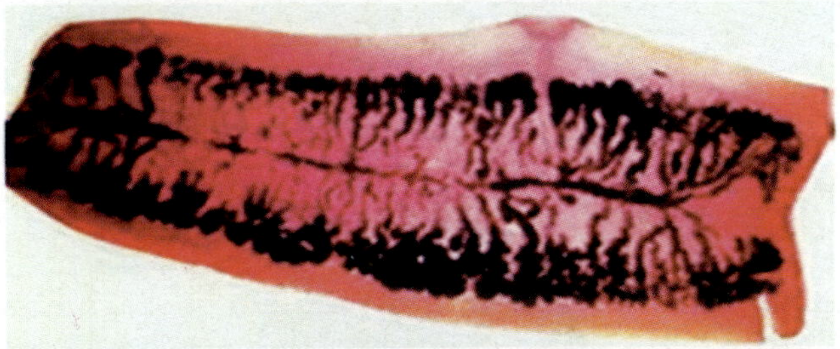

36. **Mature proglottid of T. solium, stained with carmine.**

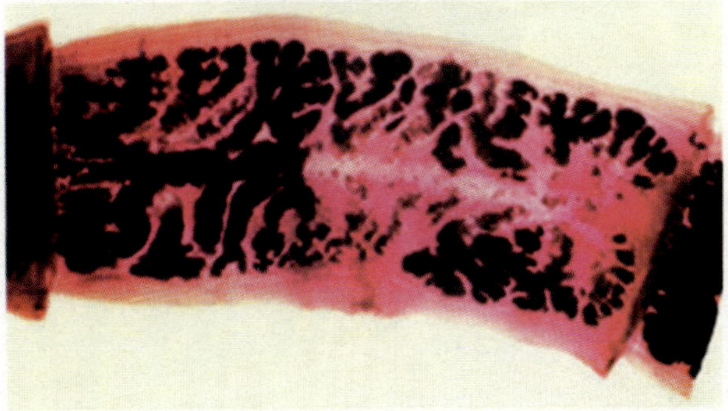

37. **Wet mount of a Taenia sp. Egg containing egg shell and onchosphere with three pairs of hooklets.**

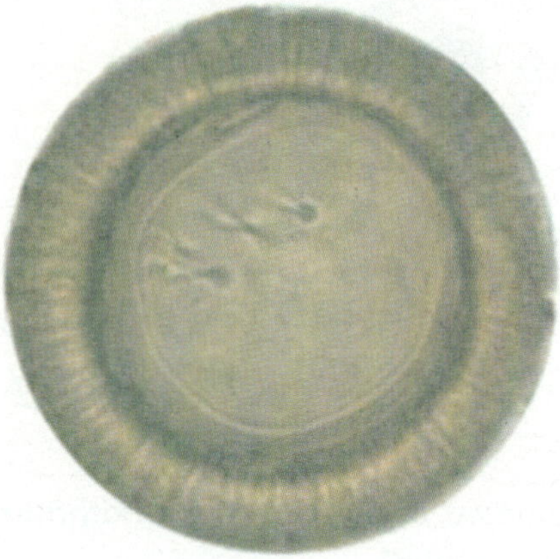

38. **Section through tissue infected with a bladderworm or cysticercus of Taenia solium. Skeletal muscle can be seen to the upper right and lower right.**

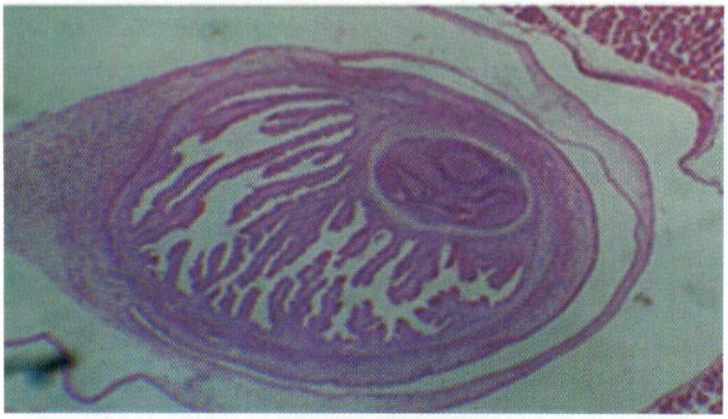

39. **Scolex of Taenia saginata (No rostellum or hooklets).**

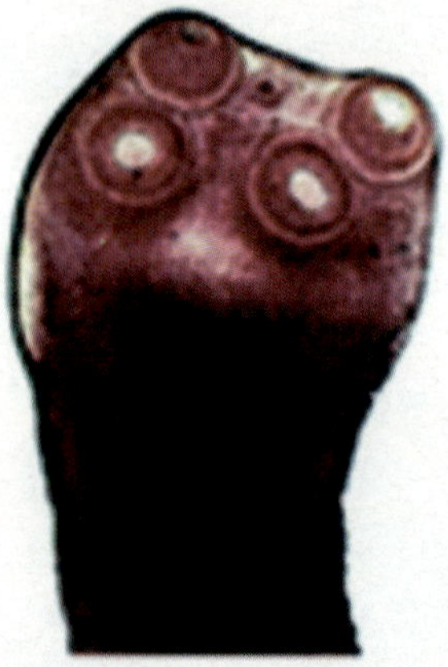

40. **Scolex of Taenia solium (Rostellum with hooklets present).**

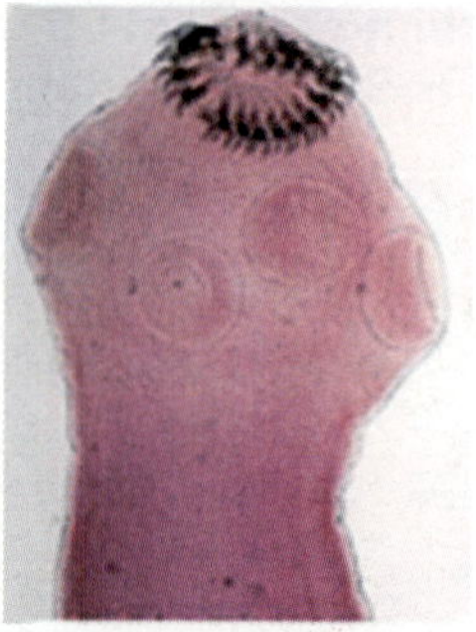

41. **Morphology of Echinococcus granulosus.**

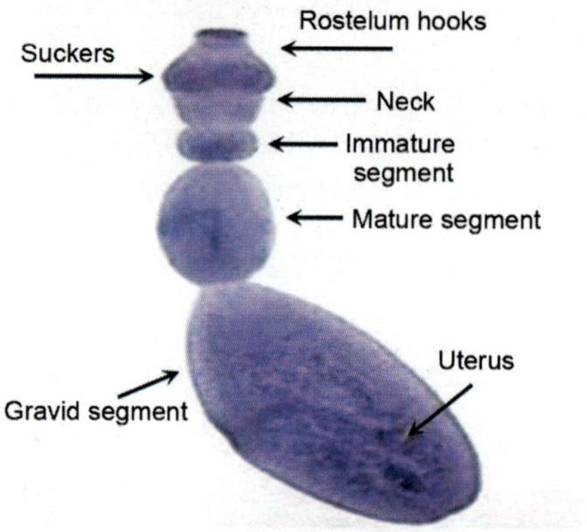

42. **Hydatid Cyst: Cystic echinococcosis in human liver: mother cyst of E. granulosus with daughter cysts.**

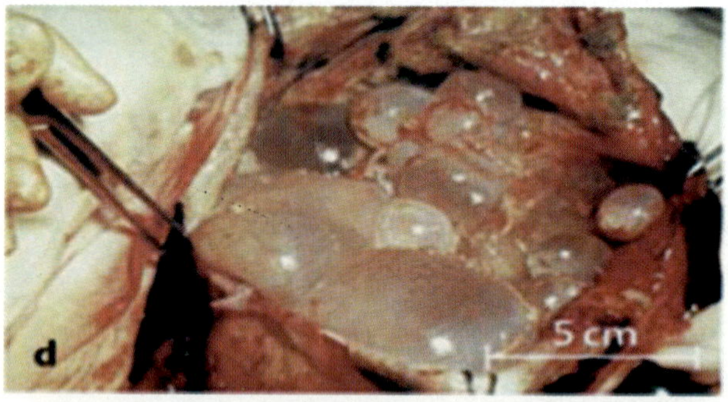

43. **Histopathological section (H and E satin) of Hydatid cysts.**

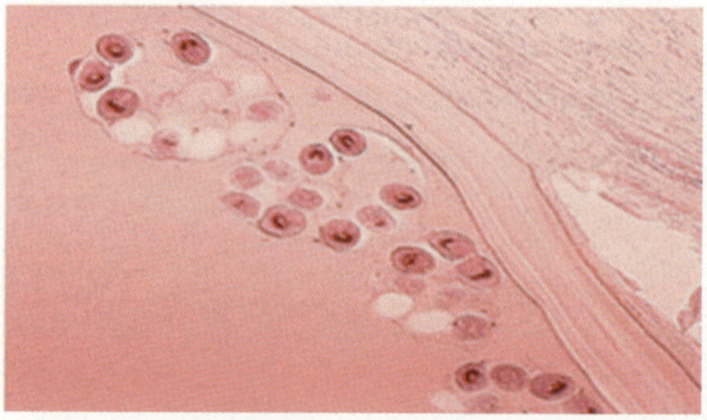

44. Hymenolepis nana egg: Non bile stained, contains polar filaments and oncosphere with three pairs of hooklets.

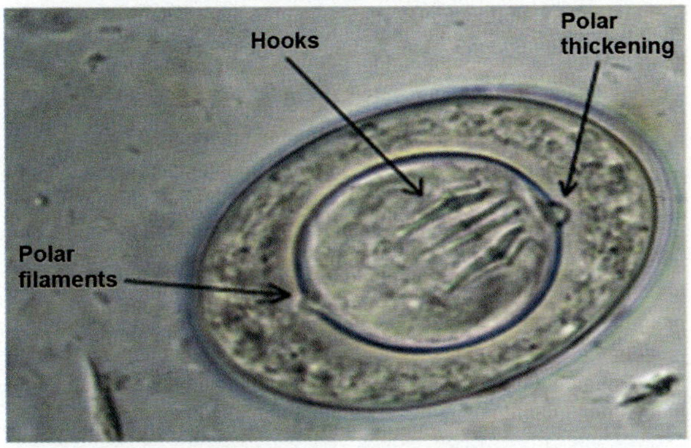

45. Schistosomes adult worms (thin female resides in gynecophoric canal of thicker male).

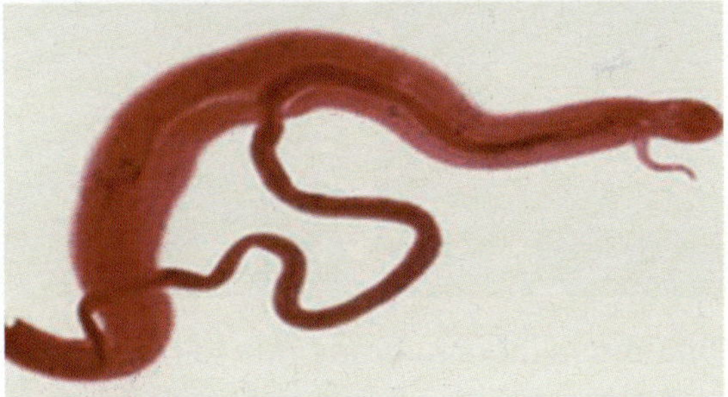

46. Eggs of Schistosoma.

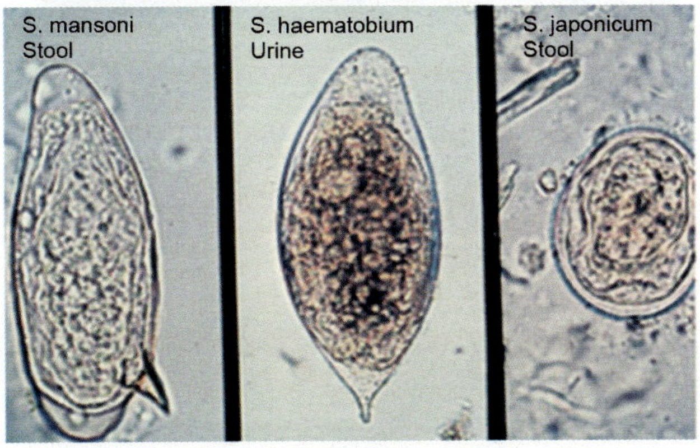

47. Morphology of Fasciola hepatica.

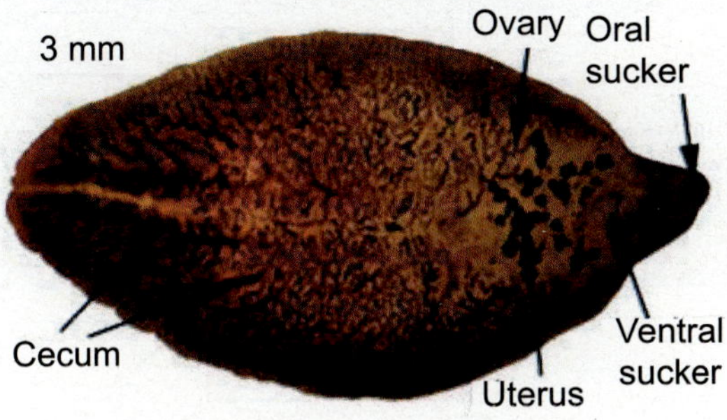

48. Fasciola hepatica egg in an unstained wet mount: Eggs are broadly ellipsoidal, operculated.

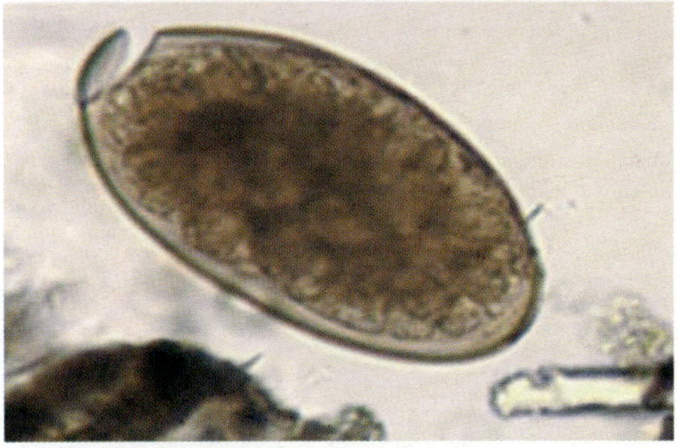

49. Paragonimus westermani adult worm.

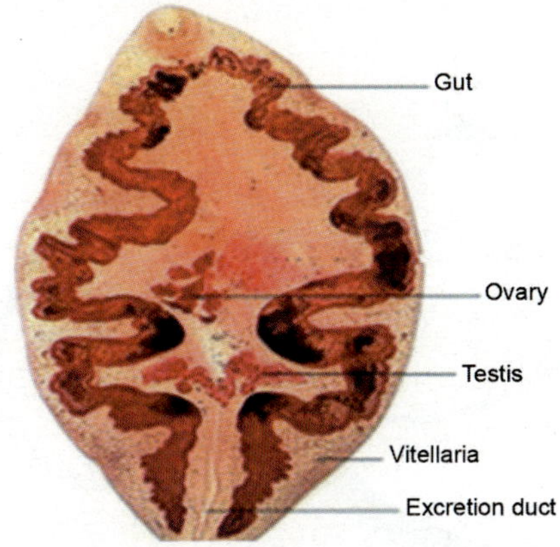

50. Paragonimus westermani egg in wet mount.

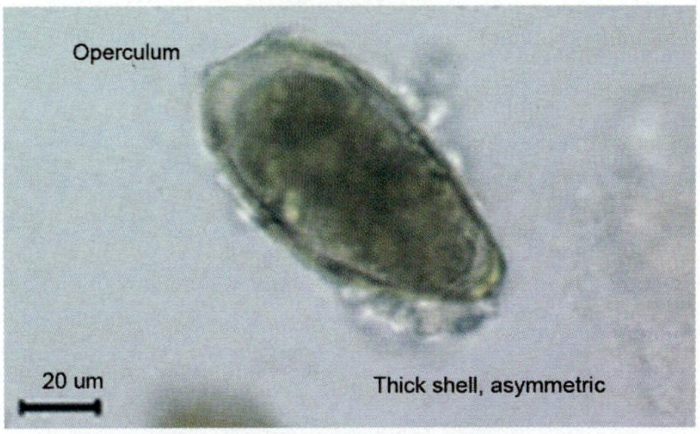

51. Egg of paragonimus sp. taken from a lung biopsy stained with hematoxylin and eosin.

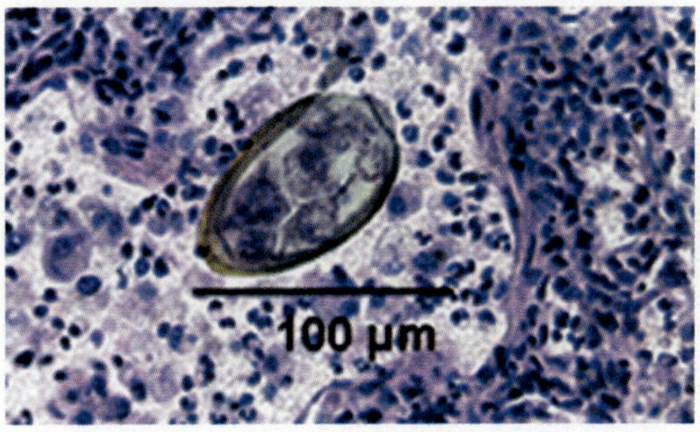

52. Trichuris trichiura egg (barrel shaped) in wet mount with mucus plugs at both ends.

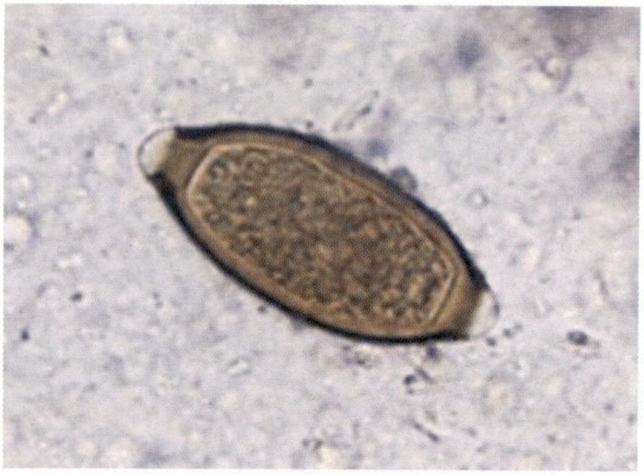

53. Adult worm of T. trichiura.

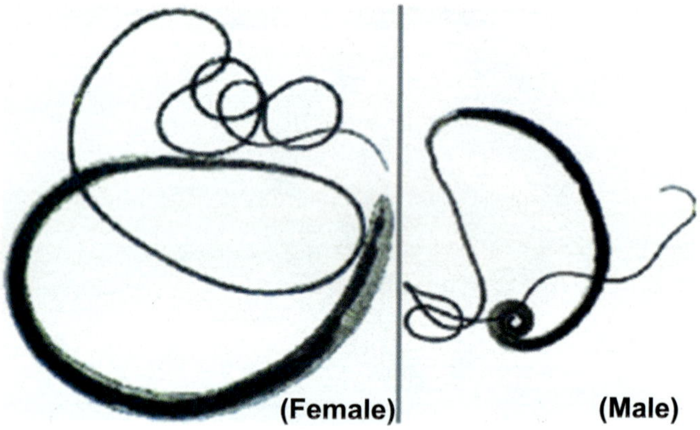

54. Enterobius vermicularis egg in saline mount.

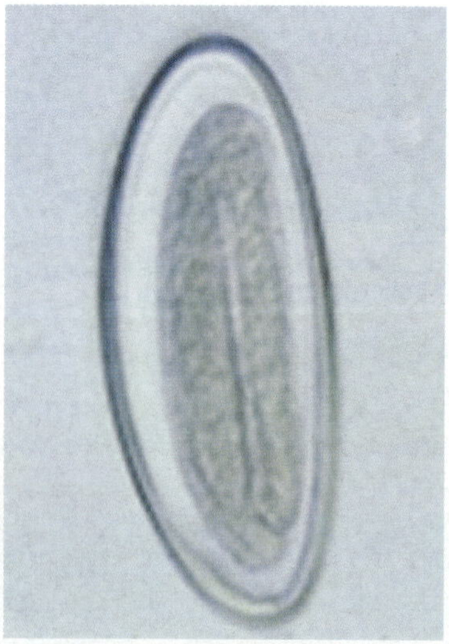

55. Hookworm egg with four blastomeres in an unstained wet mount.

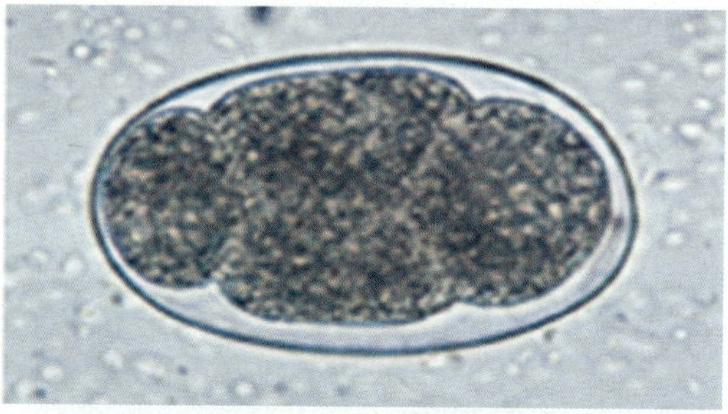

56. Hookworm rhabditiform larva (wet preparation).

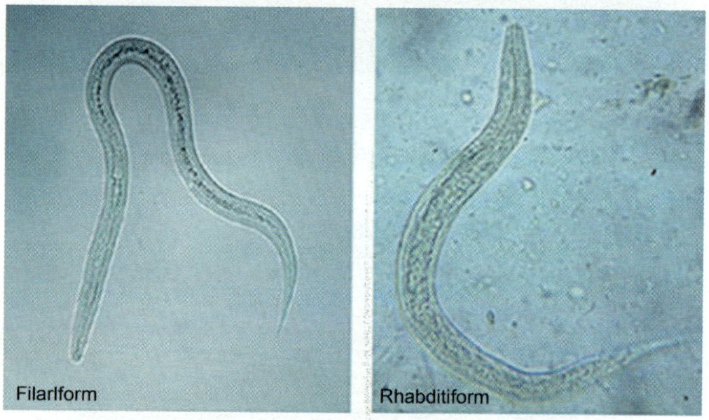

57. Cutaneous larva migrans due to hookworm.

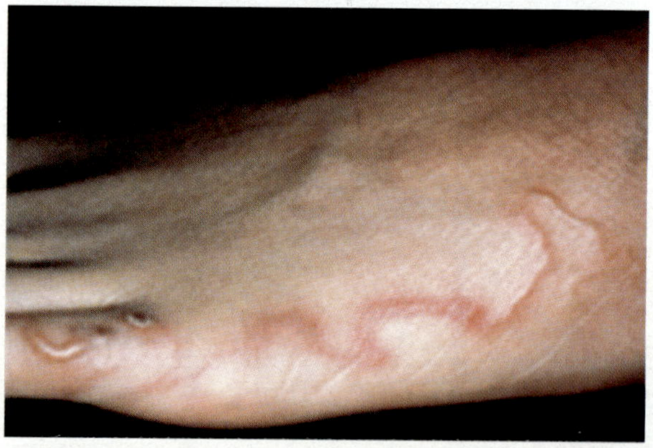

58. Ascaris adult worm.

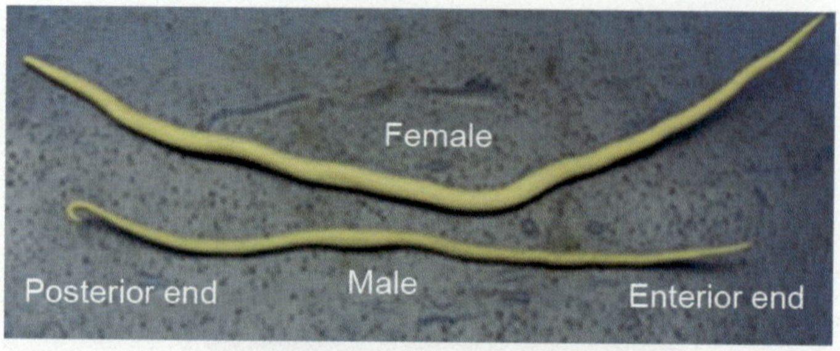

59. Eggs of different parasites.

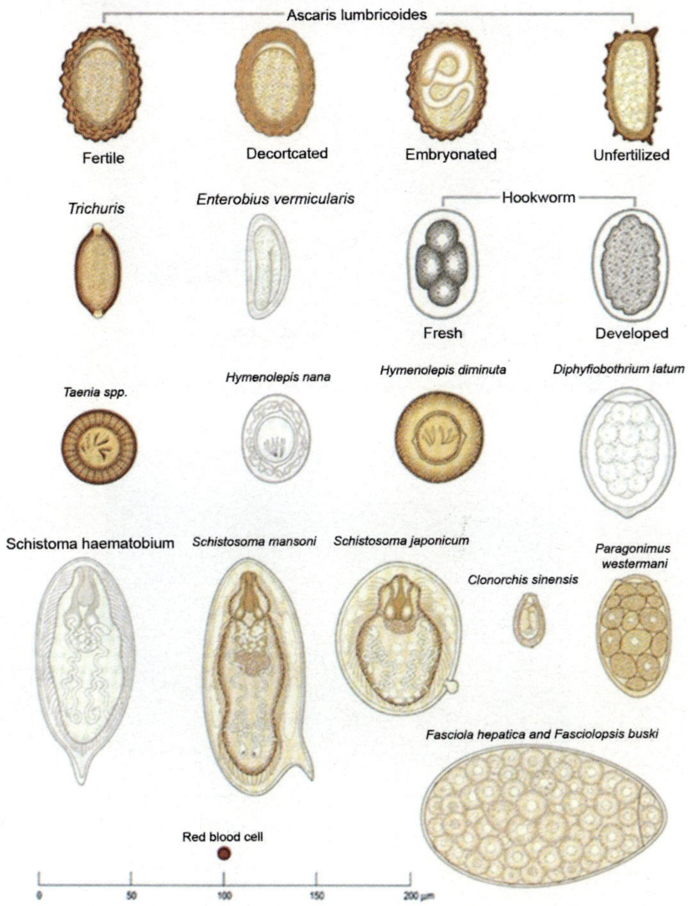

60. Unfertilised and fertilised eggs of Ascaris lumbricoides.

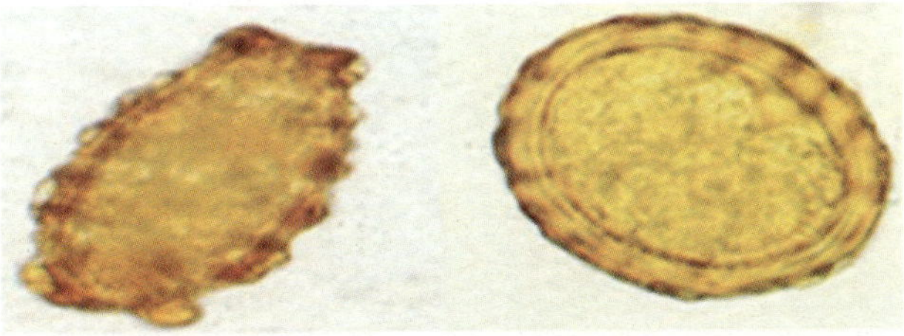

61. Microfilaria.

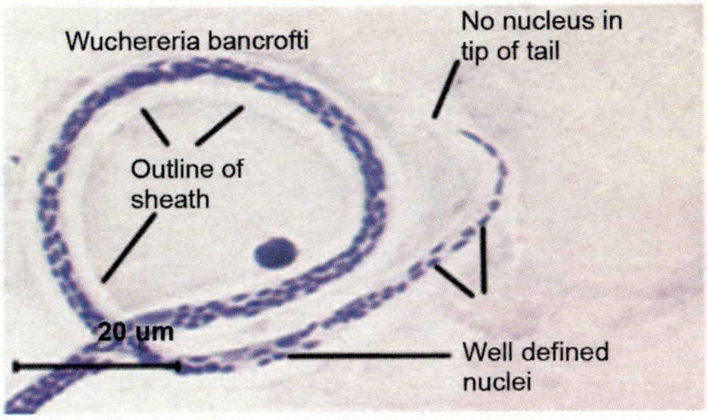

62. Microfilaria found in blood.

Sheathed			*Unsheathed*	
Tail tip free from nuclei	*Nuclei up to tail tip*		*Tail tip free from nuclei*	*Nuclei up to taif tip*
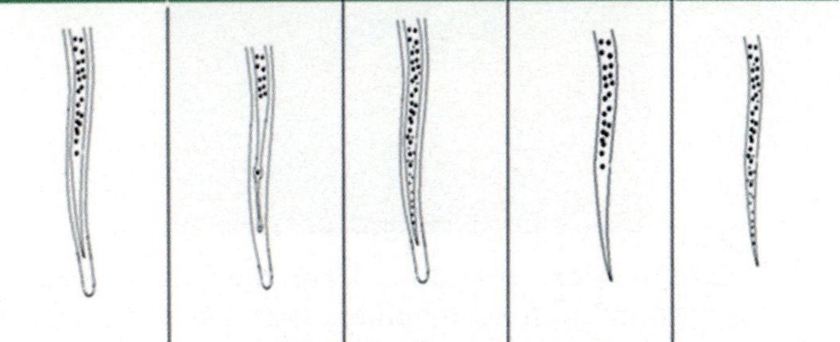				
Mf. bancrofti	Mf. malayi	Mf. loa	Mf.ozzardi	Mf. perstans

63. Elephantiasis.

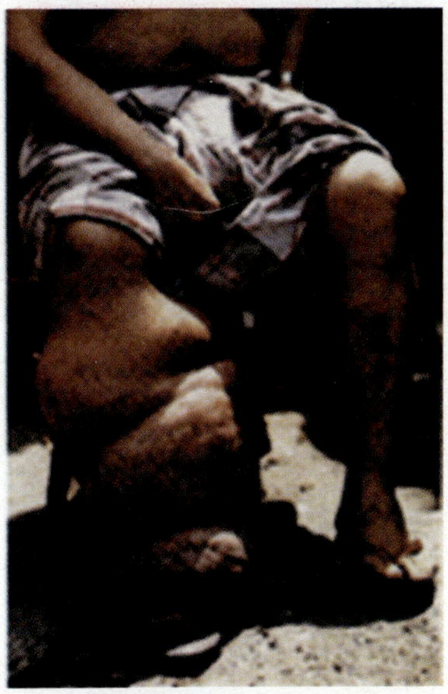

64. Hydrocele of scrotum.

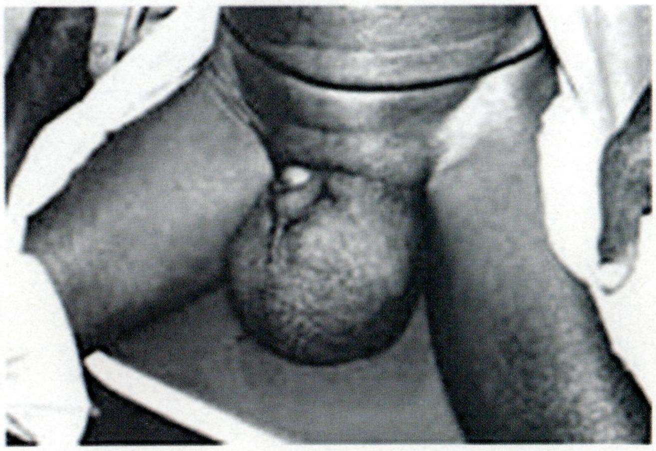

65. Using a matchstick to wind up and remove a guinea worm (Dracunculus medinensis) from the leg of a human.

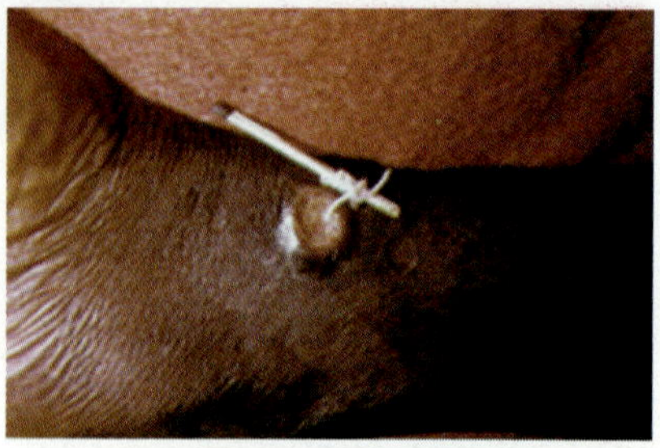

66. Onchocerca volvulus: Palpation of a subcutaneous nodule. Nodules that were surgically removed contain coiled adult worms.

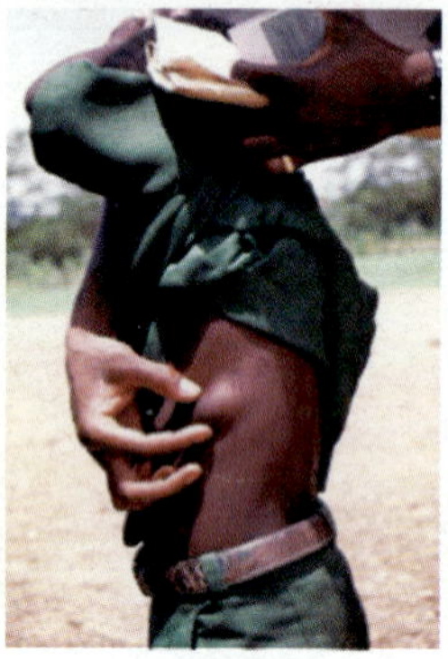

67. Infective first stage larva of Trichinella spiralis in its Nurse cell in muscle tissue.

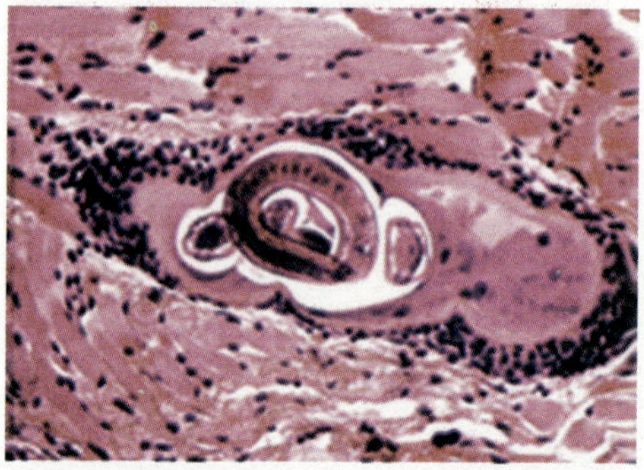

68. Strongyloides stercoralis larvae from a bronchiolar lavage.

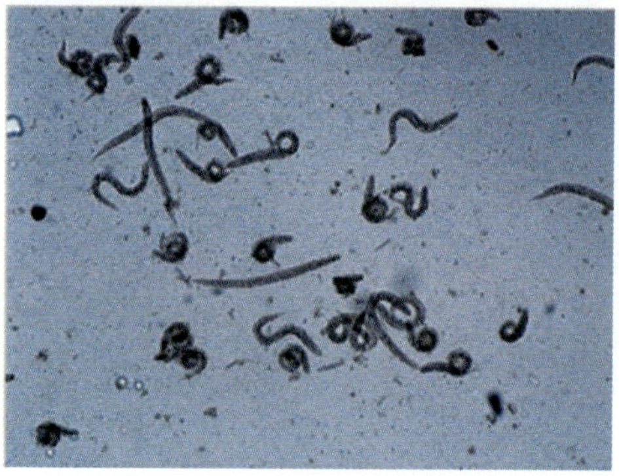

RECENTLY ASKED IMAGES

1. HBV replication

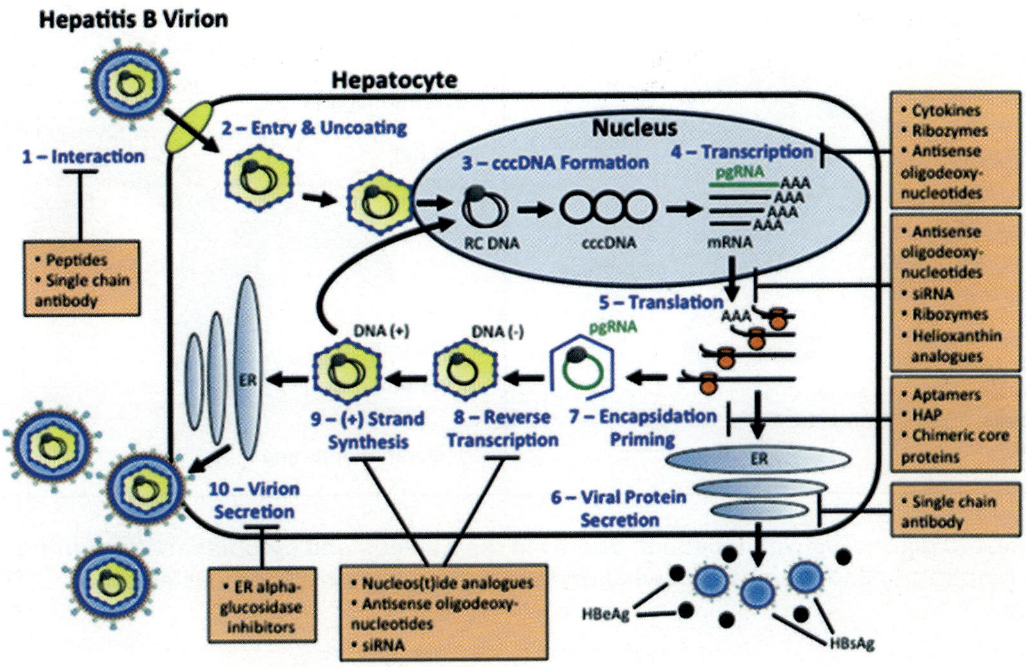

2.

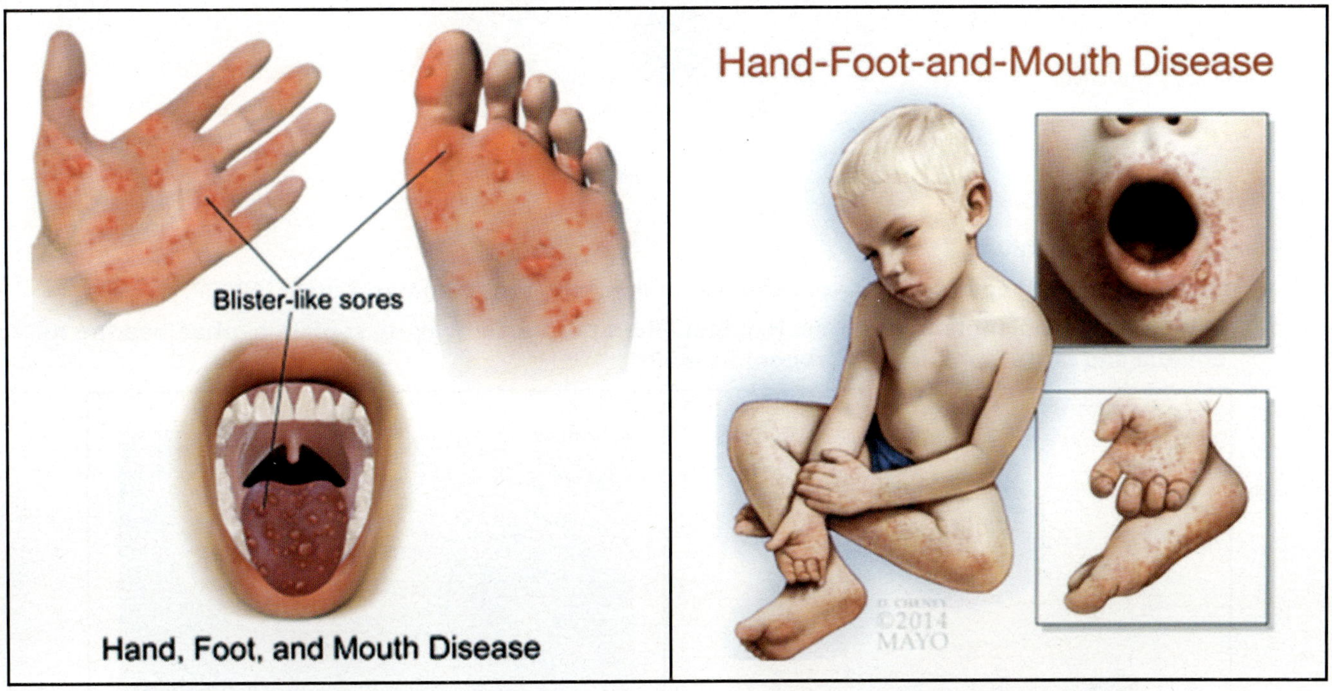

3. **Spirochetes - gram-negative, helical bacteria that move by means of axial filaments (endoflagella). Several species are associated with disease, including Treponema pallidum, the agent of syphilis and and Borrelia bergdorfi, the agent of Lyme's disease.**

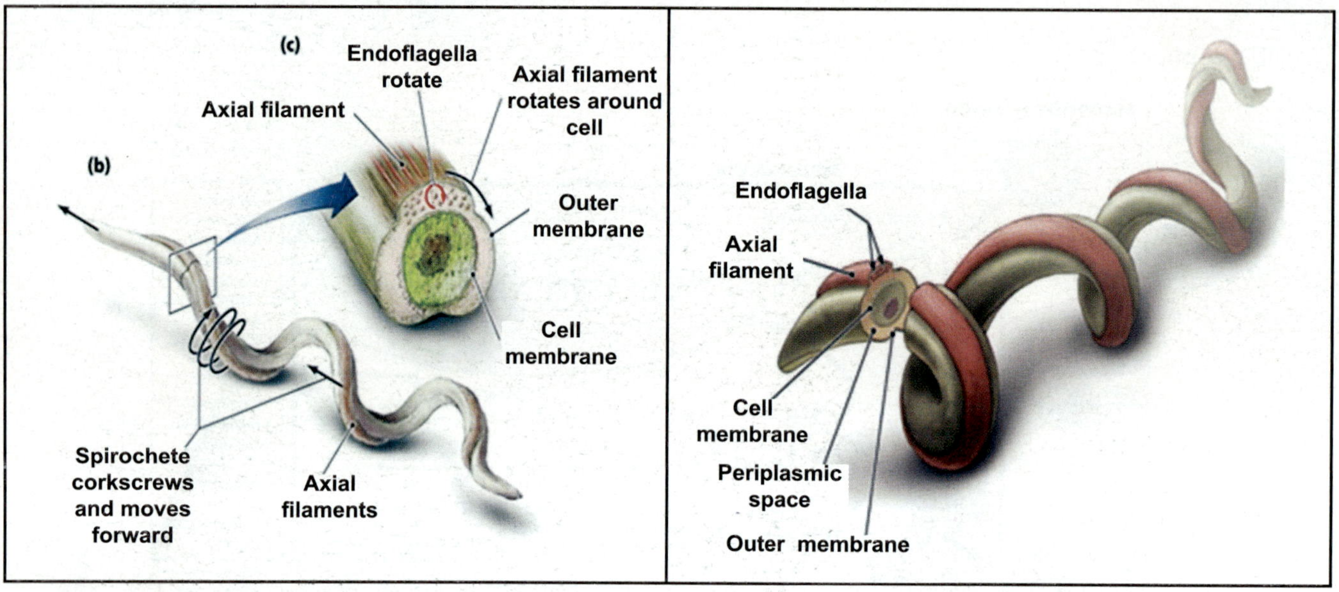

4. **Multinucleated giant cells with inclusion bodies in the nucleus and cytoplasm (Warthin-Finkeldey cells) are found in respiratory and lymphoid tissues and are pathognomonic for measles.**

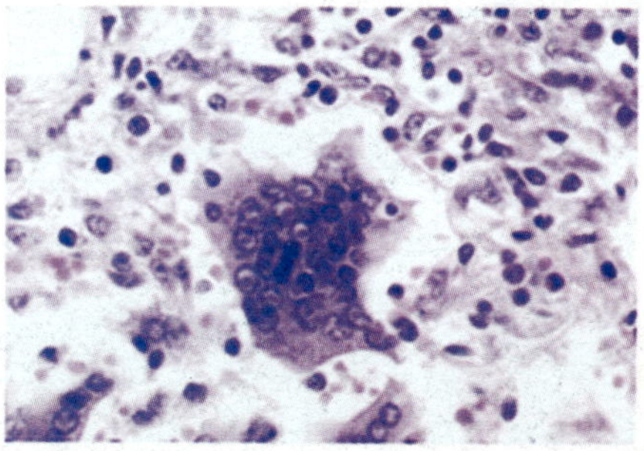

5. **Histoplasma capsulatum:**

   A: **Small, oval yeast cells (2–4 μm) packed within macrophages. Giemsa's stain. 1000×.**

   B: **In culture at ambient temperatures, H. capsulatum produces hyaline, septate hyphae bearing micro-conidia and large, spherical macroconidia. 400×.**

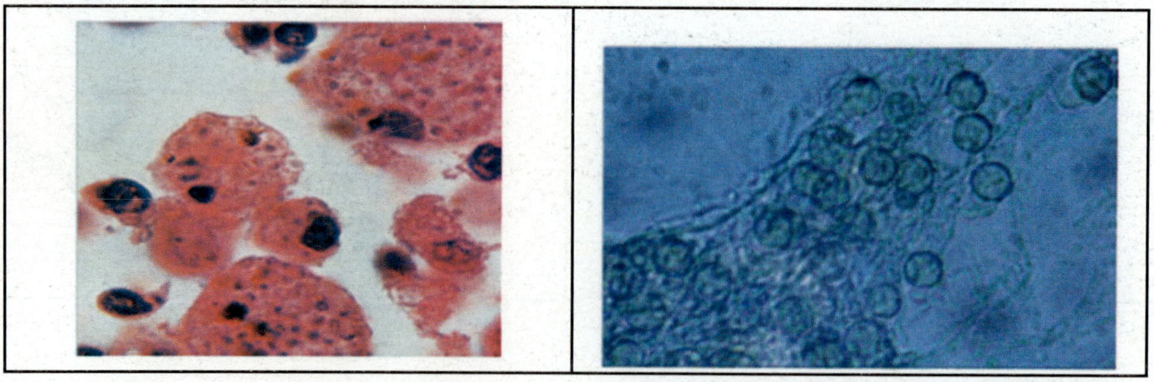